INDIGENOUS PEOPLES AND DIABETES

Carolina Academic Press
Medical Anthropology Series

Pamela J. Stewart *and* Andrew Strathern
Series Editors

Curing and Healing
Medical Anthropology in Global Perspective
Andrew Strathern *and* Pamela Stewart

Physicians at Work, Patients in Pain, 2nd Edition
Biomedical Practice and Patient Response in Mexico
Kaja Finkler

Healing the Modern in a Central Javanese City
Steve Ferzacca

Elusive Fragments
Making Power, Propriety and Health in Samoa
Douglass D. Drozdow-St. Christian

Endangered Species
Health, Illness, and Death Among Madagascar's People of the Forest
Janice Harper

The Practice of Concern
Ritual, Well-Being, and Aging in Rural Japan
John W. Traphagan

The Gene and the Genie
Tradition, Medicalization and Genetic Counseling
in a Bedouin Community in Israel
Aviad E. Raz

Social Discord and Bodily Disorders
Healing Among the Yupno of Papua New Guinea
Verena Keck

Indigenous Peoples and Diabetes
Community Empowerment and Wellness
Mariana Leal Ferreira *and* Gretchen Chesley Lang

INDIGENOUS PEOPLES AND DIABETES

Community Empowerment and Wellness

Edited by

Mariana Leal Ferreira
SAN FRANCISCO STATE UNIVERSITY

and

Gretchen Chesley Lang
UNIVERSITY OF NORTH DAKOTA

CAROLINA ACADEMIC PRESS
Durham, North Carolina

Copyright © 2006
Mariana Leal Ferreira and Gretchen Chesley Lang
All Rights Reserved

Library of Congress Cataloging-in-Publication Data

Indigenous peoples and diabetes : community empowerment and wellness / by Mariana
Leal Ferreira and Gretchen Chesley Lang.
   p. cm.
  ISBN 10: 0-89089-580-5   ISBN 13: 978-0-89089-580-1
  1. Diabetes--Social aspects. 2. Indians of North America--Diseases. I. Ferreira,
Mariana K. Leal (Mariana Kawall Leal). II. Lang, Gretchen Chesley.

  RA645.D5I53 2005
  362.196'462'008997--dc22

2005007639

CAROLINA ACADEMIC PRESS
700 Kent Street
Durham, NC 27701
Telephone (919) 489-7486
Fax (919) 493-5668
www.cap-press.com

Printed in the United States of America
Cover design: Erin M. Ehman

To all our relations!

and

To the Seven Generations!

CONTENTS

Foreword, *Nancy Scheper-Hughes*   xvii

Series Editors' Preface, *Pamela J. Stewart and Andrew Strathern*   xxiii

Acknowledgments   xxvii

Introduction   Deconstructing Diabetes, *Mariana Leal Ferreira
      and Gretchen Chesley Lang*   3

  Who are Indigenous Peoples and Where Do They Live ?   8

   What is Type 2 Diabetes? Expanding the Biomedical Point of View   9

   Indigenous, the United Nations' Definition   10

   Who is Indigenous? Territory, Politics and Identity   10

  A Worldwide Epidemic   11

   Biomedical Diagnosis and Treatment of Diabetes Type 2   12

  Racializing Diabetes, Disempowering the People   12

   Century of the Gene Becomes Century of Genetic Determinism   13

  The Politics of Indigenous Identity: Consequences of the Once-Popular
   'Thrifty Gene' Hypothesis   14

   The Gene as Culprit   15

  Linking Diabetes, Social Inequality, and Trauma   16

  Outline of the Book   17

  Final Thoughts   25

   The International Labor Organization (ILO)   27

  References   27

Part I
Colonialism, Social Inequality, and Community Experience

**Chapter 1   Emotion, Grief, and Power: Reconsiderations
      of Hawaiian Health,** *Jo C. Scheder*   33

  Part 1. Taro Tales: Land, Power and Hawaiian Health   34

  Part 2. The Death of Health: Cosmology and Emotion
   in Colonial Depopulation   39

Why "Depopulation"?   40

In Theory: The Biology of Depopulation   41

    New Pathogens, Stress, and Immunity   42

    Novel Pathogens   42

    Chronic Stress and Immunity   42

    Changes in Status and Role Expectations   42

    Caregiving and Bereavement   43

Historical Reports and Cultural Meaning in Hawai'i   43

Meaning and Being   46

The Tenacity of an Incomplete Idea   47

Questions and What We Know   48

Acknowledgments   49

References   49

Chapter 2   **'In Their Tellings': Dakota Narratives about History
and the Body,** *Gretchen Chesley Lang*   53

Narratives   55

Theoretical Considerations   56

"Things aren't being done right around here on this reservation,
and we seem to have more and more of these problems like
diabetes."—Carl Webster   58

Community at Devil's Lake   62

"Worry makes my sugar go up."—Mary Peters   64

Ethnographic Contexts   66

Final Thoughts   67

Acknowledgments   68

References   68

Chapter 3   **Slipping Through Sky Holes: Yurok Body Imagery
in Northern California,** *Mariana Leal Ferreira*   73

Introduction   74

Mapping Lines of Life: Early Studies   75

The New Genetics and Indigenous Peoples   77

The Sick, the Insane and the Criminal: Embodying Human
Relations in Disease   80

How to Read the Genealogical Charts   82

    Sarah Tsurai   83

    Mary Wo'tek   88

    Julia Stowen   93

Curiosity in Hybrids and Monsters or "The White's Blood Obsession"   94

The Distribution of Land and "Indian Soul and Conduct"   96

Concluding Observations   98

Acknowledgments   99
References   100

Chapter 4   Diabetes in Réunion Island (Indian Ocean): From Sugar
             Plantations to Modern Society, *Muriel Roddier*   105
Historical Background: The Peopling of Réunion Island   106
   From the Relation to Sugar in the Local Context to 'Sugared Diabetes'   108
The History of Diabetes on La Réunion   110
Construction of Diabetes by Those Who Experience It   114
Conclusions   118
Acknowledgments   119
References   119

Chapter 5   Nêhinaw (Cree) Socioeconomic, Political and
             Historical Explanations about the Collective
             Diabetes Experience, *Jocelyn Bruyère*   123
Historical Background: The Disruption of Cree Traditional Life   123
Etiology: *Wāmistikosew*, *Me'chim*, and Ecological Destruction   128
Me'chim (Food), History, and Politics   132
Final Thoughts   135
Acknowledgments   135
References   135

Part II
Speaking Out about Food, Health, and Power

Chapter 6   Mino-Miijim's 'Good Food for the Future': Beyond Culturally
             Appropriate Diabetes Programs, *Emily Omura*   139
Methods   141
Mino-Miijim   141
Mino-Miijim: Margaret's Program   142
White Earth Land Recovery Project (WELRP)   143
White Earth Land Recovery Project: Addressing Structural Violence   145
Production of White Earth Traditional Food Packages   149
Traditional Food?   149
Food and Community Identity   150
History of Lifestyle Changes   153
Food Availability and Individual Choices   157
Narratives of Diabetes   160
Conclusion   162
Acknowledgments   163
References   163

**Chapter 7   Diabetes and Identity: Changes in the Food Habits
of the Innu—A Critical Look at Health Professionals'
Interventions Regarding Diet,** *Bernard Roy*   167

A Fight to the End Against "Bad Food Habits"   168

Food Guide and "Culturization" of the Message   169

Mixed Results   170

Conscious and Knowledgeable Populations   172

Why the Repeated Failures?   173

The Complexity of Food Habits   174

The Act of Eating—A Political Act   175

Recognition and Differentiation through Eating   175

Sunday Meal   177

Eating as Differentiation   178

Assertion and Withdrawal   179

Eating as a Political Act   180

Acknowledgments   183

References   183

**Chapter 8   Prenatal Mysteries and Symptomless Diabetes in the
Gila River Indian Community,** *Carolyn Smith-Morris*   187

Introduction   189

An Ethnography of Pregnancy   190

Gestational Diabetes   191

Healing Practices on the Reservation   192

Pima Women's Understandings of GDM   193

   Fluctuating Test Results   194

   Symptomless Diabetes   195

   Related Problems in Diabetes   198

Summary and Discussion   200

Acknowledgments   201

References   201

**Chapter 9   Talking about a New Illness with the Dakota: Reflections
on Diabetes, Foods, and Culture,** *Gretchen Chesley Lang*   203

Introduction   205

Theoretical Considerations   207

Diabetes from a Biomedical Perspective   209

Background: Devil's Lake Sioux Community   211

Traditional Medicine and Religion   213

Foods, Eating and the "Diabetic Diet"   214

Etiological Explanations, Experience of Illness and Efficacy of Treatments 220

Discussion and Conclusion 224

Acknowledgments 226

References 226

Chapter 10 Burying the Umbilicus: Nutrition Trauma, Diabetes
and Traditional Medicine in Rural West Mexico,
Leslie E. Korn and Rudolph C. Ryser 231

Part 1. Center for Traditional Medicine—Philosophy and Practice 232

Drugless Medicine in the Tropical Forest 236

Meaning and Success 238

A. Traditional Medicine Practices in Western Mexico 239

B. "Defective Modernization" 242

C. Imposed Development and Chronic Disease 244

D. Community Trauma 245

E. Nutrition Trauma 249

F. Intergenerational Traumatic Stress 250

G. Stress and Diabetes 252

Part 2. Metabolizing Trauma: The Case of the *Comunidad Indigena de Chacala* 253

Part 3. History of Nutrition Trauma in Mexico 256

Pre-Colonial Diet 256

NAFTA-Cized Mexico: The Global Soybean, Defective
Modernization and Diabetes 258

Part 4. The Pedagogy of the Nourished 259

Natural Medicine Health Promoter Training 262

A. Exotic Food Preparation Using Local Foods 262

B. Intergenerational Activities 263

C. Herbal Validation 263

Nutritional Protocols for the Treatment of Diabetes 266

A. Nutritional Supplementation 267

B. Essential Fatty Acids 267

C. Vitamin and Mineral Supplementation 269

Project Significance 269

Acknowledgments 270

References 270

Part III
Emotional Experience and Social Support

Chapter 11 A Sickly-Sweet Harvest: Farmworker Diabetes
and Social (In)Equality, *Jo C. Scheder* 279

Background: Social Conditions, Stress, and Diabetes 280

Psychological and Social Correlates of Diabetes   282

The Neurophysiological Link Between Stress and Glucose Intolerance   283

The Mexican-American Migrant Lifestyle, Stress, and Diabetes   283

Stressors Among Mexican-American Migrants   284

Mortality and Morbidity from Diabetes Mellitus Among
Mexican-Americans   287

Research Design   288

Results   290

Discussion   297

Models of Social Conditions and Diabetes   302

Conclusion   303

Acknowledgments   305

References   305

Chapter 12   Diabetes as a Metaphor: Symbol, Symptom, or Both?,
              Terry Raymer   313

Introduction   314

Genetics and Lifestyle   315

Taking Food for "Granted?"   318

The Greedy Father, as told by Paula Allen (Yurok, Karuk, and Hoopa)   318

Gestational Factors   322

Complex and Obscure: Stress, Depression, and Cultural Trauma   324

Conclusion?   329

Acknowledgments   330

References   330

Chapter 13   The Spirit's Cell: Reflections on Diabetes
              and Political Meaning, Jo C. Scheder   335

Prologue and Perspective   335

Paths to "Untangling"   339

The Spirit's Cell: A Physiology of Oppression   342

Native Hawaiian Health   343

Compulsory Aloha   347

Acknowledgments   349

References   350

Chapter 14   Love in Colonial Light: History of Yurok Emotions
              in Northern California, Mariana Leal Ferreira   357

Introduction   358

Mollie Ruud: "Indian people have always been closely
watched and controlled"   358

The Social and Political Context Where Diabetes Originates 362

Mollie Ruud: "I just can't handle freedom" 364

Illness Narratives, Traumatic Experience, and Type 2 Diabetes 368

Ethnographic Research Methods: Correlating Qualitative and
Quantitative Information 369

Emotional Experience and the Autonomic Nervous System 372

Recipe for Acorn Soup 373

Hitting the Jackpot: Love, Solidarity and Generosity 376

A Politically Meaningful History of Emotions 380

Acknowledgments 381

References 382

**Chapter 15 Relaxation and Stress Reduction for People with Diabetes
Mellitus,** *Angele McGrady and Kim Grower-Dowling* 387

Introduction 387

Part 1. Types of Relaxation 389

Breathing Therapy 390

Autogenic Relaxation 390

Progressive or Neuromuscular Relaxation 391

Yoga 392

Transcendental Meditation 393

Mindfulness Meditation 394

Part 2. Enhancement of the Relaxation Response 394

Healing Words 395

Imagery 395

Biofeedback 396

Part 3. Autogenic Relaxation Process and Benefits 397

Part 4. Effects of Relaxation on Diabetes Mellitus 400

Summary 401

References 402

Part IV
Community Empowerment and Wellness

**Chapter 16 Community Empowerment for the Primary Prevention
of Type 2 Diabetes: Kanien'kehá:ka (Mohawk) Ways for
the Kahnawake Schools Diabetes Prevention Project,**
*Ann C. Macaulay, Margaret Cargo, Sherri Bisset,
Treena Delormier, Lucie Lévesque, Louise Potvin
and Alex M. McComber* 407

Introduction 408

Primary Prevention of Type 2 Diabetes 410

Origins of the Kahnawake Schools Diabetes Prevention Project   412

A Participatory Approach to Community-based Research   415

KSDPP Community Advisory Board   415

The KSDPP Code of Research Ethics   417

  Kahnawake Schools Diabetes Prevention Project   419

  The KSDPP Model of Community-based Intervention   419

  Elementary Schools' Interventions to Educate Young Children   421

  Community Interventions to Promote Living in Balance   423

Reflections on the KSDPP Model   425

Challenges   426

Reflecting on Community Governance   426

Conclusion   427

Acknowledgments   428

References   429

Chapter 17   "I'm Too Young for This!": Diabetes and American
             Indian Children, *Jennie R. Joe and Sophie Frishkopf*   435

Type 2 Diabetes   437

Pediatric Type 2 Diabetes   437

Risk Factors and Complications   438

Social and Political Factors   439

Childhood/Youth Culture and Diabetes   442

Cultural Competency from Within and Without   444

Intervention/Prevention Programs for Children/Youth   444

The NARTC Summer Wellness Camp   447

Issues of Cultural Sensitivity   449

Physical Activities and Diabetes Education   450

The Campers   451

Personal and Psychosocial Consequences   452

Evaluating Outcomes   454

Campers' Opinions about the NARTC Summer Wellness Camp   454

Summary   455

Acknowledgments   455

References   456

Chapter 18   Touch the Heart of the People: Cultural Rebuilding
             at the Potawot Health Village in California,
             Mariana Leal Ferreira, Twila Sanchez and Bea Nix   459

Introduction: The Importance of Culture for a Healthy Community   460

Everyday Life and the Power of Ethnographic Fieldwork   461
Cultural Rebuilding at the Potawot Health Village   463
Touch the Heart of the People: Suggested Activities
    for a Theory of Cultural Rebuilding   473
    1. Women Support Groups   474
    2. Music Therapy: Sacred Songs and Chanted Prayers   477
       Music Therapy Websites   479
    3. Art Therapy: Basket Weaving, Beading, and Abalone Carving   480
    4. History Telling   481
    5. The Right to Food: Traditional Food Gathering and Preparation   482
       The Right to Food. Indigenous Peoples International Consultations
         on the Right to Food   483
Final Thoughts   485
Acknowledgments   486
References   486

Chapter 19   **Culture Blindness? Aboriginal Health, 'Patient Non-Compliance'**
        and the Conceptualisation of Difference in Australia's Northern
        Territory, *Kim Humphery*   493
Australian Socio-Cultural Research on Indigenous Health: Some Background   495
The Uses of Culture   497
Researching 'Patient Non-Compliance'   498
    Voicing Cultural Difference   501
The Place of 'the Cultural' in Aboriginal Health Services Provision   505
Conclusion   507
Acknowledgments   507
References   507

Chapter 20   **Striving for Healthy Lifestyles: Contributions of**
        Anthropologists to the Challenge of Diabetes in
        Indigenous Communities, *Dennis Wiedman*   511
Introduction   511
Cultural Sensitivity through Community and Clinical Collaborations   515
    Profile: Rebecca Hagey   515
Cultural Models of Diabetes   516
    Profile: Linda Garro   517
Patients and Providers   518
    Profile: Linda Hunt   520
Biomedical Domination and the World System   521
Indigenous Medicine   521
Modernization and Technological Change   523

    Profile: Joel Gittlesohn   524
Policy Develoment   526
    Profile: Cheryl Ritenbaugh   527
Anthropologist and Indigenous Community Collaborations   528
Acknowledgments   529
References   530

Contributors   535

Index   543

FOREWORD

Diabetes and Genocide—
Beyond the Thrifty Gene

*Nancy Scheper-Hughes**

"To say I am Native American means I am or will be diabetic."

"That's what the doctor told me. We Indians have bad blood. See, that's why I drank so much all my life. It's in me, in my blood. So there's not much I can do about it, either."

> Yurok individuals to Mariana Ferreira, this volume

"The tradition of the oppressed teaches us that the state of emergency in which we live is not the exception but the rule. We must attain to a conception of history that is in keeping with this insight. Then we shall clearly recognize that it is our task [as intellectuals] to bring about a real state of emergency, and this will improve our position in the struggle against Fascism. One reason why Fascism has a chance is that in the name of progress its opponents treat it as a historical norm."

> Walter Benjamin, "Theses on the Philosophy of History"

There are different ways of imagining, 'reading,' and interpreting history: bio-evolutionary history; social or collective history; individual/biographical/personal history. While all of these can offer essential insights toward understanding and responding to the particular vulnerabilities of Indigenous Peoples and communities world wide to adult onset (i.e., type 2) diabetes, this collection emphasizes the impact of social history—colonial histories and their sequelae, to be exact—on the etiology and epidemiology of diabetes today in Indigenous communities in North America, Latin America, the Arctic, Australia and the Indian Ocean.

Walter Benjamin,[1] writing on the eve of World War II, recognized an invisible feature of social and political life, which while appearing in a more exaggerated form under fascism, obtains in most societies and under various forms of governance and

---

* Nancy Scheper-Hughes, Ph.D., is a Professor of Medical Anthropology and Director of the Critical Studies in Medicine, Science, and the Body at the University of California at Berkeley.

1. Walter Benjamin. 1968 [1940]. Illuminations: Essays and Reflections, edited by Hannah Arendt. New York: Schocken.

governmentality: the tendency to 'normalize' suffering, disease, and premature death among certain excluded or marginalized classes and populations. This is what Michael Taussig[2] (reflecting on Benjamin) calls "terror as usual" and what I have called "everyday violence,"[3] though we do not usually associate disease with violence and terror, except perhaps when diseases are linked to biological warfare and other forms of blatant bio-terrorism. But violence and disease are linked in more ordinary way in social and bureaucratic indifference toward the excess morbidity and mortality of certain populations under the assumption that alarming statistics are not to be seen as alarming at all but rather as 'normal' to the population and therefore 'to be expected.' Another, is in the rush to biologize and racialize gross differences with respect to vulnerability to disease. Thus, alcoholism, depression, and suicide, obesity and diabetes in Indigenous communities have been normalized and racialized, consciously or not, in etiological theories.

To date, the prevailing medical model of diabetes etiology focuses on the 'faulty genes' of Indigenous Peoples combined with their faulty diets and other unhealthy behaviors, victim-blaming hypotheses that only serve to trap the sick person inside a cage of disease that is seemingly of their own making. Thus, some of the chapters of this new collection hark back to Susan Sontag's angry and visionary broadsheet, *Illness as Metaphor*, and refer to diabetes as symbol, as metaphor, even to diabetes as myth, in an effort to contest the view of diabetes as a plain thing, a natural fact, as disease itself.

This innovative book, a paradigm-breaking endeavor, is a creative assemblage of chapters by medical anthropologists, health professionals, nurses and doctors, Indigenous Peoples and community workers. It shifts the medical gaze from the diseased body to a diseased colonial and post-colonial history of genocide, the collective experience of trauma reproduced in the many 'small wars and invisible genocides' practiced against Indigenous Peoples to this day.

This volume is a bold attempt to reframe the meaning of diabetes as a socio-political pathology and to place the disease outside and beyond the body of the individual sufferer and to see it as the consequences of genocide and its aftermaths and in the signature that these collective losses have left on the bodies and even the physiologies and chemistries of Indigenous Peoples in the past and today. To say that diabetes is a socio-political pathology is not to deny the medical model of disease but rather to search for ultimate, rather than immediate causes and to recognize that what medical anthropologist Margaret Lock calls 'local biologies' (with reference to her comparative study of menopause among Japanese and North American women) emerge out of distinctive and collective experiences and histories of embodiment and risk producing local

2. See Michael Taussig. 1992. "Terror as Usual: Walter Benjamin's Theory of the History as State of Siege." In *The Nervous System*, esp. pp. 11–16, and 195–96. New York: Routledge.

3. See Nancy Scheper-Hughes. 1992, *Death without Weeping: The Violence of Everyday Life*. Everyday violence encompasses everything from the routinized, bureaucratized, and utterly banal violence of young children dying of hunger and maternal despair in Northeast Brazil to elderly African-Americans dying unnecessarily of heat stroke in suffocating apartments in inner city Chicago during the heat wave of 1995 . See Eric Klinenberg, 1999, "Denaturalizing Disaster: A Social Autopsy of the Chicago Heat Wave," *Theory and Society* 28: 239–92.

and even culture bound symptoms and experiences of supposedly universal illnesses and disease. These papers look at the social context of diabetes within Indigenous experiences of colonial expansions and occupation that disrupted Indigenous ways of being-in and living-in the world and of living in and experiencing their bodies.

Several chapters discuss how socio-inequality, traumatic experiences and psychosocial stress produce observable changes in the neuroendocrine system, affecting the production and circulation of hormones, including cortisol, glucagons, catecholamines and insulin itself. In the absence of protective factors, the leading symptom of diabetes mellitus, hyperglycemia or high blood sugars, sets in and its persistence brings terrifying problems for the body: blindness, poor circulation of hands and feet leading to gangrene and amputations, sexual impotence and other serious afflictions. Strong family ties, networks of social support, generosity, solidarity and love can produce what the authors here call emotional liberty. In their absence, the ability to grieve, to feel pain, and to suffer is impaired, generating intense emotional pain and suffering which pave the way for diabetes mellitus to set in.

Genocide, trauma, emotion, food, the loss of and return to hunting and gathering as cultural and biological survival are generative themes of this collection. Contributors contend that the prevailing research focusing on obesity, nutrition, and individual health behavior—although undeniably contributors to health outcomes—obscures social and historical issues that are even more fundamental to the etiology of the disease. The link between diet and diabetes is a robust one, of course, but these authors and clinicians argue from a political and human rights perspective that recognizes the devastating effects of colonization on Indigenous health and on access to abundant and nourishing food. Ferreira and her associates argue that "access to quality, nutritious food has become a human rights issue for Indigenous Peoples globally since everyone has the right to be free from hunger and undernutrition." This new civil right—a 'right to *good* food'—is enshrined in various international statutes including the Rome Declaration on World Food Security (1996), the International Covenant on Economic, Social and Cultural Rights (1966) and the Universal Declaration of Human Rights (1948). The authors note that there are profound contradictions between prevailing economic and clinical visions of what a "healthy diet" is, and the hunger and scarcity that prevails in Indigenous communities, as documented in Part 2 of this book (chapters 6 by Omura; 7 by Roy; 8 by Smith Morris; 9 by Lang; and 10 by Korn and Ryser). The healing power of traditional forms of food gathering and preparation, its highly ritualized and communal dimensions requires not only equitable and sustainable food systems, but rights to the security of Indigenous livelihoods, meaning rights to land, to labor, and to social and political security, all of which are presently lacking for most of the world's Indigenous Peoples.

I recall a visit in 1995 to a dispossessed band of Kung San people originally of the Kahahari Desert, who had resettled, for a price, on the private estate of an Afrikaner entrepreneur in the Northern Cape of South Africa. In exchange for the right to live on the estate, which was turned into a nature reserve and living cultural museum for tourists, the resident Kagga Kama had to dress traditionally in animal skins and entertain wealthy tourists with their display of traditional tools and weapons, story-telling and boasts of their hunting prowess. Back stage, however, the Kagga Kama lived in wretched pre-fabricated huts, a veritable slum in the wilderness. They were prohibited from hunting the plentiful springbok deer, rabbits and other small animals and from digging up and gathering the roots, berries, melons and eggs that had once been the mainstay of their diets. All their 'hunting and gathering' was now limited and contained to the estate-owned company store where dried corn meal, coffee, sugar, lard, flour and canned foods were the only food available to these 'faux' hunters who entertained the white tourist tribes with their displays of blow guns, darts, and digging sticks which they were prevented from using. A dietician supplied by a local university was conducting a study of the effects of 'poor dietary' habits on the Kaga Kama San who suffered inordinately from respiratory infections, tuberculosis, and, of course, diabetes. The Afrikaner student of nutritional science saw no irony in her empirical studies recording the daily caloric intake and nutritional analyses of the 'deficiencies' of Kagga Kama diets.

In this important and innovative collection the authors situate diabetes *inside* history rather than outside it, as in the shadowy, mythological and certainly myth-making anthropological and bio-evolutionary models of the prehistory of hunting and gathering peoples. James Neel, the controversial human geneticist of Yanomami fame, contributed a particularly dangerous view of Indigenous genetics around his hypothesized "thrift gene" theory of genetically-transmitted propensity to diabetes. Neel imagined Indigenous Peoples as camel-like beasts with an inherited ability to over-eat during times of plenty so as to produce a storage pouch of abdominal fat that could be drawn on during times of famine and food scarcity. Like many such hypothetical and imaginative theories ("just so stories") of bio-evolutionary and physiological adaptations, the inherited traits become liabilities and risks under new or rapidly changing circumstances. Thus, the 'thrifty gene' (a gene that has yet to materialize in the age of modern genomics) is seen as an evolutionary mechanism that back-fired once hunting and gathering peoples 'evolved' toward more 'civilized' and sedentary lives complete with cash stores and McDonalds and Kentucky Fry take-outs on or in easy reach of every reservation, not to mention every inner city neighborhood. Hunting and gathering amidst alternating periods of fast and famine disappeared, but (according to the 'thrifty gene hypothesis) the propensity to store fat lives on in Indigenous Peoples causing them to sicken from overweight and diabetes-prone sedentary habits.

The notion of the 'thrifty gene' (and the way it has been interpreted by health workers) suggests that "Indigenous blood" carries a taint—the threat of passing on an inherited risk of diabetes for which the only solution, paradoxically, is the dilution of Indigenous blood through racial intermarriage, another form of ' invisible genocide.' Thus, bad genetics combines with bad anthropology to produce a theory that put Indigenous People in their place—that is, on the margins as bio-evolutionary holdovers and deviants only capable of reproducing cycles of medical and social pathology. Despite this, the thrifty gene hypothesis has been adopted not only by doctors and other biomedical practitioners but by Indigenous Peoples themselves looking for an explanation for the ills that disproportionately beset their communities.

Like all reductionist theories, the 'thrifty gene' is nothing if not a 'thrifty'/nifty hypothesis, one that simplifies and excludes the complexities, the bio-social interactions, and the intervening variables like social class, gender, and the impact of colonial and post-colonial experiences of dispossession, forced migrations, and resettlement, chronic malnutrition, segregation and social exclusion. As Ferreira notes, the thrifty gene hypothesis erodes self-knowledge and turns sufferers into their own worst enemies as they adopt the idea that they are the heirs of faulty genetics and faulty behaviors (junk-food eaters, alcoholics, etc.) This, too, is another dimension of invisible genocide.

This volume is, therefore, more than a conventional medical anthropological presentation of illness narratives to balance the medical model of disease. Rather, the authors are engaged in taking at face value what Indigenous Peoples say, and feel, and do about the diabetes 'epidemic.' The goal is to move away from the purely medical model of diabetes and toward Indigenous models and understandings, an effort that was spearheaded not by physicians and social scientists but also by Indigenous Peoples themselves who chose to invite collaborations with clinicians, social scientists and researchers, but on their own terms. New efforts, such as the Kahnawake Schools Diabetes Prevention Project described by Ann Macaulay et al., confront the ethics of research and present a model for new partnerships among scholars, activists and community members.

The invention of new therapies in some communities include successful projects of culture restoration and rebuilding, including music therapy and relaxation, language and oral history workshops, bike paths, walking trails, summer camps for young people, providing social support and the emergence of new social movements to build solidarity. Acknowledging the role of mind-body interactions in stress reduction therapies, the editors have included a provocative chapter discussing evidence of the positive effects of relaxation techniques on the production of insulin.

Indigenous Peoples and Diabetes makes an eloquent case for a new and enlarged model and understanding of a modern epidemic on behalf of those who are doubly stigmatized by a disease that is seen as hopelessly mired in faulty adaptations (biological and cultural) to modern life. The book is inspired by a strong commitment to a liberation medicine and to the belief that access to good food, respect for cultural traditions, and integrative therapies are basic human rights.

SERIES EDITORS' PREFACE

Pamela J. Stewart and Andrew Strathern

We are pleased to see the present set of essays included in the *Ethnographic Studies in Medical Anthropology* Series. This collection is a unique set of essays that address a serious and significant medical problem, i.e., type II (also referred to as Adult Onset) diabetes. This form of diabetes is becoming an increasing problem around the world, both among wealthy populations who can buy whatever sorts of foods they wish, including healthy foods, and also among populations who may not be able to purchase, do not wish to, or do not have available to them healthy food supplies.

The approaches to the maintenance of the Type II diabetes that are discussed in the collection could profitably be applied to contexts in many geographic areas among peoples living in diverse economic situations. Diet, exercise, emotional well-being, and family support have proven to be significant factors in the proper maintenance of chronic disease states, including diabetes. Education of the individual with diabetes and their family is vitally important. Doctor-patient / health-care worker-patient communication is an important part of treatment. Since the management of diabetes is complex, requiring continuous vigilance, it is important that health-care workers and patients have an easy means to exchange information and that they rely on each other in a relationship of communication and mutual understanding (see discussions in Strathern and Stewart 1999).

The essays in this volume each have their individual strengths and the book will certainly take its place in the literature on medical anthropology. We read and commented on the Introduction and Chapters 1–20 during 2004. The topics in the essays are such that the work could be used in many different contexts and set for a variety of courses, e.g. those on critical medical anthropology, cultural identities, patient-physician communication, epidemiology, and nursing awareness, also in community educational centers and in training programs for healthcare practitioners.

The ways that Indigenous Peoples deal with health, diet, and disease are of particular interest to many scholars as they are also to ourselves in our research. In two of our recent books, *Curing and Healing: Medical Anthropology in Global Perspective* (Strathern and Stewart 1999) and *Humors and Substances: Ideas of the Body in New Guinea* (Stewart and Strathern 2001), we set out to explore how the peoples we work with in Papua New Guinea see their physical bodies and the sicknesses that influence their bodily functions as a part of their larger world-view or emplacement of themselves within their indigenous cosmology.

It is also always interesting and important to learn about how people build up their bodies through food and how they think their bodies are constituted in healthy or unhealthy ways. Here we will take an example from the Mount Hagen people of Papua New Guinea, among whom we have worked for many years and published on widely (e.g., A.J. Strathern 1971; Strathern and Stewart 2000). Historically they have had definite ideas about food and the body. For them, the sweet potato (*Ipomoea batatas*) was their staple, the focal member of a class of food sources called *röng* in the local language. This also included taro, yams, green vegetables of many kinds, bananas, sugarcane, edible ferns, shoots, and inflorescences. All of these foods were appreciated and many were planted together in complex garden areas known as *pana*, a term which later came to signify "year" in colonial times after the 1930s.

Sweet potatoes, an introduced crop, nevertheless had become, in the several hundred years after its arrival in New Guinea, the staple crop for the peoples of the Highlands region, because of its ability to grow well in mountainous conditions. For Hageners, then, sweet potato was the quintessential "food", which they even described in the 1960s, using a term from the lingua franca Tok Pisin, as their "merasin" (medicine), i.e., a food that could keep them feeling well. Taro, although a much more ancient crop, was not described in this way, but people did say of it *kun pei na petem*, "there is no hunger in it", it was very satisfying to eat and stayed off the pangs of hunger.

All categories of *röng* were contrasted, and paired, with the category of *kng/kung*, "pork", which in colonial times was expanded to include beef and mutton, introduced forms of meat. The provision, for special occasions, of *kng röng rakl*, "pork and vegetables", was seen as an important marker of hospitality; and what pork especially added to foods in general was *kopong*, "grease". In turn "grease" was a general marker of vitality, prosperity, and fertility. To have *kopong* was therefore to be vital, alive, healthy, and even influential. A body lacking *kopong* was not seen as healthy.

Hageners' ideas about bodily composition, therefore, led them to associate "fatness" with "health", a supposition that can further lead to problems for them in contexts where their dietary intake has changed. Pork was rarely eaten in the past and consumed only at special ceremonies along with vegetables, which were daily staples; the availability of fatty meat and fried food in urban stores has changed this situation radically. This observation underlines the importance of studying diet as an integral part of a people's whole set of historical and adaptive circumstances and their own ideas of ideal bodily and mental states. In Hagen a good *noman* or "mind" was also said to be reflected in a "healthy" body, i.e., one with *kopong* (grease/fat).

In thinking about the body in sickness one must also consider the body and its place within the social system at large. Many discussions on the body in anthropology have tended to oscillate between a stress on the body as a passive marker and the body as a locus of agency. Mary Douglas in her writing distinguished clearly between different social environments and their effects on perception and experience (Douglas 1966) and spoke of the "social body" as constraining the perceptions of the "individual body" (Douglas 1970: 68). Thomas Csordas, by contrast, has emphasized embodied experience as the foundation of culture (e.g. Csordas 1994).

But if one starts with a different set of propositions, i.e., looking at the emplacement of the individual body within a cosmological world-view, this opposition is itself mediated. To say that the body is a part of the cosmos implies already that it has its place in the cosmos and that the cosmos, in a sense, runs through it as well as vice-versa. To be a part of the cosmos, however, is also actively to experience life within it and to experience change and stress that evoke active and energetic responses. When disjunctions occur between a sense of "proper" cosmological emplacement it is more difficult for individuals to place their bodily well-being into a cycle of day-to-day health maintenance. This is true for those peoples classified as "indigenous" and those that are not classified in that way. Issues of this kind are explored in thoughtful, practical, and concerned ways by the contributors to this volume.

References

Csordas, Thomas (ed.) 1994. *Embodiment and Experience: The Existential Ground of Culture and Self.* Cambridge: Cambridge University Press.

Douglas, Mary 1966. *Purity and Danger: An Analysis of the Concepts of Pollution and Taboo.* London: Routledge and Kegan Paul.

_____ 1970. *Natural Symbols: Explorations in Cosmology.* New York: Pantheon Books.

Stewart, Pamela J. and Andrew Strathern 2001. *Humors and Substances: Ideas of the Body in New Guinea.* Westport, CT and London: Bergin and Garvey.

Strathern, Andrew 1971. *The Rope of Moka.* Cambridge: Cambridge University Press.

Strathern, Andrew and Pamela J. Stewart 1999. *Curing and Healing: Medical Anthropology in Global Perspective.* Durham, N.C.: Carolina Academic Press.

_____ 2000. *Arrow Talk: Transaction, Transition, and Contradiction in New Guinea Highlands History.* Kent, OH and London: The Kent State University Press.

Acknowledgments

Mariana and Gretchen would like to thank each of the authors in this anthology—it has been a pleasure to work with you! We greatly appreciate the collaborative spirit and strict work ethics in putting this exciting collection of original essays together. We especially want to thank Dr. Jo Scheder for her generous contribution to this volume, inspiring all of us to look deeply into a physiology of oppression as it relates to type 2 diabetes and the on-going process of colonization of Indigenous Peoples across the planet. The critical work of Nancy Scheper-Hughes has also stirred us toward a liberation medicine that believes access to good food, respect for cultural traditions, and integrative therapies are basic human rights. Indigenous professionals, elders and community members from different nations have provided us all with invaluable knowledges and conscientious practices for the empowerment and well-being of First Peoples worldwide. Thank you!

Our thanks to the Senior Editors of the Medical Anthropology Series, Carolina Academic Press, Pamela Stewart and Andrew Strathern, for all the encouragement and editorial advice.

Mariana Leal Ferreira would like to acknowledge all the trust and support received from United Indian Health Services in northern California, and the Yurok community in particular. Research grants were provided by the Brazilian agencies CNPQ (Conselho Nacional de Desenvolvimento Científico e Tecnológico) and FAPESP (Fundação de Amparo à Pesquisa do Estado de São Paulo), and from Graduate Programs in the United States at the University of California at Berkeley, University of Tennessee, and San Francisco State University. Gretchen Chesley Lang expresses her gratitude to the Spirit Lake Dakota community, as well as colleagues and mentors, Profs. Dorothy K. Billings, Eugene Ogan, H. Clyde Wilson and the late Bernard O'Kelly, Arts and Sciences Dean (University of North Dakota), for their encouragement of her work with Indigenous health issues over many years.

INDIGENOUS PEOPLES AND DIABETES

Introduction: Deconstructing Diabetes

Mariana Leal Ferreira and Gretchen Chesley Lang

TIKI

The legend of Creation, the children of Ranginui (sky father) and Papatuanuku (mother earth), were clothing and creating life on earth. Tane (one of the children) was one, if not the main life-bringer. Tane with his brothers created Hine Titama, the first woman, for Tane. Tumatauenga then thought he would create the first man Tiki. This is how we came to be, through the breeding of the children of Tane, Hine and Tiki. This is also how Tumatauenga became god of Man and War."

from the Opening Program of the Fifth International Conference on
Diabetes and Indigenous Peoples: 'Te Hikoi o Nga Mokopuna'—Walking
with Our Grandchildren. New Zealand, 2000.

Indigenous Peoples and Diabetes. Community Empowerment and Wellness is a call for a truly interdisciplinary and revolutionizing re-consideration of *Diabetes mellitus* in the twenty-first century. Long over-due, the call is welcomed by Indigenous Peoples, health professionals, activists, scholars and community members working toward a better quality of life for present and future generations to come. Here, we situate diabetes within a complex landscape that extends beyond conventional biomedical and clinical understandings into the realm of social justice and emotional liberty. The authors of the chapters in this anthology—anthropologists, tribal health planners, physicians, health-care givers, activists and writers—share a commitment to considering diabetes in terms of the survival and quality of life of Indigenous Peoples worldwide who are disproportionately affected by the ailment. We examine the social causes of diabetes, rather than the purely biological factors, that structure risk for type 2 diabetes in Indigenous societies, and propose innovative venues for engaged research and collaborative action that promote community empowerment and wellness.

The inspiration for this volume came, as well, from the editors' own work in medical anthropology with communities where diabetes has become widespread, as well as their participation in the International Conference on Diabetes and Indigenous Peoples at different times and places over the years. Most recently for Mariana Ferreira, in 2000 in southern New Zealand, where the idea for this book began among the Maori and other southern Pacific Peoples who organized the *Fifth International Conference on Diabetes and Indigenous Peoples,* " 'Te Hikoi o Nga Mokopuna'—Walking with Our

Grandchildren." This international conference can be characterized by participants' advocacy for community-based wellness, stemming from Indigenous knowledges and practices, both traditional and modern. *TIKI*, the first Maori man, incorporated very well this dialog between past and present in the year 2000, when he posed as the protagonist of the Diabetes Conference in New Zealand. In this collection of essays, *TIKI* conveys the significance of Indigenous theories about the world experienced as well as the importance of community-initiated programs tailored to shape a better future and produce social and emotional well-being.

The purpose underlying *Diabetes and Indigenous Peoples: Community Empowerment and Wellness* is to reframe questions regarding the dramatic increase of diabetes mellitus amongst Indigenous Peoples, with an emphasis on traditional as well as creative, innovative approaches in health care delivery for those who suffer from this chronic condition. Conceptualized as a way of initiating a much more encompassing and critical perspective on the diabetes epidemic that is challenging Indigenous Peoples world wide, the essays included here illustrate a number of directions in which research and applied efforts are going. The papers presented in this collection have emerged from their authors' scholarship, fieldwork and professional experience working with or as members of Indigenous Peoples in the United States, Canada, Australia, and South Asia. The book also bears testimony of Indigenous Peoples who have seen and experienced diabetes in their families and communities. It is both an argument and a plea for new scholarship: comprehensive analyses that situate diabetes within its historical, socioeconomic, and political context, with the hope of encouraging communities in efforts to achieve wellness in the broadest sense. Likewise, readers will learn of community-based efforts underway with Indigenous Peoples whose lives have so dramatically changed from autonomy and self-reliance, to the experience of poverty, dramatic subsistence/dietary change, and social inequality within larger state-level societies. We demonstrate some positive ways in which advances in biomedical research and clinical practice may better be realized at community and individual levels.

Contributors to this book want to shift the gaze away from the medical clinic and the physical body so as to unveil additional meanings and political implications of the discourse about diabetes. Why are there such huge disparities in the geographic distribution of diabetes? Why does this ailment affect mostly poor, migrating and traumatized populations? Why are Indigenous Peoples globally increasingly at risk? Why does current research insist on the role of genetic and cultural factors and shift away from the social causes of this devastating ailment? What are the effects of disseminating the idea that "Indian" or "Indigenous heritage" is a risk factor for diabetes, when there is no real proof of a "diabetes gene"? Why do the major governmental funding agencies and pharmaceutical companies sponsor studies that lead almost exclusively to the development of more diabetes drugs and supplies when it is obvious the solution lies elsewhere? What becomes clear to the authors of this anthology is that there is a clear convergence between political ideology and medical technology in respect to the significance of diabetes. Here, we see the real priorities currently at work in the proliferation of a huge corporate pharmacopeia via the health care industry, in relation to the social control of "native" populations.

It is obvious that solutions to the diabetes question are not coming from "above" in terms of the fashioning of federal social policies that would ameliorate the life conditions of thousands of Indigenous Peoples worldwide. On the contrary, national governments have chosen to ignore and refuse to take responsibility for the diabetes epidemic, blaming, instead, Indigenous cultures, behavior and genotype.[1] However, while no governmental action is being taken to stop the "small genocides" committed against Indigenous Peoples worldwide on a daily basis (Scheper-Hughes and Bourgois 2004), Indigenous nations themselves are actively engaged in ameliorating the everyday life conditions of their peoples and taking the diabetes problem into their own hands. Indigenous governments and tribal councils do indeed hold colonizing nation-states responsible for the structural violence that has given rise to diabetes epidemics, and therefore demand structural changes that can free social ailments from the confines of individualized medical treatments. However, social suffering and pain exist, and diabetes is known to cause intense physiological, individual and social distress, including blindness, kidney failure, gangrene, impotence and depression. Indigenous Peoples worldwide, in collaboration with health professionals, scholars and activists, have thus proposed community-based programs and ideas in this book based on millennia of wisdom and experience to alleviate emotional suffering and promote emotional liberty.

The question then becomes: What can we learn from successful, community-based and/or community-initiated programs to prevent diabetes? The authors of the chapters here and, especially, as seen in the narratives of Indigenous Peoples themselves, indicate that a critical understanding of the diabetes phenomenon ultimately depends upon taking account of factors that go beyond what biomedicine in a clinical setting can examine. We feel that it is timely—most critically so after the end of the Decade of Indigenous Peoples (1995–2004), when most of the problems affecting First Nations remain the same—to present this collection of different kinds of insights regarding the social, economic, political and historical contexts in which *Diabetes mellitus* has appeared and continues to increase as an epidemic. Social and economic realities which have been well documented and that can be easily taken into account and analyzed—such as the loss of land, relocation and confinement on reservations, forced labor, poverty and unemployment—must be within our focus as we consider the vulnerability of individuals and entire communities to this epidemic. Certainly, this includes issues of social inequality—often in conjunction with racism and ethnocentrism—and rests upon centuries of traumatic lived experience by generations of Indigenous Peoples who— in many instances—were and still are dramatically disenfranchised of their lands, sociopolitical autonomy, and for many, identity as a People or a Nation.

In an age that unabashedly places most great hope on breakthroughs in genetics and clinical medicine for curing human diseases and alleviating suffering, we argue that the dramatically increasing prevalence of diabetes type 2 that disproportionately affects Indigenous Peoples, brings up the discomforting realization that solutions will require confronting situational realities within contemporary societies and will require major collaborative efforts between Indigenous communities and public health pro-

---

1. In a 2004 article, Indian Health Service (IHS, a branch of the U.S. Department of Health and Human Services) contends that type 2 diabetes starts as insulin resistance, caused by a combination of: inherited (genetic) factors, environmental factors and behavioral factors (in this order). The only "evidence" offered for the genetic explanation is that " American Indians and Alaska Natives appear to be especially vulnerable to diabetes" (<www.ihs.gov/FacilitiesServices/AreaOffices/Phoenix/phx_feature200405.cfm>; accessed on 11.08.04).

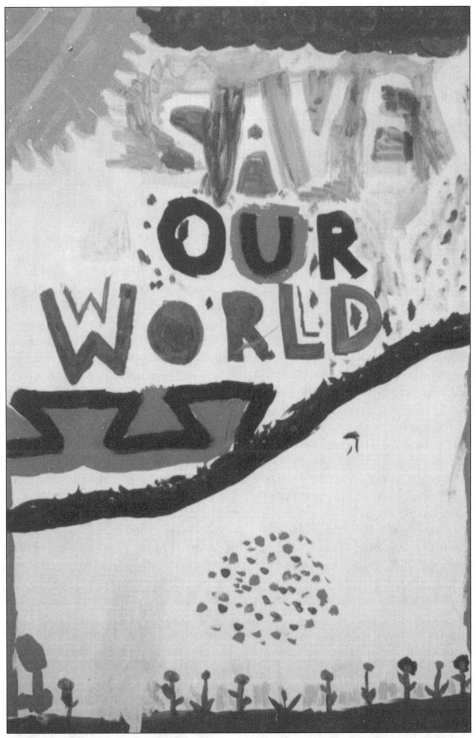

"Save Our World" is part of a collection of Yurok children's posters surrounding a toxic Cal-Trans dump site on the Yurok Indian Reservation in northern California (photo: Mariana L. Ferreira, 1996).

grams. And perhaps most importantly, solutions will require public policy measures to help empower Indigenous communities and socioeconomically disenfranchised communities within the large societies in which they find themselves—for Indigenous Peoples, illness conditions are another glaring reminder of a history of genocide and colonization that in fact continues on as social inequality appears to be increasing within the global economy (cf. Sennett 2003: 80; Wilkinson 1996). Ironically, chronic illnesses, sometimes termed "diseases of modernization" are disproportionately higher for those very people who have not necessarily benefited from modernization. A further irony is that despite intensive and continuing studies of Peoples with a high incidence of diabetes, genetically-based explanations that identify Indigenous Peoples as being more susceptible to diabetes or as having a genetic predisposition have been remarkably unsuccessful in identifying specific mechanisms through which this is alleged to happen (Park 2004). Indeed, the diabetes epidemic requires critical analyses on many levels; several contributors found that members in some Indigenous communities were troubled by health-workers statements that "Indians" were predisposed to develop diabetes "because of their genes."

The contributors to this volume want to dispel etiological explanations that adhere to a genetic determinism of diabetes—a reductionist view for a complex condition that has been virtually non-existent for many world peoples until the past 60 or 70 years. We wish to advance a call, instead, for research and clinical practice to take into consideration a much wider range of variables, including the common history of dispossession, trauma, inequality and emotional suffering that now finds Indigenous Peoples worldwide at risk for type 2 diabetes. In her recent review article, "Theories for Social Epidemiology in the 21st Century: An Ecosocial Perspective" Nancy Krieger (2001) eloquently lays out the *different kinds of explanations* for diseases that afflict groups of people disproportionately across a society or globally. Krieger (2001: 1) states:

> Grappling with notions of causation, in turn, raises not only complex philosophical issues but also, in the case of social epidemiology, issues of accountability and agency: Simply invoking abstract notions of 'society' and disembodied 'genes' will not suffice. Instead, the central question becomes: who and what is responsible for population patterns of health, disease, and well-being, as manifested in present, past and changing social inequalities in health?

The chapters in this volume range from ethnographic studies of communities in which diabetes is occurring to documenting community-based efforts to improve diabetes care, to considerations of non-conventional strategies for community involvement in their own health, to papers that argue that only a process of liberation of Indigenous Peoples, from both a macro and micro viewpoint, can give rise to a multitude of innovations to create favorable conditions for improving the quality of life and consequently the health of Indigenous Peoples in North America, Latin America, the Indian Ocean, Australia, and elsewhere in the world.

Historians of science and critical medical anthropologists have pointed out that the limited and reified scope of biological studies of many ailments has hindered a more comprehensive approach to the nature of such complex phenomena, particularly of diabetes (Canguilhem 1988, 1991; Farmer 1996, 2003; Foucault 1975; Scheper-Hughes 1993; Roy 2002; Taussig 1991; Lock et al. 2000). The papers that appear in this book take perspectives that broaden the conversation and may surprise some readers, delight others and irritate or aggravate a few!, as so much has been written about diabetes from a biomedical point of view. A radical redefinition of what *Diabetes mellitus* actually is, and what the disorder represents for Indigenous Peoples are crucial questions that need to be urgently addressed if we are to halt the perverse outcomes of such a devastating epidemic. Blindness, kidney failure, poor circulation leading to gangrene and amputations, loss of libido and sexual impotence are some of the tragic consequences. How to make sense of built-in wheel chair ramps that come with standard trailer homes built for some Indian reservations today? What to say of medical facilities and hospitals run by Indian Health Service that specialize in amputations, such as the Phoenix Indian Medical Center in Arizona?

To a great extent, the medical community and the diabetes industry encourage its members and the general public to recognize obesity, family history of the disease, and amount of Indian ancestry as risk factors for type 2 diabetes. These are the problems the literature on diabetes admits as scientific, yet from a critical perspective, could be seen as a deliberate attempt to ignore the macro-social context in which diabetes originates and the political and economic aspects of its geographic distribution across so many groups of Indigenous Peoples around the world. Variables, such as environment, culture and emotion, are often rejected as metaphysical, or else, when cited, considered "too complex" or sometimes just too problematic to be worth the time.

Who are Indigenous Peoples and Where Do They Live ?

An estimated 300 million individuals of approximately 5000 different Indigenous Peoples inhabit more than 70 countries in different parts of the globe, from the Artic to the South Pacific. More than half of this population, or 150 million people of numerous ethnic backgrounds and religious orientations are concentrated in India and China, and carry on traditional knowledges and practices within larger religious traditions of Buddhism, Hinduism, and Islam. While there is enormous cultural and linguistic diversity in these regions, Tibetan and Mongolian nomadic herders of eastern China share similar problems with isolated tribal Indigenous Peoples in South Asia, largely due to resettlement policies and the struggle for access to water and land resources. In fact, the term Indigenous or aboriginal is usually applied to Peoples who were living on their lands before the arrival of foreign settlers. From this perspective, Indigenous Peoples are the descendants of those who inhabited a country or a geographical region at the time of the arrival of colonizers. It is important to note, that the definition of Indigenous Peoples advanced by the United Nations and adopted by various international organizations today transcends territoriality and relies on ethnic and cultural identity, and political power (Ferreira 2004).

Among the Indigenous Peoples of the world are the Maya, Guarani, Mapuche, Hopi, Lakota and other Amerindians of North and South America; the Innu, Crees and Aleutians of the circumpolar region; the Sami of northern Europe; the Nanai and Taiga of northern Russia and Siberia; the !Kung, Bakgatla, and Fulani of Africa; the

What is Type 2 Diabetes? Expanding the Biomedical Point of View

The two basic types of diabetes mellitus are type 1 and type 2. In this volume, we are addressing only type 2 diabetes because it is by far the most common form of diabetes and affects Indigenous Peoples worldwide disproportionately. In the US alone, 10.3 million people have been diagnosed with diabetes and an estimated additional 5.4 million have undiagnosed diabetes. Approximately 90% have type 2 diabetes and the remainder have type 1. In type 2 diabetes, previously known as non-insulin dependent diabetes mellitus (NIDDM), either the body does not produce enough insulin or else the cells ignore the sugar brought to them by the insulin. Sugar or glucose is a basic fuel for the organism but when glucose builds up in the blood, rather than be consumed in the cells, it gives rise to "high blood glucose." Sustained high blood sugars may cause serious complications, such as kidney failure, blindness, heart disease, and sexual impotence. Diabetes is the major cause of blindness in adults aged 20–74 years, as well as the leading cause of non-traumatic lower-extremity amputation and end-stage renal disease.

Type 2 diabetes typically occurs in individuals older than 40 years who may have a "family history" of the disorder. Having diabetes in the family does not mean, however, that the ailment is hereditary or genetic, as widely believed. In this book we are critical of racist concepts, such as "Indian heritage" and "Indigenous genome," loosely and irresponsibly defined by the biomedical community as "risk factors" to help explain disparity rates in the prevalence of type 2 diabetes. Type 2 diabetes mellitus is more prevalent among American Indians (12–50%, depending on the nation), African Americans (10.8%), Hispanics (10.6%), and Asians/Pacific Islanders than in Caucasians. Type 2 diabetes is becoming increasingly common worldwide because the perverse effects of colonization and genocide in so-called developing countries are in some cases only recently being fully felt. In the so-called first world, more people are living longer and diabetes prevalence clearly increases with age. In addition, type 2 diabetes is also being seen more frequently in younger people in association with the rising prevalence of childhood obesity. Although type 2 diabetes still occurs most commonly in adults aged 40 years and older, the incidence of disease is increasing more rapidly in adolescents and young adults than in other age groups. In the United States, type 2 diabetes affects Indigenous children as young as eight or nine years of age, as discussed in this book.

Type 1 diabetes mellitus, on the other hand, accounts for only 10 percent of all diagnoses. Type 1 is not addressed in this volume because it is not known to affect Indigenous Peoples disproportionately. Type 1 diabetes was commonly referred to as juvenile diabetes, or else insulin dependent diabetes mellitus (IDDM) because of young patient's dependence on a continuous source of exogenous insulin and carbohydrates for survival. The use of terms "juvenile" and "IDDM" have been abandoned due to type 2 diabetes' current frequency in younger populations and increasing dependence on insulin (rather than diet and exercise alone). (Adapted from ADA 2004; IDF 2003; King et al. 1998; and chapters in this book.)

Ilongot of the Philippines; the Arrernte and other Aborigenes and Torres Strait Islanders of Australia; and the Maori of New Zealand. In a number of nation-states at present, such as Bolivia, Peru, Ecuador, and Guatemala, South Africa, Zimbabwe, etc., the majority of the population would be considered Indigenous.

This volume includes the voices of the Crees, Dakota (Sioux), Yurok (and members of other nations in the American Northwest), Mohawk, Navajo, Mexican-American farmworkers, the people of Reunion Island in the Indian Ocean (peopled over centuries by migrants from many world regions), Akimel O'odham (Pima of Gila River), Innu of Canada, and Aboriginal Australians of the Northern Territory. The Americas alone are the home to some 50 million Indigenous individuals. In a few regions, however, such as Brazil and the United States, less than two per cent of the residents are native to the area—between 90 and 95 per cent of these countries' original inhabitants were

Indigenous, the United Nations' Definition

"Indigenous communities, Peoples and nations are those which, having a historical continuity with pre-invasion and pre-colonial societies that developed on their territories, consider themselves distinct from other sectors of the societies now prevailing in those territories, or parts of them. They form at present non-dominant sectors of society and are determined to preserve, develop, and transmit to future generations their ancestral territories, and their ethnic identity, as the basis of their continued existence as Peoples, in accordance with their own cultural patterns, social institutions, and legal systems." (United Nations 1983)

decimated during the colonial period, which clearly amounts to genocide according to the United Nations Genocide Convention (1946). Surprisingly, but probably not for long, about 50 Indigenous Peoples still live in isolation in Central Brazil; that is, without systematic contact with the broader Brazilian society.

Epidemiologists and medical geographers would agree, that it is imperative to look at the geographical distribution and demographics of who suffers from diabetes, type 2. Recent studies in the 1980s and 90s reveal that diabetes is most prevalent among migrating, traumatized and socioeconomically disadvantaged populations in Australia, Brazil, Canada, Ethiopia, India, Japan, New Guinea and Tanzania (Famuyiwa et al. 1990, 1985; King et al. 1998; Smide et al. 1999; O'Nell 1996; Oyewole and Johnson 1980) and in many other countries. In the United States, a disparity also exists

Who is Indigenous? Territory, Politics and Identity

The problem of who is Indigenous and who is not, however, remains largely controversial. Defining how the term Indigenous applies to African, European and Asian Peoples is not as clear cut as it is to Amerindians, Canadian First Nations and Australian Aborigines. In New Zealand, "brown faces" are distinguished from Europeans, or "whites." In the Americas, "Indians" are those of non-European ancestry and non-African descent. This is not to say that the question of "who is an Indian" has been resolved in these regions—in the United States, for instance, Indianess has been defined biologically since the Dawes Act (also known as the General Allotment Act) of 1887 was enacted. One-quarter was the minimum fraction of blood allowing federally recognized Indians to claim possession of land allotments, when their own ancestral territories were opened to American citizens for homesteading. Following the US Indian Reorganization Act of 1934, blood quantum requirements were relegated to the tribal level, and today standards vary from one-quarter (among the Pima of Arizona, for instance) to open enrollment, which requires tracing descent from an Indian ancestor, however remote (the case of the Cherokee Tribe of Oklahoma). Nearly 300 native Peoples in the US are currently seeking federal recognition as American Indians, and question blood as a measure of Indigenous identity. In Brazil, while Indianess is a matter of self-definition, various groups struggle to obtain official identification because of their mixed European and/or African, and Amerindian ancestry. The purity of blood lines, and consequently individuals' appearances, still function, in most cases, as the defining criteria (Ferreira 2004).

It is also important to point out the relevance of using the term Indigenous "Peoples," rather than populations, according to international law. In general, population refers to a group of individuals, which may be of relevance for the domestic law of a particular state. Peoples, however, have the right to self-determination, that is, the right to manage local and internal affairs, including economic, social and cultural matters. This right is one of the basic principles of international law, and the consequences of the acceptance of the character of "Peoples" are far reaching (Hans-Joachim Heintze 1993).

when we compare prevalence rates for African-Americans and for Hispanics, and the population of the United States as a whole. Among Mexican farmworkers in the southern U.S. working in a debt-peonage system and living below the poverty line, the prevalence of type 2 diabetes is also 2 to 3 times higher than national average—currently at 6.5% (Scheder 1988 and in this volume). Morever, certain aspects of the disorder have been emphasized to the detriment of others. As mentioned above, the focus of current research and therapy has been on the relation between the endocrine system (the system of glands and other structures that produce hormones—such as insulin—which are released directly into the circulatory system, influencing metabolism and other bodily processes) and the digestive system (the organs concerned with ingestion, digestion and absorption of food or nutritional elements). The nervous system, which, along with the endocrine system, correlates the adjustments and reactions of the organism to its internal and external environment, has been greatly neglected, in spite of the evidence that systematic exposure to stressors such as trauma and other kinds of nervous stimuli play an important role in the onset of diabetes mellitus (Cf. Bernard 1877; Canguilhem 1991; Ferreira 1998, 1999, 2003 and in this volume; Lustman et al. 1981; Mullen et al. 1996; Roy 2002; Scheder 1988; Surwit & Feinglos 1983, 1988).

A Worldwide Epidemic

Diabetes mellitus is now a worldwide epidemic. The impact on Indigenous Peoples is far from being fully documented, though epidemiological studies show a high prevalence of diabetes began for most groups around mid-20th Century (cf. reviews, including Wiedman 2002; K.Young et al. 2000; K.Young 1993; Joe and Young 1994; Rokala et al., 1991; Szathmary 1987; Weiss et al. 1984; West 1974, 1978). In the United States alone, the share of the population diagnosed with diabetes jumped 33% nationally, to 6.5%, between 1990 and 1998 (CDC 2000). The prevalence of diabetes in adults worldwide was estimated to be 4% in 1995 and predicted to be 5.4% by the year 2025. A recent study (King et al. 1998) shows that the number of adults with diabetes in the world will rise from 135 million in 1995 to 300 million in the year 2025. The major part of this numerical increase will occur in developing countries and among the socio-economically disadvantaged in the so-called First World. There will be a 42% increase, from 51 to 72 million, in the developed countries and a 170% increase, from 84 to 228 million, in the developing countries. Thus, by the year 2025, more than 75% of people with diabetes will reside in developing countries, as compared with 62% in 1995. The countries with the largest number of people with diabetes are, and will be in the year 2025, India, China and, interestingly enough, the United States. In the current situation of globality, however, this comes at no surprise: the wealth gap between the rich and the poor in the US and all over the world, broadly speaking, sharply increased in the 1990s. With unemployment on the rise the situation tends to get worse because employment is a key driver of income, especially at the lower end of the economic ladder (*Federal Reserve Report*, Jan 22, 2003. Meanwhile, governmental health organizations associate themselves with pharmaceutical companies, ensuring enormous

---

Biomedical Diagnosis and Treatment of Diabetes Type 2

The clinical diagnosis of diabetes type 2 involves blood glucose tests and urine analysis. The treatment requires the patient to self-monitor blood glucose levels two to four times a day and follow prescriptions for food and exercise. If these fail, oral agents and insulin are added. Patients' meals are supervised by a dietician and exercises are monitored by a physical therapist. Indigenous Peoples often describe the prescribed meals as "Everything you don't want to eat: raw vegetables, fruit and lean meat." Clinicians know that a recently diagnosed patient has not been following the prescribed diet if the level of his or her blood sugar does not go down. High blood pressure and high levels of protein in the urinalysis also indicate non-compliance with the prescribed treatment. Repeated urinary tract infections and vaginal yeast infections are also associated with diabetes, thus screening for these disorders also take place. Indigenous Peoples see the diagnoses and treatment of diabetes as yet another form of social control because the biomedical rationale mimics the ideology of governmental Indian policies—based on tight scrutiny of the "quality" and "quantity" of what qualifies as "Indian blood" (Ferreira 1998, 1999).

---

financial and political gains for both sides by profiting on human suffering, as mentioned above. Such is the case of the well-known association between the National Institutes of Health (NIH) and pharmaceutical companies in the United States (Angell 2004; Steinbrook 2004). Many of the chapters here presented use diabetes as a model to examine the links among political ideology, social inequality, and health outcome.

Consequently, diabetes is *increasing* in prevalence among all American Indian and Alaska Native populations in the United States. Indian Health Services (IHS) studies show that between 1991 and 1997, the prevalence of diabetes increased in all major regions served by the agency. The prevalence ranged from 17% among nations in the Northern Plains to 80% in Alaska. Two Indigenous Peoples in the IHS Nashville Area, the Choctaw and Cherokee, had a 30% increase in diabetes prevalence in those 6 years. Earlier, in 1989, a survey among the Mississippi Choctaw showed that more than one-third of the 638 adults from ages 45 to 64 years had diabetes, and there were almost as many cases in the younger age group from ages 15 to 44 years (IHS National Diabetes Program—*Special Diabetes Program for Indians Interim Report to Congress,* Jan. 2000).

Racializing Diabetes, Disempowering the People

Important questions thus remain: How can a genetic cause be applied across the borders to 300 million people divided into thousands of ethnic groups, living across the planet under strikingly different circumstances? What do these people have in common? Their genes? What is the meaning of "Indian heritage" as a risk factor for diabetes? The current debate regarding genetic discrimination and stigmatization of groups is certainly not new to Indigenous Peoples, dating back over hundreds of colonizing years. Finally in 2001, the Human Genome Project was able to demonstrate that 94 percent of DNA variation occurs within groups, and that the DNA of two unrelated, same-sex individuals, regardless of ethnicity, is more than 99.5 percent identical (Royal and Dunston 2004). Therefore, there is no biologic basis for "race" or for any claim of a hypothetical Indian or Indigenous genome. Nonetheless, the reality is that racism exists, and In-

---

Century of the Gene Becomes Century of Genetic Determinism

"By the end of the Nineties, the century of the gene had become the century of genetic determinism. So far, the new century looks like being even more of the same. Popularized by Richard Dawkins, the notion of 'selfish genery' is a particular take on Darwin's theory of evolution. According to this twist, bodies are just 'lumbering robots' for the transmission of the all-important genes. Conversely, then, genes must be the essence of a person. Maybe there are genes for intelligence and beauty, genes for alcoholism and criminality: if it is not in your genes, you do not have it, and if it is, you have and always will.

The trouble with this view is that its meaning is as much political as scientific... [As] Steve Rose says: 'Part of the reason [genetic determinism] has been so popular is people have despaired of social solutions to problems... Now people are fatalistic, there is no way to change things, which fits with genetic determinism....'"

Mike Bygrave, "False Dawns in the Brave New World of New Genetics," *The Guardian* (UK), 22 December 2002.

---

digenous Peoples have been systematically blamed for their bad genes, blood or even pancreatic characteristics by the medical community.

The irresponsible ways, for example, in which the concept of "Indian heritage" has been applied to determine the causes of diabetes qualifies both the concept and its use as a form of "scientific racism." To say that "Indian heritage" is a risk factor for diabetes mellitus because Indians have a "defective" or "thrifty" gene sends out a very perverse message to Indigenous Peoples all over the planet: "If it's in your genes, there is nothing you can do about it." In this book we challenge this form of stereotyping and genetic reductionism by showing, with concrete examples, the ways in which specific health effects relate to macro-level politics and economics. The contributors situate diabetes within a broader debate that encompasses power relations in the process of diagnosis, treatment, and in the delivery of health services. In this respect, many of the chapters here support the small, but growing evidence that diabetes may be understood as a physiological response to adverse, traumatic or stressful life experiences, rather than as a disease in itself. On the other hand, we have also found evidence that those families and individuals who are engaged in networks of social support can manage their sentiments more effectively and are thus able to assure emotional liberty—a protective factor against diabetes. Physiologically speaking, some of our authors support the claim that type 2 diabetes is an outcome of emotionally stimulating claims in terms of the arousal of the autonomic nervous system and the endocrine system. Emotional suffering and emotional liberty are here proposed as conceptual ideas that can help redefine the diabetes question in terms of what the authors call a politically meaningful history of emotions.

Despite all the technological advances in biomedicine, the etiology of diabetes remains elusive. Earlier genetically-based hypotheses are being gradually cast aside, yet in the 'popular culture' as well as amongst a great number of practicing health professionals, these ideas retain a firm foothold, as discussed below. Moreover, favoring biologic and genetic characteristics when explaining why diabetes is so prevalent among certain Peoples has had the effect of making the intense suffering experienced by Indigenous nations seem more distant and therefore less affective, because it is imputed to "otherness." Both well-intentioned care givers as well as Indigenous Peoples themselves often make statements that directly illustrate this:

- "Indians have diabetes because they eat poorly and don't exercise enough, and many are obese."

- "Indians and other tribal Peoples are predisposed genetically to diabetes and other diseases."

- "Indigenous Peoples have a defective gene that has become maladaptive."

Such statements have the effect of lowering self-esteem dramatically, disempowering the people and rendering them unable and unwilling to change the situation. Patients often ask: "Why follow diets and do all that exercise if it's *in* us?"

The Politics of Indigenous Identity: Consequences of the Once-Popular 'Thrifty Gene' Hypothesis

The "thrifty gene theory" (Neel 1962, 1982) is, in reality, a hypothesis that never did become a theory, because it failed to show the mechanisms through which a hypothetical thrifty gene, which protected the body against starvation in times of great seasonal fluctuation, became maladaptive with modern patterns of food consumption and the ability to store fat, leading to diabetes. While conventional biomedical thinking has primarily considered diabetes to have a strong genetic predisposition—the "thrifty genotype" was once part of every medical student's training—to date, no specific understanding of the genes involved has been uncovered. In an era where genetic research is so much in the foreground, it becomes more important than ever to consider very carefully if the assumptions and questions about diabetes, themselves, are at least partly shaped by the larger culture's conviction of a genetic basis producing "conditions" that have been difficult to "cure." Alan Petersen (2001) has addressed this in a fascinating paper entitled "Biofantasies: Genetics and Medicine in the Print News Media," in which the virtues of genetic research are seen to outweigh the far more realistic and needed message that diseases occur within a complex dynamic of many kinds of variables. Peterson found that "non-genetic factors" and "multifactorial" interactions on disorders, are rarely mentioned in the media. Most recently, Daniel C. Dennett (2003: 1–3) reviews and critiques the complex issues involved in Nature vs. Nurture arguments, the controversy of "genetic determinism" vs. "environmental determinism" as explanations for human behaviour or predispositions for illnesses, by stating that the real issue really is "what we can change whether or not our world is deterministic."

From the 1930s to the 1960s, biomedical science bore some resemblance to an integrated whole (cf. Canguilhem 1988, 1991; Capra 2002; Kuhn 1962). At this point, there were researchers working at every level of biological organization—from subcellular biochemistry, to whole cells, to organs, to the whole organism. Solutions came from many different levels. For example, public health specialists looked at social, cultural, economic and public education as crucial variables in their efforts to control malaria. Cell culture specialists working with clinicians solved polio. Microbiologists working with chemists and clinicians eliminated the threats posed by most bacterial infections. Clinicians and pharmacologists working with biochemists produced the

---

The Gene as Culprit

Those familiar with medical research funding know the disgraceful campaigns waged in the 70's and 80's by scientists hunting the genes for such diseases as cystic fibrosis. Give us the money, we'll find the gene and then your problems will be solved, was the message. The money was found, the genes were found—and then came nothing but a stunned contemplation of the complexity of the problem, which many clinicians had understood all along...But the tragedy is that the whole-organism biologists and clinicians who might have helped to unravel the complexity have almost all gone, destroyed by the reductionists.

David Horrobin, "Not in the Genes," *The Guardian* (UK), 12 February 2003

---

revolution in psychiatry which enabled so many patients to leave hospitals. In every field, progress depended on a constant exchange of knowledge.

But starting in the 1960's, molecular biologists and genomics specialists rose to prominence within the biomedical sciences, where everything was to be understood completely at the molecular genomic level.

The implications of these assumptions cannot be underestimated. Reductionist, genetic explanations are very different from explanations that involve situational, environmental, sociopolitical factors. Adherence to this once highly-regarded "thrifty gene" and other genetic theories on the prevention, diagnosis and treatment of diabetes and other degenerative diseases among Indigenous Peoples, has had some perverse consequences.

The message that 'being Indian means to be diabetic' can lead to devastating consequences, such as what Kozak (1997) refers to as "an attitude of 'surrender.'" This message disempowers individuals and their communities because it blames them for being who they are, rendering them inactive: "nothing can be done about it." We suggest that such a notion can be considered another stereotype that should be of great concern to those working with communities to achieve healthy lifestyles. For example, in a recent paper, "Sickening Bodies: How Racism and Essentialism Feature in Aboriginal [Australian] Women's Discourse about Health" (1996: 258), Dundi Mitchell looks at "the meanings of illness as expressed at the level of community and as a form of embodiment associated with unequal colonial relations...individual exegeses which articulate Aboriginal women's experience of illness and their sense of identity." Mitchell (1996: 272) found that Aboriginal women "appropriate white constructs of Aboriginal bodies as sick and spreading disease," so that "well-being cannot be restored except by the acknowledgement of racism and by caring and supportive relationships." Authors in this anthology have addressed the devastating ways in which Indigenous self-knowledge becomes vulnerable to genetic stereotypes, conveyed in concepts such as "Indian heritage," as mentioned earlier.

At the epicenter of this difficulty is the politics of Indian identity, explored in several chapters of this book, starting with the definition of who "Indians" are, and the "natural" tendency to link them all together biologically or genetically due to the fact that some of these nations have the highest rates of diabetes in the world. Although recent data (Williams et al. 2000) collected among the Pima Indians of the Gila River Indian Community in Arizona (who reportedly have the highest rate of type 2 diabetes in the world) suggest "strong genetic components" in type 2 diabetes, the authors state that the nature of such genetic components have not been determined. In other words, a genetic basis

has not been established. In this respect, and under its mandate to eliminate health disparities, HEALTHY PEOPLE 2010, a national health promotion and disease prevention
initiative of the U.S. Department of Health, makes the following statement:

> "Current information about the biologic and genetic characteristics of African
> Americans, Hispanics, American Indians, Alaska Natives, Asians, Native
> Hawaiians, and Pacific Islanders does not explain the health disparities expe-
> rienced by these groups compared with the white, non-Hispanic population
> in the United States. These disparities are believed to be the result of the com-
> plex interaction among genetic variations, environmental factors, and specific
> health behaviors (US Dept. of Health and Human Services 2000: 12–13).

Linking Diabetes, Social Inequality, and Trauma

In order to elucidate some of the perverse effects of domination, demoralization and
poverty, which afflict Indigenous Peoples all over the world, the papers in this volume
suggest that we 1) reconsider the diabetes epidemic within a broader semantic domain
that extends well beyond the narrowly defined biologic and genetic condition into the
realms of social relations, history and the politics of Indigenous identity, which can lead
us to 2) consider diabetes as a *reaction of the organism* to adverse life conditions, rather
than a morbid or pathological phenomenon superimposed on the organism. This is
what the French physiologist Claude Bernard (1877) proposed more than 100 years ago,
when he went against theories of his day and argued that the symptoms of diabetes (excessive urination, thirst, and sugar in both the blood and the urine), save for their *intensity*, are known to the normal, physiological state. Stressful, traumatic situations aggravate the symptoms, causing, among other effects, blood sugars to rise. A growing
literature reflects new directions in research on the relationship between stress/trauma
and diabetes, including papers by clinical psychologist Richard Surwit (2004), British
environmental epidemiologist David Barker (2002); historian of science George Canguilhem (1991) and medical anthropologists Jo Scheder (1988; Chapter 11 in this volume) and Mariana Ferreira (1996, 1998, 1999, 2003; Chapters 3 and 14 in this volume).

Drawing upon growing understandings within neuroendochronology of how stress
and trauma may affect an individual's health, especially in the development of chronic
conditions such as diabetes, our authors here have shown a positive correlation between individuals who have experienced trauma and individuals who have been diagnosed with diabetes.

If there is plenty of evidence that trauma and stress do indeed place Indigenous Peoples worldwide at high risk for type 2 diabetes, why have biomedical studies given so
little attention to the obvious links between social inequality and the global diabetes
epidemic? In addition, structured clinical trials focusing on lifestyle interventions, such
as changing dietary and exercise patterns, have proven largely ineffective (Narayan et
al. 1997). As we see it, part of the reason lies in the use of a dated, and quite restrictive concept of "culture," focused on behaviors and used by health professionals and
the medical community at large (Stocking 1963). The authors of this book take issue,
for instance, with the public health emphasis on identifying cultural factors to explain

Indigenous Peoples' (usually poor) "choices" in reference to food and exercise, while situational and historical factors are ignored.

If, in turn, we adopt a modern concept of culture whose prototype is *knowledge*, rather than cultural norms and behaviors, emotional experience becomes variably important in structuring risk for diabetes, as discussed in this book. Macro-level changes needed to prevent or reduce the prevalence of diabetes come to the forefront of our debate, as well as Indigenous Peoples' traditional knowledges and modern everyday practices in and outside of the clinical setting. Electing knowledge as the major modality of culture promotes an understanding of how culturally distinct Peoples experience the world and act upon it, including their feelings and thoughts about health and illness (Barth 1995). Here, we argue that knowledge brings visibility to the cognitive, emotional, and psychoneuroimmunological effects of colonialism and genocide that link Indigenous Peoples worldwide. Broadening the scope of our inquiries so as to include knowledge as a major modality of culture can help Indigenous Peoples themselves devise analytic models with explanatory and predictive power, for understanding what are the factors that play a role in rendering Indigenous Peoples vulnerable to type 2 diabetes. In this respect, and if we consider emotional experience—especially traumatic memory—as variably important for placing individuals at risk for type 2 diabetes, we suggest that it will take *emotional liberty* , among other things, to free Indigenous Peoples from the deleterious effects of the diabetes epidemic. As defined by anthropologist W. Reddy (1999), emotional liberty is the freedom to change goals in response to bewildering, ambivalent situations, and to undergo conversion experiences and life-course changes involving numerous contrasting incommensurable factors. What emotional liberty means for Indigenous individuals and communities on this planet, however, will depend on what each and every one of them define as social and emotional well-being.

Outline of the Book

The chapters in *Indigenous Peoples and Diabetes* are grouped into four interrelated parts.

Part I, *Colonialism, Social Inequality, and Community Experience*, explores diabetes within Indigenous experiences of cultural expansionism and colonial occupation in Canada and the United States, including Hawai'i, and Réunion Island located in the southern Indian Ocean. Authors situate diabetes within First Nations' histories of dispossession, demoralization and oppression of distinct peoples across the globe, bridging key aspects of the health and colonialism debates.

In **Chapter 1**, "Emotion, Grief, and Power. Reconsiderations of Hawaiian Health," Jo Scheder focuses on "the physiological potency of social and political power." She argues against conventional explanatory models of Indigenous health and racial/ethnic health disparities, that in her words "confuse injury with failure, vulnerability with weakness, and that readily accept decontextualized epidemiology while they fragment lives from their surrounding life worlds." Scheder states that in populations where diabetes has reached epidemic levels, there is most often a "legacy of trauma as a structuring of experience." Rather than a biological disease in itself, Scheder suggests that diabetes is a component "in an interplay of mind, immunity, and social inequality." To explain diabetes epidemics in Indigenous communities as primarily due to "genetic" or "cultural" susceptibility to Western lifestyle factors (e.g., high fat diet and sedentism) can be seen as "racist" in that sufferers are stereotyped as having an inevitable biological predisposition for a complex condition, which in turn limits macro-level changes needed to prevent or reduce this condition. In taking issue with etiological explanations based primarily on genetics, the author proposes that "the cognitive, emotional, and psychoneuroimmunological effects of colonialism are fundamental to immune compromise and disease susceptibility."

"'In Their Tellings.' Dakota Narratives about History and the Body," **Chapter 2**, is a consideration of ways in which narratives of illness make critical social commentary that reflect the "real" relations of power between healer and patient, and between an individual or a group and larger cultural and societal forces. Gretchen Chesley Lang suggests that "narratives provide valuable clues to the ways in which individuals are linked to the larger structure and practice of medicine." Lang takes Dakota peoples' theories of history and the body seriously in order to understand the layered meanings that emerge in layperson narratives of diabetes. Lang illustrates how two Dakota individuals reflect upon issues of concern that go far beyond particularities of their own condition, in particular, to the history of Dakota people before and since European invasion. As these examples show, people speak differently for different audiences and for different purposes—thus there is an imperative for careful consideration of the multiple levels of meanings within the contexts of the past and the present. In addition, this paper considers the challenges and responsibilities of interpreting narratives and representing narratives of others when one carries out interviews and oral history.

Chapter 3, "Slipping Through Sky Holes. Yurok Body Imagery in Northern California." is a historical and critical investigation showing how colonialism marks its power and engraves memories on individuals' bodies. Mariana Leal Ferreira explores how the Yurok People of northern California view themselves in light of the constitution of the natural and social sciences, and discusses the effects of this knowledge when implemented in Yurok country particularly after the American invasion of California and the Gold Rush in the mid 1800s. To the violence and brutality of Spaniards, fur traders, gold miners, American soldiers, and Indian policies of the US government, Yurok women attribute the high incidence of diabetes and other degenerative diseases, drug abuse and criminality in the area. The chapter contemplates the lives of eight generations of sixteen Yurok extended families, mapping intergenerational shifts in Yurok social relations and political practices. Ferreira concludes that changes in contemporary Yurok body imagery have substantially altered the relations between the individual, the social, and the Yurok body politic. As the author sees it, "Yurok current perceptions of the body have become a hybrid set of historical events, cross-cultural knowledges and interdisciplinary practices that emphasize social relationships and human reciprocity."

In **Chapter 4**, "Diabetes in Réunion Island (Indian Ocean): From Sugar Plantations to Modern Society," anthropologist Muriel Roddier analyses the way in which one illness condition—diabetes—in Réunion Island "has been constructed with reference to medical discourse." The economy of the former French colony of Reunion Island was based on sugar plantations (19th and most of the 20th centuries). Waves of immigrant workers who came to work in the sugar cane industry, from Europe, Africa and Asia, brought along their healing practices and dietary preferences. The emergence of diabetes during the 20th century as a major health condition leads Roddier to "deconstruct the dominant

biomedical model, and interpret how illness has been experienced within a specific socioeconomic context, and over time by residents of Réunion Island." Despite marked similarities between biomedical and layperson understandings of diabetes, "the latter taking
the former for their source," Roddier points out that they are also far apart because they
are founded on clearly different knowledges and practices. The author suggests that it is
essential to construct models of analysis integrating the logical system of the social group
and educational tools reflecting and taking into account existing popular or lay knowledges and practices.

In **Chapter 5**, "Nêhinaw (Cree) Socioeconomic, Political and Historical Explanations
about the Collective Diabetes Experience," Bruyére draws upon her interviews with members of Nêhinaw of Opaskwayak Cree Nation of The Pas, Manitoba, Canada, focusing
on individuals' etiological (causal) explanations for diabetes; many community members have personal experience with this condition; her chapter is framed within the historical and cultural context of Cree—European relations. According to Bruyere, Cree
place diabetes in "a broad, and profound sociohistoric perspective reflecting the destruction of the environment, the inequitable treatment that tribal peoples have experienced, and subsequent changes in the traditional way of life." Community member's reflections regarding this new, initially unfamiliar, chronic condition sheds light on ways
in which medical knowledge is constructed; she suggests that interpretation of illness is
inextricably bound up with identity, history and culture, following Kleinman (1979) and
Garro (1990). As evidenced here, talking about illness is one way for people to share their
deeper critical thinking about their own lives in the lived world (their experience) and
of their concerns for the future for their relatives and communities. This chapter's considerations of changes in foodways, diet and the environment closely links this essay with
those in Part II.

The five case studies in **Part II**. *Speaking Out about Food, Health, and Power* reflect
different approaches involving foodways, the act of eating, dietary preferences and pa-
tient/community views on suggested diets for those suffering from diabetes. When
asked for ideas about the causes or prevention of the ailment, people not surprisingly,
bring up food and diet, following the biomedical emphasis on these risk factors. Indigenous narratives, more significantly, provide powerful, reflective critiques regarding the politics of identity in view of sociocultural changes experienced by their communities during the process of colonialism.

In **Chapter 6**, Mino-Miijim's "'Good Food for the Future'. Beyond Culturally Appropriate Diabetes Programs," Omura recounts her experience with one part of the White
Earth Land Recovery Project in a Chippewa community in northwestern Minnesota, USA,
focusing here on her summer internship with the Mino-Miijim Program. Mino-Miniijim
is attempting to revitalize residents' appreciation for traditional subsistence patterns and
healthful lifeways, in an effort to promote community-wide steps to achieve wellness in
the broadest sense. Omura recognizes the powerful symbolic dimension of packets of lo-
cally-harvested wild rice and buffalo meat, delivered each month to the homes of people
with diabetes. She describes the meanings attributed to foods and categories of foods,
within the ethnographic context of everyday life in this community. The essay also describes the organization and operation of this program, documenting the roles of key individuals in this effort, within the larger historical and socioeconomic context.

Chapter 7, "Diabetes and Identity. Changes in the Food Habits of the Innu. A Critical Look at Health Professionals' Interventions Regarding Diet," is based on ethnographic fieldwork in Innu First Nations communities of northern Quebec, Canada. Bernard Roy brings a critical gaze to bear on apparent Innu resistance to changing their present-day diet, one that includes many Western, introduced foods, despite public health efforts in nutrition education. In Roy's analysis, the "act of eating" (sharing food with others) is a key "social and political act," a powerful way of symbolizing boundaries, of affirming solidarity within a group, and of signaling differences with "others." As Humphery (Ch. 19), Roy takes issue with the public health emphasis on identifying cultural factors to explain why people make choices or do not change their behavior ("culturization"), while situational and historical factors are ignored. Roy states that "the second half of the 20th century was a time of increasing exclusion of the Innu from the production process of Quebec's market economy," the repercussions of which find Innu today in a situation of "deep poverty." While it may seem "irrational" to healthworkers that Innu often disregard suggested dietary changes, Roy argues that Innu health reflects a history of "colonialism, oppression and of a contemporary context where racism and intolerance occur daily in Innu society."

Carolyn Smith-Morris brings in the voices of pregnant Pima women about diabetes in **Chapter 8**. "Prenatal Mysteries and Symptomless Diabetes in the Gila River Indian Community." The author addresses the relationship between narratives and personal experience, unveiling the complex ways in which Pima women understand gestational diabetes and its screening process, the risk factors involved, and their reactions to the co-morbid problems related to the current diabetes epidemic in the community. The largely symptomless nature of gestational diabetes contributes to a "sense of mystery" about the ailment, at times limited by Pima women's comprehension of and responsiveness to biomedical testing and surveillance data. Smith-Morris highlights the importance of addressing the political economy of health on American Indian reservations and the position of Indian women vis-à-vis current biomedical practices in order to promote community empowerment and wellness.

Chapter 9, Talking about a New Illness with the Dakota: Reflections on Diabetes, Foods, and Culture by Gretchen Chesley Lang, is based on conversations and observations carried out in a Dakota community in the 1980s when diabetes had emerged as a major health concern. Foods and diet are central images in Dakota etiological explanations and their ideas about preventing or controlling this chronic condition. As Roddier noted in Reunion Island (Chapter 4), Dakota individuals' etiological explanations and views of efficacious treatment for diabetes differ markedly from biomedical explanations and therapies, yet incorporate biomedical understandings. Lang found that when people talked about health, and specifically diabetes, "most individuals turned the conversation to the discussion of foods and eating, a recalled traditional lifestyle, and at times to a commentary upon their political history." Present-day Dakota foodways reflect the drastic changes in subsistence, beginning with confinement on reservations in mid-19th century to the situational realities of on-going poverty in recent years. Lang's chapter documents these changes as a backdrop for understanding the place of specific foods in different social occasions (including the summer powwow and a one-year memorial feast for a deceased elder), and to provide the context for peoples' reflective narratives that make connections between history, food, and health.

In **Chapter 10**, "Burying the Umbilicus. Nutrition Trauma, Diabetes and Traditional medicine in Rural West Mexico," co-authors Leslie E. Korn and Rudolph C. Ryser address the consequences of "nutritional trauma" experienced by many Indigenous Peoples as their lifeways have been radically transformed over the recent century. Here, the authors focus on Korn's efforts over several decades in Western rural Mexico to develop a training center that advocates for a "community-determined model of healing and education…and integrates local indigenous knowledge and use of traditional medicine with complementary healing methods and activities." This in-depth case study is presented as one example of a community trying to draw upon their traditional resources and knowledge to prevent or intervene in the recent emergence of type 2 diabetes. It is also a broad-based analysis of the devastating effects for many Indigenous Peoples of rapid "modernization" or Westernization, which so often includes loss of autonomy, methods of subsistence, breakdown of community structure, and changes in worldview.

In Part III. *Emotional Experience and Social Support*, the political dimension of emotional experience helps reconsider diabetes mellitus as a disease of colonialism in light of a physiology of oppression. Authors in this part of the book discuss the ways in which type 2 diabetes relates to macro-level politics and economics as they affect and shape the mediating micro-level experiences of Indigenous Peoples and migrant farmworkers. The re-creation of networks of social support and relaxation therapies are proposed to help counteract the effects of stress and emotional suffering, empowering individuals to regain control of their health, spiritual knowledge, and emotional liberty.

Chapter 11, "A Sickly Sweet Harvest: Farmworker Diabetes and Social (In)Equality" is a pioneer essay relating type 2 diabetes to macro-level politics and economics. Jo Scheder broke new ground in 1988, when the essay was first published, by showing the neuroendocrine and experiential linkages between social inequality and diabetes. Using ethnographic, psychosocial, and biochemical data collected among Mexican-American migrant farmworkers in Wisconsin, the author demonstrates that "the frequent adjustment to stressful life events and change, compounded by social inequality and psychosocial stress inherent in the migrant lifestyle, act via a series of physiological responses to culminate in hyperglycemia." In addition, seasonal migration promotes separation from home and family, disrupting social networks that serve as buffers for life events. Scheder contends that migration "affects the meanings of social support, marginality, and ostracism, and limits access to coping resources."

Terry Raymer is a practicing physician and writer who has worked with Northern California Indigenous Peoples for many years, well aware of the diabetes "epidemic." In **Chapter 12**, "Diabetes as a Metaphor. Symbol, Symptom, or Both?" Raymer acknowledges the humanistic side of medicine, paying homage to the stories and histories of his patients and the communities in which he has worked. The chapter title is derived from Susan Sontag's essay, "Illness as Metaphor," so that while he makes reference to the vast biomedical literature regarding cause and characteristics of diabetes type 2 (and does not dismiss the contribution of lifestyle factors in diabetes prevention and treatment), he argues that these explanations and statistics do not tell the whole story of affliction nor of its causation. Raymer's account considers the central theme of a traditional story, the importance of sharing food. He ponders the role of trauma experienced by his patients and their ancestors over generations that he cannot help but consider, yet (as a scientist) cannot easily "prove." In thinking about diabetes as a symptom of this devastation, Raymer asserts that approaches to diabetes must also support what he cautiously ventures as "spiritual knowledge (for lack of a better term) of one's place in their world" for a revitalization of community well-being.

Diabetes is a "disease of colonialism," rather than of civilization—"and that's a very big difference," says Jo Scheder in **Chapter 13**, "The Spirit's Cell. Critical Analysis in Diabetes Theory." Scheder advances an ideology of illness causation related to what she calls a physiology of oppression, an investigative tool and a conceptual framework that focuses on "structural, macro processes including the individual's conditions of existence, while remaining equally concerned with experience, phenomenology and hormones." Scheder's research in stress, neuroimmunology, endocrinology, and psychophysiology proposes we recognize "it is the constant, lived experience of oppression that erodes the body as well as the spirit." The Spirit's Cell refers to what the author calls "the neuroendocrine cell biology of emotional life, to the spirit of a people as played out in cellular processes underlying joy, anger, triumph, grief, trust, fear, stress, health, to political awareness and the imprisonments of colonialism, and to the intangible substance of traumatic memory."

Chapter 14, "Love in Colonial Light. A History of Yurok Emotions in Northern California" unveils intrinsic links between diabetes and oppression. Mariana Ferreira points to the perverse ways in which colonialism and genocide have placed Indigenous Peoples at heightened risk for the disorder. The life history of Yurok elder Mollie Ruud (1928-2004) illuminates local perceptions of the strong relationship between diabetes and emotional suffering, placing Yurok individuals who experienced a major traumatic event at much higher risk for type 2 diabetes. On the other hand, those families and individuals who are engaged in networks of social support can manage their sentiments more effectively and are thus able to assure emotional liberty—a protective factor against diabetes. Physiologically speaking, Ferreira contends that type 2 diabetes is an outcome of emotionally stimulating claims in terms of the arousal of the autonomic nervous system and the endocrine system. Emotional suffering and emotional liberty are proposed as conceptual ideas that can help redefine the diabetes question in terms of what the author calls a politically meaningful history of emotions.

Chapter 15, "Relaxation and Stress Reduction for Peoples with Diabetes Mellitus (DM)" proposes various relaxation methods that help relax the body, mind, and spirit. Angele McGrady and Kim Gower-Dowling discuss mind-body interventions that include a broad spectrum of therapies based on the premise that thoughts, emotions, and beliefs can influence physiological function. The authors suggest that the regular use of relaxation methods and techniques, such as autogenic, progressive, transcendental, and mindfulness relaxation, including breathing therapy and Yoga, can counteract the effects of stress, thus helping people with diabetes lower blood glucose levels or glycohemoglobin in type 2 diabetes. McGrady and Gower-Dowling explain in detail the process and benefits of autogenic relaxation, presenting a script of phrases that can be used to prompt a sense of deep relaxation through physical feelings of heaviness, warmth or floating. Relaxation-based therapies can also bring physiological and psychological benefits to individuals suffering from disorders often co-existing with diabetes mellitus, such as essential hypertension.

Authors of chapters in **Part IV**. *Community Empowerment and Wellness* have initiated or have worked in various capacities with community-based grass-roots programs, either non-governmental or government health services in the southwestern U.S., Northern California, Australia, and Canada. In addition to being a historical overview of anthropological contributions to the challenge of diabetes across world societies, the final chapter by Dennis Wiedman reviews research and applied community health efforts of five anthropologists along with reference to the work of many others.

Chapter 16, "Community Empowerment for the Primary Prevention of Type II diabetes: Kanien'kehá:ka (Mohawk) Ways for the Kahnawake Schools Diabetes Prevention Project" was co-authored by Ann C. Macaulay, Margaret Cargo, Sherri Bisset, Treena Delormier, Lucie Lévesque, Louise Potvin and Alex M. McComber. They are participants in The Kahnawake Schools Diabetes Prevention Project" (KSDPP) in this First Nations community near Montreal. Chapter 16 describes this community-based participatory-research program to promote wellness and the reduction of diabetes. KSDPP is notable for its *Code of Research Ethics* that "guide this partnership from intervention to dissemination of results, ensuring community members are equal partners with the researchers, integration of intervention and evaluation teams to create synergy, being responsive to changes with organisational and programmatic flexibility, and building local capacity by making the project a learning opportunity for all." The Community Advisory Board approves research proposals and determines which researchers may conduct studies to benefit the community; research findings undergo community review before dissemination/publication. According to the authors, the KSDPP model "converged with a longstanding tradition of consensus decision-making by the Kanien'kehá:ka," to foster trust and partnerships between health personnel, health researchers and community members that may benefit similar efforts across many Indigenous communities. This case study includes narrative insights of community members, board members, researchers and healthworkers.

In **Chapter 17**, " 'I'm Too Young for This!' Diabetes and American Indian Children," Jennie Joe and Sophie Frishkopf describe their involvement, since 1991, with the Summer Wellness Camp for Indian children who suffer from type 2 diabetes. They document the rapid increase in diabetes type 2 among children, once found only among adults and now a devastating intergenerational disease. The authors review studies showing the relationship between childhood diabetes with social and political factors, emphasizing links between poverty, nutrition and obesity, along with the paucity of organized exercise programs or dietary counseling in rural communities. They also review studies of other community-based prevention/intervention programs designed for children and teen-agers. The chapter highlights the Summer Wellness Camp, a university and tribal community partnership designed to help children prevent or delay complications of diabetes, type 2. Joe and Frishkopf emphasize the need, as do other summer camp programs that target a specific health condition, for parent and community support after the initial camp experience. Dr. Jennie R. Joe, a medical anthropologist with training in public health, and Director of the Native American Research and Training Center at the University of Arizona, has long been an advocate for effective community-based programs.

Chapter 18 discusses the history and therapeutic activities of the Potawot Health Village, a tribally owned and operated health facility in northern California. Potawot provides health care to more than 13 thousand Indigenous patients from the following nations: Yurok, Karuk, Wiyot, Tolowa, Wylacki, Siletz, Hupa, Smith River, and Mattole. Twila Sanchez and Bea Nix bring in their sophisticated expertise as health professionals and members of the Yurok Tribe in order to discuss the process of cultural rebuilding launched at the newly built Potawot Village in 2001. Located in Arcata, in the Humboldt County, Potawot is now the main headquarter of a complex of 12 health clinics owned and operated by the Yurok, Wiyot and Tolowa nations, and administered by United Indian Health Services (UIHS). Ferreira, Sanchez and Nix propose that paying close attention to Indigenous conceptions of culture allows community members, health professionals, administrators and policy makers to tackle more efficiently the social and emotional dimensions of diabetes mellitus. Empowering ideas and activities that can help prevent and treat diabetes, such as women support groups, music and art therapy, and the right to food are discussed in the essay.

Chapter 19, "Culture Blindness? Aboriginal Health, 'Patient Non-Compliance' and the Conceptualisation of Difference in Australia's Northern Territory," probes even further into how "culture" is put into discourse and practice in a health setting, but this time by non-indigenous professionals. Based on his extensive research and fieldwork in Australia over many years, Kim Humphrey brings to light how health professionals exaggerate the importance of 'the cultural' in relation to what they perceive as Aboriginal "health beliefs and practices." Indigenous "culture" is understood as a largely homogenous set of ideas universally evident within all remote Aboriginal communities. Ironically, as Humphrey sees it, this process of exaggeration "both underestimates the importance of developing more sophisticated understandings of cultural disjunction and eclipses an attention to other possible factors underlying the difficulties of successful service provision and uptake, such as poverty, the institutional frameworks of medical provision, and the ramifications of a history of colonial dispossession."

Chapter 20, "Striving for Healthy Lifestyles: Contributions of Anthropologists to the Challenge of Diabetes in Indigenous Communities," by Dennis Wiedman, reflects his long-time role of documenting anthropologists' focus on diabetes from many perspectives within cultural, biological and medical anthropology. Along with his own ethnohistorical and ethnographic research efforts, Wiedman has devoted several decades to compiling information regarding the diabetes "epidemic" (cf. reference to Working Bibliography in his chapter). This chapter is an excursion into intellectual history noting anthropologists' efforts with many world Peoples to uncover factors that may be responsible for the dramatic increase in diabetes, type 2 and the significance of anthropological contributions to the design of collaborative efforts in health care. He discusses early contributions by Kelly West and James Neel, questions that remain regarding the role of genetic vs. non-genetic factors in the etiology (causes) of diabetes, type 2, and current directions in anthropologists' basic and applied research. Medical anthropologists of many different specialties (e.g., nutrition, human genetics, epidemiology) have contributed to public health and clinical understandings to date. Wiedman highlights five anthropologists whose theoretical and methodological approaches are widely respected. His chapter is a valuable backdrop for the many topics and issues addressed in this book.

Final Thoughts

The organizers of this volume suggest that there are theoretical and methodological challenges for health professionals at all levels, epidemiologists, medical anthropologists, tribal leaders (or tribal health directors), and public policy advisors to examine links between macro-level factors, such as social inequality, and micro-level individual or community health outcomes that ultimately need to be addressed if Indigenous Peoples across the globe are to regain and achieve control of their health or what we might call "wellness." And, let us not forget or downplay the real experience of diabetes and its complications if it is not controlled! The serious consequences of the signs and symptoms of diabetes, including blindness, kidney failure, impotence and amputations do exist and cause intense physical, social, and emotional suffering.

Most importantly, the recognition that rather than one's "genes," "Indian heritage," or simply "bad eating habits," it is the dramatic conditions of existence that trigger the emergence of type 2 diabetes, and this, in turn, can empower Indigenous Peoples. This approach lifts the blame from bodies, minds and spirits that have been historically stigmatized as "naturally" prone to sicken and die, signaling that *yes*, these Indigenous nations' current struggles to regain sovereign control of their land and environmental resources, religious freedom and spiritual well-being, is no doubt the best strategy to halt the diabetes epidemic. Several chapters here portrayed show in detail how some preventive programs and strategies can transcend the exclusive biomedical focus on the physiological body, so as to include aspects of the social and political bodies as well. Diabetes is a battleground with many facets—many different kinds of on-the-ground day-to-day efforts for treating individuals are taking place, as the contributors to this book have shown. Relaxation methods, music therapy, community support groups, and wellness gardens, among others, are no doubt invaluable therapeutic techniques to lower blood sugars, as contributors to this volume clearly demonstrate.

Health and health policy are inextricably linked, as Lynn Freedman, Professor of Clinical Public Health, Columbia University states:

> I view health and human rights advocacy as an essentially subversive activity, in the sense that my vision of "defining and advancing human well-being" ultimately requires overturning deeply-rooted social and political structures that produce ill health and that prevent all people—women and men—from fulfilling their highest potential as human beings. But the goal is not to destroy; it is to transform and create. The structures that now obstruct human well-being must be changed into modes of social organization and interaction that will promote and support it (Freedman 1995).

It should be noted that both Indigenous and non-Indigenous scholars, health professionals and activists represented here fiercely defend the idea that it is a *radical change in the overall conditions of existence* of Indigenous Peoples that needs to be put into effect in order to ensure good health for present and future generations. The ratification of the United Nations Draft Declaration of the Rights of Indigenous Peoples by the United States and other countries by the end of the Decade of Indigenous Peoples in December 2004 would certainly have been a great start. The Working Group on Indigenous Populations met again in New York to discuss the Declaration, for (the second part of) its 10th Session from November 29 through December 3, 2004. As the American Indian Law Alliance in the United States sees it,

> The Draft Declaration must preserve the right of self-determination for Indigenous peoples in compliance with both our own objectives and the tenants of existing international law. It has the added advantage of also permitting the evolution of international law to be more just and equitable for all the world's peoples. This is the amazing legacy that Indigenous peoples can leave for our descendants and the world as a whole. The "Package" proposal presented by the vast majority of Indigenous nations, organizations and peoples [at the first part of its 10th Session in September, 2004], along with the support of many States, represents a major breakthrough in advancing the aspirations of Indigenous peoples and moving the Declaration into the body of international law and standards that govern our relations with one another and with the environment upon which we all depend (AILA 2004).

Ellen Lutz (2004: 6), Executive Director of Cultural Survival, is looking ahead to a 2nd Decade of Indigenous Peoples: "Most of all, Indigenous Peoples hope that the sovereign states that govern the territories on which they live will honor their obligations to indigenous peoples including (1) respecting their basic human rights including their right to self-determination; (2) ensuring that they have the means to participate fully and permanently as citizens in local and national political processes that impact their lives; (3) providing them with the opportunity to give—or not give—their free, prior, and informed consent before development projects are foisted upon them or resources are extracted from their lands; and (4) making available to them the education and training they need to defend their rights, participate in civil society, and make informed decisions about their futures."

Ultimately, a reconsideration of what diabetes mellitus type 2 represents to Indigenous Peoples in the United States, and all over the world for that matter, depends on the full recognition by the US and other nation-states that Indigenous Peoples are *Peoples* in their own rights, according to international laws and conventions. The United States has developed an embarrassing record of refusing to ratify international laws and conventions, including the UN Genocide Convention, The Convention on the Rights of the Child, and the Draft Declaration of Indigenous Peoples' Rights, among many others. Such a bad record has placed the United States as one of the four worst abusers of Indigenous Peoples' Rights in the world (Amnesty International 2003).

The terrain covered in this volume has always been the most difficult to incorporate into biomedical models, clinical studies, and health-care delivery systems, as it inevitably must address the extermination of entire populations, the rights of genocide survivors, and racial discrimination, and ultimately social inequality. Critical medical and anthropological approaches try to take account of more, rather than fewer, human rights and socio-economic considerations.

As each author has brought to bear her or his particular skills and experiences, we remain challenged by a chronic illness that has increasingly affected great numbers of Indigenous Peoples, one which appears to be linked with so many contributing factors

---

The International Labor Organization (ILO)

Since its creation in 1919, the International Labor Organization (ILO) has studied the living and working conditions of Indigenous and Tribal Peoples, who are generally reduced to situations of extreme poverty. Convention Number 169 (replacing Convention 107 in 1989), recognizes the aspiration of Indigenous Peoples to control their own institutions, their way of life and economic development and to preserve and develop their identity, language, and religion. It demands full recognition of and respect for the values, social, cultural, religious and spiritual practices and institutions of Indigenous Peoples. It introduces the principle of consultation with institutions which are representative of Indigenous Peoples and communities with regard to legislation and administrative measures of concern to them and encourages their participation in decision-making at a local, regional and national level. ILO 169 includes the recognition of Indigenous Peoples' traditional and economic activities, as well as the provision of adequate health services (Roulet 1999).

---

from centuries of European expansion, conquest and colonialism, with huge technological changes that only continue as part of the on-going over-all globalization process. The critical approach here conveyed, however, clearly indicates that community-based participatory programs and research have the greatest analytic and preventive power, since such initiatives are grounded on the ethics of social justice. This means, among many other things, recognizing and respecting the rights and dignity of all Indigenous Peoples around the world.

References

American Diabetes Association (ADA). 2004. Educational Information. American Diabetes Association, 1701 North Beauregard Street, Alexandria, VA 22311 <www.diabetes.org>.

American Indian Law Alliance (AILA). 2004. Report of the American Indian Law Alliance on the Xth Session of the Working Group on the Draft Declaration— New York. September 2004. 8 Nov 2004.

Amnesty International (AI). 2003. Indigenous Rights are Human Rights: Four Cases of Rights Violations in the Americas. Washington DC: The Just Earth! Program.

Angell, Marcia. 2004. Truth About Drug Companies: How They Deceive Us And What To Do About It. New York: Random House.

Barker, David J.P., ed. 2001. Type 2 Diabetes: The Thrifty Phenotype. London: Oxford University Press.

Barth, Fredrik. 1995. Other Knowledge and Other Ways of Knowing. Journal of Anthropological Research 51: 65–67.

Bernard, Claude. 1877. *Leçons sur le Diabète et la Glycogenèse Animale* Londres; Madrid: Librairie J.-B. Baillière et Fils.

Bygrave, Mike. 2002. False Dawns in the Brave World of New Genetics. The Observer, 22 December 2002.

Canguilhem, G. 1988. Ideology and Rationality in the History of the Life Sciences. Cambridge: The MIT Press.

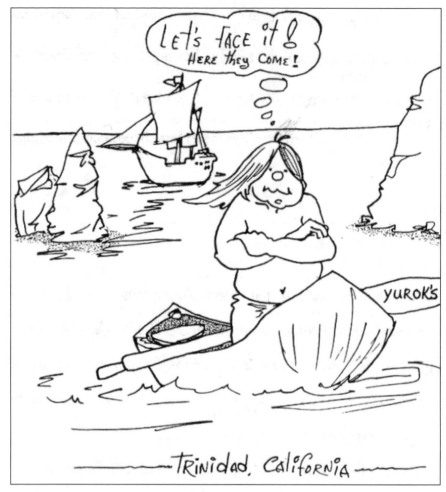

Drawing by Yurok artist, Sammy Gensaw (reproduced with permission of artist).

_____1991. The Normal and the Pathological. New York: Zone Books.

Capra, Fritjof. 2002. The Hidden Connections: A Science for Sustainable Living. pp. 158–206. New York: Anchor Books (Random House).

Dennett, Daniel C. 2003. The Mythical Threat of Genetic Determinism. The Chronicle of Higher Education 49(21): B7.

Famuyiwa, O.O., et al. 1985. Social, Cultural and Economic Factors in the Management of Diabetes mellitus in Nigeria. African Journal of Medical Science 14(3-4): 145–54.

_____1990. Important Considerations in the Care of Diabetic Patients in a Developing Country (Nigeria)". Diabetes Medica 7(10): 927–30.

Farmer, Paul. 2003. Pathologies of Power. Health, Human Rights, and The New War on the Poor. Berkeley: University of California Press.

_____1996. On Suffering and Structural Violence: A View from Below. Daedalus Special Issue on Social Suffering. 125(1): 261–83.

Federal Reserve. 2003 Report. January 22, 2003.

Ferreira, Mariana Leal. 2004. Indigenous Peoples. *In* Encyclopedia of the World's Minorities. Volume 2., Carl Skutsch, ed. Independence, KY: Routledge.

_____2003. Diabetes Tipo 2 e povos indígenas no Brasil e nos Estados Unidos. In: *Cultura, Saúde e Doenca.* [Universidade Estadual de Londrina] 2: 15–33.

_____1999. Corpo e História do Povo Yurok. *Revista de Antropologia* [Universidade de São Paulo] 41(2): 17–39.

_____1998. Slipping through Sky Holes: Yurok Body Imagery in Northern California" Culture, Medicine and Psychiatry 22: 171–202.

_____1996. Sweet Tears and Bitter Pills. The Politics of Health Among the Yuroks of Northern California. Unpublished PhD Dissertation, UC Berkeley and UC San Francisco.

Foucault, Michael. 1975. The Birth of the Clinic. An Archaeology of Medical Perception. New York: Vintage Books.

Freedman, Lynn P. 1995. Reflections on Emerging Frameworks of Health and Human Rights. Health and Human Rights Journal 1(4). <www.hsph.harvard.edu/Organizations/healthnet/reprorights/docs/freedman.html>.

Heintze, Hans Joachim. 1993. The Protection of Indigenous Peoples under the ILO Convention." *In* Amazonia and Siberia: Legal Aspects of the Preservation of the Environment and Development in the Last Open Spaces. Michael Bothe, Thomas Kurzidem and Christian Schmidt, eds. London: Graham & Trotman.

Horrobin, David. 2003. Not in the Genes. The Guardian, 12 Feb. 2003.

Indian Health Service National Diabetes Program. 2000. Special Diabetes Program for Indians Interim Report to Congress. Jan. 2000.

International Diabetes Federation (IDF). 2003. Educational Materials. International Diabetes Federation (IDF), Avenue Emile De Mot 19, B-1000 Brussels, Belgium <www.idf.org>.

Joe, Jennie R. and Robert. S. Young, eds. 1994. Diabetes as a Disease of Civilization: The Impact of Culture Change on Indigenous Peoples. Berlin: Mouton de Gruter

King, H., R.E. Aubert and W.H. Herman. 1998. Global Burden of Diabetes, 1995-2025: Prevalence, Numerical Estimates, and Projections. Diabetes Care 21(9): 1414–31.

Kozak David. 1997. Surrendering to Diabetes: An Embodied Response to Perceptions of Diabetes and Death in the Gila River Indian Community. Omega, Journal of Death and Dying 35(4): 347–59.

Krieger, Nancy. 2001. Theories for Social Epidemiology in the 21st Century: An Ecosocial Perspective. International Journal of Epidemiology 30: 668–77.

Kuhn, Thomas. 1962. The Structure of Scientific Revolutions. Source: The Structure of Scientific Revolutions. Chicago, IL: University of Chicago Press.

Lang, Gretchen Chesley. 1985. Diabetics and Health Care in a Sioux Community. Human Organization 44(3): 251–60.

_____1989 'Making Sense' About Diabetes: Dakota Narratives of Illness. Medical Anthropology 11(3): 305–27.

Lock, Margaret, Alan Young and Alberto Cambrosio, eds. 2000. Living and Working with the New Medical Technologies: Intersections of Inquiry. Cambridge, UK; New York, NY, USA: Cambridge University Press.

Lutz, Ellen. 2004. Measuring the Success of the International Decade. Cultural Survival Quarterly 28(3): 5–6.

Medvei, Victor Cornelius. 1993. The History of Clinical Endocrinology: A Comprehensive Account of Endocrinology from the Earliest Times to the Present Day. NY: Taylor and Francis Group.

Mitchell, Dundi. 1996. Sickening Bodies: How Racism and Essentialism Feature in Aboriginal Women's Discourse about Health. 7(3): 258–74.

Mullen P.E., J. Martin and J. Anderson. 1996. The Long-Term Impact of the Physical, Emotional, and Sexual Abuse of Children: A Community Study. Child Abuse and Neglect 20: 7-2.

Narayan, K.M., M. Venkat, D. Hoskin, A.M. Kozak, R.L. Krishka, D.J. Hanson, D.K.Pettitt, Nagi, P.H. Bennett and W.C. Knowler. 1997. Randomized Clinical Trial of Lifestyle Interventions in Pima Indians: A Pilot Study. Diabetic Medicine 15: 66–72.

Neel, James. 1962. Diabetes Mellitus: A "thrifty" Genotype Rendered Detrimental by "Progress"? American Journal of Human Genetics 14: 353–62.

_____1982. Thrifty Gene Revisited. In The Genetics of Diabetes Mellitus. J. Kobberling and R Tattersall, eds. pp. 283–93. NY: Academic Press.

O'Nell, Theresa. 1996. Disciplined Hearts. History, Identity and Depression in an American Indian Community. Berkeley: University of California Press.

Oyewole and Johnson. 1980. Social-Cultural Problems Affecting Management of Diabetes mellitus in Nigerian Children. Tropical Geographic Medicine 32(1): 77–81.

Park, K. S. 2004. Prevention of type 2 Diabetes mellitus from the Viewpoint of Genetics. Diabetes Research and Clinical Practice 66(Suppl): S33–S35.

Peterson, Alan. 2001. Biofantasies: Genetics and Medicine in the Print News Media. Social Science and Medicine 2(8): 1255–68.

Reddy, W. 1999. Emotional Liberty: Politics and History in the Anthropology of Emotions. Cultural Anthropology. 14(2): 256–88.

Rokala, Dwight A., Sharon G. Bruce and C.Micklejohn. 1991. Diabetes Mellitus in Native Populations of North America: An Annotated Bibliography. Monograph Series No. 4. Northern Health Research Unit. Winnipeg: University of Manitoba.

Roulet, Florence. 1999. Human Rights and Indigenous Peoples. A Handbook on the UN System. International Working Group on Indigenous Affairs (IWIGIA), Document No. 2. Copenhagen: IWIGIA.

Roy, Bernard. 2002. Sang, sucré, pouvoirs codés, médecine amère. Québec: Presses de l'Université Laval.

Royal C.D. and G. M. Dunston. 2004. Changing the Paradigm from 'Race' to Human Genome Variation. Nature Genetics 36(11 Suppl): S5-7.

Scheder, Jo C. 1988. A Sickly-Sweet Harvest: Farmworker Diabetes and Social Equality. Medical Anthropology Quarterly 2: 251–77.

Scheper-Hughes, Nancy. 1993. Death Without Weeping. The Violence of Everyday Life in Brazil. Berkeley: University of California Press.

Scheper-Hughes, Nancy and Philip Bourgois, eds. 2004. Violence in War and Peace. An Anthology. Malden, MA: Blackwell Publishing Ltd.

Sennett, Richard. 2003. Respect in a World of Inequality. New York: W.W. Norton and Co., Inc.

Smide, B., D. Whiting, F. Mugusi, L. Felten and K. Wikblad. 1999. Self-Perceived Health in Urban Diabetic Patients in Tanzania. East African Medical Journal 76(2): 67–70.

Steinbrook, Robert. 2004. Financial Conflicts of Interest and the NIH. The New England Journal of Medicine. 350(4): 327–30.

Stocking, George. 1963. Franz Boas and the Culture Concept in Historical Perspective. Race, Culture and Evolution. Chicago, Illinois: University of Chicago Press.

Surwit, Richard S. 2004. The Mind-Body Diabetes Revolution. New York: The Free Press.

Szathmary, Emöke J. E. 1985. Search for Genetic Factors Controlling Plasma Glucose Levels in Dogrib Indians. In Diseases of Complex Etiology in Small Populations. E. Ranajit Chakraborty and Emöke J. E. Szathmary, eds. pp. 199–225. New York: Alan R. Liss.

_____1994. Non-Insulin Dependent Diabetes Mellitus among Aboriginal North Americans. Annual Review of Anthropology (23): 457–82.

Taussig, Michael. 1992. Reification and the Consciousness of the Patient. In The Nervous System. Michael Taussig, ed. New York and London: Routledge.

United Nations Economic and Social Council's Sub-Commission on the Prevention of Discrimination and Protection of Minorities. 1983. Working Group on Indigenous Populations. E/CN.4/Sub.2/1983/21/Add.8, para.369.

United Nations. 1946. Genocide Convention. UN General Assembly, Resolution 96 (1) of 11 December 1946.

United States Dept. of Health and Human Services. 2000. Healthy People 2010. US DHHS 2000: 12–13.

Weiss, Kenneth M., Peter R. Cavanagh, Anne V. Buchanan and Jan S. Ulbrecht. 1984. Diabetes Mellitus in American Indians: Characteristics, Origins and Preventive Health Care Implications. Medical Anthropology 11(3): 283–304.

West, Kelly. 1974. Diabetes in American Indians and Other Native Populations in the New World. Diabetes 23(10): 841–55.

_____1978. Diabetes in American Indians. Advances in Metabolic Disorders 9: 29–48.

Wiedman, Dennis. 2002. Anthropological Contributions to Diabetes Research and Interventions: A Working Bibliography. Webpage: <www.fiu.edu/~wiedmand>.

Wilkinson, Richard. 1996. Unhealthy Societies: The Afflictions of Inequality. NY: Routledge.

Williams, Robert, Jeffrey Long, Robert Hanson, Maurice Sievers and William Knowler. 2000. Individual Estimates of European Genetic Admixture Associated with Lower Body-Mass Index, Plasma Glucose, and Prevelence of Type 2 Diabetes in Pima Indians. American Journal of Human Genetics 66: 527–38.

Young, T. Kue. 1993. Diabetes-Mellitus among Native Americans in Canada and the United States: An Epidemiologic Review. American Journal of Human Biology 5(4): 399–413.

Young, T. Kue, et al. 2000. Type 2 Diabetes mellitus in Canada's First Nations. Status of an Epidemic in Progress. Canadian Medical Association Journal 163(5): 561–66.

Chapter 1

Emotion, Grief, and Power: Reconsiderations of Hawaiian Health

Jo C. Scheder

Why do Native Hawaiians have the poorest health of anyone in the Islands? Some health experts and Hawaiian activists reject the notion that it's simply a matter of diet.

Editor, *Honolulu Weekly*, 1993

Summary of Chapter 1. This chapter focuses on the physiological potency of social and political power. I argue that colonial depopulation and contemporary chronic disease involve the interplay of consciousness, cultural meanings, neuroimmunity and stress physiology. I argue against conventional explanatory models of Indigenous health and racial/ethnic health disparities, explanations that confuse injury with failure, vulnerability with weakness, and that readily accept decontextualized epidemiology while they fragment lives from their surrounding life worlds. The chapter instead recognizes the legacy of historical trauma in the structure of experience, the generational aftermath for families and cultures, and the persistence of underlying biopsychosocial stress exposures coexisting in the ordinary and the extreme. Conventional health models ignore the daily nature of empire, then and now, and the cumulative biological risks of discrimination and daily micro-aggressions. I regard the shift from recurrent epidemic infections to chronic metabolic, cellular and immune conditions as a continuum of illness, built on the back of everyday mind-body experiences of inequality, temporally unbound from colonial to contemporary eras.

ð ð ð

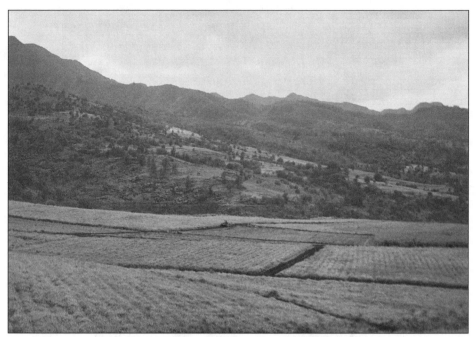

Commercial pineapple fields of central O'ahu, late 1990s.

Part 1. Taro Tales: Land, Power and Hawaiian Health[1]

In virtually every colonized corner of the planet, Indigenous People have been decimated—by violence, by disease, by loss of spirit. This so-called "post-contact decline"
has been of genocidal proportions: Roughly 90% of native populations have been eliminated within the first half-century of colonization.

That this happened in Hawai'i is a well-known historical fact. Less well known, or
perhaps overlooked, is the fact that the deleterious health effects of Hawaii's colonization continue today.

Native Hawaiians have a notoriously poor health profile, the worst of any ethnic
group in the Islands. Most of their illness is due to chronic conditions such as diabetes,
heart disease, and cancer—considered by health scientists to be diseases of "modernization," which is another way of saying that they are diseases of Western cultural expansion. On the surface these diseases are diet-related; this is the official health-pro-
motion approach. Look beneath the surface, however, and the root cause appears:
Health is inseparable from political and economic equality. In particular, Native Hawaiian health is a matter of land and power.

Enter the sovereignty movement. For Kekuni Blaisdell, indigenous rights activist
and physician, health is enmeshed in social and demographic realities. "It is not a separate issue at all. Therefore, there's no point in focusing on health alone. It stems from
the basic fabric of the colonial establishment."

---

1. Part 1 of the present chapter, Taro Tales, was originally published in *The Honolulu Weekly*, December 29, 1993, pp. 4–5. Reprinted with permission.

Terry Shintani, a physician and advocate of a traditional Hawaiian diet as crucial to reversing morbidity and restoring robust healthiness, essentially agrees: "It is important for all Hawaiian people to look at health as a result of adopting Western ways and forgetting the cultural ways of their ancestors."

"Sovereignty is how to address getting back to life," says Ku'umeaaloha Gomes, an activist and doctoral student in political science who holds a master's degree in public health. "We cannot isolate health from socioeconomic status and government issues. The policy arena is where change will happen. We must address land issues, access to land." Blaisdell agrees: "Land is basic. Without it we cannot be *kanaka maoli* (native people)."

Gomes makes clear the connection between land and health: "In talking about health, you must talk about food, so you must talk *lo'i* (gardens)—and so you've got to talk golf courses, and so you've got to talk foreign investment." She sees it as a major conceptual shift for bureaucrats and academics to think of health in a Hawaiian way. "It's not just a 'cultural perspective'; it's who we are as a people, as political and socioeconomic thinkers."

Shintani understands. His book, *The Wai'anae Book of Hawaiian Health,* he discusses Papa (Earth Mother) and Wakea (Sky Father), history, politics and the overthrow before he gets around to diet. He advocates the healing philosophy of "whole person, whole community." He says, "All of these things are interconnected. For years Hawaiians felt ashamed to be Hawaiian. That was the result of years of racism. Cultural pride was destroyed, so there came a sense of helplessness. There is no need for that."

If such a position is unexpected from a nutrition-minded physician who holds that "the No. 1 killer is diet-related disease," Shintani's background is similarly unusual. An old-time activist who worked with political action groups in college (including the Black Panthers), he also holds a law degree and retains membership in the state bar. He went into law looking for truth, justice and, he says, "to do some good. But I got out of law because I hate politics."

This is an ironic sentiment for a person whose life's work is fundamentally political. Shintani works in Waianae because that community has the lowest socioeconomic status and the poorest health statistics in the state, if not the nation. "In Waianae," he says, "people die in their late 40s or early 50s of heart disease, diabetes, and cancer."

With a need that is obvious and this extreme, and with clinical evidence of the healthfulness of Hawaiian cultural foods, what is blocking a concerted effort to change this horrendous situation? The obstacles come down to basic socioeconomic control. "It is essential that adequate resources be provided to produce proper foods: taro, sweet potato and fish," says Blaisdell. "But gardens are displaced by golf courses, and there is a constant struggle for adequate water." Hawaiians who try to hold onto the land and exist as Hawaiians tend to be portrayed by the establishment as "radicals" who belong in jail. On Molokai, for example, a Hawaiian man restored a fishpond and was arrested for trespassing.

"For so many years Hawaiians have been discriminated against and left on the lowest rung socioeconomically," says Shintani. "There is an attitude that Hawaiians are lazy and not interested in their own health, and they can't agree among themselves. That is unfair. Does the Legislature agree? Does Congress agree? If you work with any social movement, that's human nature. People say, 'They can't get it together,' but who the hell can? Agree to disagree and move forward. That's what's happening."

Herbert Hoe is among those moving forward, contributing his expertise in cultural food by working with farmers in the community and teaching an evening class at Kamehameha Schools. He agrees with Shintani: "When Hawaiians argue, people say that Hawaiians cannot get along. But for others to argue, they say that's a debate. Hawaiians are like everyone else. We have a right to have different opinions. It's healthy to have many groups."

Hoe, too, connects food with politics. "The limited availability of Hawaiian cultural food products becomes a political issue because the availability is directly tied to the land and to water resources."

The focus is on taro in particular. "About 200 years ago an estimated 8,000 acres were in taro cultivation, but today there are less than 500," says Hoe. "We continually hear 'no more poi' and blame the weather—like Iniki—but the numbers speak for themselves. Five hundred acres is nothing."

"Why not give up ten golf courses—or even one golf course—to put into taro? 'No more land for taro' is completely false. There are people who want to raise it; they're just not given the chance. Many things are connected. Is the state allowing others to benefit by long-term leases and tax breaks? It goes back to the sovereignty issue. Get lands back into these kinds of usage." Hoe talks of the millions of tax dollars being spent on a losing effort at Hamakua Sugar. "What is the state planning to do with the land? It was taro before sugar, so will the state release water from sugar to taro?"

That brings up the question of water rights and private access to water by special interests. "The key to any development is water—who owns the land, who has the say—it all ties to water." Hoe observes that in central Oahu sugar is down, but water still is diverted from Waiahole to the Ewa plain. Waiahole now has four or five acres in taro cultivation. "It used to be the whole valley. Will the water go back into agriculture?"

"It's easy to run over a taro farmer, so you can plant heliconias instead. What is more important," Hoe asks, " a complex of condos or a few acres of taro? That's the issue."

In all of this, Hawaiians feel the brunt of the decisions. The water is not going to lo'i and taro, and "Once no more taro, no more Hawaiians," says Hoe. "The taro plant has significance to Hawaiian culture; taro has meaning. To say, 'Broccoli is just as good as luau leaf, so why grow luau leaf?' is the colonial mentality."

When it comes to exploitation of Hawaiian culture, even food can be co-opted. The state, scientists, and foreign businesspeople are investigating the economic value of taro, wanting to use sugar and pineapple lands for taro for flour and other products. Commercial development and large-scale marketing can be damaging because, says Hoe, "while they can say that they are saving the taro, the foods culturally have no value." And Hawaiians are not the beneficiaries. Hoe thinks it is appropriate, however, to adapt Hawaiian foods to the world today—taro pizza for starters. "But have enough taro for poi first, then make pasta and flour." The irony of taro attaining value as a corporate commodity, where it never had value when Hawaiian farmers controlled it, is not lost on Hoe: "This is one more way of stealing."

Gomes extends the analysis to *la'au lapa'au* (plant medicine): "There is a yearning for the native medicine, but it is contaminated. Again the issue of land comes up: We cannot be healthy because things are not *pono* (right). The medicine cabinets—the forests—are being destroyed by development and golf courses, so Hawaiian pharmacies are being destroyed. It goes back to policy again. Who is making land policy and by whose principles? We Hawaiians relate to the land in lots of ways. Symbolically, land equals life. Period. Not land equals money."

Gomes talks about *lokahi*, unity or connection, the balance between all things. "The Department of Health perspective, which is the health promotion perspective, sees diabetes and other disorders as matters of personal risk and so implicitly blames the patient. But the lokahi way asks how policy—national and international—places people at risk for disease." Shintani also criticizes the standard approach to health education as being written for a Caucasian, middle-class, middle-American audience. "And the approach to weight control is so negative. Eating is not a bad habit. You have to eat. We're in an environment of bad food. Take a no-fault attitude; don't blame the patient like most professionals do."

Blaisdell feels that even Native Hawaiian health professionals are replicating the Western bureaucracy while using Hawaiian labels. "Nothing new has been going on," he says, "and nothing significant has been done to help." Instead, consider the Native Hawaiian Health Systems, which were established after a long struggle for federal recognition of Hawaiian health problems. The models presented in official government-supported program proposals (such as *Ke Ola Mamo: A Health Care System for Native Hawaiians on the Island of O'ahu*, July 1991) continue to focus on health risk behaviors, not on health risk exposures, thereby parroting the public health/medical model and the attendant bureaucratic perspective. They add a cultural sensitivity clause, effectively perpetuating the idea that it is culture and not political economy that creates and continually re-creates barriers to improved health. Nowhere do they deal with land and its availability or how it came to be that the Hawaiian diet has changed for the worse. Why? "Because that would require an admission of cultural imperialism," says Gomes. "And if you look only at individual health risk behaviors, you don't have to look at environmental issues.

"We have to ask what is behind the statistics," Gomes continues. "Who is choosing the direction of research and data collection and policy advising? How are definitions made? The DOH, which is, after all, an arm of the state, can control the information going out and can control the extent to which questions are asked. It can control the conferences, the themes, the resource people and, therefore, public thought."

Is this conscious on the Department of Health's (DOH) part? "Are they purposely out to kill all the Hawaiians?" Gomes asks rhetorically. "Of course not. But you've got to push and push and say this is what you are doing, keep saying that you are stepping on my foot, but your money belt is in the way of seeing it."

The sovereignty movement is involved in rethinking the system. "Why replicate the monster?" asks Gomes. "It is interested in being fed, in eating us, not in healing us." Government-sponsored health programs are not likely to talk land. Their language rarely gets past the slogan of "Eat right, exercise, get plenty of rest." But each of those three idols of contemporary health promotion is cloaked in political assumptions. All imply access to resources and the luxuries of time and energy. The reality is that those things are not readily available. Beyond that, a focus on diet alone is a focus on appearances, not on underlying causes. "It doesn't matter if everybody gets free Reeboks and free health care, because those things still only address the symptoms," says Gomes. "How do you stay healthy if 7-Eleven is there instead of a *lo'i kalo* (taro garden)?"

Claire Hughes, chief of the nutrition branch of the state Department of Health, agrees that the shortage of cultural foods makes it difficult for Native Hawaiians to maintain good health. But, she says, "All across the country it's difficult to promote sound nutrition in general. As a nutritionist, I would like to get all people to eat more of their cultural foods, especially more complex carbohydrates. But as an educator I'm working with the equivalent of 2 dollars compared to the advertisers on national television who are spending millions promoting the wrong foods. How many commercials on TV do you see that tell you to eat more vegetables and fruit? We need to get across a health message to everyone: Reduce your fat and sugar consumption. All Americans need to go back to the foods they used to eat."

Hughes acknowledges that the shortage of taro products is a big problem in Hawaii. "Poi doesn't come into the supermarkets every day of the week," she says. "If you're not there early in the morning, you don't get it. I know because I spend a lot of time chasing around for it, and I don't always get it."

Hoe would like to see 7-Eleven Stores stock taro, along with the school cafeterias and McDonald's. "People must demand the food; we have to be vocal." He cites a report from the Marriott food service saying that they would serve Hawaiian food if there were a demand—and if they knew how to prepare it.

"I'm afraid to say this sometimes," Shintani adds, "but eating right is important not only for physical health but also spiritual health. Because when you are eating right... In the old days, when you wanted to reach spiritual enlightenment, a dietary regimen was always prescribed. It kept individuals close to the land, kept the life force in the food. I'm not sure people are ready to hear this: Diet influences spiritual development. That's just the way it is."

"What is required is a drastic restructuring of thought and attitude," says Gomes. In the Summer Youth Program, she suggests "Why not have the youth work with *kupuna* (elders) instead of training as clerks? Why not job-train them to be marketable in the health system?" And as for the DOH's Office of Hawaiian Health, "Why not hire people to become practitioners of *ho'oponopono* (group dispute resolution)? It's a viable program to relieve stress, but why is it not being talked about? And why is ho'oponopono not part of the cultural curriculum in medicine, social work and psychology?" Because, says Gomes, "it's not a reality in the sense that it's not perceived as a real, proven—in the Western sense—methodology."

Shintani stresses that it's important for the kupuna to survive and share their wisdom with newly interested people. "A lot of folks and some Hawaiian leaders say, 'When the lands are returned, health will return.' I see it as, when Hawaiians regain health, they will regain the land. They will be a spiritually connected and unified force. Injustices will be righted."

Hoe is helping to fuel this renewal. In teaching about the value of Hawaiian cultural foods, his emphasis extends beyond nutrition to the more fundamental goals of perpetuating cultural values and elevating pride in being Hawaiian. Pride is also an emphasis for Shintani. "Look at the ancestors. They were healthy and athletic. People ought to be proud of that. Every Hawaiian ought to know that."

"Hawaiians need to have a firm personal conviction," Blaisdell says. "We are part of the earth. We belong to it, not vice versa. It is sacred and must be treated as such. Take a stand. There has to be a place for native people—for *ahupua'a*, for fishponds—not a place for blowing up reefs for marinas."

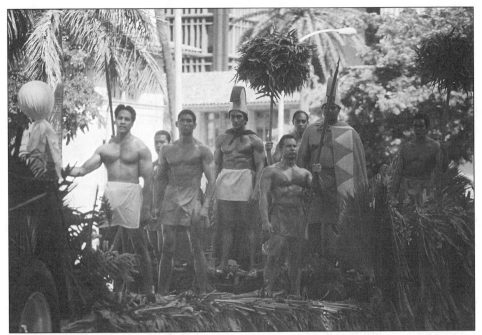

Native Hawaiian men in 1995 Kamehameha Day parade, honoring the first king of the Hawaiian Islands.

"The state is moving in a direction which is not really in the interests of Hawaiians," says Hoe. "It is very important that we be heard as Hawaiians. Water is the key to the survival of the Hawaiian nation, along with land. We gotta get involved."

"Our own people are so colonized, so afraid to face up to the situation," says Blaisdell. "This is part of a bigger problem: oppression and exploitation. Therefore, those on top have to yield. But they won't yield unless they are pushed. So Hawaiians have to push."

Given the political history of these Islands and the apparent efforts on the part of those in power to either subvert or co-opt the sovereignty struggle, how is it that the Hawaiian people are not exploding against the state? "Maybe," Gomes suggests, "because we are exploding inside."

Part 2. The Death of Health: Cosmology and Emotion in Colonial Depopulation[2]

This has been a year of colonial sesquicentennials, including the Treaty of Guadalupe Hidalgo, and statehood for my home state of Wisconsin. In 1848 Hawai'i, American

2. Prologue to the presentation of an earlier version of this paper, under the same title, at the 1998 Annual Meetings of the American Anthropological Association, Philadelphia, PA.

missionaries and colonials promulgated the Mahele, a transformation of land tenure colloquially recognized now as a pre-meditated land grab, which alienated Native Hawaiians from not only their land, but also their genealogy. It occurred during a time of epidemic deaths. There was a specific day in 1848 set aside because "So many Hawaiians died during this period that the Privy Council set [it] aside as a day of fasting and prayer for the entire nation to ask Jehovah to end the pestilence" (Kame'eleihiwa 1992:38, citing PCR Vol. 3A: 147). That day was December 6, today.

Why "Depopulation"?

"Depopulation" is the term that academics have adopted to describe the massive loss of life that occurred with colonization. Its formality lends a distance from the indigenous experience of cultural expansionism, masking the emotional and cognitive embroilments of explorer, trader, missionary, and colonial occupations. It suggests a seemingly natural history, an innocent inevitability of the epidemic deaths.

The aim of this paper is to cross that formal distance: to examine colonial-era depopulation in the Pacific, and specifically Hawai'i, from a perspective of the interactions among cultural meanings, consciousness, and neuroimmunity. Overt physical agents, such as European diseases, are viewed here as components in an interplay of mind, immunity, and social inequality.[3]

What I am questioning is the conventional idea that the epidemic deaths were due to a genetic susceptibility to novel pathogens. What I am proposing is that the cognitive, emotional, and psychoneuroimmunological effects of colonialism were fundamental to immune compromise and disease susceptibility, which then facilitated the epidemics and depopulation.

This is, of course, a sketch. I draw on various sources for the larger analysis, among them: Epidemiological and ethnographic histories of Hawai'i and the trajectory of death; the literature on colonialism and resistance; the historical accounts of daily life and performed emotion; the literatures on psychoneuroimmunology (PNI), emotion and health; the varied discourses in the histories of science, medicine, biological anthropology and the construction of knowledge; the ethnopsychological literature on Oceania; and my own ethnographic understanding from 15 years of living and working in Hawai'i during a robust period in the indigenous rights movement.

Depopulation was geographically widespread and catastrophic, but it was neither a uniform nor inevitable companion to colonization. Epidemics tore through certain populations, but spared others. Explanations for these differences, as I argue here, must consider the particulars of the contact experiences, the forms of colonial occupation and usurpation of power, and the consequences for daily lives, human rela-

---

3. Part 2 of this chapter originated with a focus on Melanesia, and was conceived as a term paper for Professor William Elmendorf's course, "Peoples and Cultures of the Pacific" (Scheder 1976). The current revision focuses on Native Hawaiian depopulation in particular, but the argument applies to Indigenous population decline across Oceania, native North America, Amazonia, and elsewhere, in the aftermath of cultural expansionism.

tionships, subsistence, worldviews, and control of cultural integrity of the respective host societies.[4]

Despite the enormous recent interest in the effects of disease in the New World following European contact,[5] the question of why so many died so fast, and for so many decades, remains.

In Theory: The Biology of Depopulation

The standard conception regarding depopulation is repeated in a host of works; that is, that population collapse was largely due to a native susceptibility to introduced pathogens.

It is an old model. Hiram Paulding, who visited the Hawaiian Islands in 1826, expressed in his 1831 *Journal of a Cruise of the United States Schooner Dolphin*, his belief that the chief cause of Hawaiian depopulation was a lack of immunity to introduced diseases (1970: 231; cited in Linnekin 1990: 209). The notion took hold in the early 1930s, an era of eugenicist thought. There has been little diversion from this model, as it has become a scientific "given" and insinuated its way into historical analyses, largely unquestioned by even the most vigorous and critical indigenous scholars.

This standard perspective on depopulation comes from acceptance of a particular view about the body and about "natives", and a readiness to accept decontextualized epidemiological models. The standard model ignores the colonizer and the nature of empire, the emotional life attendant on the political economy of colonialism. It ignores the fact that colonial rule permeated everyday life, impinging on belief systems, values and knowledge, from subsistence, land tenure, and means of production to biospheric and cosmological foundations. It ignores the question of psychobiological responses to all this—emotion, loss, grief—and their action in accelerating or prolonging the epidemics.

In effect, the standard disease resistance model reduces human beings to their immune "maladaptation" while simultaneously side-stepping a different set of biological processes that, in effect, exemplify the depths of emotionality, spirituality and nuanced consciousness of the colonized peoples. It is a convenient denial of humanity.

As we became enamored in this past century with the privileged knowledge of science and biomedicine, we came to embrace the particularistic explanations—the magic—of genetics and germ theory, while the importance of emotional experience, inequality, and powerlessness became, for a time, peripheral (cf. Kunitz 1987). The *physical* importance of cognitive and emotional meaning in health and illness — for the germs and the genes as well as the whole person—has only recently re-emerged, with extensive growth in the

---

4. Stephen Kunitz (1994) presents a compelling example of this approach, in his analysis of differential mortality in Samoa and the respective colonial styles imposed by European and American colonial administrations on what are now Western and American Samoa, and the stark contrast in depopulation between these political entities.

5. Some examples are: Verano and Ubelaker 1992; Stannard 1992; Bushnell 1993; Jackson 1994; Waldram, Herring and Young 1995.

fields of emotion and health, behavioral neuroscience, immunology, and mind-body medicine.

New Pathogens, Stress, and Immunity

Advances in psychoneuroimmunology (PNI) research leave little doubt about the active physiologic roles of stress and emotion in immune function (cf. Ader 1995). Stress, anxiety, and personal relationships interact with specific, measurable immune responses. Social and psychological stresses undermine the immune system's ability to suppress an infection, even before it produces symptoms (Glaser et al. 1999).

These findings are a small sample of the extensive PNI literature, which parses stress and emotion into their more complex and subtle components. Four components pertinent to colonial occupation, prolonged epidemics, and depopulation are: the immune response to new pathogens; the continued immune effects of chronic stress; immune effects of changes in role and status expectations in the face of a social system in collapse; and the immune consequences of caregiving, bereavement and survivor stress, of parental loss in childhood and developmental impairment of immune function.

The PNI literature provides insight to each of areas, and I offer a mere glimpse here.

Novel Pathogens

PNI pioneer Janet Kiecolt-Glaser (1996) poses a question that inadvertently cuts to the core of the depopulation question: "When you meet a new antigen, does stress alter your ability to respond to that new antigen?" Her elaboration, which describes a contemporary investigation, reveals fundamental parallels to the colonial situation in terms of stress, disturbed personal relationships, and duration of immune effects. She continues, "An experimental study with Hepatitis-B vaccine suggests yes. Students who developed measurable antibody were those who were less stressed and less anxious; at six months, the students who had an improved response to the vaccine also reported the more satisfying personal relationships; this correlated with higher antibody titers and enhanced T-cell immunity."

Chronic Stress and Immunity

Chronic stress inhibits natural killer lymphocytes that detect and destroy infected cells; it also suppresses anti-bodies and T-lymphocytes that detect and destroy the pathogens (Littrell 1996).

Changes in Status and Role Expectations

The concepts of "cultural consonance" and "status incongruence" (cf. Dressler and Bindon 2000), describe the shifting of social status markers, and may be useful analytic pry-bars for considering the immune effects of colonialism as it disrupts social status expectations and role fulfillment. McDade (2002), in an excellent example of psychoneuroimmunological work in anthropology, found immune function to be reduced in "status incongruent" Samoan youth.

Caregiving and Bereavement

Contemporary knowledge on the immune effects of caregiving, bereavement, and loss are particularly pertinent to depopulation, and provide bases for speculation on their comparable actions during the epidemics.

Caregiving is now clearly understood as a potent stressor across age, gender, ethnicity, and illness type, at least in contemporary American society. The stress of caregiving is a process involving the primary as well as secondary stressors, including strain on roles and activities outside of care-giving and including a diminishing sense of control or mastery over life (Pearlin et al. 1997). For example, Latina caregivers experienced higher rates of chronic illness and mortality than the norm for Latinas; many of these caregivers were themselves a bereaved partner or parent as they continued to provide care for others (Land et al. 2002). Latina AIDS caregivers' own HIV disease accelerated as they attended others (Black et al. 1994). Immune suppression continues with repeated bereavement (Kemeny et al. 1994).

Loss and grief can suppress immune function. As people die and support networks disappear, especially extended family and group support systems, there are consequential losses of companionship, assistance, and mutual understanding. The loss of buffers brings greater stress exposure, and continued immune effects. In depopulation, the capacity to mobilize other resources is presumably compromised: there are no other resources left. What are the consequences for the performance of ritual caring for the souls of the dead, and how do those consequences affect the emotional and spiritual life of the survivors?

Are the situations of the caregivers and the bereaved in these studies comparable to that of Hawaiian caregivers and bereaved during the colonial-era epidemics? Continuity of bonds, attachment, and a continued relationship with the deceased, are described across the anthropological literature (e.g., Bonanno 1998, 1999; Kastenbaum 1995; Opoku 1981). Cross-cultural variation in caregiving and mourning is virtually unplumbed with regard to immune function or moderation of the loss and grieving experience. How did missionary and trader activities interfere with these bonds and ancestral beliefs, and undermine culturally-defined coping processes? How did the epidemics affect understandings of the meaning of illness and healing, confidence in native healing, the power of treatment in affecting how a person feels, and the physiological cascade the belongs with feeling? How is the cultural processing of death affected by the loss of so many members? Ceremonies and rites of passage were curtailed or abandoned because of the losses, including ritual offerings to ensure the souls of the dead would go on to live together with their ancestral gods (Kamakau 1964: 33–34). What might be the immune consequences of the cultural and social losses wrought by the new illnesses?

Let's turn to the historical and cultural record of colonization and depopulation.

Historical Reports and Cultural Meaning in Hawai'i

What was the temporal trajectory of colonialism and disease in Hawai'i? The death of health for Hawaiians began with contact and colonial encounters, commencing with the voyages of Captain James Cook and others following in the late 1770s.

From the 1780s to the early 1800s, a raft of new animals, plants, fruit trees, vegetables —and fleas, centipedes and scorpions—were introduced by trading ships, and upset the

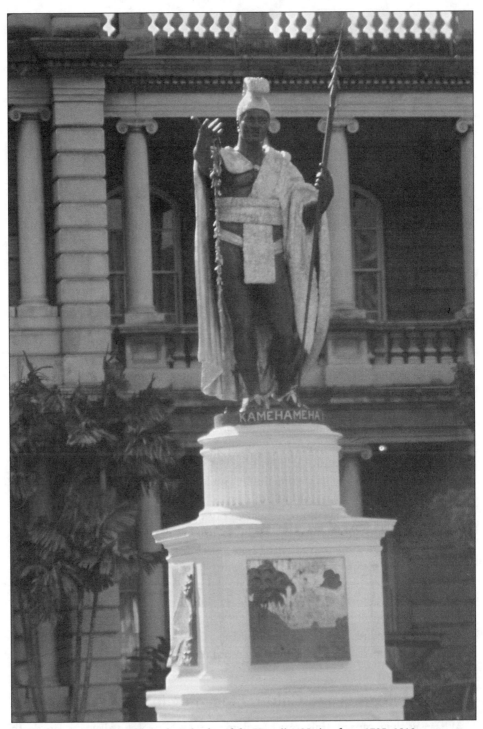

Statue of Kamehameha I, leader of the Hawaiian Nation from 1795–1819.

natural balance in the islands. This was a balance keenly cultivated by Hawaiians, who saw themselves as a familial part of the environment.

In the realm of ideas, "new concepts and different ways of interpreting the phenomena of nature, new points of view in regard to the relationship between social classes and in regard to the position of women, and the new economic practices inevitably raised questions and generated a skeptical attitude which weakened the foundation of the old system and prepared the way for its collapse" (Kuykendal 1938: 28).

The initial deaths happened in new and grotesquely frightening ways. Led by venereal disease introduced by Cook's crew during the initial European encounter in the islands at Kaua'i in 1778, varied epidemics ensued. Their peaks included: 1803–04 typhoid-like illness; 1826 influenza; 1839, 1844, 1848–49 combined influenza, measles, mumps, whooping cough; 1853 smallpox; 1860s leprosy; 1882 smallpox again; 1895 cholera; 1899 bubonic plague; and various influenza epidemics throughout the 1800s.[6] The extremes of population decline were in the late 18th and early 19th Centuries. By 1878, 100 years after first contact, the population collapse reached 90%.[7]

"Hawaiians saw their society falling apart as their friends and loved ones died around them" (Kame'eleihiwa 1992: 20). How did witnessing the illness and death of loved ones, crucial members in an eco-psychology of relationships, prime the population for continued spread of these new pathogens? More was lost than these specific lives: at stake was community, cosmology, formulations of self and being.

This was an era of terror (Obeyesekere 1992: xv), a pervasive terror, different from the culture of terror in which we now live, but a terror constructed by cultural intrusion and cosmological grief.

But what constitutes spiritual and psychological experience? How is it formed and supported, and how did colonized Hawaiians experience it during the 18th and 19th Centuries?

Colonial ethnographic descriptions from elsewhere in the Pacific, of anguish, of grieving, of despair, of giving up, are bridges to current literature on bereavement, fear, anger, and immune suppression, and on generational effects of childhood stress.

In the late 19th and early 20th Centuries, several writers turned to questions of psychological distress and social disintegration as a contributor to Pacific depopulation. Their descriptions were couched in the ethnocentrism of their times. Rivers (1922: 84–113) proposed that a loss of interest in life, what he called 'giving up', was a major factor in depopulation in Melanesia. Durrad referred to "loss of vitality…stagnation and lifelessness…utter depression and abandonment of all idea of fighting an illness…" (1922: 11–12, 17–18). Keesing (1945: 59) mentioned a "sense of hopelessness in the force of the new order," and echoed the observations that "demoralized" individuals were more susceptible to disease. Roberts (1927: 59–60, 72) described a "general lassitude," despair and melancholia, and stated bluntly what has come to be a common interpretation among Pacific scholars: "when the native saw the white man violate these *tapus* (the most vital element in his religion) with impunity, his inherited house of faith came crashing down".

---

6. See Ito (1999: 39) for a concise chronological summary of the epidemic tolls.

7. Estimates vary between 85–95% depending on the pre-contact population figure used. By 1878, the full-Hawaiian population was 44,088 (Schmitt 1968: 74).

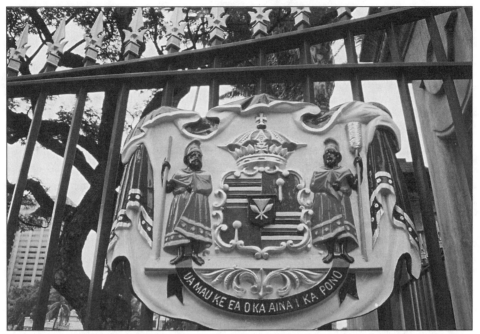

Crest of the Hawaiian Nation: "The life of the land is perpetuated in righteousness."

These descriptions are, certainly, the "other's gaze." By comparison, Native Hawaiian historian Lilikala Kame'eleihiwa provides an indigenous view of the psychological response to colonialism and epidemic disease: "In traditional Hawaiian society...when disaster struck, it was because the *Mo'i* [the paramount chief] was no longer *pono* [in a state of perfect harmony]. Certainly epidemic disease and massive death were signs of loss of *pono*..." (1992: 81). Kame'eleihiwa (1992: 203) further questions the interpretation of the "indolence" described by Calvinist missionaries: "This reported 'indolence' may have been a sign of psychological malaise resulting from terrible disease, serious depopulation, and excessive taxation. Or it might have been a kind of cultural schizophrenia engendered by the Christian *kapu* that condemned the Hawaiian celebration of life. Or perhaps, having lost the great *Akua* [god] Lono, the *maka'ainana* [commoners] had no grand purposes to work toward as a whole community.".[8]

Meaning and Being

Hawaiians understood life as "a relationship between the spirit of the land and the people of the land, between material survival and cultural expression...this structured the core of Hawaiian kinship" (Trask 1984/85: 120). Daily activities "...expressed spiritual as well as physical aspects of being" (Trask 1984/85: 120). Interpersonal values, kinship relations and the emotional ties binding kin together were linked in *Aloha 'aina*, love of the land; Hawaiian culture then and now resided in social interactions, emo-

---

8. Fijian, Tahitian and Hawaiian writers of the time also wrote of the peoples' grief and loss of spirit (cf. Roberts 1927: 58, 74–75).

tional relationships, and shared meanings of those relationships (Ito 1999). How are relationships altered by epidemic illness and death?

Questions about the self implicitly permeate these relationships. Hawaiians interact with their natural and social environment as part of their social world, and depend on these interactions for the maintenance of the self. As Ito (1985: 301–2) describes it, "The Hawaiian concept of the self is grounded in affective social relations (which) are not confined to humans but include the spiritual and natural worlds as well. [It is] highly interpersonal...based on...dynamic bonds of emotional exchange and reciprocity... Self and Other, person and group, people and environment, are inseparable...Inexplicable illness, injury, misfortune, or even death are public evidence of negative acts of self-retention...interpreted as warnings...of violations of the Hawaiian ethos."

In this world, what is the meaning of mass death? How are beliefs about life and its meaning, about religion, spirit worlds, and the workings of the cosmos, challenged or undermined by the epidemics? How much rethinking of relationships to gods and cosmology? Ka'ahumanu (c. 1768–1832), along with other *Ali'i Nui* [High Chiefs and Chiefesses], abandoned the *'Aikapu* religion in an effort to stop the dying (cf., Kame'eleihiwa 1992: 82, 141, 316).

In essence, stress and the quality of personal relationships have immune impacts. Relationships are of paramount importance to Hawaiians and other Indigenous Peoples, having instrumental social support components, as well as emotional bonds, symbolic meaning, and status definitions.

What this implicitly argues is that "social forces mediated between newly introduced infective organisms and their human hosts" (cf. Oliver 1951: 115–19; Kunitz 1994: 73), upsetting the balances among kin, and between humans and the environment. Subsequent missionary and settler activity operated on these disturbed spiritual relationships.

Colonialism brought disruption to the relational worlds of Native Hawaiians. What did disruption to these social worlds mean to the 19th Century Hawaiians, to the experience of grief and loss, and how was this meaning processed neuroimmunologically? I suggest that these disruptions and losses had reverberations in the cellular physiology of bereavement, in an organic toll of chronic grief.

Ultimately, the epidemics and depopulation served the commercial, territorial, and ecclesiastical aims of Empire.

The Tenacity of an Incomplete Idea

Epidemics occur because pathogens or toxins are present in highly susceptible populations. What makes for this susceptibility? The popular explanation, novelty of the pathogen, is one factor; but does it present a full understanding? Enhanced transmission or virulence because of changing population conditions are also factors, and historical events are important shapers of illness context and disease expression.

Depopulation happened because of immune compromise, on that there is general agreement. But the form or origination of the immune compromise is the issue.

With late 19th century germ theory and changing ideas about disease causation, specific diseases needed specific causes. This occurred in the context of colonial entrenchment, post-1848, around Civil War over slavery and social control, and post-

1898 and annexations of Hawai'i, Puerto Rico, and the Philippines. The immune in-sufficiency paradigm served a purpose: it was useful to imperial pursuits for its 'oth-ering' of colonial subjects, and for reinforcing the notion of their weakness and infe-riority relative to the colonizers.

In our own era, "lifestyle" has replaced "germs." Both paradigms remove the realm of social meaning from causation, therefore objectifying illness and separating the acts and effects of the dominant society from the symbolic and emotional mediation of the disease process. Germ theory absolved colonialism of its genocidal effects because the germs and not the colonial situation caused the deaths. The effects of this reification of "germ" or "diet" as cause create a new realm of dictated experience, including guilt, blame, and deservedness of care.

The contemporary reification of lifestyle and the earlier reification of the germ the-ory both assign weakness; but where "germ" also recognized risk exposure, "lifestyle" celebrates agency. The assumptions of agency are inherently political. The ideology re-inforces the dominant ideas of the larger society, whether colonial ideas about im-mune-weakened natives or current implications that ethnic or cultural groups self-in-dulgently cause their own illnesses.

Questions and What We Know

There are many other biocultural questions to ask. Was it coincidence, for exam-ple, that there was a series of major epidemics during the period of the land division, the *mahele*, 1848-1849? Why was the death toll at this time apparently higher among girls and young women, who were symbolically associated with land, having a spiri-tual and cosmological connection through Papa (Earth Mother), the progenitor of the Hawaiian people (cf. Linnekin 1990: 208, 238)? Are there PNI effects of gender and the distribution of power, changing with the missionaries' introduction of Christian patriarchy, causing another level of disruption, and collective frustration and loss for women and girls in particular, while the land was being taken away by American men? This is pure speculation, admittedly, but a challenge to think more deeply and cre-atively about meaning and illness.

What we do know today is this: links among loss, depression, grief, and immune sup-pression are documented, and rigorous research continues to confirm the potency of emotion and symbolic meaning in physical vulnerability to pathogenic processes. So-cial networks, social embeddedness, perceived social support resources, and self-con-cept are important to immune responsiveness. There can be later, delayed effects of un-expressed grief on endocrine and immune function (cf. Kiecolt-Glaser 1996).

Those research findings are consonant with the colonial experience. But this paper is not simply an academic reverie about the past. The principle applies to the illness patterns now, such as the continued high rates of infectious disease that persist today for many American Indian communities (cf. Rhoades 2000), no longer subject to facile explanations of a lack of immune preparedness for novel pathogens. The principle ap-plies to the particular pattern in which AIDS established itself, first among communi-ties whose members were culturally or politically marginalized. The principle applies to neocolonialism, and the utility of immune function as a biomarker for the stress of changing cultural dynamics (McDade 2002).[9]

Granted, this entire concept is speculative and suffers from the absence of biological evidence from the period. Historical records and ethnographic documents can provide windows, and osteological data, where available, can provide some evidence of disease states, but these data have not been assessed from a stress perspective.

We don't have an archeology of biopsychology—yet. We do know, however, that epidemics and illness susceptibilities are shaped by their contexts. We know that contexts include emotion and consciousness, the force of the experiential and the political, of collective emotions and individual biochemistries. We know that contexts—histories and meanings—can bridge the distance between appearances and understanding. We have the contexts and a bridge. Perhaps crossing that bridge could change the appearance of "depopulation" and enrich our understanding of contemporary infectious disease.

Acknowledgments

My respectful appreciation and thanks to Professor Daniel Muller, University of Wisconsin-Madison Institute on Aging and Mind/Body Center, for his interest in this perspective on depopulation, consciousness and PNI, his thoughts on the 1998 version, and his encouragement to revive the argument.

References

Ader, Robert. 1995. Foreword. *In* Stress, the Immune System and Psychiatry. B. Leonard and K. Miller, eds. pp. ix-xiii. New York, NY: John Wiley and Sons.

Black, M., P. Nair and D. Harrington. 1994. Maternal HIV Infection: Parenting and Early Child Development. Journal of Pediatric Psychology 19: 595–616.

Bonanno, G.A. 1998. The Concept of "Working Through" Loss: A Critical Evaluation of the Cultural, Historical, and Empirical Evidence. *In* Posttraumatic Stress Disorder: Vulnerability and Resilience in the Life-Span. A. Maercker, M. Schuetzwohl and Z. Solomon, eds. pp. 221–47. Gottingen, Germany: Hogrefe and Huber.

_____ 1999. Factors Associated with the Effective Accommodation to Loss. *In* The Traumatology of Grieving. C. Figley, ed. pp. 37–52. Tallahassee, FL: Taylor and Francis.

Bushnell, O.A. 1993. The Gifts of Civilization: Germs and Genocide in Hawai'i. Honolulu, HI: University of Hawai'i Press.

Dressler, William W. and James R. Bindon. 2000. The Health Consequences of Cultural Consonance: Cultural Dimensions of Lifestyle, Social Support, and

---

9. McDade (2002) presents a lucid overview of medical and biological anthropologists' approaches to stress and culture change research, the common quest to understand the contexts that give meaning to change, and the models used to explain these processes.

Arterial Blood Pressure in an African American Community. American Anthropologist 102: 244–60.

Durrad, W.J. 1922. The Depopulation of Melanesia. *In* Essays on the Depopulation of Melanesia. W.H.R. Rivers, ed. London: Cambridge University Press.

Ito, Karen L. 1999. Lady Friends: Hawaiian Ways and the Ties that Define. Ithaca. NY: Cornell University Press.

———1985. Affective Bonds: Hawaiian Interrelationships of Self. *In* Person, Self and Experience: Exploring Pacific Ethnopsychologies. Geoffrey M. White and John Kirkpatrick, eds. Berkeley, CA: University of California Press.

Jackson, Robert H. 1994. Indian Population Decline: The Missions of Northwestern New Spain, 1687–1840. Albuquerque, NM: University of New Mexico Press.

Kamakau, Samuel M. 1991. Ka Po'e Kahiko: The People of Old. Translated by Mary Kawena Pukui from the Newspaper Ke Au 'Oko'a, 1866–1871. Special Publication 51. Honolulu, HI: Bernice Pauahi Bishop Museum.

Kame'eleihiwa, Lilikala. 1992. Native Land and Foreign Desires. Honolulu, HI: Bishop Museum Press.

Kastenbaum, R.J. 1995. Death, Society, and Human Experience. 5th Edition. Needham Heights, MA: Allyn and Bacon.

Keesing, Felix M. 1945. The South Seas in the Modern World. Revised Edition. New York, NY: John Day Company.

Kemeny, M.E., H. Weineer, S.W. Taylor, S. Chneider, B. Visscher and J.L. Fahey. 1994. Repeated Bereavement, Depressed Mood, and Immune Parameters in HIV Seropositive and Seronegative Gay Men. Health Psychology 13: 14–24.

Kiecolt-Glaser, J. 1996. Immunologic Changes in Alzheimer Caregivers. *In* Mind-Body Interactions and Disease, and Psychoneuroimmunological Aspects of Health and Disease. Proceedings of a Conference on Stress, Immunity and Health. N.R.S. Hall, F. Altman and S.J. Blumenthal, eds. pp. 125–33. Rockville, MD: National Institutes of Health.

Kunitz, Stephen J. 1987. Explanations and Ideologies of Mortality Patterns. *Population Development* 13: 379–408.

———1994. Disease and Social Diversity: The European Impact on the Health of Non-Europeans. New York, NY: Oxford University Press.

Kuykendal, Ralph S. 1938. The Hawaiian Kingdom, Volume I: 1778–1854, Foundation and Transformation. Honolulu, HI: University of Hawaii Press.

Land, Helen and Sharon Hudson. 2002. HIV Serostatus and Factors Related to Physical and Mental Well-being in Latina Family AIDS Caregivers. Social Science and Medicine 54(1): 147–59.

Linnekin, Jocelyn. 1990. Sacred Queens and Women of Consequence: Rank, Gender, and Colonialism in the Hawaiian Islands. Ann Arbor, MI: University of Michigan Press.

Littrell, J. 1996. How Psychological States Affect the Immune System: Implications for Interventions in the Context of HIV. Health and Social Work 21: 287–95.

McDade, Thomas W. 2002. Status Incongruity in Samoan Youth: A Biocultural Analysis of Culture Change, Stress, and Immune Function. Medical Anthropology Quarterly 16(2): 123–50.

Obeyesekere, Gananath. 1992. The Apotheosis of Captain Cook: European Mythmaking in the Pacific. Princeton, NJ: Princeton University Press.

Oliver, Douglas L. 1951. The Pacific Islands. Cambridge, MA: Harvard University Press.

O'Nell, Theresa D. 1996. Disciplined Hearts: History, Identity, and Depression in an American Indian Community. Berkeley, CA: University of California Press.

Opoku, K.A. 1989. African Perspectives on Death and Dying. In Perspectives on Death and Dying. A. Berger, P. Badham, A.H. Kutscher, J. Berger, M. Perry and J. Beloft, Eds. pp. 14–23. Philadelphia, PA: Charles Press.

Pearlin, Leonard I., C.S. Aneshensel and A.J. LeBlanc. 1997. The Forms and Mechanisms of Stress Proliferation: The Case of AIDS Caregivers. Journal of Health and Social Behavior 38(3): 223–36.

Prigerson, H.G., A.J. Bierhals, S.V. Kasl, C.F. Reynolds, M.K. Shear, N. Day, L.C. Berry, J.T. Newsom and S. Jacobs. 1997. Traumatic Grief as a Risk Factor for Mental and Physical Morbidity. American Journal of Psychiatry 154: 616–23.

Rhoades, Everett R. 2000. American Indian Health: Innovations in Health Care, Promotion and Policy. Baltimore, MD: Johns Hopkins University Press.

Rivers, William Halse Rivers. 1922. The Psychological Factor. In Essays on the Depopulation of Melanesia. W.H.R. Rivers, ed. London: Cambridge University Press.

Roberts, Stephen H. 1927. Population Problems of the Pacific. London: George Routledge and Sons, Ltd.

Scheder, Jo C. 1976. Biopsychology and Pacific Depopulation. Unpublished manuscript, Department of Anthropology, University of Wisconsin-Madison.

Schmitt, Robert C. 1968. Demographic Statistics of Hawai'i: 1778–1965. Honolulu, HI: University of Hawai'i Press.

Stannard, David E. 1989. Before the Horror: The Population of Hawai'i on the Eve of Contact. Honolulu, HI: University of Hawai'i Press.

_____1992. American Holocaust: Columbus and the Conquest of the New World. New York, NY: Oxford University Press.

Trask, Haunani-Kay. 1984–85. Hawaiians, American Colonialism, and the Quest for Independence. Special Issue: The Political-Economy of Hawaii: Social Process in Hawaii 31: 101–36.

Verano, John W. and Douglas H. Ubelaker. 1992. Disease and Demography in the Americas. Washington, DC: Smithsonian Institution Press.

Waldram, James B., D. Ann Herring and T. Kue Young. 1995. Aboriginal Health in Canada: Historical, Cultural, and Epidemiological Perspectives. Toronto: University of Toronto Press.

Chapter 2

'In Their Tellings': Dakota Narratives about History and the Body[1]

Gretchen Chesley Lang

> *You don't have anything if you don't have the stories.*
>
> Leslie Marmon Silko, *Ceremony* (1977: 2)

> *Thus we may say, more generally, that we all come to know each other by asking for accounts, by giving accounts, by believing or disbelieving stories about each other's pasts and identities.*
>
> Paul Connerton (1989: 21)

Summary of Chapter 2. Anthropologists have given increasing attention to peoples' narratives of illness experience and theories of health and illness, oftentimes referred to as "layperson" or "commonsense" accounts. The focus in this chapter is on narrating or the "telling" of stories and the giving of accounts, as well as the importance of understanding contexts *within which* and *with which* these accounts are presented. Anthropological study traditionally involves in-depth, and often lengthy, ethnographic fieldwork. Collection of narrative material—as for other information and observations—requires care in interpretation and representation, not only to better grasp its meanings, but also in respect of the thoughts and experiences shared with the listener. This chapter expresses my thoughts about conversations with Dakota (Siouan) people carried out in the 1980s who shared stories about their lives and, specifically, their ideas regarding a new illness, type 2 diabetes (see Lang, Ch. 9, this volume). Dakota people "make sense"—in complex ways —in their talk about illness and health, and speak differently at different times and in varied settings, making reference—on multiple levels—to larger issues in their history and present-day community. To illustrate the variation and scope of the narrative process, I have drawn upon the statements of one

---

1. Portions of this chapter were presented as part of the Invited Session organized by Drs. Linda C. Garro and Cheryl Mattingly: Narrative Representations of Illness: Stories of Sickness and Stories of Healing, Annual Mtgs. of the American Anthropological Association, New Orleans, 28 Nov. – 2 Dec., 1990]

individual made at different times in the context of a life history project, and through the accounts of another individual crafted for different audiences.

ᴥ ᴥ ᴥ

I first visited Mr. Carl Webster,[2] a noted Dakota elder in his early 60s, at his small frame house on a back road at Spirit Lake (formerly Devil's Lake Reservation),[3] in late 1981. Housebound on this freezingly cold December day, one foot propped up on a kitchen chair, he was talkative about the diabetes that "has laid me up with numbness in my feet and hands." "I don't like to use a cane, so I hobble around and my legs hurt. Last summer I had to stay in the drumming circle while everyone else was up and down between playing, visiting their friends. I just had to sit there and have people visit me…I didn't see lots of people because of this." He often spoke of what his disability was keeping him from doing, which he described as not being able to attend celebrations and occasions in his own and other communities. He had invitations to perform naming ceremonies, to be an announcer—an "Emcee"—at powwows, to sing at memorials; these were "obligations" that he said he was now often unable to meet.

The occasion of my visit to Carl Webster and his wife was to carry out a series of interviews as part of a wider ethnographic consideration of foodways, diet and health.[4] These interviews focused on perspectives of persons with diabetes regarding the etiology (cause) of their condition, their illness experience, and ideas about treatments. Though Carl Webster had suffered from this condition for many years and was afflicted with a number of complications, for many residents, type 2 diabetes was a relatively "new" illness at Spirit Lake[5] in the early 1980s, as it is for other American Indian communities. Carl Webster and a second individual, Mary Peters, whose talk about diabetes will also be considered in this paper, were two older individuals among the 23 people initially visited in their homes; both individuals were well-known to many others in the community with whom I also talked about diabetes and other matters during the 1980's. The initial interviews carried out in people's homes, included an open-ended question format based on Kleinman's (1980) "explanatory model" ("EM"); these discussions subsequently developed into a life history project with Mr. Webster, and several additional visits with Mrs. Peters to ex-

---

2. Names used here are pseudonyms.

3. Devil's Lake Sioux Tribe has changed its name to Spirit Lake Nation; the new name is used in this chapter.

4. For more background information about the Dakota experience with diabetes at Spirit Lake, see Ch. 9 in this volume, "Talking about a New Illness with the Dakota: Reflections on Diabetes, Foods, and Culture" (also Lang 1985, 1987, 1989). This essay focuses on the complexity and meaningfulness of narrative accounts and what such accounts may contribute to fuller understandings of what individuals choose to convey about their lives and experience. Here, I try to emphasize the importance of making a serious effort to grasp the historical and ethnographic contexts in which peoples' ideas and feelings are expressed. This is especially valuable for health planners, care-givers, as well as those carrying out many projects related to health and well-being.

5. In 1981, residents at Spirit Lake were becoming aware from biomedical screening and health education programs of the newly-incepted Indian Health Service "Five Sites" Diabetes Program that type 2 diabetes was an increasing presence in their community, and being diagnosed among elderly people as well as their middle-aged children at approximately the same time (see Lang 1985, 1989).

plore ideas about foods, diet, medications and additional topics that came up after our earlier conversation.

As elders, each with many responsibilities for three generations of their families and to whom many turned for advice, assistance and direction, in a community of approximately 2800 people, it is likely that pronouncements of these two individuals may have influenced, as well as reflected, views held by others in this Dakota community. In the following vignettes, I will attempt to first portray my understandings of Mr. Webster's efforts to represent the contexts of his life as a "traditional" Dakota person while he talked about a particular illness, and secondly, to portray my understandings of Mrs. Peters' efforts to tell others about Dakota history by talking about this illness as a symptom. The objective here is not to summarize or "typify" Dakota health and illness beliefs, but rather to examine the relationship between representation and context for one illness condition by two unique individuals, who, in their role as elders— were considering many factors and thinking along many lines in their concern about the emergence of a new threat to health.

Narratives

One of the hallmarks of cultural anthropology is in-depth ethnographic study within communities or settings in which the anthropologist spends a significant amount of time, and depending upon the specific topic or domain under investigation, attempts to gain understanding of the "insider" point of view. Cultural anthropologists—as other social scientists—have increasingly turned their attention to narratives of health and illness and illness experience. This chapter is concerned specifically with the act of *narrating*, or the "telling" of stories and the giving of accounts of illness experience.[6] While an interest in the "insider" point of view is not new to anthropology, the current focus on layperson (or 'commonsense') views regarding causes of illness (etiology) and experience of illness reflects, a larger shift during the past three decades within anthropology to a more interpretive approach (Geertz 1973; Kleinman 1988, among others). Narrative accounts, themselves, are peoples' representations and interpretations and, in turn, attempts by social science writers to write about these accounts involve further representation and interpretation. And, here, one might suggest that narratives may only "make sense" for the listener if he or she is aware of the many layers or kinds of contexts within which nar-

---

6. Narrating, following literary theorist Genette's (1980: 27) distinction between different meanings of the term *narrative*, is the enunciating, or the "telling," of narrative statements. Genette's clarification of terms are useful for the present discussion; he proposes to "use the word *story* for the signified or narrative content (even if this content turns out, in a given case, to be low in dramatic intensity or fullness of incident), to use the word *narrative* for the signifier, statement, discourse or narrative text itself, and to use the word *narrating* for the producing narrative action and, by extension, the whole of the real or fictional situation in which that action takes place." While Genette (190: 26) suggests that an interest in the event that consists of someone recounting something has been somewhat neglected by analysts of literary texts, it should be noted that anthropologists have long been concerned with the relation between story (narrative content) and context in which narrating— the "telling"—takes place, a relationship examined in different ways by Hymes (1977), Tedlock (1977, 1983) Bruner 1986b) and Frankenberg (1988), among others.

ratives are produced, including the one-to-one relationship of the speaker with an interviewer, local social, political, economic, and historical contexts, and larger institutional and structural contexts as well as popular culture (Mattingly and Garro 2000; Lang 1989; Williams 2004). Anthropologists, as other qualitative researchers, face special challenges in communicating their results to audiences of health planners, policy-makers, and public health professionals who are generally more familiar with studies of health and health care presented and described in conventional—and often statistical—formats (Williams 2000).

Theoretical Considerations

Efforts to achieve clearer understandings of what Good and Good (1980) refer to as "meanings of symptoms" and Kleinman (1988) calls "the personal and social meanings of illness" have increasingly focused upon "narratives" of illness and suffering (cf. Williams 1984, 2000; Kleinman 1988: 3; Frankenberg 1987; Mattingly and Garro 2000). The study of health, illness and healing from the layperson or "native" point of view is hardly a new tradition in anthropology. The rationale for studying this topic was set forth quite explicitly by W.H.R. Rivers in the early part of the 20th C. who described local medical beliefs and practices as "a social institution, one as worthy of study as any of a people's institutions" (Wellin 1977: 27); the subsequent history of anthropological approaches to health beliefs and practices have involved both quantitative as well as quantitative methods too extensive to review here. However, the more recent attention directed towards "narratives" or "narrative accounts" appears to have developed, in part, within the wider discourse regarding representations of experience as discussed by Bruner (1986a) and the complex issue of how ethnographers work their interpretations of patient/layperson representations into an anthropological text (cf. Geertz 1973; Tedlock 1977, 1983).

Anthropologists, in their role as ethnographers, must necessarily attempt to "ground" such accounts—and the occasion of their *telling*—not only in the context of interview or conversation but with consideration to the social, cultural and historical context for narrative statements, issues discussed by Taussig (1980) Young (1982) and Connerton (1989), and others. As sociologist Claudine Herzlich (1979: vii) noted in her study of lay health beliefs in France, narratives of illness and suffering may also—and often, indeed, do—make critical social commentary that reflect the "real" relations of power between healer and patient, and between an individual [or a group] and larger cultural and societal forces. On a more strident note, Michael Taussig (1980: 3) has cautioned medical anthropologists and clinicians to take into consideration what Young (1982) calls the "social relations of sickness", for to neglect the "human relations embodied in symptoms, signs, and therapy, we not only mystify them but we also reproduce a political ideology in the guise of a science of (apparently) "real things..." Physician-anthropologist Paul Farmer (1990: 23), with reference to his well-known work on HIV/AIDS in Haiti points out that "When the illness under consideration is a new one, it is clear that our ethnography must be not only alive to the importance of change but also accountable to history and political economy..." Farmer has documented the changing imagery through which AIDS is deliberated upon by Haitians, as the affliction has moved from the urban area to the village, from the anonymous city-dweller to the local villager.

British medical sociologist Gareth Williams (2004) explores the "use of narratives to inform our understanding of the dynamics of health inequalities;" drawing upon reflections of residents regarding the closure of a steelworks in an already economically stressed area of South Wales. In describing the response of local people to the closing of the steelworks, Williams emphasizes that narrative accounts—even narrative 'snippets'—are a "window" (2004: 2) through which one may glimpse the many personal and often subtle ways in which people experience deprivation and disruption of social relations, individual and community identity, as well as their physical environment itself, in statements that go far beyond conventional descriptions of economic difficulties. Williams (2004: 1) develops the argument "that narrative accounts illuminate how "social conditions are experienced, perceived, and handled and how they constrain the freedom of people to act in such a way that those conditions could be transformed, adapted or avoided in different in different ways." In an earlier essay, Williams (2000: 135) discussed "knowledgeable narratives"—with respect to patients' "detailed descriptions of symptoms and critical assessments of clinical care." Narratives provide valuable clues to the ways in which individuals are linked to the larger structure and practice of medicine, and often "are important points of resistance to doctors, even—or especially—where the need for these doctor's skills is very great."

Narrative accounts of illness may be presented in quite different ways as Cornwell (1984: 15–16) found in her study of health beliefs in an East London neighborhood. She identified a dichotomy between "public accounts" as "sets of meanings in common social currency that reproduce and legitimate the larger assumptions people hold about the nature of social reality" and "private accounts" which "spring directly from personal experience and from the thoughts and feelings accompanying it." In her interviews with East Londoners, she found that public accounts generally preceded private accounts, and reflected a "subtle shift of power" between interviewer and interviewee. In a somewhat similar vein, Davis (1989: 69) described what she terms as "idiosyncratic" (or "individual") and "collective" features of the health condition that local residents of a Newfoundland fishing village categorize as "nerves." Attributes of nerves and the reference to nerves in everyday conversation are varied; for example, Davis (1989: 74) observed that "How a woman presents her nerves varies with the circumstance and the person to whom she is speaking."

Dakota accounts also illustrate Cornwall's observation, where answers to specific questions seemed to invite public accounts, while peoples' "telling stories" resulted in more private accounts; public accounts tended to be more general, referring to the larger collective, "Indian people" (and drew upon larger themes of historical change and disenfranchisement, loss of traditional subsistence and relocation to reservation lands, issues of concern at present, such as 'cluster housing' or political/human rights issues) while private accounts disclosed specific details and circumstances in which personal theories of an individual's explanation of etiology (cause) or ideas about efficacious treatment regarding diabetes would emerge (Lang 1989). Dakota deliberations about a "new illness"—diabetes—through often subtle shifts in context, often vary in their "tellings," so that statements of "collective autobiography" may be juxtaposed with idiosyncratic considerations regarding etiology, illness experience, and efficacy of treatments. Reflections about a new illness also make commentary on Dakota culture history and identity. Representations of experience with diabetes are examined in accounts given by an individual within the context of a life history project, and through the accounts of one individual crafted for different audiences.

As illustrated by a number of chapters in this volume, ethnographic research is a valuable component of studies or applied projects regarding health, health care, and experience of illness. In their introduction to *Narrative and the Cultural Construction of Illness and Healing*, co-editors Mattingly and Garro (2000: 5) discuss many ways in which a focus on narratives may "illuminate aspects of practices and experiences that surround illness but might not otherwise be recognized." While research protocols increasingly include narrative material, such as responses to open-ended, yet specific questions, I would strongly suggest that there is a concomitant responsibility by those privileged to listen to narratives of life experience to also engage in the personal and time-consuming work of ethnography (and the often extensive, rich conversations that this involves) to do justice to what has been offered—the "tellings."

* * * *

"Things aren't being done right around here on this reservation, and we seem to have more and more of these problems like diabetes".—Carl Webster

In talking about his illness, Carl's etiological explanation interwove biomedical details (often quoting the physician's pronouncements) into stories involving other kinds of explanations and ideas about a range of possible effective treatments. These deliberations were phrased in what fluctuated between an idiosyncratic and what can be called a "collective autobiographical" voice.

> I was a lot heavier then, which may be why I got diabetes, that was about nineteen years ago now. These days I have been losing weight, and the doctor says my vision is going. This is a new disease for us Indian people you know; we didn't have this in the old days, and I think it has to be treated by white man medicine—I don't think traditional medicine will work for this...I have been considering trying something besides the clinic...they say that there is a medicine man out at Ft. Smith that can cure diabetes, but I'm not so sure. I used to know this man when we were young. But then lately I've heard that he lost his "power."[7]

Carl also brought up many instances in which illness or other misfortune had befallen persons or their families who did not carry out their "obligations" to living persons or the deceased. Such responsibilities included the necessity of adhering to the

---

7. Considerations of the current "status" of particular medicine men's "power" are on-going among many individuals at Spirit Lake, as well as in other Native American communities (Lame Deer and Erdoes 1972; DeMaille and Lavenda 1977) for analysis of Siouan concepts of power). An extensive ethnographic and historical literature on the Dakota has primarily focused upon the more well-known Western Division or Teton Dakota; valuable accounts of Dakota religious beliefs and practices, including healing are found in Kemnitzer (1976); W. Powers 1982); and writings by the physician Walker (1980) who recorded accounts of healing among the Oglala (Sioux).

one-year restrictions on a mourner for a deceased relative, or taking up a calling when "one has been told something" (in a vision),… The repercussions of not following tradition… may affect the individual's entire family into the future."

Times of sickness or death, he explained in speaking of his recently-widowed "aunt," require certain actions by others for the afflicted individual or the (soul of the) deceased, and for the family:

> …right after she lost Jim we invited her over. Something like that, it bothers you, you know…Sometimes, when somebody dies seems like I'm pulled over there, or I want to do something. I think of the person and think of their lives, and I've just got to go and take stuff to them…If somebody is sick, they remember him, they honor him with a song at a celebration. A member of the family would give [a gift in a "give-away"] for that…If my uncle came over and told me George was pretty sick and they'd like an honor song for him, then you [as an announcer at a celebration, or a powwow] have to go back just a ways about George, because you have to bring out things about his life. You can go back further, too, and then all the way to his kids. You have to explain the main parts of his life.

Though Carl never directly attributed supernatural causes to the origin of his own illness,[8] he referred to the accidents and illnesses of others as "coming to people who aren't living their life the right way." "You know the goings on around here these days makes them under these hills restless," he said, "lately around here, people have been seeing things at their windows at night." Many of his stories also implied sorcery as an existent force within the community and as being directed into the community particularly from Ojibway communities to the east. He generally gave examples in which "medicine" or "power" (either "bad" or "good") was used to determine the outcome in gambling, romantic pursuits and sexual manipulation, and at times in causing a person to be susceptible to illness, and failing in energy or "wasting" which referred to unexplained weight loss.

Carl talked about the cause of diabetes on several levels—one incorporated biomedical explanations as he had been told at the clinic (cf. Roddier, Ch. 4, this volume, describing how lay accounts may draw upon biomedical knowledge.) He was precise in describing his prescribed medications, his ideal body weight (at this time he was not considered overweight), the suggested diet that he said that he did not follow and the doctor's advice that he should not smoke cigarettes. On another level, he told many stories in which "something was sent to a person to make them ill." In these references to sorcery, he most frequently described instances in which someone was incapacitated to keep them singing or dancing at a celebration, but other examples included the onset of generalized weakness and "doing poorly" as he referred to it; in these instances, a medicine man must be consulted to counteract the effect of such "bad medicine." Carl also made more veiled suggestions that problems such as diabetes may result from unhappiness of the deceased (ancestors) with the way people at the present time were living their lives (as not following Dakota "tradition") or a more diffuse spiritual punishment for particular families or the community for moral transgressions.

---

8. Black-Rogers (1989: 231) in her work with Ojibway spiritual leader and medicine man Dan Raincloud, found that he "set limits" on talk of his own powers: "His lesson was clear: a person speaks of his or her powers and their acquisition only while using them. *The telling is part of the doing.*" [italics mine].

In these conversations, Carl did not choose to settle upon a single etiological explanation, and while he was not a medicine man himself, he (and other "traditional" people in his personal network whose ideas he often referred to) appeared to be continually sifting through the misfortunes of others in an on-going effort to diagnose and to come to a consensus on probable causes. Carl also recounted examples that covered a range of possible treatments, discounting as much as praising various methods (he discussed possible benefits for some people through the use of *peyote* as practiced by members of the Native American Church in his community, participation in the *Yuwipi* Healing Ceremony held in communities to the west though rarely at Devil's Lake, the ingestion of various herbal remedies such as those known by his paternal grandmother, and individual consultations with a medicine man, *wicasa wakan*). He also made frequent comments upon the current status of various known healers' "power", substantiating his judgments with stories about others' claims—persons whom he said knew more directly than he through their personal experience with a particular healer (cf. Kemnitzer 1977; W. Powers 1982).

In discussing these possibilities, Carl told stories about people who had tried this remedy or that for various ailments, explaining the relationships of these individuals to himself and his family, in the past and in the present. This form of "telling" was best described by Carl himself as he talked about our doing his "life story" as he referred to it. During the spring of 1982, he had broached the possibility of my assisting him with a project that he had had in mind for some time, mainly he said to help "keep the tradition" that he said he understood.

> These are the things that we're standing with now-a-days, and it's all coming back, no matter where you go on the reservation, they keep saying that, they're trying to revive tradition, trying to bring it back to life. I notice at these pow-wows they've been doing for the past three years…like us traditional persons, if you happen to do anything at a powwow or anyplace [teenagers] laugh at you. I was talking to Blaine, and he said… "I've been thinking. What's going to become of the reservation when you and I die? Who's going to carry on the tradition? Singing? All the young guys we have, they're not interested in these songs—traditional songs, veteran's songs, victory songs, flag songs. Seems like if you and I die every thing is going to die off."

We continued to discuss his experience with diabetes along with his ideas about illness and misfortune within this life-history project from early 1982 until shortly before his death four years later in October, 1986. Early on, he brought out notebooks in which he kept his writings and described how he envisioned this project, and also, I think, his way of "telling."

> I'd like to talk about some of my family affairs, and the history part. And then remember when I told a story about my friend Sam Bear? Friends like that I like to bring in there…I like to bring in something that I've been involved in with other people, I don't like to have too much on me in there…Read those three poems I wrote about my son—the one I lost. A lot of this stuff [in these notebooks] I got off magazines or books, and paper. Sometimes you just don't realize what you pick up in those celebrations—some people just throw away papers, and you pick it up and realize it was something worthwhile.

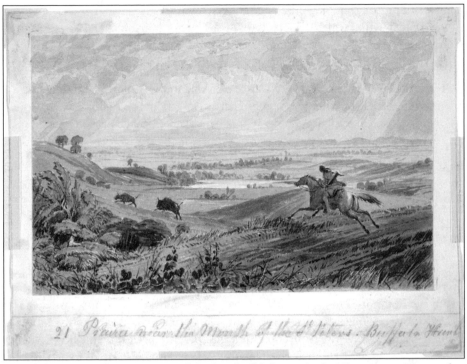

Seth Eastman watercolor, 1846–1848, of a Dakota buffalo hunter in the Minnesota prairies, southeast of Spirit Lake, ND. The original title (as seen on the painting) is "Prairie near the Mouth of the St. Peters—Buffalo Hunting." Minnesota Historical Society Photographic Collection.

These are some of my feelings about my son. I started a little history of my friend Virgil, too, and then I went into his life and our lives together.

Carl planned in advance for what he wanted to talk about at the tape-recording sessions, and would generally begin by speaking about a particular friend or relative and his relationship with this individual. One major theme that emerged was a recounting of the hardships he had been faced with as a young husband and father after W.W.II in the late 1940's when he had difficulty finding any steady employment. He detailed at some length his being hired for seasonal work on nearby (non-Indian) farms. One of his recollections was focused on trips in severe weather to obtain government rations, "and when I got home, I just went around the next day, passing sugar out to my grandfather, aunt. This is the way we helped each other out a long time ago…but my family had hard times…I could feel like crying at times. There wasn't a thing I had that I could sell…I had to make my own homemade beds."

Carl's stories were framed in his representations of relationships between people and the consequences of people's actions over a genealogically-measured time and across the social landscape. The socioeconomic factors of poverty, unemployment, and social problems are part of this landscape, but were not directly implicated. Illness, as Carl implied in these deliberations, emerged as an indicator of an individual's or the community's spiritual and moral lack of wellness (as a weakness of tradition); his representations of his own experience with diabetes combined biomedical understandings with an explanation of how his life (as a "traditional" person who had an obligation to convey traditional knowledge) had been altered by its restrictions. This brief vignette of the context within which diabetes is discussed by one individual illustrates, perhaps, Connerton's (1989: 21) observation:

> In successfully identifying and understanding what someone else is doing we set a particular event or episode or way of behaving in the context of a number of narrative histories. Thus we identify a particular action by recalling at least two types of context for that action. We situate the agents' behaviour with reference to its place in their life history; and we situate that behaviour also with reference to its place in the history of the social settings to which they belong. The narrative of one life is part of an interconnecting set of narratives; it is embedded in the story of those groups from which individuals derive their identity.

Community at Devil's Lake

In her book *Oglala Women*, Marla Powers (1986) remarked that Oglala Sioux are "very clear about what is 'traditional' and what is 'modern'; individuals move easily between such categories in their daily life." Listening to narrative accounts would appear essential for grasping such eclecticism in people representations of identity. Likewise, statements that draw upon or combine quite distinct bodies of medical/religious knowledge and practice in their considerations of, and in their actions to do with, the relief of illness and disability may also be understood as an extension of such representations for particular contexts (cf. Cohen 1986; Kleinman 1980; Helman 1984).

Diabetes was talked about at Spirit Lake in varied ways: as a "new disease that has come to us," as something that "runs in my family, but everybody seems to have it now." "In the old days we used to live to an old age, but now there are all these diseases you hear about, like cancer and diabetes." "It is the foods we eat now that make us sick. We used to eat fresh food, wild game and all the plants that used to grow around here." "It is all this canned food that gives us diabetes." "I think it is the worry that brought it on, all the stress we have now." "I have worked hard all my life and I have a lot of worries—I worry about my children. I think that's what has caused my diabetes to be so bad." "I think diabetes has to be treated by white man's medicine. We don't have treatments for this." Or, conversely, that "I have heard there's a medicine man out west who can cure you with traditional medicine, and I might try this." These fragments suggest that diabetes is being represented in ways that involve personal or idiosyncratic experience, along with an implied collective experience of the "Dakota" or "Indian" people. (cf. Lang, Ch. 9, this volume).

When people were asked for their ideas about the dietary modifications prescribed at the clinic for diabetes treatment, conversations most frequently shifted into a discussion of foods of the past and a recollection (as they had heard it from their elders) of a lifestyle in a distant past that was centered around the strength and healthfulness of a diet of wild plant foods and game. Foods—as they are linked to aspects of health and illness—provided a rich imagery for demarcating cultural boundaries: the disjunction of a "way back" past with present, and also between Dakota-non-Dakota, between Dakota-Euroamerican (cf. Lang 1989). Ideas about attributes of foods emerged as an area of marked convergence or "collective representation." In talking about the past, one also may be talking about the present. Anthony P. Cohen (1985) has observed

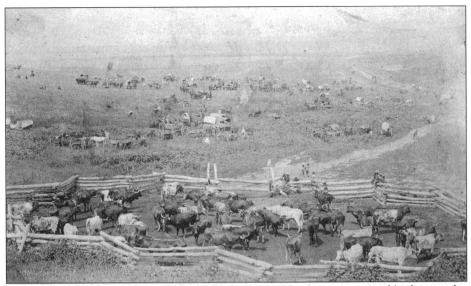

Cattle that will be butchered and distributed as beef rations by the government; this photograph was taken in Dakota Territory by Gilbert ca 1880, likely to the west of the Spirit Lake Nation, perhaps at Standing Rock. (Minnesota Historical Society Photographic Collection).

that "the manner in which the past is invoked is strongly indicative of the kinds of circumstances which makes such a past reference salient. It is a selective construction of the past which resonates with contemporary influences."

Spirit Lake cannot be easily characterized as a single community in terms of cultural orientation or ethnic identity (cf. Albers 1982; Albers and James 1984). Outsiders are frequently struck with contrasting images of everyday life at Spirit Lake. Spirit Lake Nation is a community of strong extended family loyalties and intense community involvement as well as a community with shared experience of rural poverty (Lang 1985). Statements of identity that drew upon an image of a collectivity arose in relation to a speaker's *audience* and *purpose* —these references may be developed to fit with commentary upon family, kin group, tribe, or Dakota vis-à-vis others. Cohen remarks in his book *Symbolic Construction of Community* (1985: 81) that "we find symbolism reinforcing the cultural boundaries of the community by reconstituting its tradition." Without meaning to underplay the personal experience of this illness and the day-to-day challenges in following prescribed treatments, it would appear that diabetes—its diffuse symptoms, its rapid appearance in the community, and especially (as biomedical treatment has drawn attention to foodways) prescribed dietary regimens—has provided Dakota with imagery through which to reflect upon their distinctiveness in the past and present, and likewise, upon the hardships that they have endured during the past century and more. As diabetes has become a major health concern, subject to varying lay interpretations with respect to its possible etiology and considerations regarding efficaciousness of treatments for its many symptoms, its has been drawn upon by some individuals as an way *though which* other issues of concern could be represented. And just as 'nerves' described by Davis (1989), diabetes may serve as a symbol; Cohen (1985: 55) states that "it is the very ambigu-

ity of symbols which makes them so effective as boundary markers of community."
Herzlich's (1973: vii) observation, in her study of French layperson beliefs, that
"When an individual talks about health and illness, he also talks about something else:
the nature of his links with his environment, physical and social, as well as aspects of
social organization" is somewhat similar. In the following vignette, Mrs. Peters, a
woman respected as an informal spokesperson in this community has talked about
diabetes differently in different contexts.

* * * *

"Worry makes my sugar go up."—Mary Peters

In May 1982 at a university conference on health issues sponsored by Native American medical students, in between speakers' presentations of health statistics and profiles of health care delivery in remote reservation settings, a slight and somewhat frail-
appearing Dakota woman in her late sixties moved forward to speak about community
perspectives regarding health issues. Mrs. Peters began in a soft-spoken voice to tell
what became a long recollection of her mother's life and subsequently her own childhood at Spirit Lake in the early 1900. Her description was detailed, referring to specific foods they were able to procure, and of frequent periods of hardship in their log
house. She recalled that their diet at times primarily consisted of potatoes and somewhat erratic government handouts of flour, sugar, lard, and green coffee. She continued, eloquently, to describe the challenges in later years of raising a large family. She
also referred to a longer time ago—to the pre-reservation days before 1867, portraying a lifestyle centered upon the buffalo and prairie plants, when people were actively
engaged in "traditional" methods of making a living.

> We once ate the right foods and lived the right way as *Wakantanka* intended us
> to do. People used to live to a very old age, before we were put onto reservations.
> Today we have these diseases like cancer and heart disease and now we all seem
> to be coming down with diabetes. I remember when my father was told that he
> had "sugar"—it was about 1952. There was little they could do at the clinic. They
> couldn't stop the sugar from building up in him. He was the first person at Devil
> Lake to get diabetes. It is all the foods we eat now—they make us sick—all the
> sugar in these junk foods that everyone is eating around here that don't agree
> with us. For me, I think it is the stress from living all bunched together in these
> new housing projects that I think keeps my sugar up. Some days I just know it
> is high when I am worried about things. Everyone seems to have it. It used to be
> tuberculosis and other diseases that were brought to us, and now it is diabetes.

This speech was more than nostalgia. I had heard similar etiological explanations
and commentaries interwoven in other autobiographies. For her presentation, Mrs.
Peters chose diabetes as a way to talk publicly and persuasively about specific issues
that were on her mind, including on-going difficulties of the Dakota as she continually reflects upon them.

Seven months before her public speech —in the autumn of 1981—I talked with
Mrs. Peters at her house; on this day, she attributed the cause of her diabetic condi-

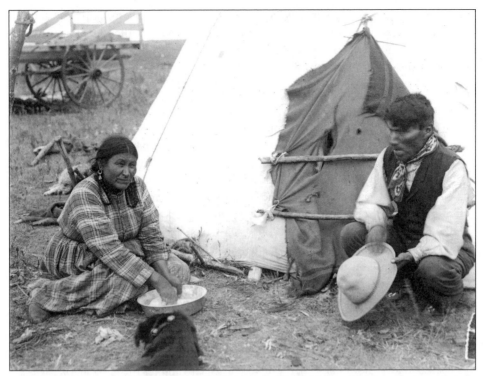

A photo taken in 1920 at Ft. Totten, ND (Spirit Lake Nation) by an unknown photographer. The photograph reflects both the traditional and the new elements in Dakota everyday life; neither the names of these individuals nor the exact context for this photograph are known. I should like to note that in his recent book, *The Sioux: The Dakota and Lakota Nations,* Guy Gibbon (2003: 1–16; 120–25) has shared valuable insights (and cautionary notes) regarding historical bias and photographic representation. Minnesota Historical Society Photographic Collection.

tion to "stress" that everyone was experiencing in the community. She said "all this diabetes around here and I think cancer, too, is caused by stress." Mrs. Peters explained her thinking in some detail:

> The cause of many sicknesses can be from things like germs and viruses — these take over when our inner peace is weakened. For diabetes, it is not the diet that keeps us well, but our state of mind. For me, my sugar is low when I am feeling good and I eat all kinds of things that we aren't supposed to eat. They tell us at the clinic not to have sugar, but I have coca-cola, cookies, fruits and my blood sugar still is low... Other times, this insulin gives me diarrhea. I get depressed. I have been in the hospital for sores that don't heal up, and for the diarrhea. You know, I drink a coca-cola every afternoon about 4:00 — then I don't feel so weak. I don't think this does any harm.

As Carl, Mrs. Peters brought in personal theories and practices that she had developed to deal with her health condition, drawing upon biomedical knowledge but also emphasizing that she was in charge of regulating how she felt, even if it went against "doctor orders."

In the spring of 1982, perhaps in preparation for her upcoming public speech, Mary Peters showed me what she had written down about her thoughts regarding diabetes. In this account, the events culminating in the recent "epidemic" of diabetes began at a specific time and from a number of oppressions:

> The American Indian had to fight for survival from the earliest times, which was several hundred years ago. They had to make do with whatever was at hand. It took a lot of energy with the result that Indian people used every calorie taken into their system and turned it into energy. As the Whiteman came and coveted the land, the Indians and his way of life were threatened with extinction. As a way of assuaging the pangs of conscience, the white through the Congress and Government began to "pray" for the lands taken. By giving the Indian annuities in the form of foods and outmoded clothing. The food by the time it reached the Indian was sometimes unfit to eat. However, the Indian having been deprived of the honorable pursuit of survival had to *sit* and wait on the whims of Congress. I think that is where the beginnings of diabetes were. There were other diseases like tuberculosis which took many Indians to the better hunting ground. There probably is a correlation between the types of food eaten in the period before the Whiteman came and when the Indian had to eat whatever was given to him. That and the fact that he could not expend his energy as in the old days. No where to go and nothing to do. So much for that. The food he ate could be classed as low calorie-high energy or was his system and his mental outlook such that he could turn all his calories into energy? Being his own boss in other words. Not depending on anyone except himself and his immediate family.

> Now, knowing about diabetes has made us more conscious of our diets and we do not have to eat everything before us as we were made to do in School. It has been a hard road for the Indian, especially the children now, as they have to reap the fruits of years of guiding and guarding the parents of these children. Guiding them in ways alien to their nature and guarding them from their true instincts that the Great Spirit instilled in them or did he make the Indian and forget him?

Mary Peters' oratory and writing are evidence for her ability to persuasively make a point, within her community and well as to an outside audience. In her public narratives, Mrs. Peters uses diabetes as a touchstone for her representation of the loss of "wellness" in Indian society due to the history of Indian-white relations.

Ethnographic Contexts

As the study of the experience of illness (and suffering) has increasingly shifted from the context of clinic to the context of home and community, the recognition of the richness of narrative representations for attempts to comprehend and portray this complex, emotionally-charged aspect of human life has come to the foreground. For example, in her study of health beliefs in an East London working class neighborhood, Cornwell (1985) has noted that the ways people talk in their community and in their homes—to each other and to outsiders— reveal the difficulties inherent in generalizing to a set of underlying principles, or to a single cultural model, difficulties also discussed by Garro (1988), Dingwall (1976), and Farmer (1990), among others. Calnan (1986: 8), suggesting a greater interest on the part of health professionals to understand the "lay perspective" of patients and community members, highlights the value of an interpretive approach where "... emphasis is placed on understanding lay people's actions in terms of the meaning that they place on these actions. The meaning is in itself derived from peoples own complex body of knowledge and beliefs, which is closely linked with the social context in which they live their daily lives." Likewise, Williams and Wood (1986: 1435) have drawn attention to the layperson's "making sense" of illness etiology in terms significantly different from a biomedical explanation for their diagnosed condition. From an ethnographic perspective, a layperson's presentation of symptoms, explanations of possible etiology, and deliberations regarding treatments for various illness conditions are conceptualized as interwoven with other social and cultural factors in the fabric of everyday life. Such a conceptualization is consistent with the larger anthropological "goal" of understanding phenomena—beliefs and behaviors— within their social and cultural *context*, and offers a humanistic and powerful means of communicating meaningfully the experience of social inequalities, social conditions, and historical experience that is often represented in more abstract or dispassionate formats.

The context in which representations of experience, such as illness, are expressed—their "tellings"—includes the *relation* between narrator and the interviewer or audience. Williams (1984: 181) has noted that narratives occurring in the context of interviews, no matter how open-ended and lengthy, are *co-authored* enterprises. The relation between narrator and listener (in the context of a structured interview or in a more loosely-constructed fieldwork encounter) is of perennial interest to anthropologists. It is of particular significance for those who sense changes in the "boundaries" between the "field" and "home." In her Frazer Lecture regarding major shifts in the writing of ethnography, Strathern (1987: 269) made the point that "If anthropologists write now about 'other peoples' they are writing for subjects who have become an audience...this makes problematic the previously established distinction between writer and subject. *I must know on whose behalf and to what end I write.*" [italics mine]. It would appear that from the ethnographer's perspective, as interpreter of other people representations, awareness of this "newer" audience has stimulated reflection within anthropology about representation and about the relationship between the anthropologist and people with whom they work. The anthropologist now writes about him or herself in an ethnographic text, setting forth the context of their relationship with the people and community with whom they are engaged. Anthropologists are often advocates for the people with whom they work, and some anthropologists are members of communities in which they do research. Anthropological research brings a valuable dimension to team efforts (cf. Wiedman, Ch. 20, this volume)—perhaps especially with regard to health issues—and may strengthen collaborative efforts towards community empowerment.

Final Thoughts

In her provocative essay entitled "Who Gets to Tell the Stories?" Lakota novelist and essayist Elizabeth Cook-Lynn (1993: 64) states the answer to her question at the outset of her essay: "Those who get to tell the stories are the people that America wants to listen to." Cook-Lynn discusses both American Indian writers and others who write about American Indians, with a particularly strong critique of "as-told-to" biographies of American Indians written by non-American Indians (1995: 117). Cook-Lynn introduces a cautionary note that might also be considered by those who work with narrative material. This goes beyond issues of privacy, which is of course critically important. Representing and offering interpretations of the utterances of "others," with all good intentions to bring attention to terrible problems, inequalities, injustices, alternative histories, especially statements made in times of grief, pain, illness, and deprivation is no small charge. Those who are entrusted with these stories share with journalists and other writers, photographers, filmmakers, and artists a responsibility not to be carried lightly.

The oral history of subordinate groups will produce another type of history: one in which not only will most of the details be different, but in which the very construction of meaningful shapes will obey a different principle. Different details will emerge because they are inserted, as it were, into a different kind of narrative home.

        Paul Connerton (1989: 19)

> *I will tell you something about stories,*
>   *[he said]*
> *They aren't just entertainment.*
>   *Don't be fooled.*

        Leslie Marmon Silko, *Ceremony* (1977: 2)

Acknowledgments

Most of the fieldwork on which this paper is based was carried out between 1981–1984 as part of a larger study of community perspectives on health care, diabetes and diabetes treatment, cf. Lang, Ch. 9, this volume, 1985, 1989; Garro and Lang 1993), but I continued my involvement in this community for nearly a decade. I am grateful to the many individuals who talked with me about diabetes, foodways, and many other topics, tribal health committee members who introduced me to some of these individuals, and the staff of the Diabetes Program at the Indian Health Service Clinic, Ft. Totten, ND (Devil Lake Sioux Reservation, now the Spirit Lake Nation). The Diabetes Program was initiated in late 1979 as part of the Five Sites IHS Diabetes Project headed by Dorothy Gohdes, M.D., IHS Hospital, Albuquerque, NM, whose objectives included the development of models for diabetes education and treatment in Native American communities.

References

Albers, Patricia C. 1982. Sioux Kinship in a Colonial Setting. *Dialectical Anthropology* 6: 253–69.

Albers, Patricia C. and William R. James. 1984. On the Dialectics of Ethnicity: To Be or Not to be Santee Sioux. *Journal of Ethnic Studies* 14: 1–27.

Black-Rogers, Mary. 1989. Dan Raincloud: "Keeping our Indian Way." *In* Being and Becoming Indian: Biographical Studies of North American Frontier. James A. Clifton, ed. pp. 226–48. Chicago: The Dorsey Press.

Bruner, Edward M. 1986a. Introduction. *In* The Anthropology of Experience. Victor W. Turner and Edward M. Bruner , eds. pp. 3–30. Urbana, IL: University of Illinois Press.

_____1986b. Ethnography as Narrative. *In* The Anthropology of Experience. Victor W. Turner and Edward M. Bruner, eds. Urbana, IL: University of Illinois Press.

_____1990. Introduction: Experiments in Ethnographic Writing. *In* Conversations in Anthropology: Anthropology and Literature. P. J. Benson, ed. Journal of the Steward Anthropological Society 17: 1 and 2, 1–19 (1987–88).

Calnan, Michael. 1986. Health and Illness: The Lay Perspective. London: Tavistock Publications.

Clifford, James and George E. Marcus, Eds. 1986. Writing Culture, The Poetics and Politics of Ethnography. Berkeley, CA: University of California.

Clifton, James A. 1989. Alternative Identities and Cultural Frontiers. *In* Being and Becoming Indian: Biographical Studies of North American Frontiers. James A. Clifton, ed. pp. 1–37. Chicago, IL: The Dorsey Press.

Cohen, Anthony P. 1986. Of Symbols and Boundaries. *In* Symbolising Boundaries: Identity and Diversity in British Cultures. Anthony P. Cohen, ed. pp. 1–19. Manchester, UK: University of Manchester Press.

_____1985. Symbolic Construction of Community. London: Tavistock Publications.

Cook-Lynn, Elizabeth. 1993. Who Gets to Tell the Stories? Wicazo Sa Review, 10(1): 64.

Connerton, Paul. 1989. How Societies Remember. New York: Cambridge University Press.

Cornwell, J. 1984. Hard-Earned Lives: Accounts of Health and Illness from East London. New York: Tavistock Publ.

Davis, Dona L. 1989. The Variable Character of Nerves in a Newfoundland Fishing Village. Medical Anthropology 11: 63–78.

DeMallie, Jr., R.J. and R.H. Lavenda. 1977. *Wakan*: Plains Siouan Concepts of Power. *In* The Anthropology of Power: Ethnographic Studies from Asia, Oceania, and the New World. Raymond D. Fogelson, and R. N. Adams, eds. pp. 153–65. NY: Academic Press.

Dingwall, R. 1976. Aspects of Illness. London: Martin Robertson and Co., Ltd.

Farmer, Paul. 1990. Sending Sickness: Sorcery, Politics, and Changing Concepts of AIDS in Rural Haiti. Medical Anthropology Quarterly 4: 6–27.

Fitzpatrick, R. 1984. Lay Concepts of Illness. *In* The Experience of Illness. R. Fitzpatrick, J. Hinton, S. Newman, G. Scambler, and J. Thompson, eds. pp. 11–31. London: Tavistock Publ.

Frankenberg, Ronald. 1987. Narratives of Healing and Suffering: A Paradigmic Presentation. Paper presented at the American Anthropological Association Annual Meetings, 1987. Chicago, IL.

_____1988. Your Time or Mine? An Anthropological View of the Tragic Temporal Contradictions of Biomedical Practice. Int. J. Health Services 18:1, 11–34.

Garro, Linda C. 1988. Explaining High Blood Pressure: Variation in Knowledge about Illness. American Ethnologist 15: 98–119.

_____2000. Cultural Knowledge as Resource in Illness Narratives: Remembering through Accounts of Illness. In Narrative and the Cultural Construction of Illness and Healing. Cheryl Mattingly and Linda C. Garro, eds. pp. 70–87. Berkeley, CA: University of California Press.

Garro, Linda C. and Gretchen Chesley Lang. 1993. Explanations of Diabetes: Ojibway and Dakota Deliberations Upon a New Illness. In Diabetes and Native Americans: The Impact of Lifestyle and Cultural Changes on the Health of Indigenous Peoples. Jennie R. Joe and Robert Young, eds. pp. 293–327. Berlin: Mouton Press.

Geertz, Clifford. 1973. The Interpretation of Cultures. New York: Basic Books.

Genette, G. 1979. Narrative Discourse: An Essay in Method. Ithaca, NY: Cornell University Press.

Gibbon, Guy. 2003. The Sioux: The Dakota and Lakota Nations. Malden, MA (USA): Blackwell Publishers, Ltd.

Good, Byron J. and Mary Jo Delvecchio Good. 1980. The Meaning of Symptoms: A Cultural Hermeneutic Model for Clinical Practice. In The Relevance of Social Science for Medicine. Leon Eisenberg and Arthur Kleinman, eds. pp. 165–96. Boston: D. Reidel Publ. Co.

Hagey, Rebecca. 1984. The Phenomenon, the Explanations, and the Responses: Metaphors Surrounding Diabetes in Urban Canadian Indians. Social Science and Medicine 18: 265–72.

Helman, Cecil. 1984. Culture, Health and Illness. Bristol, UK: Wright—PSG Publishing Company.

Herzlich, Claudine. 1973. Health and Illness: A Socio-Psychological Approach. London: Academic Press.

Hymes, Dell. 1977. Discovering Oral Performance and Measured Verse in American Indian Narrative. New Literary History 8: 431–57.

Kemnitzer, Luis S. 1976. Structure, Content, and Cultural Meaning of Yuwipi: A Modern Lakota Healing Ritual. American Ethnologist 3: 261–80.

Kleinman, Arthur. 1980. Patients and Healers in the Context of Culture. Berkeley, CA: University of California Press.

_____1988. The Illness Narratives: Suffering, Healing, and the Human Condition. NY: Basic Books, Inc.

Lame Deer and R. Erdoes. 1972. Lame Deer, Seeker of Visions. NY: Simon and Schuster.

Lang, Gretchen Chesley. 1985. Diabetics and Health Care in a Sioux Community. Human Organization 44: 251–60.

_____1987. Testimony as Expert Witness. Select Committee on Hunger, U. S. House of Representatives. 1987. Hunger and Nutrition Problems among American Indians: A Case Study of North Dakota. Hearings, New Town, ND, July 10, 1987. Serial No. 100-11. U.S. Gov. Printing Office, Washington, D.C. pp. 26–29, 62–84.

_____1989. 'Making Sense' About Diabetes: Dakota Narratives of Illness. Medical Anthropology 11: 305–27.

Mattingly, Cheryl and Linda C. Garro, Eds. 2000. Narrative and the Cultural Construction of Illness and Healing. Berkeley, CA: University of California Press.

Powers, Marla. 1986. *Oglala Women in Myth, Ritual and Reality.* Chicago, IL: University of Chicago Press.

Powers, William. 1982. Yuwipi: Vision and Experience in Oglala Ritual. Lincoln, NE: University of Nebraska Press.

Silko, Leslie Marmon. 1977. *Ceremony.* New York: Viking Penguin Books.

Strathern, Marilyn. 1987. Out of Context: The Persuasive Fictions of Anthropology. Current Anthropology 28: 251–81.

Taussig, Michael T. 1980. Reification and the Consciousness of the Patient. Social Science and Medicine B14: 3–13.

Tedlock, Dennis. 1983. Ethnography as Interaction: The Storyteller, the Audience, the Fieldworker, and the Machine. *In* The Spoken Word and the Work of Interpretation. Dennis Tedlock, ed. pp. 285–301. Philadelphia, PA: University of Pennsylvania Press.

Tedlock, Dennis. 1977. Toward an Oral Poetics. New Literary History 8: 507–19.

Walker, J.R. 1980. Lakota Belief and Ritual. Raymond. J. DeMaille and Elaine A. Jahner, eds. Lincoln, NE: University of Nebraska Press.

Wellin, Edward. 1977. Theoretical Orientations in Medical Anthropology: Continuity and Change Over the Past Half-Century. *In* Culture, Disease and Healing: Studies in Medical Anthropology. David Landy, ed. pp. 47–58. NY: Macmillan Publ. Co., New York.

Williams, Gareth. 1984. The Genesis of Chronic Illness: Narrative Reconstruction. Society, Health, and Illness 6: 175–200.

_____2000. Knowledgeable Narratives. Anthropology and Medicine 7: 135–40.

_____2004. Narratives of Health Inequality: Interpreting the Determinants of Health. Paper presented at the Annual Meetings of Sociology, San Francisco, CA. 2004.

Williams, Gareth and Wood, P. 1986. Common-Sense Beliefs about Illness: A Mediating Role for the Doctor. The Lancet, Dec. 20/27, 1986: 1435–37.

Young, Allen. 1982. The Anthropologies of Illness and Sickness. Annual Review of Anthropology. Bernard Siegel, ed. Palo Alto, CA: Annual Editions 11: 257–85.

CHAPTER 3

SLIPPING THROUGH SKY HOLES: YUROK BODY IMAGERY IN NORTHERN CALIFORNIA

Mariana Leal Ferreira

At Sherman, they'd line us girls up to check our [menstrual] pads. They wanted to know exactly when we had our periods, so they could control us and know if we were seeing any boys. Not that we were allowed to see them, but it was just like…humiliating. They'd check your pads once a month, and then check again to see if you had scrubbed them good, too. Them pads had to be white as snow, white, white. So now you go to the clinic, You get in line. They prick your finger and test your blood. You get a number and that number tells on you. If you haven't been eating good, I mean, a lot of fat, sugar, junk food, you know, the doctors can tell. If you haven't been exercising too much, watching a lot of TV, just sitting around, they know, too, because your blood sugar goes up. So your blood tells on you. Don't you see? It's the same thing!

> Sarah Horn, 85 years old, on the Yurok Indian Reservation in California, in 1994. She spent three years at the Sherman Institute Boarding School in southern California, in the 1910s. (In Ferreira 1996: 252)

Summary of Chapter 3. Yurok perceptions of the body as a surface where social and environmental change can be inscribed, are explored in this paper. To the violence and brutality of Spanish conquistadors, fur traders, gold miners, American soldiers, and Indian policies of the United States government since the eighteenth century, Yurok women attribute the high incidence of degenerative diseases, such as diabetes and cancer, drug abuse and criminality in northern California. This chapter contemplates the lives of eight generations of sixteen Yurok extended families, mapping inter-generational changes in social relations and political practices starting in the 1850s with the discovery of gold in California. The life trajectories and experiences of Yurok men, women and children in mining and logging camps, boarding schools, fish canneries, prisons, and ultimately reservations and rancherias delineate intricate connections between the classification of diseases and American family values; between the distribution of land and the transformation of "Indian" soul and conduct; between the circulation of commodities (alcohol, bullets, clothing, food and women) and the notion of civilization; and between military genocidal practices and a particular knowledge of the human body. Here, we shall see how the destruction of traditional healing and medicinal foundations of the Yurok and other Indigenous Peoples in California gave rise to fear, despair and hopelessness. Alternatively, the current operation of United Indian Health Services in northern California by the Yurok, Tolowa and Wiyot nations is regarded as a powerful way of exercising tribal sovereignty and strengthening solidarity ties among local Indigenous medical systems.

ò€ ò€ ò€

Introduction

Because there's no hard evidence on the relation between pesticide spraying and cancer, they'll just allow the spraying to go on…So now they've created cancer country up here, yes! That's how people refer to us: 'You live in cancer country'! Trees grow crooked in my backyard, ducks with their feathers growing inside out…large, huge chicken eggs being laid. My husband's got ear cancer, the neighbor dies of blood cancer, Mollie's daughter of ovarian cancer at 21. Is it in our genes?…We are mutants all right. And then we're made into interesting research objects, I guess we're really interesting…So they'll let this lawless country go on. You know, there's this saying up here that goes: 'There's no law above the Klamath.' (D.H. on the Yurok Indian Reservation, northern California, Oct. 1995)[1]

Human relationships are at the core of Yurok women's contemporary perceptions of the body. Their self-understanding—the knowledge of the sort of persons they are—and especially the ways in which they understand some of the meanings and causes of illnesses, are revealed through social relationships taking place among Yurok women and their close kin, and among Yuroks and government officials, foreign navigators, medical practitioners, and the non-Indian population at large in northern California. Connections Yurok women have made among seemingly unconnected life events, histories, practices, ideas, physical ailments and emotions add another dimension to kinship studies in anthropology, to the study of human genetics and ultimately, to socio-political understandings of the human body. The sixteen Yurok genealogies traced for a study on the politics of health among the Yuroks in northern California (Ferreira 1996, 1999), and which I here present sections of, delineate intricate connections between the classification of diseases and American family values, between the distribution of land and the transformation of "Indian" soul and conduct, between the circulation of commodi-

---

1. The present chapter is a slightly edited rendering of its original version, published in *Culture Medicine and Psychiatry* [Harvard School of Social Medicine] 22: 171–202, 1998. A Portuguese version appeared in *Revista de Antropologia* [University of São Paulo] 41(2): 54–98, 1999. Ethnographic fieldwork was conducted in northern California between 1994 and 1996 in the Humboldt and Del Norte Counties at United Indian Health Services in Trinidad and its satellite clinics, and on the Yurok Indian Reservation. The research and its publications were approved by United Indian Health Services, tribally owned and operated by the Yurok, Tolowa and Wiyot Indigenous Peoples. The Committee for Protection of Human Subjects, at the University of California, Berkeley campus, authorized the research process (protocols # 94-6-21 and # 95-6-81).

ties (alcohol, bullets, clothing, food and women) and the notion of civilization, and between military genocidal practices and a particular knowledge of the human body.

Here, the body is taken "as simultaneously a physical and symbolic artifact, as both naturally and culturally produced, and as securely anchored in a particular historical moment" (Scheper-Hughes and Lock 1987: 7). My main concern is the relationship between history and the body or, in other words, the relations among the individual, social, and political dimensions of the Yurok body. Yurok interpretations of health and sickness, which vary considerably, are at the level of the lived experience of the Yurok body-self, that is, the individual body. The social body encompasses the ways in which Yurok men and women use the body as a symbol to construct a particular world view and think of themselves and other beings within it. The political dimension of the body—the body politic—refers to the ways in which Yurok individuals have been disciplined, regulated and controlled within different institutions: boarding schools, local jails, high-tech prisons, and health clinics. While the "three bodies" represent three separate and overlapping units of analysis, Yuroks have emphasized the body politic in different aspects of the life histories they chose to tell me. Their emphasis on the body politic has illuminated why and how certain kinds of ailments, such as diabetes and alcoholism, have emerged.

In this piece, history also assumes a broader conceptualization than the one which treats the event as a material or physical process. In a comprehensive view of history, events and meanings coincide; they take place on the surface of bodies as well as on the surface of words (Foucault 1977: 175–76; Sahlins 1985: 154–56). Events can be corporeal, manifested as sicknesses, for instance, or else non-corporeal, located in sentiments that spring from relationships, or in ideas and thoughts that take place in discourse. Within this conception of history, the body emerges as "the inscribed surface of events...Genealogy, as an analysis of descent, is thus situated within the articulation of the body and history" (Foucault 1977: 148).

This historico-critical investigation is, as the philosopher Michel Foucault has defined it, "genealogical in its design and archaeological in its method" (1984: 46). Archaeological because it treats what Yurok women and men have said to me, that is, instances of their discourse that articulate what they think, say and do as so many historical events. Genealogical because, in contrast to approaches that deduce from what the Yuroks were who they now are, I focus on their present as a product of what they are doing, thinking and saying *now*. This study of descent, represented graphically in the form of genealogies, values conscious, empirical knowledge, derived from the everyday lives and mundane sentiments of human beings. I have tried to stress the importance of particular, affective and domestic aspects of Yurok social life.

Mapping Lines of Life: Early Studies

Ideas of descent and heredity have flourished within anthropology and biology since the mid 1800s. Until then, ethnological time—an idea put forth by the lawyer and anthropologist Lewis Henry Morgan, the "inventor" of kinship—had been confined within the traditional, Bible-based chronology of history since the flood. The Darwinian revolution, the discovery of fossil man and the works of Morgan himself on the human

mind spurred research on cultural and biological forms of evolutionism, often correlating the two. Lewis Henry Morgan's zoology and ethnology, for instance, placed the
American beaver at the bottom of the evolutionary scale, the complex kinship system of
the Iroquois guaranteed the nation's placement in the middle of the scale, while Europeans or Euro-Americans stood at the top, as the standard of civilization. Animal
metaphors were used to register the white's extreme distance or difference from Indigenous Peoples. The "conjugal life" of the Yuroks "is very chaste," wrote gold miner Carl
Meyer in 1851, upon visiting the Tsurai village in Trinidad Bay, northern California. "As
in the case of all other wild creatures, they mate only in spring" (Vaaren 1855, in Heizer
and Mills 1991: 128). "It is remarkable that…one of the lowest tribes on Earth…has a
widespread tradition of its derivation from animals," reported Charles Brace, after noting that skulls of California Indians had an enlarged cerebellum "making the animal organs prominent" (Brace 1869, in Rawls 1986: 200). Evolutionist ideology was used to
justify industrial society as against traditional society. It gave meaning to the word *primitive* and salved the conscience of colonialists (Canguilhem 1988: 37).

In *League of the Iroquois* (1851), *The American Beaver and his Works* (1868), *Systems
of Consanguinity and Affinity of the Human Family* (1871) and *Ancient Society* (1877),
Morgan developed his ideas on family, family relationships, modes of descent and rules
of marriage. Over a network of biological ties, Morgan interpreted the complexity of
the Iroquois social organization. "The Iroquois mode of computing degrees of consanguinity was unlike that of the civil or canon law; but was yet a clear and definite
system" (1962[1851]: 85).

Tables of systems of consanguinity and affinity, later called genealogical charts (from
the Greek *genea* race, family), have since become an instrument for anthropology. In
fact, the possibility of submitting kinship systems or simply "marriage laws" to math-
ematical analyses helped "reduce contemporary societies to those cases favourable to
the inquiry" (Lévi-Strauss (1969[1949]): xxxv), elevating the status of the discipline to
that of science. A relationship is established between the biological system of relations
(the biological father or mother, for example), and the social or cultural aspects of kin
relations—the fact the Yuroks call their biological aunts "mother," for instance (Kroeber 1917, 1934). Morgan's genealogies also showed—and this was crucial at that
time—the genetic connection of all peoples to one another in opposition to poly-
genism or the separate creation of the races. His writings launched an ethnological career best represented in the works of anthropologists Radcliffe-Brown (1924), Evans-
Pritchard (1940), and Lévi-Strauss (1969), among many others.

The birth of the field of genetics also dates back to the 1850s and 60s with the works
of the Augustinian monk Gregor Mendel on pea plants. But it was only in the early
1900s, with the gene theory in 1911 and developments in the fields of agriculture and
eugenics, that genetics gained importance as a discipline of its own. Human genetics
has, especially after the 1980s, produced information on genes that individuals share
with ancestors, siblings, and children, diagnosing genetic disorders that run through
certain families. Pedigrees map the lines of an individual's ancestors, calculating his or
her risk of being a carrier for a defective gene. Individuals whose mother or father are
affected with Huntington disease (HD), for example, have a 50 per cent chance of carrying the gene and, therefore, of developing the disorder at some point in their lives.
An estimated 125,000 people are at risk for HD in the United States (Quaid 1994: 4).

Defects in the BRCA1—the "breast cancer gene" —-are responsible for half of the inherited cases of breast and ovarian cancer (Chang 1995). Genetic diseases have become a family affair, "with all the attendant problems of family interactions" (Quaid 1994: 6). In a recent survey conducted by the Alzheimer's Association, which involved 146 people in New York City with at least one close relative affected with the disorder or who died of it, 81 said they wanted the test because they wanted to "make plans for the future" (Gilbert 1995).

At the time of this writing, research on the contribution of genes to aggressive and criminal conduct, rapidly extrapolating from rodents to colored people, especially the mentally ill and imprisoned populations, was being debated by socio-biologists at the Conference on Genetics and Crime, held in San Francisco, California, in 1995 (Angier 1995). Claiming that certain "races" are more vulnerable to both biological diseases (diabetes, cancer) and social ailments (alcoholism, violence), socio-biologists have helped attribute putative genetic markers to African-Americans and "Indians." This is the case of the "thrifty gene theory," to which I now turn.

The New Genetics and Indigenous Peoples

The analysis of Indigenous Peoples' "pedigrees," traced from information gathered in California Indian Rolls, the Indian Health Services (IHS) database system and hospital records, indicate, according to various studies, that diabetes is directly related to Indian heritage because of the thrifty genotype Indigenous Peoples in North America carry (Knowler et al. 1993, Bogardus 1993). The thrifty gene theory contends that a thrifty gene, which protected the body against starvation in times of great seasonal fluctuation, has now become maladaptive; that is, the ability to store fat has become a disadvantage with modern patterns of food consumption, leading to diabetes (Neel 1962, 1982). The recent discovery of a mutation in a gene involved in the body's response to insulin, enhancing the accumulation of abdominal fat and therefore speeding the adult-onset of diabetes, has "confirmed" the thrifty gene theory (San Francisco Chronicle 1995). In a similar vein, the "firewater theory" claims that "Indians" cannot hold their liquor and are uniquely vulnerable to alcohol abuse. Ninety-four percent of Navajo adults agreed that Indians have a problem with alcohol, and 63% went on to say that "Indians have a 'physical weakness to alcohol that non-Indians do not'" (Bernstein 1989: 328, in Sigelman et al. 1992: 266).

Based on these so-called genetic theories, Yurok individuals diagnosed as "diabetic," for example, or else who are "at risk" for the disorder because family members are affected or have died of it, decide which risks to take and which to ignore. As will be seen ahead, while local physicians complain of "non-compliance," some Yuroks reason that if diabetes is "in their blood, there's nothing that can be done about it." Such theories thus acquire facticity, that is, they turn into facts, shaping the self-knowledge of patients, clinicians and researchers. The genealogies traced for this study reveal that Yuroks do recognize diabetes, alcoholism and drug addiction as potential dangers that they should guard themselves against. However, their narratives consider the social aspects of risk, revealing, among other things, connections between perceived risk and moral blame, and between Yurok body imagery and changing historical conditions.

The psychological impact of the diabetes epidemic on Indigenous communities is tremendous. The apparently simple and innocuous statement that "Indian heritage" is a risk factor for diabetes is emotionally charged because it touches deeply upon issues of self-knowledge, body-imagery and social identity. As a Yurok outreach worker at United Indian Health Services in California recently put it, "To say I am Native American means I am or will be diabetic." A recent statistical analysis of the Yurok database (see Chapter 18 in this volume), however, reveals that there is a weak, negative correlation (-.223) between diabetes and quantum of Indian blood. This finding demonstrates, among other things, that the concept of "Indian heritage" cannot be used as a general risk factor for Indigenous Peoples. Yurok tribal leaders in northern California feel that blaming "Indian blood" is a pretext for discrimination, because the whole notion of "Indian heritage" is not explicitly defined. They repudiate this novel and genetically based form of colonial control, which mimics the tight scrutiny carried out in boarding schools, reservations, high-tech prisons and mental homes they were, and still have been, confined to.

In fact, few medical studies actually correlate individual genetic admixture with the occurrence of diabetes, when stating that Indian blood quantum structures risk for diabetes. Most studies take "Indian heritage" for granted, and use it as a major variable to establish genetic causative links for the diabetes epidemic. The problem here is, of course, one of social identity, because it is closely related to the question "Who is an Indian"?—which appears as the most frequently asked question in the Bureau of Indian Affairs' website. While there are nations, such as the Pima of the Gila River Indian Community, which require a minimum of 25% (one quarter) "Indian blood" for tribal membership, in other groups, such as the Cherokee Tribe of Oklahoma, there are members who are 1/2048 Cherokee because ancestry can be traced back to Indian rolls of the 1800s. Genetically speaking, "Indian heritage" has different meanings for enrolled members of the Pima and Cherokee tribes.

It should also be noted that while genetic testing for other degenerative ailments that are most prevalent among Caucasian populations, such as Alzheimer and Huntington Disease (HD), are carefully divulged, the medical community has no reservations about advertising "Indian heritage", however loosely defined, as a risk factor for diabetes. There is concern that genetic testing, in the case of Alzheimer and HD, can produce "genetic social outcastes" because issues involving health insurance, life insurance policies, employee discrimination and negative social stigma are at stake. No such concern is addressed regarding the disclosure of information regarding a putative "flawed" genotype of American Indians, as well as Indigenous Peoples worldwide, who hold the highest rates of type 2 diabetes globally.

The ways in which Yurok women and men, who I worked closely with during the course of my doctoral research in Northern California between 1994 and 1996, mapped their lines of life, transcend common associations made between "Indian heritage" and diabetes, alcoholism, obesity, and sedentary lifestyle. The "Strong Heart Study" (Howard et al. 1992; Lee et al. 1995), for example, "the first study of CVD [cardiovascular disease] and its risk factors, including diabetes, in American Indians using a standardized protocol in several geographic areas" associates "diabetes with… age, obesity, family history of diabetes, and amount of Indian ancestry" (Lee et al. 1995: 599). Such studies strip diabetes, its risk factors and other aliments of their social contexts, denying the human relations embodied in symptoms, signs and ther-

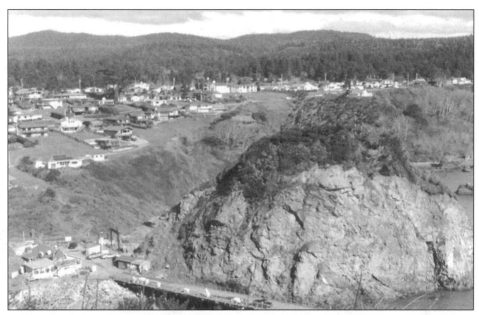

The Trinidad Bay in northern California. Note the Trinidad Head in the foreground and city of Trinidad in the background, which replaced the Yurok Village of Tsurai, where the Spaniards first arrived in 1775. (Photo: Mariana L. Ferreira, 2000)

apy. By doing so, "we not only mystify [human relations] but we also reproduce a political ideology in the guise of a science of (apparently) 'real things'—biological and physical thinghood" (Taussig 1992: 84). In other words, we purposely ignore the evidence that poverty, scarcity, violence, relocation and confinement are largely responsible for the epidemics of both infecto-contagious and degenerative illnesses that have decimated Indigenous Peoples in California and all over the world largely speaking. In doing so, we comfortably seclude ourselves in a medicalized—and highly profitable!—world of individual treatments, thus secluding social suffering from the potentially disruptive political arena.

Yurok men and women, of varying ages and professions, have correlated the manifestation of signs and symptoms of several illnesses, including diabetes mellitus type 2, alongside individuals' outstanding achievements and changes in occupations, marriage arrangements, economic situation and causes of death. The Yurok people whose pseudonyms appear in this chapter have constructed these genealogies through a filter of the mostly pathological in an attempt to point to the different contexts where "disease" originates. Their life histories speak of misfortunes, traumatic events, violence and despair. Diabetes, hypertension, depression, drug addiction and domestic violence appear side by side with confinement in boarding schools, state prisons, metal homes and foster homes, war experiences, and so forth. The genealogical charts thus correlate, in a summarized way, these traumatic experiences within Yurok extended families.[2]

2. The 1852 census made available by Kroeber (1974 [1925]: 16) identified Yurok "houses" and "villages". The term "house" referred to the physical building, the redwood plank house, while "village" was defined as a "cluster of houses." Waterman (1993 [1920]) and Kroeber (1974) wrote of

Sarah Tsurai, Mary Wo'tek and Julia Stowen are the three Yurok women whose life histories appear in this piece. They have traced the genealogies of their extended families back to the mid-1800s, when gold was first discovered in northern California. Gold miners and other immigrants then poured into the area, pushing the Yuroks and other populations inland, while exterminating several others (Rawls 1986). Aside from memory itself, the Yuroks also relied on government censuses elaborated in this period—the first census was compiled in 1852 (Kroeber 1976 [1952]: 16)—and other documents—California Indian Rolls, court cases and land allotment papers. I myself obtained some information, mostly birth and death dates of the late 1800s and 1900s, at the National Archives in San Bruno, California, where I had access to Health and Sanitary Records of the United States Indian Service, and school records of the Hoopa Valley Agency. The Hoopa Valley Agency was the subdivision of the United States Indian Service that was responsible for the Yuroks, Karuks, and Hupas confined inside the Hoopa Valley Reservation in Northern California in the late 1800s and early 1900s.

The Sick, the Insane and the Criminal: Embodying Human Relations in Disease

Sarah Tsurai's, Mary Wo'tek's and Julia Stowen's parents, grandparents and great-grandparents were treated for a variety of ailments by physicians in charge of the Hoopa Valley Agency. The names of these women's ancestors can be found in "Quarterly Sanitary Report of Diseases and Injuries" of the United States Indian Service, Hoopa Valley Agency, for the period 1886–1912, listed under various disease categories, such as tuberculosis, whooping cough, superfluous hair, freckles, syphilis, gonorrhea and seminal emissions. The "Special Notice" of the September 30, 1904 edition offered a "One dose at bedtime" of the compound "anaphrodisiac in Gonorrhea" was used to "repress the sexual instinct" of the Indians in order to combat the outbreak of venereal diseases in 1893 (Ferreira 1996: 254).

Anaphrodisiac in Gonorrhea

"Ext. ergotae fluidi…m. xv 1; Tinct. Gelsemii…m. v; Potassi bromidi…gr. xx 1; Tinct. Hyoscyami…m. xxx2; Syrupi aurantii, q. s. ad…3ss 16. Sig. Shake. One Dose at bedtime".

Source: "Quarterly Sanitary Report of Diseases and Injuries" of the United States Indian Service, Hoopa Valley Agency, for the period 1886–1912.

"house" as a descent group. By 1925 Kroeber (1974: 19) was already using the term "family" to designate individuals who lived in the same "household": "It was customary, by this time [1895], for a family to have two or three houses." Yuroks who have participated in this study referred to individuals as "family" members when these individuals belonged to the maternal, paternal, and sometimes both descent groups.

The same "Special Notice" of 1904 also included instructions on how to make Indians adopt "rational medical methods" and "elementary principles of physiology and hygiene":

In connection with the sanitary report, AT THE END OF EACH QUARTER, the physician must note the progress the Indians are making in abandoning medicine men and adopting rational medical methods, the proportional number of Indians who seek his service and those whom he seeks for treatment, what proportion he visits at their homes, and what proportion come to his office or dispensary…He will also endeavor to improve sanitary and hygienic condition generally and instruct the Indians how to do so. He should do his best, with tact and firmness, to induce the Indians to discard the practices of their native medicine men and to substitute civilized treatment for superstitions and barbarous rites and customs…In addition to his professional duties a school physician shall give the pupils at Government boarding schools appropriate talks, at least as often as once a week, on the elementary principles of physiology and hygiene, explaining particularly the necessity for proper habits in eating and drinking, cleanliness, ventilation, and other hygienic conditions.

Source: "Quarterly Sanitary Report of Diseases and Injuries" of the United States Indian Service, Hoopa Valley Agency, 1904.

The way in which these sanitary reports were organized and the ways in which Indigenous patients were classified inform how the medical discourse about individuals has been structured since the eighteenth century, with the emergence of the field of pathological anatomy and the advent of the clinical experience. Much like their ancestors, Sarah Tsurai, Mary Wo'tek and Julia Stowen have also been diagnosed for several ailments, including diabetes, obesity, depression and alcoholism. Their names can be found in various diabetes registries, including the 1996 diabetes registry of 215 patients at United Indian Health Services (UIHS), a tribally owned and operated set of health clinics operating under Congressional Act 638, which provides primary health care for the American Indian population in Northern California. The Potawot Health Village, inaugurated in 2001 in the Humboldt Bay Area is the main site and there are another nine satellite clinics in Humboldt and Del Norte Counties that assist approximately 13,000 local American Indians (see Chapter 18 in this volume on Cultural Rebuilding).

The diagnoses made at UIHS and at other health facilities in Northern California usually follow the medical tradition of the eighteenth century, that is, the disease is observed in terms of symptoms and signs. " The symptom—hence its uniquely privileged position—is the form in which the disease is presented" of all that is visible, it is closest to the essential.…The symptoms allow the invariable form of the disease—set back somewhat, visible and invisible—to show through" (Foucault 1975: 90). Transformed into diagnostic criteria—fasting plasma glucose and oral glucose tolerance test results, for example—the signs and symptoms of diabetes, among other ailments, say nothing about the world in which the Yuroks live and help create at the same time.

The system of correspondences or "network of analogies" (Foucault 1970: xi) Yurok individuals have recreated—diseases/family values::land/Indian soul and conduct::commodities/civilization::genocide/human body—reveal much more about diabetes and its related illnesses. That is, the critical correlations Yurok individuals have created when

talking about their lives and identities transcend the traditional proximities (the most obvious connections) between signs, symptoms and therapy of biomedical disease categories. Rather than relate the disorder exclusively to diet, exercise and "Indian heritage,"
Yurok women transform diabetes into a much more encompassing ailment category, incorporating emotional experience, mostly trauma, as its social cause (see also Ferreira
2003 and in this volume). Their narratives shed light on the role of social, political and
economic factors that link together depression, substance abuse, violence, diabetes, and
other disorders that are common to Indigenous Peoples. High unemployment and ar-
rests rates, extensive use of boarding schools, lower educational levels, malnutrition, and
migration from reservation to cities, for instance, have increasingly been identified as
"stressor" or "risk factors" for co-morbid disorders (Westermeyer et al. 1993; Brown et
al. 1993).

A number of studies on the manifestations of psychiatric disorders among Indigenous Peoples has looked into the correlation between mental health and social,
political and contextual factors, including racial discrimination. High rates of foster
placement and adoption, less access to medical treatment, lower education levels,
high unemployment, as well as a high number of potentially addicting sedative drugs
(prescribed in some Indian Heath Service settings), are possible sources for a "different distribution of psychiatric disorders" among Indigenous Peoples (Westermeyer
et al. 1993: 519–20; see also in this volume chapters by Bruyère, Joe & Frishkopf,
Macaulay et al., Roy, and Scheder). Other studies have linked poor living conditions
in childhood to cancer and heart disease (Michalek and Mahoney 1994; Fennerty et
al. 1992), as well as stressful life situations to the concentration of blood glucose in
individuals with diabetes(see chapters by Bruyère, Scheder, and Ferreira in this volume). In fact, most scholars in this volume use diabetes mellitus as a model in examining links between social inequality and health outcome, rather than view it as a
disease in itself.

How to Read the Genealogical Charts

When looking at the genealogies presented ahead, the reader should first look for the
protagonist of each narrative—Sarah Tsurai, Mary Wo'tek or Julia Stowen—identified
by an arrow ↘. Each one of these women is our point of reference, from which the narrative unfolds. The symbol for women is a circle ○, while men are designated by a square
❑. Relationships are represented as follows:

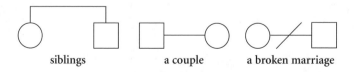

A couple with three kids (two girls and one deceased boy) is thus:

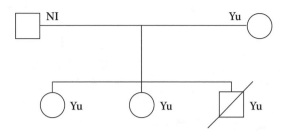

Each generation covers approximately 20 years. The original diagrams (Ferreira 1996) include approximately 1700 individuals, most of whom are Yuroks, but a small number of whom are Karuks (KA), Hupas (HU), Tolowas (TO), Wiyots (WI), Sioux (SI) and non-Indians (NI). Tribal affiliation, as shown above, is abbreviated outside each ❑ or ◯; if unknown, the information is not given. In the example above, a Yurok woman married a non-Indian, a very common occurrence after the gold rush and the American invasion of California. Their three children "claimed their Yurok blood" and are, therefore, members of the Yurok Tribe (YU; individuals must have at least 1/8 Yurok blood in order to be eligible for enrollment in the Yurok Tribe). Immediately below each man or woman comes his or her date of birth and death, if known, main occupation and other pieces of information the protagonist of that particular family history considered relevant to display. Causes of death are preceded by a "+", as in "+ car accident".

Within each ❑ or ◯, there are markers for ailments that are associated with changing life conditions and Yurok body imagery. These ailments are designated as:

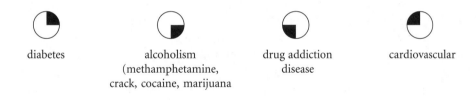

| diabetes | alcoholism (methamphetamine, crack, cocaine, marijuana | drug addiction disease | cardiovascular |

These markers can be associated, as in:

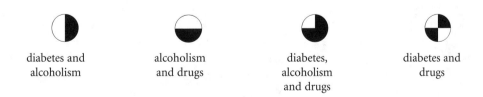

| diabetes and alcoholism | alcoholism and drugs | diabetes, alcoholism and drugs | diabetes and drugs |

Sarah Tsurai

Let us consider how Sarah Tsurai brought together physical manifestations of illness and their social contexts. Born in 1932, Sarah married a non-Indian, who worked as a

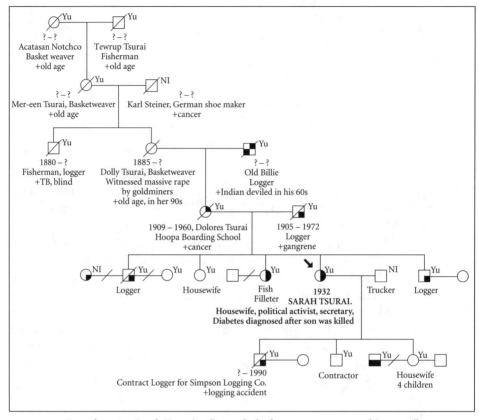

Genealogy 1   Sarah Tsurai—"A symbol of status to marry a white man."

trucker, with whom she had three children, two boys and a girl. In her early 40s, after divorcing her husband, the woman began working as a secretary and became deeply involved in political activities in northern California. Her name can be found in several court cases involving Yurok Indians and the United States government, and today she is a member of several Indigenous rights organizations and Indigenous health committees. Sarah and I met once or twice a month between 1994 and 1996 at her home in northern California, at social events sponsored by the Yurok Tribe and at the United Indian Health Services Tsurai clinic in Trinidad, where she sought treatment for diabetes.

   Sarah Tsurai spoke to me at length on many different occasions, between August 1994 and November 1996, about changes brought about by marriage arrangements between Yurok women and non-Indian men. Going through a picture album that portrayed Yurok coastal villages in the 1910s, 20s and 30s, Sarah traced the descent in her family through the maternal line, starting with her great-great-grandparents, Acatasan Notchko and Tewrup Tsurai, who were born in the 1840s or 50s. (The couple is at the top of the page on Genealogy 1.) At that time, most Yurok women, like Acatasan, married into their husbands' households, and children inherited names and goods mostly from their paternal relatives (Waterman and Kroeber 1934). However, fur-trading in the late eighteenth century, and especially gold mining and the invasion of American soldiers in the mid nineteenth, brought thousands of immigrants to northern California. Yurok country—located on the Pacific Coast north of Humboldt Bay and spread inland along the Klamath River—swarmed with English, Irish, Portuguese, Swedish, German and Spanish men, among other nationalities, who "jumped ship" in San Francisco, or else that came from the eastern coast in search of riches. One of these men was Karl Steinen, a German shoemaker who paid Tewrup Tsurai the sum of sixty dollars for the hand of Mer-een Tsurai, Sarah's maternal great-grandmother.[3] According to Sarah Tsurai,

> Marrying white men had a lot of implications. See, my [great-]grandfather was white, and he didn't want my father to learn to be an Indian. So he didn't want him to learn the [Yurok] language, didn't want him to sing or dance…Most white men didn't want their Indian wives to act Indian either. They punished them if they did. Since the women couldn't really be white the whole way, men would abandon them for some white lady who they'd run off with…they wanted to have sex all the time. That means kids and more kids to come; it got out of control. The whites observed no taboos, neither did they respect our moon time. The 111 tattoos, too, on the women's chins were considered ugly, so we stopped doing that. Only very few women still carry that around. Did you read *The Four Ages of Tsurai*?[4] There's a great passage about our 'pretensions to beauty.' Those who didn't turn into real nice white ladies were abandoned, left alone with all these kids to raise on their own.…That's why you have so many grandparents adopting their grandkids. The mother had to leave the house to work and her parents had to raise her kids. And sometimes the grandmother herself was a single mother, making things even more difficult.…But it was a symbol of status to marry a white man, and you wanted to be respected, anyway.

Foreigners moved into Yurok households because they had no homes in the area to which to take their Yurok wives. More than half (67%) of the non-Indian husbands abandoned their Yurok wives, seeking non-Indian wives in San Francisco or else sending for their fiancées overseas. Yurok women were left with the responsibil-

---

3. Of the 108 marriages that took place between 1850 and 1889 and were recalled members of the 16 Yurok families here considered, 30 (27.7%) were between Yurok women and non-Indian men (Ferreira 1996: 83). In 1852, the Yurok population was estimated as 1052 individuals. Of the 16 families under consideration, only one did not arrange marriages with non-Indians until the 1970s. Within 15 families, the remaining marriages were between Yuroks (57%), between Yuroks and Tolowas (11%), Yuroks and Karuks (2%), and Yuroks and Hupas (2%). There were no recorded marriages between Yurok men and non-Indian women at the time.

4. On his visit to Trinidad Bay in May 1793, Captain George Vancouver wrote in his journal: "Amongst these people, as with the generality of Indians I had met, some mutilation, or disfiguring of their persons is practiced, either as being ornamental, or of religious institution, or possibly to answer some purpose of which we remain ignorant.…All the teeth of both sexes were, by some process, ground uniformly down, horizontally, to the gums; the women…ornamented their lower lip with three perpendicular columns of punctuation, one from each corner of the mouth, and one in the middle, occupying three fifths of the lip and chin. Had it not been for these frightful customs, I was informed that amongst those who visited our party on shore the last day, there were, amongst the younger females, some who might have been considered as having pretensions to beauty. The men had also some punctuations about them and scars on their arms and bodies…[so] our curiosity could only be indulged in those few respects that inspection gratified" (Heizer and Mills 1991: 67).

ity of raising a number of children that was unusually high for the average Yurok family—11, 12, or 13—against an average of 4 or 5 before 1850 (Ferreira 1996: 84). Yurok women became the heads of huge households and this shift in the form of residence—from patrilocal to matrilocal—brought many transformations to the lives of Yurok women, as well as to the lives of their close kin. The inheritance of family names and goods, especially houses and regalia, also changed its course. Most Yurok extended families or "houses" became matrilineal. Yurok men had either been killed in local conflicts with the newcomers or were themselves lured into the mining business and logging enterprise, which has predominated in the area well into the twentieth century.

Sarah Tsusai's maternal grandmother, Dolly Tsurai, was born in 1885. The elder, who had 12 children herself (only one daughter is shown in Genealogy 1), often reminded her kin of the acts of violence she had witnessed as a child:

> My grandmother would tell me of the horrors, of the time the white men first came. Nobody could sleep at night from the screaming that went on, night after night, the men raping our women and children. No one was spared. It was horrible. The women were so frightened that to avoid being raped again and again, they would stuff themselves with sand from the [Trinidad] beach. No one was spared, not even the little girls. My grandmother only escaped because she was small and was able to hide.

Like most of the Yurok children born in the first half of the twentieth century, Sarah Tsurai's mother, Dolores Tsurai, was confined in a governmental boarding school for eight years and later worked shifts of twelve to fourteen hours a day as a fish filleter in local salmon canneries. She was one of the first Yurok women of her generation to develop diabetes and cancer (as shown in the diagram). Sarah attributes the onset of her mother's and her own heightened blood sugars to their adverse life conditions and to traumas they both suffered witnessing premature death and disablement of their close kin in alcoholic brawls, logging disasters and car accidents:

> My diabetes acted up yesterday. Way up there in the 250s or something. Guess it was the bad news again. It's a hard thing when your mind is 20 and your body doesn't correspond. I feel so young and yet look at me. I'm overweight, my eyes are failing on me…That's when it all happened. An Indian doctor came when my son was killed. His spirit said: 'Mom, mourn me, I'll be OK.' I had a war dance to overcome my enemy, my bad feelings. I thought I was OK but my body let me know I wasn't. It started acting up on me. Feeling thirsty, sleepy, and craving for junk food, fat, sugar.…Sugar diabetes! Just like my mother, she couldn't take those memories either. Boarding Schools, you know what that's all about? Being kicked around like a dog, slapped across the face for saying one little word in Yurok, feeling guilty about the very color of your skin. We, the redskins! You feel like giving up. No wonder your blood sugars go way up there!…Just name the people around here whose kids have been killed, whose husbands abuse them, who have no hope left at all. You know who I'm talking about. Aren't they all on your list? Don't they all have diabetes? Aren't most of them blind or almost blind, sitting on a wheelchair,

with a foot or two missing, pricking their fingers all day long, trying to figure out which medicine they're suppose to take every two, three hours?

According to the American Diabetes Association (ADA 1996: 14), an individual is diagnosed as diabetic if the level of plasma glucose in the fasting state is equal to or about 6.9mM (125 mg/dl). ADA has also eliminated the terms insulin dependent diabetes mellitus (IDDM) and non-insulin dependent diabetes mellitus (NIDDM), retaining the terms Type 1 and Type 2 diabetes, respectively.

When I asked Sarah Tsurai how her ancestors dealt with misfortune, whether there was some social mechanism Yuroks resorted to when they faced traumatic and stressful events, memories and emotions, she replied:

> Long ago when people were in a situation like this, I mean, when things got out of control, you knew an Indian devil would take care of it. Like Grandpa Billie, Old Billie, he was Indian deviled. The Indian doctor said he was Indian deviled. See, when you go somewhere, you never accept anything to drink. And if you do, you're supposed to spit out the first sip. But he didn't.... He was in his 60s, and I guess he had a stroke or heart attack or something. That's what the doctors tell me today: 'There's no such thing as Indian devils!' But I think it's just a manner of how you look at things. Being Indian deviled is just like receiving a death sentence: 'You are doing to die.' And you do, because you believe in it. So now the death sentence is: 'You've got diabetes' or 'You've got cancer' or something like that. So if you accept the diagnosis, you're dead. I like to think I don't have diabetes. Doctors say they can prove it. When I think that way, I feel the sentence. I feel I'm being Indian deviled, too.

"Devils' were described to me an entities who possess the power to destroy or harm individuals whom they envy or hate. Indian devils manifest themselves in a variety of ways. They can take the form of animals, people, or objects. A Yurok man who would not accept a biomedical diagnosis of cancer and hypertension in 1995 told me that "once you and others around you believe that you have been deviled, that's it: your body acts up on you and before you realize it your dead" (Ferreira 1996: 95). Here, both witchcraft and biomedical diagnoses are metaphors for social relations. The psycho-physiological mechanisms underlying death by exorcism and the casting of spells have been the object of several studies since the early 1940s (Cannon 1942 in Lévi-Strauss 1963: 167).

> On every occasion and by every action, the social body suggests death to the unfortunate victim, who no longer hopes to escape what he considers to be his ineluctable fate....First brutally torn from all his family and social ties and excluded from all functions and activities through which he experienced self-awareness, then banished by the same forces from the world of the living, the victim yields to the combined effect of intense terror, the sudden withdrawal of the multiple reference systems provided by the support of the group, and, fi-

nally, to the group's decisive reversal in reclaiming him—once a living man, with rights and obligations—and an object of fear, ritual and taboo. Physical integrity cannot withstand the dissolution of the social personality (Lévi-Strauss 1963: 167–68).[5]

Medical practitioners at United Indian Health Services (all of whom were non-Indians in the 1990s) were initially taken back by the comparison Sarah and other Yuroks traced between clinicians and Indian devils, as well as by other issues I have raised, when the first version of this essay was presented to then in 1996. How could the Yuroks be talking about "Indian devils" and "bad blood" when the Diabetes Awareness Program at UIHS, a model for the state of California, was a collaborating site of the International Diabetes Center's Staged Diabetes Management Program? How could I be talking about diabetes without even mentioning laboratory measurements of glycosylated hemoglobin and microalbuminuria values of Yurok patients? Why was I questioning genetic theories if they have been "scientifically" proved? The "data" I worked with—life experiences, emotions and cultural "factors"—were too subjective and metaphysical to be translated into clinical practice, too problematic to be worth the time. I was adding too many pieces to a puzzle the medical team already know how to solve, "predicated on the assumption that the scientific community knows what the world is like" (Kuhn 1970: 5).

Sarah Tsurai's articulation of history and the body, the ways in which she places physical manifestations of illness in their social contexts, questions the epistemological tradition that separates mind from body, natural from supernatural, seen from unseen, spirit from matter and magical from rational. This epistemological tradition is a cultural and historical construction and not one that is universally shared. The system of relations the Yurok elder constructs by articulating aspects of the individual body, the social body and the body politic subverts existing paradigms about Indigenous health, suggesting new ways of ordering knowledge about diabetes and other illnesses.

Mary Wo'tek

Mary Wo'tek is a small frail woman who lives alone in a small motor home on the banks of the Klamath River on the Yurok Indian Reservation. When I first visited her, in the winter of 1995, Mary was curled up against the gas stove in a corner of the kitchen, "trying to warm up." Empty beer cans and wine bottles trashed the floor, as

---

5. Citing Cannon (1942), Lévi-Strauss (1963: 168) explains how the complex phenomena of exorcism and the casting of spells are expressed on the physiological level: "Cannon showed that fear, like rage, is associated with a particular intense activity of the sympathetic nervous system...if the individual cannot avail himself of any intensive or acquired response to an extraordinary situation (or to one which he conceives as such), the activity of the sympathetic nervous system becomes intensified and disorganized; it may, sometimes within a few hours, lead to a decrease in the volume of blood pressure, which result in irreparable damage to the circulatory organs....These hypotheses were confirmed by the study of several cases of trauma resulting from bombings, battle shock, and even surgical operations; death results, yet the autopsy reveals no lesions."

well as the small flat area outside where the motor home was parked. When I asked Mary how she was doing, she answered back: "Cold, cold, and very, very depressed."

The history of the Wo'tek household portrayed in Genealogy 2 resembles the trajectories of Yurok individuals traced in Genealogy 1. An Englishman, Brian Williams, became a part of the Wo'tek household when he married, in the late 1980s, Mary's grandmother, Ya-ter Wo'tek, a basket weaver born in 1886. Between 1902 and 1916 the Yurok-English couple had 11 children (only Mary's father, Old Mack, is shown in the diagram). Soon after, the Englishman "disappeared," that is, he moved to San Francisco where he opened an upholstery store and married an Irish lady. With the help of her parents, Ya-ter Wo'tek raised her 11 children. Mary's father, Old Mack, returned from World War II as an alcoholic. In 1975 he was murdered in an alcohol-related brawl. Mary Wo'tek introduced me to her ancestors in the following way:

> We're pretty ugly people, Indians are ugly people. You take Grandma Ya-ter, she was pretty lucky Grandpa Brian chose to marry her. She knew nothing about knitting or sewing, let alone acting like a decent white lady. She was pretty healthy I guess, but you think an Englishman is interested in that crap? Basket making, singing. I bet you he got tired of all that Indian stuff....He took off. I would, too. Now my Mom had a better start, she got to work as a maid in San Francisco. She learned to cook good, make fancy cakes and pies. And clean real good. Some whites would come over and say: 'Now that's a clean Indian family!' They'd even eat out of our plates! Now Dad was a drunken Indian all the way. Got back from the war on the bottle, never let it go. It's true what people say, Indians can't drink liquor. But he did and he got killed. Just like my husband, he had Indian blood, too. He was on the bottle forever....Come to think of it, all of us, my brother and sister and I, we all like the bottle a lot. Samuel plunged into the Klamath river. He never liked being an Indian, either. Both him and Maggie went to Carson Indian School in Oregon, but that didn't straighten them out at all. They never liked school. Samuel's been sober for almost a year....Now I don't know what it is with the young kids today. They're into sexing and drugging all the time. I don't know if it's about being Indian, you know. Jim's a jail bird, now he's in Pelican Bay. It was a hit and run type of thing, he killed some white girl on the road. He'll be in there for a while, you know, he's an Indian. Jackie was in and out of rehab until she passed out in '87. She didn't like me. My kids blamed me for being Indian and for marrying an Indian. But George didn't look like one, he was so handsome! I thought Rita was going to do better cause she married a Mexican. Turned out the guy was even worse than an Indian, he did all kids of drugs and abused his kids, too. Their kids? They're all into trouble big time. Only Nora's doing good. She doesn't look too dark, she's got pretty skin and nice looking feet. She's studying at College of the Redwoods. I hope she marries a nice, decent white man.

By the turn of the century, the widespread consumption of alcohol helped weaken Yurok social structure and deteriorate the relationship between Indigenous Peoples in California and the general non-Indigenous population. The genealogies show Yurok individuals born in the 1890s, as well as non-Indians, Karuks, Tolowas, Wiyots and other Northern California nations, already deeply troubled by alcoholism in the early

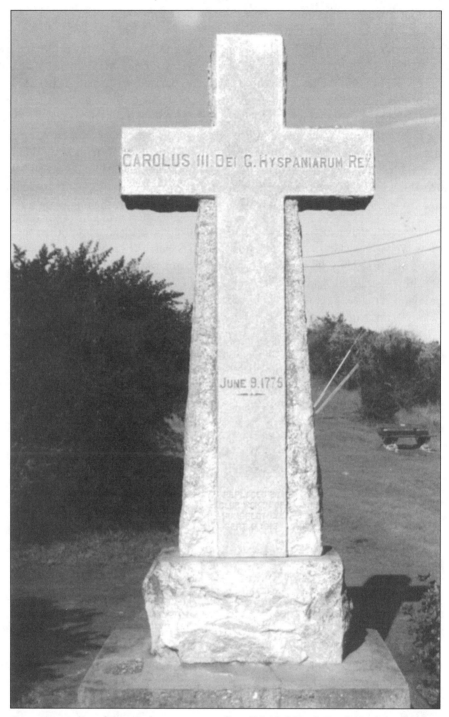

A concrete replica of the wooden cross, erected on Trinidad Head, Yurok Territory, by the Spaniards in 1775. (Photo: Mariana L. Ferreira, 1996)

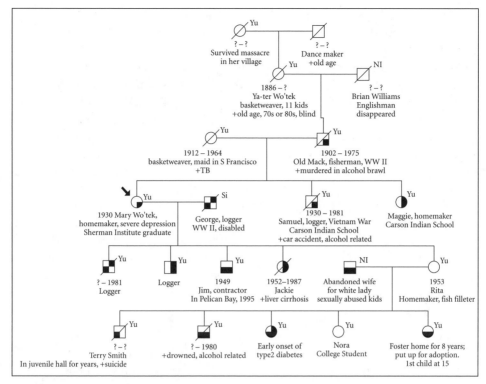

Genealogy 2 Mary Wo'tek—"Indians are ugly people."

1900s. Alcoholism was defined to me by a Yurok elder as "a drinking problem, when people drink heavy, on a dialy basis" (Ferreira 1996: 102). Other Yuroks, however, related "alcoholism" to individuals' behavior, rather than to the amount or frequency of alcohol consumed. In the genealogies, family members were identified as having a "drinking problem" if drinking interfered with their work and social relationships, or caused them to frequently engage in "brawls" or to withdraw from social gatherings and ceremonial dances. As of the 1960s and 70s, marijuana, crack, cocaine, and different kids of "speed' or methamphetamines (usually in this order of preference) have also been incorporated into the lives of most Yurok families I met.

What intrigued me the most about Mary Wo'tek, however, was her body imagery, that is, the self-knowledge she constructed about herself. Not only did she "enjoy" her boarding school experience, but she actually believes she and other "Indians" deserve the punishment and prejudice they have faced.

> I cried the first few nights and the Sherman Institute, but I soon got over it. I really loved the school. The matrons were very involved with the children, they really wanted to teach us good habits, how to be clean and neat, how to do all the house chores. It was so lovely! They made sure we knew that god is our father in heaven, that we understood what Jesus Christ our Lord did for us. And why the Holy Spirit is so important in our lives. We prayed when we got out of bed, we drilled before breakfast, we said 'grace' before we ate....I felt very lucky that people cared about me.

The picture of the "drunken Indian," as well as the "primitive," "oversexed," "lazy," and now "diabetic Indian," is a cultural and historical product, rather than a natural fact. Mary Wo'tek and other Yuroks confirm empirically the reality of this picture because of the place these perceptions occupy in their lives, by their experiences and convictions, and by the personal and collective investments that have been made in it. Backed up by genetic theories, these images become "facts" and shape individual's self-knowledge. When I presented a draft of my doctoral research on Yurok health to members of the Diabetes Awareness Program at United Indian Health Services in July 1995, I was told by a Yurok health professional that she had "found a better diagnosis for Indian people…post-traumatic stress disorder [PTSD] is, in my opinion, a diagnosis that fits most Indian people for everything we have gone through." I responded that a recent study shows that much like the figure of the "drunken Indian," the "generally accepted picture of PTSD, and the traumatic memory that underlies it, is mistaken. The disorder is not timeless, nor does it possess an intrinsic unity" (Young 1995: 5). When I argued that labeling Yuroks as suffering from PTSD would be yet another way of medicalizing community distress, Bea Nix, a member of the Diabetes Team at UIHS who introduced me to most of the Yurok individuals I met during the course of my research, said out loud:

> Medicalized or not medicalized, what's the point? I'd much rather be diagnosed, and I bet so would most of people around here, as having this post-traumatic stress disorder, than being blamed for what I eat, drink or do. You know how they blame us drunken Indians, whatever goes wrong they'll say 'Oh, it's just some drunken Indian!'. At least there's more dignity in a category like PTSD, because it doesn't blame our genes, our bad habits, or our lack of education (Ferreira 1996: 196).

I then realized how acts of violence and terrible personal losses that stand behind traumatic memories are trivialized by diagnostic categories such as PTSD and by genetic theories such as the thrifty gene. Furthermore, the reification of such disease categories goes as far as "insulat[ing] the community from those socially important problems that are not reducible to the puzzle form, because they cannot be stated in terms of the conceptual and instrumental tools" the diagnosis supplies (Kuhn 1970: 35). By assigning the source of disease exclusively to pathogenic or related factors, social distress "is secluded from the potentially disruptive political arena and secured within the safer medical world of individualized treatment" (Baer et al. 1986: 97).

The relationship Mary Wo'tek establishes between the individual and social body illuminates aspects of the Yurok body politic because it involves issues of power and control. If we divert our attention from the strictly repressive faces of power to its positive attributes, as the philosopher Michel Foucault has taught us to do, we learn that the regulation, surveillance and control of the Yurok body has singularized certain desires and pleasures. From within power relations that have scrutinized, classified, monitored, invaded and scandalized the Yurok body, the most repressive and deadly forms of pleasures and desires have been multiplied to include a "craze for junk food, alcohol, sex, drugs and violence, everything you wouldn't ever think of wanting so bad," as a 50-year old Yurok who lives in a trailer park on the outskirt of the Yurok Indian Reservation recently put it.

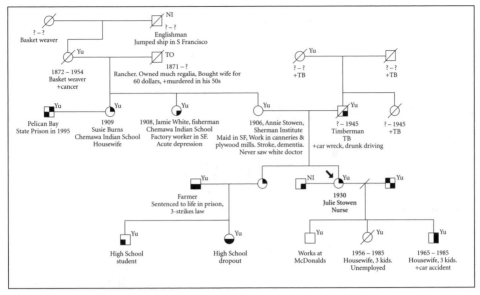

Genealogy 3   Julia Stowen—"Your blood tells on you."

Julia Stowen

Julia Stowen is a Yurok nurse in her 60s whom I met at a Brush Dance on the Yurok Indian Reservation in August 1995. Like other Yuroks, Julia also pointed to confinement in off-reservation boarding schools, state prisons, and forced labor in canneries, plywood mills, rich homes and factories in San Francisco as centers of illness production and distribution. In establishing such connections, Julia Stowen delineated a circuit of disciplinary mechanisms and establishments that extends itself beyond the most common associations made between elements of the American penal system (Ferreira 1996: 234–51).

Boarding schools were a product of the great nineteenth-century effort in discipline and normalization. Boarding schools for Indigenous Peoples in the United States were fashioned after the Auburn solitary and silent system of hard labor, devised for the country's penitentiaries by Indian superintendent Edward F. Beale in 1852 (Ferreira 1996: 185, 2000). Beale proposed a system of military posts on reservations to enforce a program of " discipline and instruction" in which the category of "Indian blood" appeared as a marker for various diseases.

Julia Stowen's mother, Annie Stowen, was born in 1906 on the Yurok Indian Reservation. The years she spent at the Sherman Institute, a boarding school for Indigenous children in southern California, gave her the necessary skills—sewing, cooking and cleaning—to become a house servant in San Francisco. A stroke in her early 60s prevented Julia's mother form working simultaneously in salmon canneries and plywood mills to "make ends meet." When I asked Annie Stowen why, in her opinion, there were so many people in the area suffering from diabetes—including one of her sisters, her two daughters, two nieces and grandson (all shown in Genealogy 3), she answered:

> It's all one and the same thing. When I went to boarding school, more than 70 years ago, they'd line us girls up to check our [menstrual] pads. They wanted to know exactly when we had our periods, so they could control us and know

> **The biomedical diagnosis of type 2 diabetes** involves blood glucose tests and urine analyses. The treatment requires the patient to self-monitor blood glucose levels two to four times a day and follow prescriptions for food and exercise. If these fail, oral agents and insulin are added. Patients' meals are closely supervised by a dietitian and exercises are monitored by a physical therapist. Yuroks described the prescribed meals to me as "everything you don't want to eat: raw vegetables, fruit and lean meat." Clinicians know that a recently diagnosed patient has not been following the prescribed diet if the level of his or her blood sugar does not go down. High blood pressure and high levels of protein in the urinalysis also indicate non-compliance with the prescribed treatment. Repeated urinary tract infections and vaginal yeast infections are associated with diabetes, thus screening for these disorders also take place.

if we were seeing any boys. Not that we were allowed to see them, but it was just like…humiliating. They'd check our pads once a month, and then check again to see if you had scrubbed them good, too. Them pads had to be white as snow, white, white. So now you go to the clinic, you get in line. They prick your finger and test our blood. You get a number and that number tells on you. If you haven't been eating good, I mean, eating a lot of fat, sugar, junk food, you know, the doctors can tell. If you haven't been exercising too much, watching a lot of TV, just sitting around, they know, too, because your blood sugar goes up. So your blood tells on you. Don't you see? It's the same thing!

Annie Stowen and other Yuroks I had the opportunity to meet were constantly trying to figure out ways of "cheating": they sometimes took their blood test before eating (fasting blood glucose) to get a low test result (saved in the memory of their blood testing machines), and entered the information as if they had already eaten (random blood glucose). A 62-year-old woman confessed to me that she would provide the clinicians with urine from her non-diabetic daughter because she "[couldn't] stand all that control. What I like the most is to eat salmon, deer meat, milk, cheese. And doctors say it's too much protein. I just can't help leaking all that protein." These individuals that were constantly trying to "cheat" had been previously labeled as "non-compliant" or "in denial" by their doctors. The rules provided to the clinicians by the *Stage Diabetes Management Guide* (Mazze et al. 1995) did not allow them to see beyond the common associations made between the signs and symptoms of diabetes, limiting the acceptable solutions they eventually came up with.

Curiosity in Hybrids and Monsters or "The White's Blood Obsession"

Blood has served several purposes for the whites. The seventeenth century ideology of hereditary transmission, spurred by the curiosity in animal and plant hybrids and monsters, was "useful in resolving legal questions concerning the subordination of sexes, paternity, purity of blood lines, and the legitimacy of the aristocracy" (Canguilhem

1988: 35). "Half-breed", "quarter blood," "full blood," "real Indian" and other similar expressions are still current today among Indigenous Peoples in northern California, reflecting what some Yuroks call "the white's blood obsession." The place this obsession occupies in the lives, experiences and convictions of several Yurok individuals denotes the extent to which it has penetrated people's life worlds, shaping their self-knowledge and the perceptions they create of individuals they relate to. Julia Stowen's first cousin, Jamie White, speaks of himself and of his close relatives evoking their blood quantum. Julia showed me a picture of Jamie as a young boy, proudly holding one of the first king salmon he caught on the Klamath River.

> Here's Jamie, when he was only eleven or twelve, his mother was still alive then....Everybody talked trash about this boy, nobody gave him any credit. He was bad, I guess, but I still loved him. I could see all this hate locked up inside him, that's what they did to him at Pelican Bay [State Prison]. He was in the hole so many times; to him life was a hole, that's what he used to say. Jamie had this way of talking about people, about Indian people. What he hated most, he said, was being an Indian. He never forgave his mother for that, even blamed his grandmother! He said we were all dirty, we were Indians, that his grandma married a half-breed. 'If Mom had only married a white man,' said Jamie, 'I'd be only an eighth, rather than a quarter-blood.'[6]

"Pure," "half-breed," "quarter-blood" and other fractions of Indianess are common identifiers used by Indigenous Peoples and non-Indigenous populations alike, used to include or exclude individuals from certain social groups, and to assess different dangers Indigenous Peoples are at risk for. In certain situations, a high amount of "Indian blood" is desirable, while in others it is not. Hundreds of individuals are trying to prove they have at least 1/8 Yurok blood in order to become a member of the Yurok Tribe. According to a Yurok teenager whom I met in 1996, "Some are lucky enough to have the blood but not the looks," thus allowing them to be a member of the Yurok Tribe or to be eligible for health care at UIHS, while avoiding racial discrimination. As the so-called Indian blood "thins out," however, one also runs the risk of becoming "white trash," a category that is obviously undesirable for Yuroks and non-Yuroks alike.

An aristocratic society in itself, the Yurok have, since times immemorial, defined their belonging to the *Talth* or "people of the great houses" as the owners of a major dance, a ritual or a ritual prayer, and regalia (Thompson 1991; Pilling 1989), and not to blood quantum or type. Blood occupied a very specific place in Yurok life; it was understood exclusively as a purifying substance for women and men. Despite all the changes the concept of blood has undergone, several Yuroks I met still conceive that the blood which flows from menstruating women serves to purify the women, preparing them for spiritual accomplishment (Buckley 1988: 190). Men in training for wealth acquisition, in order to ascend to higher status in Yurok hierarchy, "gashed their legs with flakes of white quartz, the flowing blood being thought to carry off psychic im-

---

6. The "hole" is what inmates call the solitary cell at Pelican Bay State Prison in Del Norte County, Northern California.

purity, preparing one for spiritual attainment" (Buckley 1988: 195). Although this practice has been largely abandoned, two Yurok men reported to me that they gash their legs before hunting or fishing. Al Gray, a Yurok elder who died in 1996 at 83 years of age, told me that when he received a diagnosis of cancer, he "scratched his legs and thighs with a paring knife, to get all that bad blood out."

The Distribution of Land and "Indian Soul and Conduct"

Until the mid 1800s, Yuroks did not use the quality of ones blood as the primary diagnostic sign of health and illness, nor was its quantity used as criteria for inclusion or exclusion in social groups. Following the General Allotment Act of 1887 (when California Indian reservations were broken into individual parcels and opened for homesteading), Yuroks were introduced to the landholding system of private property. "Indian kinship" was then redefined in terms of the "quantity" of Indian blood. American kinship values outlined the symbolic ground according to which the legal status of the American Indian was defined. A very specific order of nature which invokes a shared substance of blood, was associated with a precise order of law, based upon a customary code for conduct (Schneider 1968, 1989). Julia Stowen explains:

> Allotment did much more than just strip us of our land and make us use English names. It made us start fighting among ourselves over the distribution of land, who paid taxes, who's whose relations....You know, they figured your right to each fraction of a piece of land, based on your percentage of Indian blood. Kids who were adopted out still got their share while those who were adopted into families didn't get anything. Sometimes Indian marriages weren't recognized. All of this created a lot of tension among our own people (Ferreira 1996: 99).

Julia later explained that her parents had been involved in a court suit in the late 1920s over a piece of land on the Yurok Indian Reservation. The 64-acre tract, appraised at $1,000.00 in 1942, was arbitrarily divided into 14 smaller lots. One of her aunts, the allottee's wife, received 13/39ths of the parcel, while their 13 children got 2/39ths each.[7] "Claiming one's Indian blood," as the Yuroks put it, has since been a requirement for enrollment in federal assistance programs for Indigenous Peoples in the United States. The Governing Council of the Yurok Tribe, organized under a Constitution since 1993, established a minimum of 1/8 Yurok blood for enrollment.

The emphasis on the quality or quantity of Indian blood on the part of health practitioners who indiscriminately subscribe to genetic theories also help shape Yurok perceptions of the body. The belief that alcoholism is genetic and, therefore, an uncontrollable disease that leads to liver cirrhosis or degeneration and eventually death is also common among the Yurok community. So is their belief that other degenerative dis-

---

7. Data for heirship finding of the Office of Indian Affairs, 1942. Probate case number 6890-44.

eases like diabetes and cancer are also uncontrollable, "in their bodies" or "genetic." This is precisely what a physician in Eureka, Northern California, told an 80-year-old Yurok woman who has been diagnosed as "diabetic." Her blindness and amputation of her right foot are because of

> …my bad blood. That's what the doctor told me. We Indians have bad blood. See, that's why I drank so much all my life. It's in me, in my blood. So there's not much I can do about it, either. I tell my kids: 'watch out for drinking 'cause it's in your blood.' You think I'm going to follow some diet, not eat all the good stuff I crave for if it's in my blood? You know, it's like they want to kill you over and over. First they give you whiskey, then when they've got you hooked on it they say you can't drink it. Then they put you on commodities, give you sugar and fat, you get to liking it, and they say it is bad for you. But if diabetes is in us, and there's nothing we can do, why bother with diet this and that, exercising and stuff? I just can't believe in anything anymore…My alcoholic son's now gambling like crazy. He spends all his welfare at the casino [in Trinidad]. Now *that* they really can say is in our blood, 'cause we Indian people always used to gamble, the Indian card game, those sticks, you know.

A local physician, who has unsuccessfully tried to make Julia's maternal aunt, Susie Burns, comply with treatments for diabetes, describes his frustration in the following way:

> I almost had this patient in the net. I kept telling her that her blood sugars were high, and that she has a family history of the disease. She kept saying: "No doctor, I'm not a diabetic and I'm not taking any of those pills.' So I insisted, I showed her the results of her exams but she still wouldn't believe me.

Susie had explained to me two months earlier the reasons for her refusal to accept the physician's diagnosis:

> You see, this whole thing about diabetes. Doctors have told me about diabetes. They'll say: 'your blood sugar is high, therefore you have diabetes.' Now, I don't believe them. They say they have evidence. Then they want to check on me to recheck their evidence. The diabetes program calls me and tells me: 'you've got diabetes!' Now, that's a devastating thing to tell somebody. Everybody's walking around saying I've got diabetes. They want me to take pills. Think I'm going to pop pills into my mouth just like that? Pop? 'Cause they tell me? Just like my sister does. She's popping pills into her mouth all-the-time. She's got into the habit. It's pills, pills, pills. Now look at me…I feel young. I eat like a bird, people tell me. I exercise, trimming the ivy and the grass at home. Then the doctor asks me: Do you get up in the middle of the night to pee? No. Do you feel thirsty all the time? No. Everything they ask me is no. But then they check my urine and say there's something wrong with it. Then they check my blood and see, this one day I had it checked and the blood sugar was 175. So they told me to come in fasting and I forgot. So the blood sugar was high again, around 180, so they said: you've got diabetes! Once it's the urine, then it's the blood. Until they check me all, the whole thing and get it all down on paper; until they prove me I've

got diabetes, I just won't admit it. People say I'm tough, that I don't understand, that I wanna act up on them, but it's not being tough. I'm just healthy. How could I have diabetes? Then, you see, nobody in my family has got it either. How could it be me?

Yurok body imagery, which includes their perceptions of health and illness, are compared by a tribal medicine woman to those fostered today by medical institutions in Northern California:

> You see, medicine to us is much more than what goes on inside your body. When I'm inside that [brush dance] pit with a child, it's not all about curing a disease, but bringing strength and happiness. It's the relationship of the child with the world that matters, with the Creator, with the people around it. If people have bad feelings, they shouldn't be here. People should be clean, like myself. I fast for 10 days to go in the pit. I don't drink any water for 10 days. You see that sign over there that says "No drugs or alcohol?' Well, that's a sign of being clean....Now hospitals around here think of the body in an entirely different way. Actually, it's a different way of relating to the world, to the Creator, to everything. It's about your blood and your organs, your insides and what not. You have a number, a medical chart, a list of your diseases and a huge amount of medicine to take. Who you really are doesn't even matter. When they can't find your name, just give them your social security number or your date of birth and they'll track you down.

Concluding Observations

Changes in contemporary Yurok body imagery have substantially altered the relations between the individual, the social, and the Yurok body politic. Some men and women, like Mary Wo'tek, have both created and reproduced images about the generic "Indian," based upon the place biogenetic theories have come to occupy in their lives. Their individual body-self has incorporated a bio-identity—the drunken, diseased, criminal Indian—recognized by its probability to sicken and die. It is through these medicalized body images that Mary Wo'tek relates to society and gives meaning to the world. Others, like Sarah Tsurai, are more aware of the relationship between body and history. The connections they establish between the body and its environment, between illness and perverse social contexts, question the dualistic thinking of Western science and clinical medicine that opposes mind and body, passion and reason, nature and culture, real and unreal. Here, conceptions of health and illness do not obey exclusive laws of physiology inasmuch as they do not escape the influence of local and foreign histories.

Finally, the ways in which Julia Stowen and other Yuroks use blood as a metaphor for social relationships illuminate the convergence between the requirements of political ideology and those of medical technology (Foucault 1975: 38). The stability of the Yurok body politic now includes the manipulation of blood quantum to regulate tribal membership, a mechanism that ends up disciplining individual family arrangements, such as marriage and adoptions. Yurok current perceptions of the body have become a hybrid set of historical events, cross-cultural knowledges and interdisciplinary practices that emphasize social relationships and human reciprocity.

As Jimmy James, a Yurok singer and dance maker who lives on the Yurok Reservation, put it in January of 1995:

> You know the blood thing, how whites are obsessed with it. To be an Indian you've got to have one-fourth, one-eighth Indian blood. Even if you don't think like one, you are. It's their law. Then it's the buyouts, when they offered each Yurok, who had the required blood quantum, 15 thousand dollars to give up their Indian identities. Some people took the money, most didn't. Now it's this genetic testing, back to the blood again....But now we, the Yurok Tribe, we are in a different level, a different reality. You know that there were places the Yurok would not go even in their imagination. I'm talking about a long time age, when we believed that our world was held up by redwood trees. Well, in between the sky and the earth there were sky holes, where spirits would slip through and come onto solid land again....Places where no one dared to go, just spirits. But now things have changed so much and we've had to organize ourselves under different laws. We've had to change our way of being. But our culture, our culture has never died, as the white men think it has. Just because we ride cars, go to the supermarket and stuff? Is that really meaningful? No, we still believe that we are the Pohlik-lah, and our organization under a Constitution means we have slipped through these sky holes and come into a different level of the world where we can understand aspects of different law systems and engage fully in all those ceremonial practices—the Brush Dance, the Jump Dance and World Renewal ceremonies—that the whites once forced us to abandon.

Acknowledgments

I am indebted to the Board of Directors of United Indian Health Services (UIHS) and to Jerry Simone, Executive Director of UIHS, for their support during the research process. Without the suggestions of Yurok tribal members Bea Nix and Lavina Bowers I would not have been able to write this piece. To my colleagues Natasha Schüll and Adriana Petryna, and to Professors Nancy Scheper-Hughes and Lawrence Cohen at the University of California at Berkeley I owe critical readings of the original manuscript. Finally, to members of the Yurok community who have trusted me throughout these years I am gratefully thankful. This research was funded by the Brazilian agency CNPq (Conselho Nacional de Desenvolvimento Científico e Tecnológico), as well as by Olson Grants and a Continuing Graduate Student Fellowship provided by the UC Berkeley Anthropology Department in 1994–1995, and a UC Berkeley Vice-Chancellor for Research Fund Award in 1995.

References

American Diabetes Association (ADA). 1996. Report of the Workgroup on the Diagnosis and Classification of Diabetes Mellitus. Alexandria, VA: American Diabetes Association.

Angier, N. 1995. Gene Defect Tied to Violence in Male Mice. The New York Times. Nov. 23, 1995.

Baer, H., M. Singer and J. Johnsen. 1986. Toward a Critical Medical Anthropology. Social Science and Medicine 23(2): 95–98.

Barkow, J. 1980. Culture and Sociobiology. American Anthropologist 80(1): 5–20.

Bohman, M., S. Sigvardsson and R. Cloninger. 1981. Maternal Inheritance of Alcohol Abuse: Cross-fostering Analysis of Adopted Women. Archives of General Psychiatry 38(9): 965–69.

Bogardus, C. 1993. Insulin Resistance in the Pathogenesis of NIDDM in Pima Indians. Diabetes Care 16(1): 216–27.

Brown, G., B. Albaugh, R. Robin, S. Goodson, M. Trunzo, D. Wynne and D. Goldman. 1993. Alcoholism and Substance Abuse Among Selected Southern Cheyenne Indians. Culture, Medicine and Psychiatry 16(4): 531–42.

Buckley, T. 1988. Menstruation and the Power of Yurok Women. In Blood Magic: The Anthropology of Menstruation. T. Buckley, ed. Berkeley: University of California Press.

Buydens-Branchey, L., M. Branchey and D. Noumair. 1989. Age of Alcoholism Onset: II. Relationship to Susceptibility to Serotonin Precursor Availability. Archives of General Psychiatry 46(3): 231–36.

Canguilhem, G. 1988. Ideology and Rationality in the History of the Life Sciences. Cambridge: The MIT Press.

Chang, K. 1995. Advance in Breast Cancer Research. San Francisco Chronicle. Nov. 3, 1995.

Cowie, C. 1993. Diabetic Renal Disease: Racial and Ethnic Differences from an Epidemiologic Perspective. Transplantation Proceedings 25(4): 2426–30.

Evans-Pritchard, E. 1940. The Nuer. Oxford: Oxford University Press.

Fennerty, M., J. Emerson, R. Sampliner, D. McGee, L. Hixson and H. Garewal. 1992. Gastric Intestinal Metaplasia in Ethnic Groups in the Southwestern United States. Cancer Epidemiology, Biomarkers and Prevention 1(4): 293–96.

Ferreira, Mariana. 1996. Tears and Bitter Pills. The Politics of Health Among the Yuroks of Northern California. Unpublished doctoral dissertation, UC Berkeley.

_____1999. Corpo e História do Povo Yurok. Revista de Antropologia [Universidade de São Paulo] 41(2): 54–98.

_____2000. De puro-sangue, meia-raça a lixo branco: os internatos para índios e o sistema penal nos Estados Unidos da América. In G. Debert & D. Goldstein, eds. Políticas do Corpo e o Curso da Vida. São Paulo: Editora Sumaré.

_____2003. Diabetes tipo 2 e Povos Indígenas no Brasil e nos Estados Unidos. *Anais do Seminário Cultura, Saúde e Doença* [Universidade Estadual de Londrina], pp. 21–42.

Forsdahl, A. 1977. Are Poor Living Conditions in Childhood an Important Risk Factor for Asteriosclerotic Heart Disease? British Journal of Preventive and Social Medicine 31: 91–95.

Foucault, Michael. 1970. [1966] The Order of Things. An Archaeology of the Human Sciences. New York: Vintage Books.

_____1975. [1963] The Birth of the Clinic. An Archaeology of Medical Perception. New York: Vintage Books.

_____1977. Language, Counter-Memory, Practice. Selected Essays and Interviews by Michel Foucault. D. Bouchard, ed. Ithaca, New York: Cornell University Press.

_____1980. Power/Knowledge. Selected Interviews and Other Writings 1972–1977. C. Gordon, ed. Pantheon Books: New York.

_____1984. What is Enlightenment? *In* The Foucault Reader. P. Rabinow, ed. New York: Pantheon Books.

_____1993. The Order of Things. An Archaeology of the Human Sciences. New York: Vintage Books.

Gilbert, S. 1993. Alzheimer's Group Finds Many Members Want Test for Risk. The New York Times. Dec. 26, 1995.

Heizer, R. and J. Mills. 1991. [1952] Four Ages of Tsurai. A Documentary History of the Indian Village on Trinidad Bay. Berkeley and Los Angeles: University of California Press, and London: Cambridge University Press.

Hinkle, L. and S. Wolf. 1952. Effects of Stressful Life Situations on the Concentration of Blood Glucose in Diabetic and Nondiabetic Humans. Diabetes 1(5): 383–91.

Howard, B., T. Kelty, R. Fabsitz, L. Cowan, A. Oopik, N. Le, J. Yeh, P. Savage and E. Lee. 1991. Risk Factors for Coronary Heart Disease in Diabetic and Non-diabetic Native Americans. The Strong Heart Study. Diabetes 41(suppl. 2): 6–11.

Knowler, W. C., M. Saad, D. Pettitt, R. Nelson and P. Bennett. 1991. Determinants of Diabetes Mellitus in the Pima Indians. Diabetes Care 16(1): 216–27.

Kroeber, Alfred. 1917. California Kinship Systems. University of California Publications in American Archaeology and Ethnography 12(9): 339–96.

_____1934. Yurok and Neighboring Kin Term Systems. University of California Publications in American Archaeology and Ethnography 35(2): 15–22.

_____1948. Anthropology: Race, Language, Culture, Psychology, Prehistory. New York: Harcourt.

_____1976. [1925] Handbook of the Indians of California. New York: Dover.

_____1977. Yurok Myths. Berkeley: University of California Press.

Kuhn, Thomas. 1970. The Structure of Scientific Revolutions. Chicago: The University of Chicago Press.

Lee, E., B. Howard, P. Savage, L. Cowan, R. Fabsitz, A. Oopik, J. Yeh, O. Go, D. Robbins and T. Welty. 1995. Diabetes and Impaired Glucose Tolerance in Three

American Indian Populations Aged 45-74 Years. The Strong Heart Study. Diabetes Care 18(5): 599–610.

Lévi-Strauss, Claude. 1963. The Sorcerer and His Magic. Structural Anthropology. New York: Basic Books.

_____1969. [1949] The Elementary Structure of Kinship. Boston: Beacon Press.

Mazze, R., E. Strock and D. Etzwiler. 1995. Staged Diabetes Management Guide. Minneapolis: International Diabetes Center.

Michalek, A. and M. Mahoney. 1991. Provision of Cancer Control Services to Native Americans by State Health Departments. Journal of Cancer Education 9(3): 145–47.

Morgan, Lewis Henry. 1871. Systems of Consanguinity and Affinity of the Human Family. Smithsonian Contributions to Knowledge, Vol. 17. Washington D.C.: Smithsonian Institution.

_____1962. [1851] League of the Iroquois. New York: Corinth Books.

_____1969. [1868] The American Beaver and his Works. New York: Burt Franklin.

_____1984. [1877] Ancient Society, or Researches in the Lines of Human Progress from Savagery through Barbarism to Civilization. Tucson: University of Arizona Press.

Neel, James V. 1962. Diabetes Mellitus: A 'Thrifty' Genotype Rendered Detrimental by 'Progress'. American Journal of American Genetics 14: 353–62.

_____1982. The Thrifty Genotype Revisited. The Genetics of Diabetes Mellitus. Serono Symposium, No. 47. In J. Kobberling and R. Tattersall, eds. pp. 283–93. New York: Academic Press.

Pilling, A.1988. Yurok Aristocracy and "Great House." American Indian Quarterly, Fall 1989: 421–35.

Quaid, K. 1994. A Few Words from a 'Wise' Women. In Genes and Human Self Knowledge. Historical and Philosophical Reflections on Modern Genetics. R. Weir, S. Lawrence and E. Fales, eds. Iowa City: University of Iowa Press.

Radcliffe-Brown, A. 1924. Mother's Brother in South Africa. The South African Journal of Science 21: 542–55.

Rawls, J. 1984. Indians of California. The Changing Image. Norman and London: University of Oklahoma Press.

Rice R., P. Roberts, H. Handsfield and K. Holmes. 1991. Sociodemographic Distribution of Gonorrhea Incidence: Implications for Prevention and Behavioral Research. American Journal of Public Health 81(10): 1252–58.

Sahlins, Marshall. 1976. Use and Abuse of Biology. An Anthropological Critique of Sociobiology. Ann Arbor: The University of Michigan Press.

_____1985. Islands of History. Chicago: The University of Chicago Press.

San Francisco Chronicle. 1995. Flawed Gene Linked to Spurt in Obesity. Mutation Can also Lead to Diabetes. August 10, 1995.

Scheder, Jo C. 1988. A Sickly Sweet Harvest: Farmworker Diabetes and Social Equality. Medical Anthropology Quarterly 2: 251–77.

Scheper-Hughes, Nancy and Margaret Lock. 1987. Mindful Body: A Prolegomenon to Future Work in Medical Anthropology. Medical Anthropology
Quarterly 1(1): 6–26.

Schneider, David. 1968. American Kinship: A Cultural Account. Englewood Cliffs,
N.J.: Prentice Hall.

_____1989. A Critique of the Study of Kinship. Ann Arbor: The University of
Michigan Press.

Sigelman, C., T. Didjurgis, B. Marshall, F. Vargas and A. Stewart. 1992. Views of
Problem Drinking Among Native American, Hispanic, and Anglo Children. Child
Psychiatry and Human Development 22(4): 265–76.

Taussig, Michael. 1992. Reification and the Consciousness of the Patient. In The
Nervous System. Michael Taussig, ed. New York and London: Routledge.

Thompson, L. 1991. [1916] To the American Indian. Reminiscences of a Yurok
Woman. Berkeley: Heyday Books.

Von Knorring, A.L., M. Bohman, L. von Knorring and L. Oreland. 1975. Platelet
MAO Activity as a Biological Marker in Subgroups of Alcoholism. Acta
Psychiatrica Scandinavica 72: 51–58.

Waterman, T. and A. Kroeber. 1934. Yurok Marriages. University of California
Publications in American Archaeology and Ethnology 35(1): 1–14.

Westermeyer, Joseph., J. Neider and Michelle Westermeyer. 1993. Substance Use and
Other Psychiatric Disorders among 100 American Indian Patients. Culture,
Medicine and Psychiatry 16(4): 519–29.

Young, Alan. 1995. The Harmony of Illusions: Inventing Post-traumatic Stress
Disorder. Princeton, NJ: Princeton University Press.

CHAPTER 4

Diabetes in Réunion Island (Indian Ocean): From Sugar Plantations to Modern Society

Muriel Roddier

Thus, during the three centuries of successive waves of immigration [to Réunion Island] that preceded the 20th C. sugar played a predominant role because many of these immigrants were destined to lives of working in the cultivation of sugar cane and production of sugar. M. Marimoutou (1989) has researched the conditions surrounding the arrival of hired laborers of Indian origin in the last half of the 19th century. In 1861, these immigrants were funneled through the lazar house of Grande-Chaloupe, a kind of "sieve" of decontamination and medical examination, where they were placed in quarantine in order to avoid the possible spread of infectious diseases. The daily ration served at that time to these immigrants resembled the diet of many inhabitants of La Réunion today: rice, cod, dry grains, salt, fat, "spices" (onion, garlic, pepper, tamarind, etc.), to which were sometimes added potatoes, meat, and tobacco. Sugar was not provided; in fact, it was excluded by the local administration from what was considered the "basic food ration" of Réunion Island. It is likely that for the decision-makers, sugar represented more a substance of pleasure than a source of energy (which only later would be seen as necessary for workers).

Muriel Roddier, in her chapter presented here.

Summary of Chapter 4. Over the course of the 20th century, and especially since 1980, changes in ways of life for residents of Réunion Island have included a significant increase in the prevalence of diabetes. This remote island, situated in the Indian Ocean, has been populated by successive waves of migrants of diverse origins, who arrived from three continents with their traditional knowledges. For our focus here, we are interested in knowledge related to healing and health. It should be pointed out, that since 1946, when the long-standing French colony of Réunion Island became a French "Overseas Department," over-all indicators of public health have clearly improved.

In considering the challenges of diabetes for residents of Réunion Island, it is crucial that one take into account the interactions and exchanges between differing traditions that occurred over time. What, for example, has been the relationship of people to sugar ? Certainly this calls for an examination of social history as well as individual habits, such as food availability and food preferences, the preferential recourse to medicinal teas, or more generally, the frequent practice of drawing upon both traditional and modern therapies for the alleviation of problems.

In order to grasp the ways in which illness, diabetes in particular, has been interpreted over time, it is absolutely necessary to deconstruct the dominant biomedical model, examings how illness has been experienced within a specific socio-economic context. The differences between the two principle models of an illness—the bio-medical and the layperson's, have already been clarified many times in medical anthropology. Here we pay particular attention to showing the possible reconciliation between the dominant biomedical model and traditional layperson model, in order to construct interactions that might effectively bridge these chasms. I describe two situations to show how an individual experiencing diabetes in La Reunion may "take charge" of his or her condition.

ᔑ ᔑ ᔑ

Historical Background: The Peopling of Réunion Island

One of the historical facts about Réunion Island (La Réunion), a French Overseas Department situated in the middle of the Indian Ocean, is that it remained uninhabited until 1663. When the first inhabitants, of French or Malagasy origin, disembarked, it was named "Île Mascarin" or "Île des Mascareignes." Then in 1665 the island, baptized "Île Bourbon," was colonized by a score of Frenchmen who arrived from Madagascar on the orders of the King of France, Louis XIV.

The peopling of Réunion Island subsequently occurred by successive waves of inhabitants arriving from three continents: Europe, Africa, and Asia. Among the principal migratory movements was the arrival of other French people, notably women brought from Paris in 1674 to procreate on the island. Then the first slaves were disembarked in 1705. Coming mainly from East Africa, they were called the "*Kaffirs.*" In 1828, the first "free Indians" arrived from South India to cultivate sugarcane. But it was between 1865 and 1885 that the great period of "Engagement" took place, that is, the arrival of a great number of free Indians, coming in particular from the Southeast of India (known today as Tamil Nadu) to work under contract in the sugarcane plantations or the sugar factories. These Indians practiced a popular Hinduism, known on Réunion Island as the Tamil Cult, and they were named the "*Malbars.*" In Réunion Island's history, 1848 must be cited as an important date because it was the year that slavery was abolished and that the island received its definitive name: La Réunion.

Then other immigrants arrived: the first Chinese and Vietnamese in 1860 and, in 1875, a second more important group: the Guandong from the region of Canton, China. In 1875 and in 1910, there were also arrivals of other Indians, in particular , Muslims from the Northwest of India, nicknamed the "*Zarabes.*" The Guandong and the Indian Muslims took up positions in the tertiary sector: the Chinese in small groceries and the Muslim Indians in cloth and clothing stores.

In 1918, before the dismantling of the great sugar estates, inhabitants of the Mascarene Archipelago arrived: Malagasies, Comorians, and some Rodrigans. Finally, in

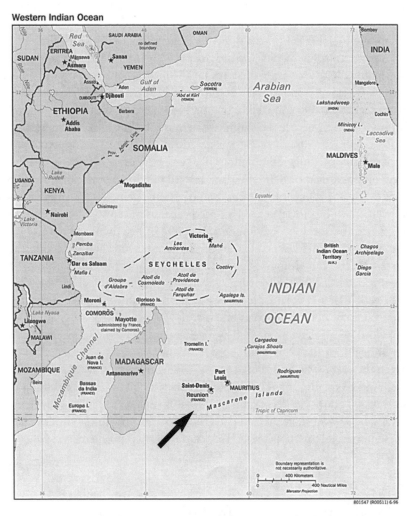

Location of Réunion Island in the Indian Ocean, south of Mauritius.

1950, a wave of metropolitan French, nicknamed the "*Zoreils*" disembarked on the island to occupy leadership positions, which unleashed at the time a press campaign
hostile to their arrival. Zoreils were to confine themselves largely to the sectors of education, health, and social services, acting as functionaries or having a liberal profession. The result of these movements of diverse peoples into Réunion Island remain
visible today in the community's social organization. In 1970, the society of Réunion
Island could be characterized as having three sectors: plantation society, peasant society, and pseudo-industrial society. Now, at the beginning of the 21st century, the first
two seem to be progressively disappearing as the third sector is continuing to expand
and develop.

Housing and pattern of residence in La Réunion reflected and still reflect the successive waves of immigration. In effect, the population remains clustered in the form
of a "horseshoe" around the island for various reasons. Some are geographic, due to
terrain and access routes. Other reasons are historical, with an organization of space

according to an administrative vision directed from the Metropole, leading to centers of concentration of workers in urban centers that grew up around sugar factories. Further reasons are sociological; with a difficulty of peopling the Heights, the rise of shantytowns on the margins of developed zones which indicate the exclusion of some groups, notably the descendents of slaves or of Malagasy and Comorian immigrants.

La Réunion passed from colonial status to that of a French Overseas Department (DOM) on March 19, 1946, and since that date the standard of living has improved, especially on the level of health. This improvement is due, above all, to an increase in education for a population that in 1954 was described as having 57% of people with a low literacy; it is also due to the elimination of a large part of unhealthy habitats, and the movement of the workers of Réunion Island toward the city to obtain better employment.

One of the great benefits of Réunion Island's having gained departmental status was an improvement in health services. Free medical assistance was extended to the DOM in 1956, as was the social protection of the regime of health and maternity insurance for wage-earners. Priority was given to the fight against a high mortality rate (estimated as 28.2% in 1935) among adults and against a catastrophic infant mortality rate (estimated in 1935 as 82.6% of births). At this time, the principal causes of mortality at all ages were infectious, parasitic illnesses, and respiratory illnesses. Until the 1970s, the society could be characterized as one marked by social inequality. Poverty was not always obvious because it was masked by a generally solid familial solidarity. However, the state of health of the population bore its stigmata.

Between the years 1980 and 2000, the telescoping of modernity and tradition, along with the rapid disruption of ways of life, are incriminated in the alarming development of non-infectious health conditions, notably metabolic diseases involving eating behaviors. One sees an increase in the diagnosis of chronic illness conditions, including diabetes, arterial hypertension (AHT), cardiovascular problems, and chronic renal insufficiency.

From the Relation to Sugar in the Local Context to 'Sugared Diabetes'

Thus, during the three centuries of successive waves of immigration that preceded the 20th Century. sugar played a predominant role because many of these immigrants were destined to lives of working in the cultivation of sugar cane and production of sugar. M. Marimoutou (1989) has researched the conditions surrounding the arrival of hired laborers of Indian origin in the last half of the 19th century. In 1861, these immigrants were funneled through the lazar house of Grande-Chaloupe, a kind of "sieve" of decontamination and medical examination, where they were placed in quarantine in order to avoid the possible spread of infectious diseases. The daily ration served at that time to these immigrants resembled the diet of many inhabitants of La Réunion today: rice, cod, dry grains, salt, fat, "spices" (onion, garlic, pepper, tamarind, etc.), to which were sometimes added potatoes, meat, and tobacco. Sugar was not provided; in fact, it was excluded by the local administration from what was considered the "basic food ration" of Réunion Island. It is likely that for the decision-makers, sugar represented more a substance of pleasure than a source of energy (which only later would be seen as necessary for workers). It also seems likely that this "official" image of sugar as a pleasurable food contrasted markedly with the dietary patterns and expectations of the Indians. Traditional foodways of Indian laborers included sweets, so it is not surprising that they were drawn to sugar, and, in addition, they had specifically come to Réunion Island to work in the sugar plantations and factories. Given this paradoxical situation, it is perhaps not surprising to read in historical writings that there were thefts of sugar on the part of these immigrants. Those who engaged in such theft risked a penalty of the same magnitude as for the theft of wine, of vegetables or fruits, likewise excluded from the daily ration.

Still today, some employees of sugar factories sometimes take to stealing sugar, despite its low price. One of them, hospitalized in 1999, had been gravely wounded by a fall, when he fled precipitously after having "borrowed," to use his word, sugar from the factory where he worked. To be precise, sugar is at the source of a system of social discrimination that was established at the beginning of the 19th century when the cultivation of cane developed on the island. The sugar factories, like the residential patterns ("habitation") analyzed by J. Benoist (1984), have long been a place where social difference in the division of labor was clearly visible. This corresponded to the ethnic differences reflected in social hierarchy that developed with respect to sugarcane, as J. and R. Potier have noted (1971), tracing a sort of "color line" according to the expression of J.L. Bonniol (1992) that marked the separation into three groups: the Whites and the halfcastes / the Malabary Indians / the Kaffirs. Each group had a place reserved with respect to the production of sugar; each occupied a position in the hierarchy, and a recognition of their abilities and degree of effort were inevitably seen as a function of their belonging to one of the three groups. As J. Benoist (1984) notes: "The economic importance of cane is not denied, but the sociological ramifications, in general, have been minimized. Everything happens as though sugar agriculture were not the basis of a social universe but merely one activity, among others, in a rural world" (p. 178). Further on he adds: "The weight of the universe of sugar makes itself felt far beyond: all global society is oriented by it, modeled by its preponderant influence" (p. 183) [editors' note: cf. Mintz 1991].

On Réunion Island, sucking on a piece of sugarcane is a customary practice, often seen in children on their way to school. While attentive mothers took care that the little stomachs were not filled exclusively with liquid sugar, staple food dishes were also sweetened. Boiled fruits or roots, like manioc, sweet potato or breadfruit, have for a long time occupied an important place in the local diet. These dishes, considered bland by many, were abundantly sweetened to enhance their taste. Sugar is still considered by some as a basic foodstuff as important as rice. The image of sugar, forbidden first by parents, by the foremen of the factory, then by doctors to prevent tooth decay and obesity, perpetuates itself in an ordinary way. But the attraction of sugar is nonetheless neither diminished, nor mastered, by the consumer—child or adult—above all if he or she is from Réunion Island.

The experience of diabetes is reflected in a discourse of common sense particular to the local context. The society of La Réunion still carries the stigmata of its history, notably marked by migration and slavery. It reflects the ambivalence between the will of migrants to form a new society with shared knowledges versus a situation in which their diverse origins inspires the construction of a plural social reality. In a situation like this, some borrowings are conserved and others are discarded as a result of community choices and individual interpretations. Here it should be pointed out that since the end of the 1970s a unifying cultural movement has developed, centered on the word "Creoleness." Creoleness was defined in 1978 by a bishop of the island, Monseigneur Aubry, as "a cultural quest for a La Réunion identity, with a view to favoring solidarities." But the notion of Creole remains relatively fluid and plural. The fragility of the foundations of the society of Réunion Island as it has been submitted to contradictory challenges is visible in numerous domains, and certainly that of health is no exception. As an increasing number of inhabitants of Réunion Island have been confronted with chronic illness, it has also become a moment of negotiating a new social identity. This new social identity—as determined by conventional biomedical practice—involves becoming a person who now needs to be in charge of his or her "diabetic condition, "and thus for those who may already be on the margins of society there is now a necessary sort of "third socialization" in which people must learn to "live with diabetes." Those who are afflicted with diabetes and who understand the requirements of a life-long regimen for a chronic condition such as diabetes, begin to view their lives as a function of their state of health and of being more or less under "normative" medical control.

The History of Diabetes on La Réunion

The local representation of diabetes on Réunion Island has been constructed by the lay person's reinterpretation of medical discourse. Medical discourse has gradually diffused and has been incorporated into lay understandings after the achievement of departmental status in 1946. This discourse was really structured at the local level during the 1980s (during which time, moreover, scientific discoveries were made about the treatment of diabetes by injections of insulin). But diabetes had already been recognized and reinterpreted by the population of Réunion Island before this recent period. One finds mention of diabetes in the phytotherapeutic notebooks of a local "tea-maker,"[1] the Catholic Father Raimbault (1944), born in Bourges in 1875, who came to the island to care for those who suffered from leprosy. Father Raimbault also collected information on medicinal plants used locally for the treatment of various illnesses. This is the oldest written tract found on the subject of diabetes in the traditional pharmacopoeia of Réunion Island. No plants with anti-diabetic applications are cited in the "Notice on La Réunion" edited under the direction of A.G. Garsault, published earlier in 1900.

It might seem contradictory to observe that in an island peopled exclusively by descendants of immigrants, the arrival of people *from outside*, to use the Creole expression, is often poorly received. The origin of the islanders' distrust of newcomers may be somewhat obscure today but, as in earlier times, this distrust appears to consistently be motivated by preoccupations of a medical order, because disease often

---

1. The tea-maker is a phytotherapist, that is, someone who recommends or prescribes and sometimes himself sells medical plants. He has precise therapeutic knowledge of medicinal plants, their harvesting, and the preparation of cold drinks called "*rafraichissants*" in Creole, or warm infusions: the teas.

is perceived as coming from "elsewhere." In Réunion Island at the beginning of the 20th century, people feared the "polluting" consequences for the local environment emanating from the waves of immigrants arriving from Africa or Asia who were suspected of bringing in smallpox, cholera, typhus, or malaria. Several generations of children have read about these diseases in the schoolbooks written about Réunion Island, including the work by P. Hermann (1920), under the rubric "climate" of the island:

> A good sky, a pure air used to make Bourbon one of the healthiest lands on earth; but since the introduction of Malagasy, Indian, African, Comorian, and Vietnamese immigrants, its so highly praised healthiness found itself sensibly modified. Let us nonetheless hope that the new illnesses and pernicious fevers imported by these foreign workers will eventually disappear on the one hand through the practice of hygienic wisdom and, on the other, under the influence of this beneficent air that not long ago cured all afflictions.

Others, from a contrasting perspective, could see a positive benefit in the arrival of immigrants who brought with them certain therapeutic knowledges. That is the case with B. Duchemann, a schoolteacher from Réunion Island, who in 1899 profited from his vacations to harvest and inventory locally-used medicinal plants; in preparation for the Universal Exposition of 1900 in Paris. Duchemann (1900: 119) wrote:

> Slavery disappeared long ago and we take an ever greater distance from the state of nature where the curing instinct manifested itself in its integrity. The plants are there...But soon we won't know how to use them, inasmuch as the rare possessors of traditions are jealous of their science and transmit it differently, some to preserve for themselves alone the benefits of this kind of heritage, others out of fear of the authorities who, thanks to progress of civilization, can prosecute them for the illegal practice of medicine.

Duchemann thought there existed among humans a sort of "instinct" for curing oneself, more or less developed, in the manner of a "science" founded—in the case of Réunion Island—on the ancestral knowledges of slaves brought to the island. He contrasted "the medicine of tropical common people [simples tropicaux]"[2] with "the official medicine of the doctors" (Duchemann 1900: 117). At the end of the report, Garsault 1990: 120) tempers the teacher's revolutionary statement in adding a *nota bene* that, according to him, in the "medicine of the Blacks," the plants indicated are in fact the same as those of "official medicine." The plants, since known to possess hypoglycemic properties: the *jamblon* or *bitter rose*, were used at the beginning of the century to treat other illnesses than diabetes. It is important to note for the discussion here that references to diabetes did not appear in this book.

The representation of diabetes on La Réunion thus began to be constructed since the end of the colonial period, not surprisingly, as a response to the needs of the population among whom some cases were diagnosed. It is quite understandable that the people were resourceful from the start in identifying curative methods that were easy to obtain and that could be incorporated into their lives. As to the choice of cur-

---

2. Medicinal plants are also called "simples."

ative plants, lay medical ideas about treatments corresponded with medical under-standings of diabetes—both were characterized by the excess of ingested sugar that must be eliminated to relieve the ill person weakened by this excess. Diabetes was viewed as directly related to a loss of equilibrium between the interior of the indi-vidual's body and one's environment, according to both lay and biomedical models of the illness. Following this logic, it is by the re-establishment of this precious equi-librium that one recovers one's health. That would seem to be why the plants used had in common a bitter taste contrary to the sweet taste[3] of urine and to the sweet-ened blood, following Hippocrates' principle of oppositions. Moreover, these me-dicinal plants often have diuretic qualities that facilitate the urinary elimination of excessive sugar and, sometimes, they would be stimulating for the ill person affected by fatigue.

Since the time of Father Raimbault's work published in 1944, the list of plants with anti-diabetic uses has grown longer. In the "Notebooks of Ariste Payet," re-transcribed by J. Benoist (1993), a range of medicinal plants considered particularly beneficial in cases of diabetes are listed under the categories of leaf, flowers, bark, grains, fruit, or juice. R. Lavergne (1989: 41) even describes a plant known on La Réunion under the vernacular name of "diabetic coffee" (*Acanthaceae*).

In 1902, almost half a century before Father Raimbault, J.M. MacAuliffe, a physi-cian on Réunion Island, made the first reference to diabetes in his writings. He was originally from Rennes in Brittany, and served as president of the association of doc-tors on Réunion Island and was the Resident Doctor at the thermal establishment of Cilaos. MacAuliffe explained that the state of health of the population of Réunion Island at the time was very bad, notably because of epidemics, with high levels of mortality especially among children; of the lack of means to care for oneself; and of the weak spread of medical or even basic hygienic knowledge. His last observation can be explained by the very small number of health professionals; by the situation of poverty extending across a large sector of the population suffering from malnu-trition and unhealthiness; as well as very few available means by which people gained information.

MacAuliffe observed that for patients stricken with what he calls "intermittent dia-betes," improvement was noted if they followed his recommendations of drinking four to six glasses of Cilaos spring water each day and taking warm baths at 36 degrees centi-grade as part of their thermal cure. He observed that urination became less frequent, that thirst and dryness of the mouth became less painful, that appetite returned, that digestion became easier, that the condition of the skin improved. He extolled the virtues of curative waters: to be taken internally (as a drink) and to be used externally (as a bath). The doctor considered that the thermal treatment recommended in the am-phitheatre of Cilaos was above all effective for obese diabetics and the "gouty" forms of diabetes, that is, among those whose diabetes was associated with "gravel" (a renal in-

---

3. Until modern means of measurement like testing-strips were available, physicians tasted the urine of their patients. In 1998 we met a thirty year old individual affected by diabetes from La Réu-nion, living in the middle of the cane fields, who still used this method as though she had need of this tangible proof of the reality of her diabetes.

sufficiency) and with "gout."[4] These forms of aggravated diabetes would be described by modern medicine as a renal attack and/or vascular distal attacks responsible for polyneuritis, associated with the initial pathology.

In return, MacAuliffe thought that these therapeutic measures were ineffective in more advanced cases of chronic illness when the ill had reached a period of "denutrition," or emaciation. He considered that it was necessary to add a nitrogenous regime and to forbid the ill to eat starchy food. MacAuliffe remarked that the general amelioration of the illness revealed itself in a feeling of well-being which had been forgotten by the ill person for a long time. The remarks of this doctor at the beginning of the century correspond, in fact, exactly to the expectation of most individuals suffering from diabetes interviewed today, who first of all hope for an easing of their malaise due to glycemic variations, as the possibility of a cure often seems to them to be a matter of chance. It appears that MacAuliffe had, in 1900, a vision of diabetes quite close to that which the French physician C. Bernard held fifty years earlier. This medical representation, which did not yet understand the role of the pancreas, was perhaps the one commonly prevalent in France during this period. Even in France there was a lag in incorporating the great discoveries of the epoch, such as those of Minkowski, in 1889, on the pancreatic function as regulator of glycemia and of Laguesse, in 1893, on the internal secretions of islets of Langerhans.

This time-lag is actually not surprising to students of medical history, especially given the geographically remote location of Réunion Island, several months' distant from metropolitan France by boat, which delayed the transmission of scientific results. Concerning the treatment of diabetes, MacAuliffe's account remains quite consistent with the standard recommendations given in the 19th century, by Rollo for a nitrogenous diet, by Trousseau for the drinking of mineral water, by Bouchardat for the suppression of starches and with the prescription of thermal baths. MacAuliffe also notes in his writings that diabetes, gout, gravel, and bladder stones were rare illnesses on Réunion Island at the end of the 19th century and the beginning of the 20th century, but were much more frequent in Mauritius. This remark is supported by the considerations of doctors of the beginning of the century concerning these conditions, the cause of which they attributed to an acquired or congenital nutritional problem. MacAuliffe explains that the Mauritians coming to visit Réunion Island had a reputation for high living, for drinking wine, tea, and for doing little physical exercise. That, according to him, is what explains the greater frequency of these illnesses, notably diabetes, on Mauritius due to what he calls "a slowing down of nutrition," in other words a hyper-caloric dietary pattern, not easily utilizable by a sedentary lifestyle. Note the persistence of this discourse on the relation between available energy and physical exercise, upon which medical logic has supported itself for at least a century now and which is not always either truly understood, or followed, by the public. The pleasures of the table remain dangerous and culpable, when they reach an excess. But numerous people, among them the chronically ill, nonetheless do not renounce them, despite a certain general awareness of the habits considered a "high risk" for health.

Thus, from the beginning of the 20th century to the recent period of the last two decades, a certain evolution of medical and lay attitudes has reinforced perceptions of

---

4. This concerns an accumulation of uric acid, characterized by painful inflammations, notably on the articulatory and renal levels.

diabetes as characterized by certain symptoms and responsive to particular treatments. Some testimonials allow the retracing of the local history of diabetes within this context. Among them, a general practitioner physician of La Réunion origin, having practiced from 1953 to 1986 in the principle town of the island, Saint-Denis, remembers that diabetes was seldom detected. For the doctors of the island, of which there were few[5] in the middle of the century, the signs of diabetes were above all furunculosis and repeated infections. The physician would then proceed to an analysis of the patient's urine to search for an eventual glycosuria. This information confirmed or disconfirmed the diagnosis of diabetes. According to this doctor, diabetes seemed apparently more frequent among the population of East Indian origin and specifically among those from the Muslim community. As a result, he and his colleagues were more attentive when these patients came to them.

This physician pointed out that in 1953 there were already lay treatments among the local population, transmitted by oral tradition, encouraging recourse to medicinal plants. It is interesting to observe that one of the warning signs of diabetes, according to the medical representation of that period, believed to be more frequent among the population of Indian origin/Islamic practice, corresponds to the popular Creole expression still used today: "*bobo zarab*," a phrase designating an ulcerous wound that does not heal, as is the case for some sufferers of diabetes.

Other signs show that popular discourse on diabetes has continued to construct itself with reference to medical discourse. Thus, the concern of doctors and nurses regarding the increase in diabetes and the broad attention to it in the media in recent years may help explain why diabetes has become today the primary reason for the purchase of medicinal plants, according to the tea-makers of Réunion Island.

Likewise, certain practices show how popular thought borrows from medical practice as well as knowledge. As a result of the local habit of searching for available means to maintain health, many people on Réunion Island who have diabetes use a biological laboratory to verify the hypoglycemic effect of absorbed medicinal teas. Some tea-makers themselves recommend this precaution. Medical discourse which invariably insists upon glycemic control has thus penetrated peoples' minds without necessarily displacing lay beliefs about therapies. This notion of control is implicit in the lay logic that has integrated, in its own way, the idea that diabetes is an excess of sugar in the body (blood) of the affected person and which must be eliminated, before verifying whether "interior harmony" has returned.

Construction of Diabetes by Those Who Experience It

Today, in order to understand the experience of the inhabitants of La Réunion who suffer from diabetes, it seems important to deconstruct the dominant medical model and to grasp the manner in which an individual reconstructs this chronic condition based on their particular knowledges. Biomedicine is supported by scientific discoveries and epidemiological evidence regarding the development of the global "epidemic"

---

5. A. Lopez (1987) notes that the number of doctors is 37 in 1946, whereas it exceeds 748 in 1985.

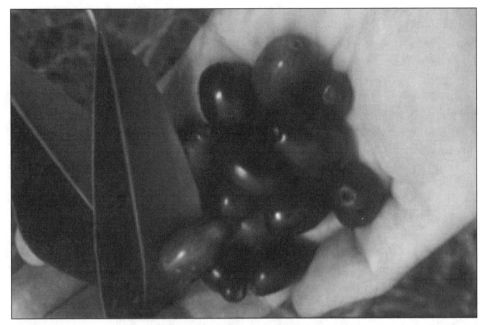

Jamblon (*Syzygium cumini, MYRTACEAE*) is widely used to treat diabetes on Réunion
Island. It is also a very well known and commonly-used plant in Madagascar; in recent times, a
Madagascan physician created a capsule (gel cap) to counter "The Great Island's" lack of
affordable medication.

of type 2 diabetes. However, those who are afflicted with this chronic condition and
those close to them usually have different explanations based on their theories of causes
of misfortune. Their interpretations often reflect the significance of their experience
with diabetes. It is necessary, however, to guard oneself from "culturalizing" behaviors
tied to health and illness. Such a viewpoint allows one to imagine that it is culture that
in a preponderant fashion accounts for reality, and may cause one to overlook other
crucial determinants of human behavior including cognitive, socio-economic, or familial conditions. As a result it is important to research the articulations of collective
and personal values that give meaning to the event of illness and that orient attitudes,
above all, amongst persons faced with a chronic condition. For that purpose we propose to examine the main steps in the course of "appropriation" of the person with diabetes. By looking at the multiple paths taken by Réunion Island residents who are afflicted with diabetes leads, for example, to the identification of four shared major
stages: 1) the posing of the diagnosis; 2) the search for causes; 3) the demand for care;
and 4) the question of a cure. These stages mark the individual's modeling of diabetes
rooted in a particular social environment. Different stances correspond to each of the
phases of the experience of the illness, and are elaborated upon in relation to lived situations and acquired knowledges. Here we will primarily address some aspects of diagnosis and etiological explanations.

     For the Réunion Island residents, diabetes is generally perceived as an illness pre-
senting itself as a common sickness, non-contagious, with which many people are

struck today. It is first of all recognized as a poorly explained event,[6] before complications and the long term nature of the condition modify this representation. The chronic aspect of this condition is not significant from the start; this is a reality that takes on meaning progressively as constraints induced by the illness and its treatments are experienced. To have diabetes on Réunion Island is generally not perceived as shameful, but there is reluctance to show oneself as weakened in front of younger people, in particular, by men proud of their position as head of the family.

The posing of the medical diagnosis does not immediately have a negative reality for those who are diagnosed as having diabetes. This illness that develops quietly, slyly inside one, is not always believable for the person who lives in the heart of a society where only external manifestations—faintness, pains, or unusual signs—attest to the presence of sickness. The afflicted individual first must understand what has happened to him in order to interiorize the change and find a strategy adapted to it. In this process, it is essential to research[7] peoples' ideas of cause (Kleinman 1992). A patient's recognition of having this chronic condition does not necessarily occur simultaneously with the moment of the medical diagnosis. A diagnosis is often a simple factual report, significant first of all for the doctor, which enters nonetheless into the memory of the patient. This dated official "beginning" will take on variable meanings according to the individual at stake, his or her own history, knowledge, as well as the context of the report and the clinical signs. Of course, the diagnosis will remain the primary reference for all health professionals involved with the patient in order to evaluate the evolution of the chronic illness, to determine the priorities of action, to establish a plan for care. The diagnosis is, as a result, the start of medical supervision to which often the patient, who is not ready and not prepared, does not adhere immediately. The anamnesis registered by the doctor never takes into account this possible time-lag between his diagnosis and conscious acceptance of the patient vis-à-vis his or her illness, no more than it does for that matter other divergences between the medical prescriptions and the therapeutic resources actually used. It is within this mutual incomprehension that the doctor-patient relationship is established, where each party develops a more or less divergent position.

For those experiencing diabetes on Réunion Island, the significant elements of diabetes onset are essentially an intense recurrent weakness, a tenacious thirst, abundant urine, a disgust with food, a suspicious emaciation, itching and, among women, the *gratèl dann ba* (vulvar pruritis). Men may experience impotence, so there is a difference between men and women's experience with this affliction. Age is equally a determining variable for the representation of diabetes, for the pairs "youth-health" and "old age-illness" constitute common images of the "natural order" of life. Other signs of a painful or limiting kind, in the eyes or the extremities of the limbs, cited as early symptoms that initially led the ill person to consult a doctor, are in fact often signs of complications. If these elements are not explained carefully by the health care-giver, the patient may not take full measure of the gravity of the situation and, in turn, may result in the doctor's judgment of the patient as irresponsible. Nonetheless, over time, those afflicted

---

6. According to Marc Auge (1984), illness is among the natural "events" of life.

7. A. Zemplini (1985) writes: "…the idea of 'cause' is constitutive of the very notion of 'illness'" (p. 20).

with diabetes often develop the widespread image of a "poison" that has invaded all the aspects of their life, and even that of their wider family and social network.

In patients' etiological models, the causes that are often identified and blamed for the onset of diabetes are principally external but individuals often bring in personal characteristics. These explanatory systems in many ways simulate biomedical models that associate environmental and behavioral factors as explanations for the occurrence of diabetes.

Among the behavioral causes, negligence notably through inactivity and through dietary abuses (sugar, alcohol) are regularly cited by those affected by diabetes. It is first of all the excess of ingested sugar that is blamed, despite scientific affirmation that sugar, per se, does not cause diabetes. In some ways this simple explanation reassures oneself about the situation, as the eater paradoxically may consider himself more a victim than a culprit. Such a behavior of excess is sometimes excused by the counter-posing view of a past of undernourishment and poverty, by a predisposing socioeconomic context (sugar factory, soft-drink factory, kitchens, food business, etc.), justified by conformity to local habits, or the ascendancy of consumer society. But such lay explanation may also be rejected by those who say they have never over-eaten. How well patients will accept a prescribed hypoglucidic regime follows directly from their etiological understandings, and thus may differ according to how a patient responds to his or her own knowledges about the cause.

The notion of fragility, used by some patients, refers to the *weak temperament* according to the Creole expression; this would appear to be a true endogenous cause, against which the person is helpless (as when faced with a hereditary factor). Fragility is associated with a state of vulnerability present especially at a very young or old age, or during a particular period for women, such as the times of pregnancy, nursing, fatigue, misfortune, or illness. Lack of personal "responsibility" does not appear to be called upon as a common explanation, except when there occurs an *imprudence*, close to the modern notion of "at-risk behaviors," such as being exposed to a draft.

The abuse of rum is a third biomedical cause re-asserted, above all, by men who suffer from diabetes, which is related to the notion of excessive intake of sugar (still cited by some physicians). This indiscretion, socially condemned (especially within the Muslim community), generally blames the individual for his or her illness. Diabetes then often has the image of a "punishment-illness" to which one must resign oneself. Such a negative interpretation may incite the affected person either to be compliant like a repentant child or to consider that the harder the torment the greater the expiation of the sin. The active participation of some individuals in their treatment is very difficult to obtain on the part of health professionals, because these patients have a devalorized vision of themselves and are often marginalized even when they benefit from a certain solidarity with others who are experiencing the same conundrum.

Obesity is perceived more as a minor or associated condition, of what popular discourse refers to as "fat diabetes," than as a true cause. The relation to the body is notably determined by the level of education, by the socio-economic category, by the adhesion to traditional or modern values, as well as by the social environment. On Réunion Island, excess weight on the part of a woman of mature age, in particular if she is a mother, is part of a "feminine ethos." This plumpness is often perceived as a "quasi natural" consequence of pregnancies and hormonal states, the image of which is sometimes reinforced by the familial maternal model.

Some etiological explanations are as common as the preceding ones, others are more personal. Among the etiological explanations for diabetes commonly expressed one finds those of illness in general: modernity and its share of nuisances like the degradation of diet, ordinary aging or the cares that render the person vulnerable to illness. For many people, anxiety may be more geared towards material concerns, and often subsumes the energy of adults who relegate health precautions to second place. Misfortune profits from these moments of lack of vigilance to infiltrate itself into a body whose defenses are weakened. For example, inactivity would be considered dangerous because it incites one to hark upon worries and not because it might facilitate gaining weight as the doctors say. While varied, individuals invoke various personal theories of causation of their illness: some people blame quitting tobacco, taking a contraceptive, a difficult pregnancy, contagion or divine will. Quitting tobacco (above all, among men) represents the rupture of a habitual equilibrium that might then have allowed the penetration of the illness into a perturbed organism. In a more complex manner, some women think that their diabetes might result from a contamination, revealing itself after the loss through death of a relative due to diabetes as the origin of their own attack. It would be a matter of a kind of "inheritance," left behind by the deceased relative, as though it were now the turn for the survivor to suffer. This knowledge perhaps corresponds to the denial of one's own aging or to the attachment to a cyclical logic, common in traditional and/or rural folk knowledge, in which the disappearance of one element, here the ill person, demands its replacement in order to assure the equilibrium of the familial system.

For many, diabetes seems to be a consequence of divine will, the sickness coming "out of the air" or from misfortune that strikes a victim by chance, the sickness is "in the air." These conceptions found what is customarily called "fatalism," here corresponding more to a feeling of profound helplessness faced with superhuman forces supposedly responsible for the illness. In popular thought, diabetes is among the "illnesses of God," which in a curious manner are physical ailments, of "natural" causes, distinct from those, with more psychic manifestations, that have "supernatural" causes.

When it comes to explaining one's own diabetes, a patient's understanding does not always correspond to the global (biomedical) representation of the illness. Common sense explanations which reflect both community understandings and personal idiosyncratic understandings may diverge significantly. Diabetes seems like an unusual illness, in that it is new and increasingly widespread on Réunion Island. In an empirical way, the person diagnosed with diabetes is drawn to considerations about many factors, as diabetes is poorly explained, remains long invisible, and becomes a chronic condition.

Conclusions

It is somewhat perplexing to observe how the medical and lay representations of diabetes are at the same time close, the latter taking the former for their source, and so far apart because they are founded on clearly different knowledges and practices. Medical representations are general and anonymous, while lay representations are often particular and personal. This makes a deconstruction of the biomedical model concerning the illness, its definition and associated symptoms, fundamental, in order to promote the valorization of empirical interpretation, as determined by the local culture and the individual experience of those afflicted by the illness.

In order to combat the current epidemic of diabetes, it is essential to construct models of analysis integrating the logical system of the social group and educational tools reflecting and taking into account existing popular or lay knowledges and practices. In Réunion Island, a few concrete applications following our discussion include: 1) Personalized consultation, including an explanation in clear and suitable terms, establishing an educational diagnosis to determine health objectives that take into consideration life circumstances; 2) Because dietary behaviors are profoundly interiorized and symbolize a particular identity, the dietary regimen should always be personalized and explained collectively; 3) It is equally important that the sufferer be supported in his or her negotiation of the management of everyday life among his relatives; and 4) Because on Réunion Island the use of medicinal plants is widespread, it would be pertinent to compare the composition of the meal to the preparation of a medicinal tea where the plants are chosen and measured precisely. Excessive and inadequate combinations are considered dangerous in both cases: phytotherapy and diet. The reconciliation of the models, medical and lay, is a truly essential step toward taking charge of a chronic illness.

Acknowledgments

The author wishes to thank all those who shared their ideas and understandings about diabetes in Réunion Island. This article was translated from the French by Owen Bradley.

References

Andoche, J. 1988. L'interprétation populaire de la maladie et de la guérison à l'île de La Réunion, *Sciences sociales et santé*, VI (3-4): 145–65.

_____1989. Partir d'une ethnographie des troubles mentaux : les représentations de la personne et du corps à l'île de La Réunion, *Nouvelle Revue d'Ethnopsychiatrie*, 14: 111–22.

Aronowitz, R. 1999. *Les maladies ont-elles un sens?*, Le Plessis-Robinson, Institut Synthélabo, 379p.

Auge M., Herzlich, C. 1984. *Le Sens du mal. Anthropologie, histoire, sociologie de la maladie*, Paris, Ed. des Archives Contemporaines, 278 p.

Baszanger, I. 1986. Les Maladies chroniques et leur ordre négocié, *Revue française de sociologie*, XXVII: 3–27.

Benoist, J. 1984. *Paysans de La Réunion*, Aix-en-Provence, PU d'Aix-Marseille, 240p.

_____1993. *Anthropologie médicale en société créole*, Paris, PUF, coll. Des champs de la santé, 215 p.

Bonnet de Paillerets, F., et al. 1998. Le Diabète : pour une meilleure prise en charge de la pathologie chronique, in *Annexes du rapport 1998 de la conférence nationale de santé du 22-23-24 juin*, Paris, DGS, II(3), 24p.

Bonnoil, J.L. 1992. Processus identitaires dans les situations de «métissage» : la logique de la partition, in J.L. ALBER et al., *Métissages. Linguistique et anthropologie*, Saint-Denis, L'Harmattan, II : 109–20.

Canguilhem, G. 1966. *Le Normal et le pathologique*, Paris, PUF.

Cohen, P. 1994. Alimentation, corps et santé à l'île de La Réunion, *Prévenir*, 26: 45–56. Collectif, 1998, *Rapport du groupe de travail. Diabètes. Prévention, dispositifs de soin et éducation du patient*, Paris, Ministère de l'Emploi et de la Solidarité - Haut Comité de la santé publique, mai, 62p.

Corin, E. 1996. La matrice sociale et culturelle de la santé et de la maladie, in EVANS R.G., BARER M.L., MARMOR T.R. (sous la direction de), 1996, *Etre ou ne pas être en bonne santé. Biologie et déterminants sociaux de la maladie*, Paris, J.L. Eurotext et P. U. de Montréal, (traduit en français par M. GIRESSE), 103–41.

Direction Générale de la Santé (DGS). 1999. *Circulaire 99/264 relative à l'organisation des soins pour la prise en charge du diabète de type 2, non-insulinidépendant*, Ministère de l'emploi et de la solidarité/DGS, 4 mai, 13p.

Duchemann, B. 1900. Les Plantes médicinales, in *Exposition universelle de 1900. Colonies françaises. La Réunion*, Paris, Librairie africaine et coloniale, 305 p.

Flick, U. (sous la direction de). 1992. *La Perception quotidienne de la santé et de la maladie. Théories subjectives et représentations sociales*, Paris, L'Harmattan, traduit de l'allemand par A. CREAU et S.VEZINA, coll. Santé, Sociétés et Cultures, 375p.

Frankenberg, R. 1988"Your Time or Mine ?" An Anthropological View of the Tragic Temporal Contradictions of Biomedical Practice. *International Journal of Health Services*, 18(1): 11–34.

Good, B.J. 1998. *Comment faire de l'anthropologie médicale ? Médecine, rationalité et vécu*, Le Plessis-Robinson, Institut Synthélabo, (traduit de l'américain par S. GLEIZE), 372 p.

Hermann, P. 1920. *Histoire et géographie de l'Ile de La Réunion*, Paris : Librairie Dela grave, 59p.

Hubert, A. 1995. Anthropologie et recherche biomédicale. De quoi parle donc l'anthropologie médicale ?, in BARE J.F. (sous la direction de), *Les Applications de l'anthropologie. Un essai de réflexion collective depuis la France*, Paris, Ed. Karthala: 221–39.

_____1997. Adaptabilité humaine : biologie et culture. Du corps pesant au corps léger : approche anthropologique des formes, *Diététique et médecine*: 83–89.

Kirchgassler, K., Matt, E. 1987. La Fragilité du quotidien : les processus de normalisation dans les maladies chroniques, *Sciences Sociales et Santé*, V(1) 93–114.

Kleinman, A. 1992. Pain and Resistance: the delegitimation and relegitimation of local worlds, in *Pain as human experience : an anthropological perspective*, Berkeley CA: University of California Press, 169–98.

Lavergne, R. 1989. *Plantes médicinales indigènes. Tisanerie et tisaneurs de La Réunion*, Doct. Bot. Trop. Appliquée, Montpellier.

Lopez, A. 1987. Le rôle de la départementalisation dans les grandes conquêtes sanitaires et sociales à l'île de La Réunion, *Bulletin de l'association géographique française*, 5, 377–94.

MacAuliffe, J.M. 1902. *Cilaos pittoresque et thermal. Guide médical des eaux thermales*, Saint-Denis, Azalées Ed.- Grand Océan : 217–18.

Marimoutou, M. 1989. *Les engagés du sucre*, Saint-Denis, éd. du Tramail, 171p.

Marzouk, Y. 1995. Fausses connivences et malentendus productifs entre patients maghrébins et praticiens hospitaliers, *Journal des anthropologues*, 60 : 41–50.

Masse, R. 1995. *Culture et santé publique. Les contributions de l'anthropologie à la prévention et à la promotion de la santé*, Montréal, Gaëtan Morin Ed., 471 p.

Massiau, C. 1990. *Les Plantes de La Réunion à visée anti-diabétique*, Doct. Pharm., Grenoble 1.

Mintz, S.W. 1991. *Sucre Blanc, misère noire. Le goût et le pouvoir*, Paris, Nathan, coll. Essais et Recherches, (traduit de l'américain par R. GHANI), 231 p.

Morgan, L.M. 1990. The Medicalization of Anthropology : A Critical Perspective on the Critical-Clinical Debate, *Social Science and Medicine* 30(9) : 945–50.

Morizot, J. 1838. *Considérations historiques et médicales sur l'état de l'esclavage à l'île Bourbon (Afrique), suivies d'un coup d'œil sur quelques-unes des maladies les plus communes chez les noirs de cette colonie*, Doct. Méd., Montpellier.

Obadia, G. et al. 1986. Prise en charge hospitalière du diabète insulino-traité chez les immigrés africains en France, *Diabète & Métabolisme*, 12: 16–20.

Potier, J.and R. Potier. 1971. *Etude anthropologique d'une zone sucrière à La Réunion : le Gol et son aire d'approvisionnement. Travail sur l'organisation sociale de la région de Saint-Louis*, Tananarive : Musée de l'université de Madagascar, 219p.

Raimbault, C. 1948. *Les Plantes médicinales de l'île de La Réunion*, Saint-Denis, Imprimerie Dieu et Patrie, 58 p.

Roddier, M. 1995. Diabète sucré et culture à l'île de La Réunion, *Cahiers d'Anthropologie et Biométrie Humaine*, XIII (3-4): 335–55.

———1998. *Enquête sur les comportements alimentaires et le mode de vie des femmes réunionnaises âgées de 20 à 59 ans. Résultats de l'enquête anthropologique*, Saint-Denis, PRS/ORS, 39 p.

———1999. *Le diabète entre culture et santé publique. Approche anthropologique des représentations du diabète de type 2 à La Réunion*, Thèse de Doctorat d'Anthropologie, La Réunion, 635p.

———2003. Plantes médicinales et diabète : des savoirs populaires qui co-existent avec la biomédecine, *La phytothérapie européenne*, 16: 11–15.

Roddier, M. and X. Debussche. 2001. La prise en compte des particularités individuelles des diabétiques. Etude anthropologique à l'île de La Réunion, *Diabète éducation*, 11 (1), 8–14.

Zempleni, A. 1985. La maladie et ses «causes», *L'Ethnographie*, LXXXI (2): 13–44.

Nêhinaw (Cree) Socioeconomic, Political and Historical Explanations about the Collective Diabetes Experience

Jocelyn Bruyère

The person must look after everything. That is the way we used to look after ourselves a long time ago. Today we are trying to be Wamistikosew (white men). I do not condone the way we are being looked after today. Ever since the white man controlled me, I am sick. Ha, ha.

> Nêhinaw Elder, Manitoba, Canada

Summary of Chapter 5. This chapter describes a project with 22 members of the Nêhinaw of Opaskwayak Cree Nation to collect their understanding of diabetes. The indepth interviews were conducted in the Cree language. This First Nation is situated on the banks of the Saskatchewan River north of the town of The Pas, Manitoba, in Canada. Explanations offered by the tribal members of this community incorporate socioeconomic, political and historical understandings about the dynamics of this illness. A pervasive theme running through personal narratives is that this ailment is new, European, and was unknown prior to colonization. The Nêhinaw of Opaskwayak view recent ecological disruptions, pollution, and hydro development as having contributed to the increase in the rates of diabetes in their community.

ﺯ ﺯ ﺯ

Historical Background: The Disruption of Cree Traditional Life

Historically, contact with the new peoples of North America brought with it contagious diseases to which North American original inhabitants were not immune, and the effect was to devastate whole populations. The First Nation people are experiencing a new assault to their well-being, this time, in the form of an epidemic of diabetes.

Type 2 diabetes mellitus and its sequelae are rapidly increasing among many First Nations people today (Young 1993; Health Canada 2000).

In contrast to the abundance of literature examining biological factors, genetic contributions, prevalence, and distribution, there are few studies which address perspectives and understandings of this disease among First Nations peoples (see Rokala et al. 1991). Yet, very little is known about collective tribal or individual understandings regarding diabetes among First Nations peoples. The emergence of type 2 diabetes has been observed amongst Indigenous Peoples who have experienced transition and change to a diet which is non-traditional to their cultures (Eaton 1977; Young 1994). However, few studies address the issue of the dynamics that sociocultural exploitation and colonization have played in the increase of this illness amongst Indigenous Peoples.

Health Canada statistics indicate type 2 diabetes to be the most prevalent chronic disease suffered by First Nations peoples (Health Canada 2000). Manitoba has the highest percentage of First Nations people with diabetes by region in the entire country (Bobet 1998). The Manitoba First Nation Regional Health Survey estimated that the overall prevalence of self-reported diabetes in the general population of Manitoba First Nations is 18% (Elias and Sanderson 1998). Further, there is evidence that type 2 diabetes occurs in Aboriginal children in Manitoba who are under the age of 15 (Dean et al. 1992; 1995).

It has long been noted that perceptions of illness, cultural norms, and individual response to illness may influence morbidity and mortality levels (Suchman 1964). Adherence to diet regimen was reported to be low among Indigenous Peoples with diabetes mellitus in several nations because of food preferences and other cultural factors (Broussard et al. 1982; Lang 1985; Tom-Orme 1994). Few studies attempt to examine First Nation socioeconomic conditions and feelings of external control which influence these conclusions regarding "noncompliance."

This project sought to document tribal perspectives about diabetes among the Nêhinaw (Cree) of Opaskwayak, a First Nation which is situated north of the town of The Pas, Manitoba. One of the investigators was a Nêhinaw from this First Nation who explored diabetes from a language speaker's "emic" viewpoint of the illness. An "emic" approach strives for a high degree of internal validity which reflects "a valid understanding of the local context in its own terms" (Kleinman 1988: 28). The site chosen for the project was the Nêhinaw community of Opaskwayak Cree Nation (OCN). The word Opaskwayak is Nêhinawawin (Cree language), meaning "wooded narrows." This term is used in Nêhinaw to describe a place for high ground with a wooded area, in comparison to the flatness of the surrounding Saskram and the Carrot River Valley areas. Opaskwayak is situated 630 kilometres on PTH 10 northwest of Winnipeg, Manitoba, a boreal forest area which borders on the Canadian Pre-Cambrian shield.

Traditionally, Opaskwayak was a site where hunting, fishing, social, and Mite'wiwin (Medewin among the Anishinaabeg) gatherings took place. The Grand Medicine Society gatherings took place amongst this group of Nêhinaw (Opaskwayak Cree Nation 1996). The Grand Medicine Society, a medicine lodge which was an hierarchical institution, is Ojibwa in origin and a "late acquisition" among the Cree (Hallowell 1936: 33).

Other history among the Nêhinaw talked about by the elders is the sacred rock of Wapasquiak (Elder George Lathlin 1996, in Constant 1996). The description of this sacred rock is not dissimilar to the "Iron Stone" described by Dempsey, who stated that this was a great monument venerated by the Plains Cree as a guardian of the Buffalo

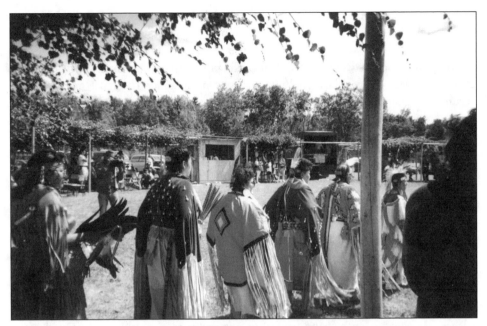

Cree Confederacy Pow Wow at the Opaskwayak Cree Nation Summer 1999 (Photo by author).

and Indian people (Dempsey 1984). According to the elders, the sacred rock was rolled into the Saskatchewan River on the urging of an Anglican missionary (Henry Budd) at that time (Constant 1996). The "Iron Stone" of Big Bear's people in Saskatchewan met a similar fate (that is, taken away) in the hands of the Methodist missionaries in 1866 (Dempsey 1984). The "shaking tent", much documented among the Ojibway and the eastern Cree, was also part of Opaskwayak Nêhinaw oral history and recently recounted and published in the OCN paper, *Natotawin* (Constant 1996). These traditions indicate that not only was the historical past of Opaskwayak shared with other tribal Cree peoples, but they also shared knowledge of concepts regarding power and spirituality. Indeed, Opaskwayak continues to be important as a gathering place. This is evidenced by the Cree Confederacy gatherings which have been a recent phenomenon (founded at Opaskwayak Cree Nation), wherein Cree peoples across Canada meet who are from locations across Canada from Quebec to Alberta and which includes the "southern Cree" of the Rocky Boy Reservation in Montana.

The language spoken by the Nêhinaw is the one known as the "n" Cree dialect. Early historical records indicate that contact in the Opaskwayak area began in the fur trade era when the Saskatchewan River delta was occupied by the Basquais, a Cree tribal people who spoke Cree with the "th" dialect. However, the Saskatchewan River delta was almost totally depopulated of the Basquais by a smallpox epidemic in the years between 1781 to 1782 (Tomison 1952, *in* Meyer 1985). The more eastern Crees then introduced the "n" dialect when they moved into the area. A century later, the area then known as Le Pas, North West Territories, experienced the impact of the joining of Manitoba to confederation. A subsequent census in 1870 records that the population of the Nêhinaw was 558. It was also noted in the same census that there were 5,757 Metis, 4,083 "English half breeds", and 1,565 "Whites," reflecting the colonization and subsequent economic activity in the area at that time (<www.nwnet.ca/thepas/hist.html>).

In 1876, Treaty Number Five was signed on behalf of the Opaskwayak Nêhinaw. Mainly, the objective of this treaty process in northern Manitoba (which was sparse of agricultural land) was related to "natural resource use" (Waldram 1988: 39). The understandings of these First Nations people regarding the treaty at that time was described by Waldram (1988: 41) as follows: "When Treaty Commissioner Thomas Howard tried to secure the signatures of Indians missed during the previous year's work, the Indians requested terms similar to those in treaty six, which had just been signed to the west of them, and whose terms they knew." The terms of this "treaty six" provided for more land (640 acres as opposed to 160 acres per family of five) and included the "medicine chest treaty." These terms were rejected by the commissioner (Waldram 1988). The population recorded at this time was 599. Following the trend of colonization at the time, several Church missions were established. No doubt the most influential among the Nêhinaw was the Anglican Church mission, which was established by Henry Budd (a Cree missionary who was educated at the Red River Settlement) in 1840 (The Pas and District Horizons c1988). During the treaty making process, commissioner Howard proposed a relocation plan for what was then and until recently, known as "The Pas Band," but this met with opposition from them (Waldram 1988). However, in 1906, the Nêhinaw occupation of the south side of the Saskatchewan River came to an end when the land for the present town site of The Pas was "bought" from the band (<www.nwnet.ca/thepas/hist.html>). The Opaskwayak Nêhinaw were then forced to relocate north of the Saskatchewan River.

In order to appreciate the impacts of relocation on the Opaskwayak Nêhinaw, a cursory look at the history of developments in the area surrounding the reserve is important. Historical records indicate that there had been flooding of the Saskatchewan River. In 1902 when "From Cedar Lake to Cumberland House the only dry land was at The Pas, and at the Barrier," and in 1948 when the effect was described as "inundating the farming area of the Carrot River Valley" (<www.nwnet.ca/thepas/hist. html>). These events led to other projects which would affect the natural environment and the Nêhinaw.

The first, the "Pasqua Reclamation Project," was initiated to protect some 138,000 acres from future flooding. The Carrot River Valley was cultivated by the non-Nêhinaw occupants of the area who were the beneficiaries of such a project. The result is 75,000 acres under cultivation because of the rich soil, and are "some of the most productive farmlands in western Canada" (The Pas Chamber of Commerce 1996). However, these dams, dykes, and drainage canals had affected trapping and hunting areas for the Nêhinaw.

The second "stage" of these developments which had an impact on the way of life for the Nêhinaw was a waterfowl conservation project. The Bracken Dam, built at the junction of the Saskram and Carrot Rivers by a water fowl conservation establishment, altered water levels of the Saskram marshes (<www.nwnet.ca/thepas/hist.html>). In addition, in 1955, the Pasqua River dam was built as well as a canal to divert the Pasqua River into the Carrot River. The resulting dams, diversions, and projects served to deplete the trapping, fishing, and fowling for the Opaskwayak Nêhinaw.

A further development, which served to disrupt the traditional life ways and ended the muskrat trapping in the area of the Nêhinaw, was when the Manitoba Hydro project at Grand Rapids was implemented in 1963. A dam was constructed on the Saskatchewan River, raising Moose Lake and Cedar Lake water levels and flooding many thousands of acres, and disrupting much wild life habitat. This project flooded 7,000 acres of land which was held in trust by Canada and belonging to The Pas, Moose

Lake, and Chemawawin Bands (Ralph Abramson, personal communication 1997). At that time, Mr. J.R. Bell, Indian superintendent, noted that "Many of the resources from which the people derived a livelihood will be lost or seriously depleted for a number of years and in some cases, possibly forever" (Waldram 1988: 97).

The process of constructing a paper mill complex north of the Saskatchewan River in The Pas began in 1967 (Economic Development, The Pas Office 1998). This development also had an impact on the environment surrounding this Nêhinaw community.

These projects all had an impact on the way of life for the Nêhinaw, who, into the 1950s and early 1960s were pursuing trapping, fishing, fowling, and hunting as a major subsistence activity. However, because of the imposed changes, subsistence activity was impacted negatively and brought about many changes to the Nêhinaw.

An example of the economic situation faced by the Nêhinaw in the early and mid-1960s reveals that this First Nation was not exceptional in its situation from those across Canada, in respect to the poverty conditions that they were forced to face. In a journal kept by a councillor at that time, the total unconditional grant budget from the government for the band was $2,376.00 for the year. There were no waterworks. The band council's priorities at this time reflected the conditions. For the year 1964, the band's projects from the grant included the repair of a tractor, two church renovations, a new road, and one person was employed at a rate of $2.00 (two dollars) a day. Mention was made that there were 17 families in 1976 who did not have "privies", and a concern regarding the water supply (Beatrice Wilson, personal communication 1996). Because of the imposed changes, subsistence activities were drastically affected.

This First Nation, among others in Canada, has undergone a rapid socioeconomic transition. The Nêhinaw subsistence economy has suffered great blows from the development of hydroelectric projects, as well as other development projects. Perhaps more profound was the aforementioned Manitoba hydroelectric project which raised water levels and flooding 7000 acres of land in the 1960s. Among other environmental disruptions, it effectively ceased muskrat trapping for the Opaskwayak Cree Nation (Ralph Abramson, personal communication August 2, 1996). Although there is still high unemployment, the Opaskwayak Cree Nation is rapidly developing projects which can alleviate this problem.

The registered population of Opaskwayak Cree Nation was 3,538 people as of October 2, 1996, at the time of this study. There were 447 housing units (OCN 1996). The sudden increase in population was, in part, attributable to the enactment of Bill C31 of the Indian Act. (This act allowed those members previously enfranchised and their children, admission to status.) Of the OCN total population, 2,298 members were on-reserve as of June, 1996, and 1139 off-reserve. Nêhinawawin (Cree) is spoken as the working language (with some mixture of English) among the people, and it is taught in school. Historically, this First Nation's people have, amongst others, experienced externally-controlled boarding schools and day schools where speaking Nêhinawawin was discouraged (Friesen et al. 1996). A one-room day school on the reserve existed prior to the construction of a four-classroom day school. After 1968 the Opaskwayak Cree Nation children were forced to attend the schools located in the town of The Pas. After a lengthy and complicated process, this First Nation now has a locally controlled school (the Joseph Albert Ross School) which offers courses to grade 12 based on culturally relevant curricula.

A look at the history of diabetes in this community reveals that there has been a steady increase of people diagnosed with diabetes, almost doubling each decade. In

1976, there were 38 people who had been diagnosed with diabetes out of a total of 1020 on-reserve members at that time (Beatrice Wilson, personal journal Sept. 1996). In 1986, there were 75 people with diabetes when the on-reserve population was 1408 (E. Personius, personal communication Sept. 1996). In 1996, approximately 176 people of the 2,399 were on the chronic list as having been diagnosed. The present estimate is 262 of the 2652 on-reserve population.

In the following section we will examine explanations and statements about diabetes in their community given by 22 Opaskwayak residents.

Etiology: *Wāmistikosew, Me'chim,* and Ecological Destruction

The Nêhinaw interviewees see diabetes as a new, or a European disease which was not experienced until recent times. Their perceptions encompass understandings that the Nêhinaw were a strong people in the past who related to and depended on nature and wildlife for sustenance. However, the changes and environmental destruction they see around them are witness to the disruption of their way of life. This threat was expressed eloquently by a woman, who stated her understanding of the sudden increase of diabetes in the community. The explanations include not only change in diet as a factor, but also include the socioeconomic and political realities which she feels that the Nêhinaw had to face in recent years. I include a substantial amount of her account, as it provides a picture on the recent past for the Nêhinaw and allows for a better appreciation of their experience and relationship with food and the environment. It also expresses the meaning and importance of *Me'chim* to the Nêhinaw. She relates her own experience, and draws an eloquent picture of the recent past of Opaskwayak.

> We didn't eat that way long ago…And…we had duck, moose, eggs…we used to go by canoe to pick eggs, we did not buy them from the store. And we used to have our own chickens. My late father had his own. We ate chicken from there too. Also in the store we did not even buy our own gum from the store. A tree from the bush…we looked for it…and we used to dig our own gum from there. We also got our tea from the tree. Leaves, green; we used to use wood to make fire to make our own bannock. We used to use a tilted frying pan or even used heated rocks to bake bannock. The bannock used to cook there. They also made these smoke tents (*akowana*) from sticks. To smoke fish and sometimes they used to mince the fish. And also meat was dried there… crushed and also made *moosopimii* (sometimes called *pemmican*), they used to call it. And we hung ducks and geese in the shed. We ate them in the winter…beaver, grouse [partridge], rabbits. We never bought anything from the store. When we had a lot of meat we…*aki ne ke monipimichankanan* (foraged) *Ni ke monipitenan*. Water…they used to go and we used to go to the wilds..and we used to get fish and water. I don't know…we used berries, we used to pick all the time and make jam. We never used to use the store too much. I think that is where it (*sôkkawaspinewin*) comes from. We eat store-bought food… even sardine. Fish was smoked hung upside down…in clearwater lake and we

used horses in winter to get it. We ate that [fish] in the winter. Even potatoes. They made a hole…we had put them in a hole. Even carrots, rhubarbs, corn, onions, they grew. We used to use the cows milk from a cow who had a calf… we used to use the milk from that. Nothing from the store. It worked right a long time ago. Now we go to the store and this is where we are very much sick from. Also the power we use, if we put this in the fridge or the deep freeze, we freeze the food…freeze it. We don't know if it is spoiled. Then we thaw it and we don't know if it has spoiled. Even if you find that the meat looks green the storekeeper will get mad if you take it back. This has happened to me many times, green meat, when I returned it. Even…the vegetables we buy, they also spoil from the store. They did not spoil. We kept them ourselves…our grand-father…they used to keep them and we also knew that they were not spoiled. We used wood to burn and we used ice from the river. It is only recently that we have begun to use this [technology]. In the winter we used to use ice, blocks of ice. We used to drag the ice from the river. Not like these things— it is only now that we are beginning to use these things (*Pise'wiskwāō*).

This account is drawn from a Nêhinaw woman's own life experience and how the relationship with the environment has changed over the recent past. She relates the ill-ness to changes in technology, the modern way of life for the Nêhinaw, and the in-creased reliance on store bought foods. The woman concluded:

A kee meecheeak uskeek ochi [We ate from the land]. *We were rich in the past, now we are poor.* We were able to have everything from the earth. We didn't take anything to buy.

Although her views about changes in diet and food preparation agree with the An-ishinaabe (Garro 1996) as well as other interpretations (Lang 1986), this woman's nar-rative about the recent past vividly draws a picture of Opaskwayak Nêhinaw practices relating to the sources of *Me'chim* (food) as well as their procurement, preservation, and preparation. Indeed, Cree rituals have been described by Rogers as revolving mainly about the food quest, and that it was "uppermost in the minds and thoughts of the Mistassini Cree" (Rogers 1969). However, the loss of hunting and gathering tra-ditions is pervasive in the understandings of the individuals I interviewed about the increased incidence of diabetes in the community.

These understandings reflect cultural and socioeconomic realities. Although there are a few individual idiosyncratic explanatory models, in large part most of the Nêhi-naw explanations complement each other. There is agreement about the causes and ef-fects of diabetes, not unlike other Indigenous Peoples, such as the Dakota (Lang 1986) and the Anishinaabe (Garro 1996), for whom diabetes is a relatively recent phenome-non related to the change from traditional to "modern" life ways. However, for the Nêhinaw these explanations are specifically related to the more recent developments and resultant decrease in the trapping, fishing, gathering, and hunting traditions due to environmental disruptions. One individual stated:

I don't know, maybe it is something we eat…using too much chemicals, they are killing our…like the fish used to taste good but now they do not. Since they had that sawmill (pulp and paper mill), when it started…that is when

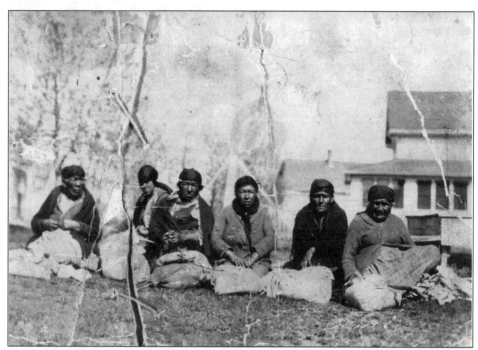

A group of women with rations taken in late 1930 near the nursing station that was known locally as "the little medicine house." Contents of ration allotment: Flour, salt pork, white beans, and tallow. It is not only the change in food but indeed the abject poverty under which many first Nations were forced to live. (Courtesy: B. Wilson)

> people got sick. Because a long time ago nobody used to get sick. Too much pollution…they are killing our wild meat, too (*Pinā'ses*).

The loss of the traditional food is also related to the loss of traditional medicines (herbal) and the way of life, with subsequent reliance on store-bought food, as seen in the narrative below:

> Because we eat differently. We eat like the white man. This is what I think. Because a long time ago we did not open anything in a can. I remember when I was a child. Everything was grown, or people hunted. This is where we ate from. Today we just go and buy everything. We do not know what is in it. This is where it comes from, I think (*Nis'ku*).

> Because there was not anything like we have. Well, the way Indians used to live, they did not get no sugar or nothing to cause diabetes (*Sese'p*).

> *Mache maka* [as you know], they did not have it…long ago…the food was very good…but now, "Ducks Unlimited" is spoiling (destroying) everything… he destroyed the ducks also…yeah (*Mu'skwa*).

The majority of the interviewees (20 out of 22) viewed the increase in diabetes in the community as a consequence of the destruction of the environment which until recent times had provided sustenance. The *Wāmistikosew* (white man) is seen to have effected the destruction which the Nêhinaw see around them. One individual put it more succinctly as a political statement: there is a threat to the very identity of the Nêhinaw. The following statement reveals some power relations which operate today in the area:

> ...even a plane, CFI [pulp and paper mill situated north of the reserve], cars... they are beginning to destroy the plants and leaves, the wild animals cannot eat. They are the ones who are doing this. "Ducks Unlimited" also are drying up the lakes and the wild animals do not have a place to drink. They are starting to die out because they are being killed by the white men. It was very bad (*pakotigon*) when the white man first came. He is destroying everything. He (*Wāmistikosew*—the white man) will even begin to take us out of our homes...evict us from our homes. He will vie for the reserve here. He will try to take this reserve here (*Pise'wiskwāo*).

> I have come to see this. And all these planes and cars that are becoming ubiquitous? That is what they used to tell us about. They (the elders) used to say that they would not see this but now I see that the white man (*Wāmistikosew*) is taking everything over. That they really control us. Even if there is a house being opened, I see a white man already working there. Take, for example, at the old folks home, all you see is white women working there. They will not make room for you. If you apply, you will not be chosen...they will take an outsider, a white person. They will be chosen because these people in the office are afraid of the white man. Those are the ones who are doing these things (*Pise'wiskwāo*).

The "store bought food" model has been discussed by other Indigenous Peoples in their accounts of diabetes (Garro 1996; Lang 1986 and Ch. 9 in this volume). A Nêhinaw woman, however, offered a more elaborate explanation. She suggests that the change in diet for the Nêhinaw has many meanings. Although she did not have the appropriate terminology for the concept of what has often been termed as "internal neo-colonialism" (O'Neil 1986), her theory explains the effects of European encroachment and external control, revealing historical changes in the Nêhinaw way of life. The woman also warns us that if the people are not careful, they will " lose" their culture and identity. It is a commentary which reveals the inequitable relationship with the non-Nêhinaw population. "We are going to lose everything" is a profound statement and a clear warning that external control will eventually destroy the Nêhinaw. It reveals the socioeconomic and political changes which have resulted in the increase in diabetes within the community. Another Nêhinaw woman noted that the changes and the destruction of the environment are being caused by the *Wāmistikosew*, leading to less wild food for the Nêhinaw.

> Maybe...I don't know what we can attribute it to, blame it on. I have never heard of people talking about it. But they cannot blame it on the medicine. Only that. They are eating too much from the store. Today there is very little Indian food available. The way the people used to live. They used to talk about using a lot of fish and also moose, duck, rabbit. I heard one man talking: "Just outside my door...I do not walk far to get my snare and I can have a rabbit to eat." I believe him. It is true. There used to be a lot of bush here. You did not have to go far to go to the bush here. That was the extent of the amount of bush that was here. Today, one has to go far. You must ride to get that far...when you want to go

snaring [rabbits], or when you want to go and do your stuff in the bush…to get good food. Or fish. Today you can't take it from the river, to eat fish…so many things are being destroyed. Because the white man, *Wāmistikosew*, is pulling everything to himself to make money for himself from our land here (*Pinā'ses*).

Her explanation touched on the theme about environmental destruction and external control. In total, the majority of informants attributed the increase in diabetes in the community to the sometimes narrowly described "change in diet" from a traditional to a modern one. The sociohistoric explanations mean many things to the Nêhinaw: The loss of control, the loss of the way of life due to external control, and destruction of the hunting way of life. It is not my intent here to expound on neo-colonialism, which has greatly affected the Nêhinaw. Neither do I suggest that every Nêhinaw feels this way. However, the discussion on the causation of diabetes evoked an explanatory model which has wide cultural, historic, and political associations for the people, who see it also as an issue of "class and power" (Scheper-Hughes 1988). Similarly, other studies have found that diabetes is often seen as the result of the white man's destruction of tribal society and culture (Tom-Orme 1994; Lang 1986; Garro 1996). The " white man" or *W_mistikosew* which is talked about here is a concept which gives meaning to the political control exercised over the Nêhinaw. The concept also serves to differentiate between "others" who have the power to effect those changes, and the Nêhinaw, who do not. Indeed, Adelson (2000) found that the Cree meaning of health was tied into politics.

Me'chim (Food), History, and Politics

Nêhinaw ancestors are seen to have been a strong People because of the hunting lifestyle they led. The way they lived off the land and the use they made of plants and animals around them gave them power. "They ate right" is often a phrase used, perhaps reflecting the value placed on *Me'chim*, in view of previous and present understandings of Nêhinaw culture. Indeed, Adelson (2000) aptly described the Cree concept of "*miyopimatiseewin*," which she translated into English as "being alive well." A Cree hunter's attributes is being able to eat the right food, as an individualt succinctly clarified: "They had wild food..they were very strong. There was not much that could destroy them" (*Penā'o*). Other interviewees agreed:

> …I listen to the elders…a long time ago…I hear the elders…because they never had this illness. They had to do without [modern conveniences] each day. And the way that they cooked for themselves a long time ago…they boiled everything…that is what they think is where we get this diabetes, this food, the canned food…and foods we rush to eat [fast foods]. This is where they think it comes from…this diabetes (*U'misk*).

> Not as much [diabetes], I guess. They had wild food. They did not have salt (*Numā'o*).

Other explanations given by the Nêhinaw discuss individual responsibility and biomedical information. According to Adelson, "Eating well for the Cree incorporates notions of living well that are rooted in Cree life and practice. Being Alive well is ultimately

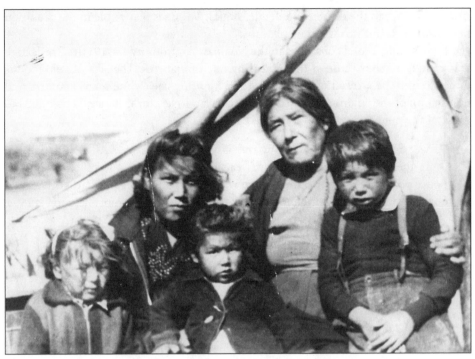

A "Kookum"spring camp with the grandchildren in Opaskwayak Cree Nation Traditional lands. This is taken in the late 1940s. (Courtesy of Gladys Munro, granddaughter).

tied to all that it means to be Cree and thus eat cultural food" (Adelson 2000). This understanding may translate into food now being considered a locus of control exercised by foreign populations over the Nêhinaw. Indeed, as Lang and Garro observed, "Foods and food ways constitute complex codes for social relations and symbols of cultural identity and change and as they are linked to aspects to health and illness provide salient imagery in which to demarcate community and cultural boundaries" (Garro & Lang 1993: 322).

Nêhinaw men's understandings of diabetes integrates many cultural issues and white/Indian differences in his explanation. His narrative demonstrates that multiple explanations can be held by one person. He stated it this way:

> What I think is...my life...They took the children to the camp...and they were frying food all the time...and that is fried food that brings your sugar up. And then that is what happens to us...but not these young kids, they don't go to the camp any more. They are not doing their culture. Then some of them will not be diabetic. But then some of them will be...because they eat a lot of junk food. But even the white man when he is hunting...he takes a lot of junk food to the camp. But they don't have problems like this. We have more problems like this than the white man (*Wu'chusk*).

This is a complex explanation of causation. Although his initial explanation appears to be extremely idiosyncratic in that he blames his diabetes on "fried moose meat" and his experience with going to camp with his parents, he goes on to elaborate and infer many meanings to the diabetes epidemic."Junk food" does play a role in the causation of the disorder, but it is not the only cause.

There is almost total consensus in the Nêhinaw community (n=19) that the lack of wild food is a major cause of the increasing rate of diabetes. The lack of wild food is understood to be a result of pollution, the *W_mistikosew* (white man's) control and destruction of the environment. The Saskatchewan River, for instance, is polluted because of the pulp and paper mill in The Pas.

> Those things that are there along the Saskatchewan River...All the sewage come there...You know...you can't eat fish from there...too much pollution...you cannot eat fish from there when it is polluted. And that is all...I don't know about Grand Rapids...I don't like to eat fish any more...I am very afraid of it...(*Mooswu*).

> Maybe...REPAP (TOLKO) has lots to do with it...because when that smoke comes out, it always comes out when it's cloudy. When it's a nice day they won't let that smoke come out. Because...someone told me that they saved $20 thousand a day when it's cloudy (*Okimaw*).

Inactivity due to the resulting decrease in wildlife and accompanying traditional activities, and the increased amounts of technology in the form of modern vehicles and technology are also seen as a causal factors. Junk food and sweets, which are considered "*pikonata kekona*," as well as the increased reliance on store bought food are also seen by more than half of the informants as being causal factors for diabetes. There was total consensus among the women, and seven out of the ten men informants, that one of the causes of diabetes in the community was the change from a traditional diet to a modern one, attributed to the increasing lack of wild foods. For these and other tribal peoples, diabetes is known to be new to them, and that understanding of this illness is placed in a broad, and profound sociohistoric perspective reflecting the destruction of the environment, the inequitable treatment that tribal peoples have experienced, and subsequent changes in the traditional way of life (Bruyère 1998; Garro 1999; Lang 1986).

Diabetes stands as a powerful metaphor for the loss of the way of life for the Nêhinaw, in the form of profound socioeconomic and environmental changes to their traditional culture. Opaskwayak Nêhinaw individuals described the destruction of the plant and wildlife of the surrounding area and the traditional hunting territories. Many referred to the smoke that permeates the community on some cloudy days when the wind comes from the northeast. They also talk about "Ducks Unlimited," an institution which has often been seen as being in conflict with Nêhinaw interests regarding hunting and trapping territory. One informant pointed to one of the consequences of the developments: "The people say that the fish do not taste the same, neither do the rabbits down river who eat the bark off the trees." He attributes the latter to the paper mill. There is also a sense that there is a decrease in quality and quantity of wildlife because of increased control by *Wāmistikosew*. There is an understanding that a direct relationship exists between diabetes and the decline of available wildlife for food. There is also a perception that in the past, the human beings (*ininiwuk*) were strong (*ke muskawatiseewak*), and "there was not much that could destroy them" (*Pinā'sew*). This model is drawn from understandings regarding traditional food (*Me'chim*), wildlife, and environment.

The Nêhinaw understandings of diabetes have to do with issues of power, identity, political, and economic control. This becomes clear in the expression used when speaking of external control by *Wāmistikosew*. The following quote perhaps describes best the meaning given to politics and health.

> The person must look after everything. That is the way we used to look after ourselves a long time ago. Today we are trying to be white men. I do not condone the way we are being looked after today. Ever since the white man controlled me, I am sick. Ha, ha (*Pise'wiskwāo*).

Further, the woman stated: "We are going to lose everything." The message is strong and warns us that the Nêhinaw will be destroyed. The very identity of the Nêhinaw is threatened.

Final Thoughts

The broad purpose of the study was to identify Nêhinaw ways of talking about diabetes, and the impact that language has on these understandings. Research directed at understandings of health and illness among North American Indigenous Peoples reveals that these interpretations do not take the form of "impoverished biomedical accounts," but reflect, instead, issues of identity, history, and culture (Garro 1990). This is most certainly true of the accounts of the Nêhinaw informants in this study. Further, the Nêhinaw maintain that "being alive well" among the Cree is deeply rooted in identity and politics, as described in the study conducted by Adelson (2000) among the Whapmagoostui Cree. The concept of power and wellness among the Ojibwa was also described by Black (1977). These themes are clarified in the explanatory models of the Nêhinaw, reflecting profound changes in culture, language, politics and history. Studies directed at how medical knowledge is constructed indicate that social, cultural, economic, political experience and history interacts with interpretations of illness (Kleinman 1979; Garro 1996; Farmer 1996). Broad dimensions about health and wellness must be inclusive of cultural experiences and of the broader historical context.

Acknowledgments

Many thanks to my Opaskwayak Cree Nation collaborators, some of whom have now gone to join the Creator. I also want to thank Linda Garro for advising me on the thesis from which this material is drawn. Thanks to Gretchen Lang, who patiently guided preparation of this document for publication. To all my relations…

References

Adelson, N. 2000. Being Alive Well: Health and the Politics of Cree Well-Being. Toronto, Canada: University of Toronto Press.

Batchelar, T. 1997. The Pas' History. Electronic Document, <www.nwnet.ca/thepas/hist.html>, accessed December 1997.

Black, Mary B. 1977. Ojibwa Power Belief System. *In* The Anthropology of Power. Raymond D. Fogelson and Richard N. Adams, eds. pp. 141–51. New York: Academic Press Inc.

Bobet, E. 1997. Diabetes among First Nations People: Information from the 1991 Aboriginal Peoples Survey carried out by Statistics Canada. Final Draft, July 23, 1997. Ottawa: Health Canada.

Broussard, B. A., M. A. Bass and M. Y. Jackson. 1982. Reasons for Diabetic Diet Non-compliance Among Cherokee Indians. Journal of Nutritional Education. 14(2): 56–57.

Constant, E. 1996. Legend of the Shaking Tent. Opaskwayak Cree Nation: Natotawin. The Pas, Manitoba. September 13.

Dean, H. J., R. L. Mundy and M. Moffatt. 1992. Non-insulin Diabetes Mellitus in Indian Children in Manitoba. Canadian Medical Association Journal 147(1): 52–57.

Dean, H., W. Degroot, A. Henderson and F. Friesen. 1992. NIDDM in Aboriginal Youth. Diabetes News 3(1): 1–11.

Dempsey, H.A. 1984. Big Bear: The End of Freedom. Toronto, Canada: Douglas.

Eaton, Cynthia. 1977. Diabetes, Culture Change, and Acculturation: A Biocultural Analysis. *In* R. Ness, G. H. Pelto, and P .J. Pelto, eds. Medical Anthropology 1(2). New York: Redgrave Publishing Company.

Economic Development, The Pas Office. 1998. Town of The Pas: Community Profile. The Pas: Economic Development Office.

Elias, B. and D. Sanderson. 1999. Preliminary Report on Diabetes: Manitoba First Nation Regional Health Survey. Assembly of Manitoba Chiefs: Manitoba First Nations Health, Information, and Research Committee with the University of Manitoba: Northern Health Research Unit. Winnipeg, Manitoba.

Farmer, Paul. 1992. Aids and Accusation: Haiti and the Geography of Blame. Berkeley: University of California Press.

Friesen, G., A.C. Hamilton and C.M. Sinclair. 1996. Justice Systems and Manitoba's Aboriginal People: An Historical Survey. *In* River Road: Essays in Manitoba And Prairie History Review. G. Freisen, ed. p. 49. Winnipeg: University of Manitoba Press.

Garro, Linda C. 1990. Continuity and Change: The Interpretation of Illness in an Anishinaabe (Ojibway) Community. Culture, Medicine and Psychiatry 14(1): 417–54.

_____1995 Individual or Societal Responsibility? Explanations of Diabetes in an Anishinaabe (Ojibway) Community. Social Science and Medicine 40(1): 37–46.

_____1996. Intracultural Variation in Causal Accounts of Diabetes: A Comparison of Three Canadian Anishinaabe (Ojibway) Communities. Culture, Medicine and Psychiatry 20: 381–420.

Garro, Linda C. and Gretchen Chesley Lang. 1994. Explanations of Diabetes: Anishinaabeg and Dakota Deliberate upon a New Illness. *In* Diabetes as a Disease of Civilization: The Impact of Culture Change on Indigenous Peoples. Jenny R. Joe and Robert S. Young, eds. pp. 293–327. New York: Mouton de Gruyter.

Hahn, R.A. and A. Kleinman. 1983. Biomedical Practice and Anthropological Theory: Frameworks and Directions. Annual Review of Anthropology 12: 305–33.

Hallowell, A.I. 1936. The Passing of the Medewiwin in the Lake Winnipeg Region. American Anthropologist 38: 32–51.

Health and Welfare Canada. 1991. Health Status of Canadian Indians and Inuit— 1990. Ottawa: Minister of National Health and Welfare. Health Canada.

_____2000 Diabetes Among Aboriginal People in Canada: The Evidence. Ottawa: Minister of Health, Canada.

Kleinman, Arthur M. 1978. Concepts and a Model for the Comparison of Medical Systems as Cultural Systems. Social Science and Medicine 12: 85–93.

_____1988. Rethinking Psychiatry: From Cultural Category to Personal Experience. New York: The Free Press.

Kleinman, Arthur M., Leon Eisenberg and Byron Good. 1978. Culture, Illness and Care: Clinical Lessons from Anthropologic and Cross-Cultural Research. Annals of Internal Medicine 88: 251–58.

Lang, Gretchen Chesley. 1989. Making Sense about Diabetes: Dakota Narratives of Illness. Special issue: Anthropological Approaches to Diabetes. Maria Luisa Urdaneta, ed. Medical Anthropology 11:3: 305–27.

_____1986. Diabetes and Health Care in a Sioux Community. Human Organization 44: 251–60.

Lathlin, G. 1996. Opaskwayak Elder Interview. Natotawin, Sept. 1996.

Mandelbaum, D.G. 1979. The Plains Cree: An Ethnographic, Historical, and Comparative Study. Regina: Canadian Plains Research Center.

Meyer, D. 1985. The Red Earth Crees, 1860–1960. Canadian Ethnology Service Paper No. 100. National Museum of Man Mercury Series. Canada: National Museums of Canada.

O'Neil, John D. 1986. Colonial Stress in The Canadian Arctic: An Ethnography of Young Adults Changing. In Anthroplogy and Epidemiology. Craig R. Janes et al., eds. pp. 249–74. Boston: D. Reidel Publishing Company.

Opaskwayak Cree Nation. 1996 Sacred Rock of Wapasquiak. September 13. Opaskwayak Cree Nation.

_____1996 Legend of the Shaking Tent. September 13. Opaskwayak Cree Nation.

_____1996 A Community in Transition Opaskwayak Cree Nation: OCN Communications.

_____1995 Report of the Second Elders' Conference of the Opaskwayak Cree Nation. Elk's Hall, The Pas, Manitoba, July 26 and 27.

Personius, E. 1996. Personal Communication, September 1996.

Rate, RG., W.C. Knowler, H.G. Morse, M.D. Bonnet, J. McVey, C.L. Chervenak, M.G. Smith and G. Pananich. 1983. Diabetes Mellitus in Hopi and Navajo Indians: Prevalence of Microvascular Complications. Diabetes 32: 894–99.

Rogers, E.S. 1969. Natural Environment—Social Organization—Witchcraft: Cree versus Ojibwa—A Test Case. *In* Contributions to Anthropology: Ecological Essays. David Damas, ed. National Museum of Canada Bulletin #230. Anthropological Series No. 86. pp. 24–39. Ottawa: Queen's Printer.

Rokala, D.A., S.G. Bruce and C. Micklejohn. 1991. Diabetes Mellitus in Native Populations of North America: An Annotated Bibliography. Monograph Series No. 4. Northern Health Research Unit. Winnipeg: University of Manitoba.

Scheper-Hughes, Nancy. 1988. The Madness of Hunger: Sickness, Delirium and Human Needs. Culture, Medicine and Psychiatry 12: 429–58.

Sinclair, V. 1994. 'Agreement...Double What We Would Accept'. Friday, September 30. P. 2. Opaskwayak Cree Nation Natotawin.

Suchman, E.A. 1964. Sociomedical Variations among Ethnic Groups. American Journal of Sociology 70: 319–31.

The Pas and District Horizons. 1988. A Brief History of The Pas Indian Band. The Pas and District Horizons (a Special Newspaper Publication). The Pas, Manitoba, pp. 17–18.

Tom-Orme, L. 1994. Traditional Beliefs and Attitudes about Diabetes among Navajos and Utes. *In* Diabetes as a Disease of Civilization: The Impact of Culture Change on Indigenous Peoples. Jenny R. Joe and Robert S. Young, eds. pp. 271–328. New York: Mouton de Gruyter.

Tomison, W. 1952. "Cumberland House Journal, 1781–82". Cumberland and Hudson Bay Journals, 1775–82. E. E. Rich, ed. London: Hudson's Bay Record Society Vol. 15 (Series 2): 1779–82.

Waldram, J.B. 1988. As Long as the Rivers Run: Hydroelectric Development and Native Communities in Western Canada. Winnipeg: University of Manitoba Press.

Young, T. Kue. 1993. Diabetes Mellitus among Native Americans in Canada and the United States: An Epidemiological Overview. American Journal of Human Biology 5: 399–413.

_____1994. The Health of Native Americans: Towards a Biocultural Epidemiology. Oxford: Oxford University Press.

CHAPTER 6

MINO-MIIJIM'S 'GOOD FOOD FOR THE FUTURE': BEYOND CULTURALLY APPROPRIATE DIABETES PROGRAMS

Emily Omura

The White Earth Land Recovery Program seeks to build a good food program to service those who suffer from diabetes, elders and at-risk populations on our reservation through increasing local production and distribution of traditional foods. The project seeks to address the epidemic levels of diabetes in our reservation community, which destroys our people, devastates our communities, taxes our health resource base, and is perhaps the largest health threat to our community. Diabetes is a symptom of the larger loss of our community, and needs to be redressed through the holistic approach of recovery of food production (The White Earth Land Recovery Project, Grant Proposal for Mino-Miijim 2002).

Summary of Chapter 6. During the fall of 2001, the White Earth Land Recovery Project (WELRP), a community-based organization, started the Mino-Miijim program to address epidemic levels of type 2 diabetes on the White Earth Reservation in Northwestern Minnesota. The Mino-Miijim program is an example of the recent movements in community building and wellness taking place in Indigenous communities. Mino-Miijim represents efforts to change the structural violence that perpetuates unhealthy lifestyles within the community, rather than simply treating the "cultural factors" often associated with diseases of modernization like diabetes. This chapter will describe Mino-Miijim and the experiences of the author working with the WELRP.

⟠ ⟠ ⟠

During the third week of each month residents of the White Earth Reservation of Ojibwe in Northern Minnesota can see Mino-Miijim's spectacular blue-green mini-van flying down the back roads of the reservation. Margaret Smith is out delivering, and delivering much more valuable commodities than frozen meat and dried corn. This is no ordinary food; rather, it is a collection of indigenously produced, locally grown and processed, organic traditional food. And perhaps even more importantly, these foods are imbued with special significance to residents of this remote Northern Minnesota community. Even though there is only enough food in each package to

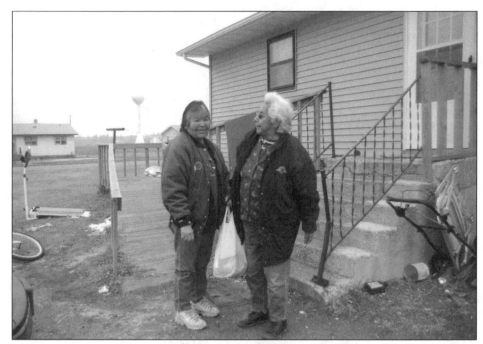

Margaret on deliveries.

make a meal or two, this traditional food could be key to the community's survival. The Mino-Miijim ("Good Food") program delivers these packages to elderly Anishi-naabeg (Ojibwe) suffering from diabetes.

The simple phrase "you are what you eat," has been given extensive meaning by an-thropologists examining the symbolism and aspects of identity that are often found in food. The community at White Earth is no exception, and conceptions of traditional food, while not always strictly from the pre-European contact period, are generally conceived of as idyllic alternatives to the current diet. Food preferences, identity and narratives have an undeniable connection with diabetes; the Mino-Miijim program uses valuations placed on traditional food to promote alternatives in diet, and create a more healthful lifestyle.

Reclamation of resources, gifts of tangible pieces of community identity, and the control over sustainable production are the prescriptions that a traditional food pro-gram like Mino-Miijim can offer.

> "It's not just a medical program, and it's not just a preventative health pro-gram...it's a cultural restoration program" (Interview with the Minneapolis Star Tribune, Winona LaDuke, Oct. 16, 2002).

Mino-Miijim goes beyond superficial notions of being a culturally appropriate pro-gram that treats the "cultural factors" of lifestyle disease. Rather, Winona LaDuke, the Founding Director of Mino-Miijim, and Margaret Smith, an elder and the Program Director of the Mino-Miijim Project, acknowledge a past that has left the community disconnected from resources and dependent on unhealthy systems, much like the sit-uation faced by many other Indigenous Peoples.

The Mino-Miijim Program views diabetes not as a disease, but as a symptom of larger societal problems. Margaret Smith, the Program Director, is a major voice in delivering a powerful and positive message. With the delivery van she takes small steps toward changing huge social structures and redirecting recent history that support lifestyle ailments like diabetes. Within the program diabetes is viewed as part of a historical legacy, with an acknowledgement of the changes to Anishinaabeg connection to resources and sustenance over time. The Mino-Miijim program works to change the underlying causes of the "diabetes lifestyle" through a recovery of resources and control over processes of production. The hope of the program founders is that type 2 diabetes will be given greater dimension than its clinical risk factors, especially in the intersection of community interactions, knowledges, and health. The traditional food approach at Mino-Miijim involves objects, symbols, production processes and ideals that converge to combat type 2 diabetes. The philosophy and implementation of an anti-colonial ideology by a community-based sustainable development project like Mino-Miijim provides a unique demonstration of community empowerment, cultural revitalization, and a repossession of resources.

Methods

This chapter reports on a collaborative effort that reflects my position as a former employee of the Mino-Miijim Project (summer of 2002) and student of my co-workers. Before the final version of this paper was complete, the people I learned from at White Earth had the opportunity to edit content and presentations of themselves within the paper. In this sense, the information in this chapter emerges from a participatory research process as discussed in detail by others in this volume, especially in chapter 16. As an "intern," I assisted with the gathering of food stuffs, the deliveries and on other assorted projects that the White Earth Project and Mino-Miijim sponsored. During the next academic year, with the support of my professors and the hospitality of Margaret Smith and the WELRP staff, I continued to visit, volunteer, and spend time at the White Earth office. The year I spent on the White Earth reservation culminated in the production of my senior thesis, from which this chapter is taken.

Mino-Miijim

We are starting a new food program-and we hope to bring traditional foods to the people-our elders, those who are diabetic and those who need the foods the Creator gave us. Food is a spiritual and physical medicine provided from the Creator, that will keep us well and healthy, as long as we use it in a balanced and respectful way. (Mino-Miijim Brochure 2001)

Mino-Miijim is a grassroots, community based-program, administered through the White Earth Land Recovery Project (WELRP). Mino-Miijim's aim is to promote the delivery of traditional foods to over 150 elders who suffer from diabetes on the reservation every month. The third week of every month, the blue-green tax-exempt van travels all over the reservation delivering packets of buffalo meat, hominy, wild rice, coffee, jam, maple syrup, and broken rice (*mazon*). Its other programs are aimed at a wider population, from school children to adults selling berries. Mino-Miijim's most publicized purpose is to promote the consumption of traditional foods as medicine for the increasing numbers of people who suffer from diabetes on the reservation (cf. LaDuke and Alexander 2004). This mission is complementary to the White Earth Land Recovery Project's goals of producing the traditional food or buying it locally to promote economic development within the community.

Mino-Miijim: Margaret's Program

> I thought of this program because of the high diabetes on White Earth. People are not eating properly. The poor can't even afford to buy hominy. We live on a budget that doesn't last and some people can't get by. I talked with Winona and she figured that we could get money through some foundation to buy our first buffalo. (Personal Communication, Margaret Smith, June 14, 2003)

Informally known around the office and the reservation as "Margaret's food program," Mino-Miijim is successful because of the efforts of this 84-year-old program director. Margaret Smith is a prominent figure in the community, an "honored elder," a great-grandmother several times over, and a recipient of a 2002 McKnight Service Award. She is active in the support of reservation policies and programs, and runs Christmas toy programs out of her own home. Not only was she the impetus for the formation of the program, she is the one who organizes the services of Mino-Miijim around the elders' abilities and desires, inserting the invaluable perspective of an elder with diabetes into the structure of the services which Mino-Miijim offers. An example of the utility of this information is her choice of the third week of every month to deliver food because that "is around when the elders run out of money."

> I love visiting the people because I know, looking at them, I would be lonely if I wasn't out; so I know they are. I can get to see the people. They really need somebody to come in. A lot of them are lonesome. They're really happy when I come. (Personal Communication, Margaret Smith, Oct. 20, 2002)

Margaret has been privately delivering supplemental food for many years and has only recently gained the backing of WELRP to fund her deliveries. Her participation as the program director is essential for the functioning of the program itself, because she is the only one who knows the houses of the elders, the relatives they might be staying with, and all of the back roads of the reservation.

> When me and Paul [her husband] moved back up here from the Cities, we would go and shoot deer and rabbit, then give it to the elders who couldn't go out anymore. (Personal Communication, Margaret Smith, Oct. 20, 2002)

Margaret's participation perpetuates the idea that diabetes is not an isolated individual's disease, but is a community ailment. According to Margaret, solutions to the

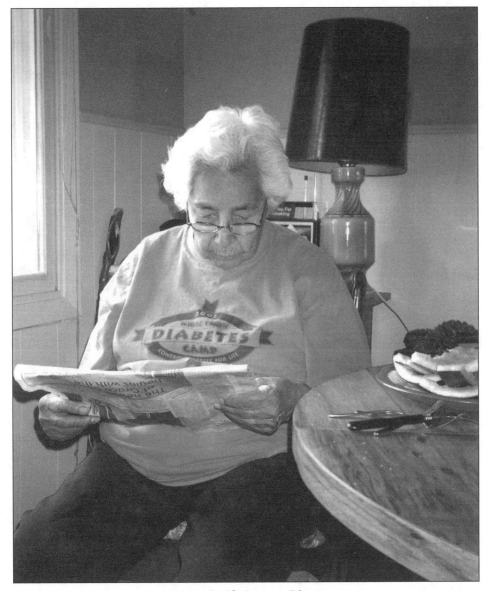

Margaret Smith: Program Director

problem cannot be sought solely in biomedicine, but in larger community changes and actions.

White Earth Land Recovery Project (WELRP)

The Mino-Miijim program is based out of the WELRP office. The closest town is Ponsford, Minnesota, just south of the White Earth Reservation. White Earth Reservation is located in Becker, Clearwater, and Mahnomen counties in north-central Minnesota. Created in 1867 by a treaty between the United States and the Mississippi Band

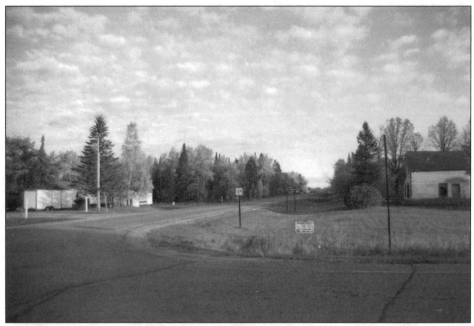

Delivering in Ponsford.

of Chippewa/Ojibwe Indians, it is one of the seven Chippewa/Ojibwe reservations in Minnesota. The White Earth Band of Ojibwe constitutes an amalgam of different clans that go by the overarching designation of Ojibwe. The term "Ojibwe" is preferred over "Chippewa" in designating tribal affiliation. "Anishinaabe" and its plural "Anishnaabeg" are the Ojibwe words for "original people" and are used often by community members to refer to themselves.

Currently the White Earth Reservation is 20,225 members strong, and approximately 4000 of those enrolled members live on the reservation itself. The diabetes epidemic is present on the White Earth Reservation, and becoming a growing concern. On the reservation the White Earth Health Services treats approximately 860 people with diabetes. The number of people who have not been diagnosed is unknown. Some informal estimates put the percentage of diabetes patients as more than 27 percent (Centers of Disease Control website 2003). This is even more alarming when the average age on the reservation, 18 years, is factored into the statistics.

About ten minutes outside of Ponsford on Highway 35, the WELRP's office is located at the end of East Round Lake Road. It is impossible to discuss the Mino-Miijim Program separately from the WELRP. Mino-Miijim is one of the numerous projects that exist under the White Earth Land Recovery Project (WELRP). Mino-Miijim is part of the WELRP in ideology and operation and was designed as a sub-organization of the WELRP, described in WELRP Report for Year 2000 (p. 1):

> The White Earth Land Recovery Project is a grassroots Native environmental, educational, and advocacy organization based at the White Earth reservation in northern Minnesota. Our mission is to facilitate recovery of the original land base of the White Earth Indian Reservation to preserve and restore traditional Native practices of sound land stewardship; to support

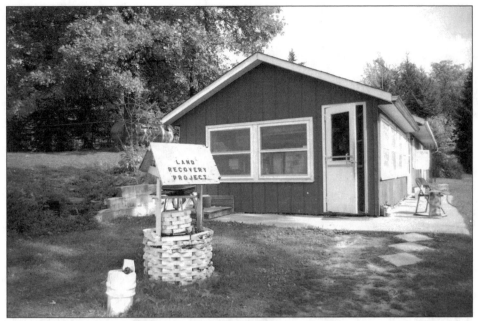

The WELRP Office.

community development and language fluency; and to strengthen our spiritual and cultural heritage. The White Earth Land Recovery project was founded in 1989.

The Founding Director of the WELRP is Winona LaDuke, an Anishinaabeg member and charismatic political figure. She founded the organization over 13 years ago to buy back the 97 percent of White Earth Reservation land that was privately held. Today among her many accomplishments, she leads one of the largest reservation nonprofits in Minnesota and has added a plethora of integrated programs, projects and events.

All of the White Earth sponsored and housed programs work towards the ideals of sustainable communities and spiritual and cultural wellness. In addition to the community projects the WELRP has a business subsection called Native Harvest, where community members bring their crafts, fruit harvests and rice to be sold to a national market. "Native Harvest is a community development project that tries to capture a fair market price for traditionally and organically grown foods" (LaDuke 1999: 130). Of all the small programs and projects the WELRP supports, Native Harvest is the most closely tied to Mino-Miijim, both in goals of production and the finished food products. The project and all of its smaller programs are aimed towards the promotion of a healthy and self-sustaining future for the community.

White Earth Land Recovery Project: Addressing Structural Violence

The WELRP uses the cohesive force of traditional food as a cultural symbol to promote long-term goals of sustainability and community control over resources, such

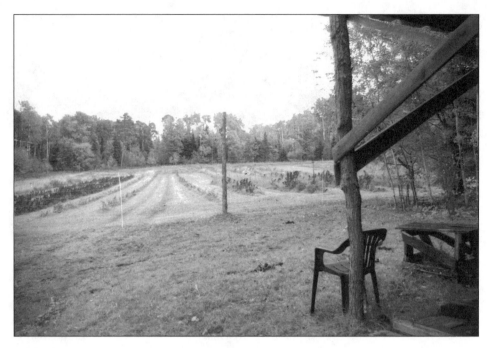

The berry field.

as wild rice and buffalo meat. By viewing diabetes as a symptom of poverty and oppression, Mino-Miijim is able to address the roots of many problems within the community by recognizing and incorporating an ideology which differentiates between
structural violence and cultural factors.

Paul Farmer is a medical anthropologist and physician who has dealt extensively
with HIV/AIDS and tuberculosis. In his recent edition of *Infections and Inequalities:
the Modern Plagues* (1999), he discusses the confusion of structural violence and cultural difference in the context of disease causation, diagnosis and treatment.

> Their sickness is a result of structural violence: neither cultural nor pure in-
> dividual will is at fault; rather, historically given (and often economically
> driven) processes and forces conspire to constrain individual agency. Struc-
> tural violence is visited upon all those whose social status denies them access
> to the fruits of scientific and social progress (Farmer 1999: 79).

Paul Farmer cautions against attributing differences in disease prevalence between
groups to differences based on cultural practices rather than to structural violence. This
is a crucial analysis for the diabetes epidemic which now confronts many minority and
Indigenous Peoples.

The far-reaching and devastating implications of the overuse of so-called cultural
factors in the examination of diabetes is also explored by medical anthropologist Mariana Ferreira:.

> Coupled with the accepted biomedical data about the disease, which gravi-
> tates around diet, sedentary lifestyle and genetics, "cultural" norms and val-
> ues are reduced to nutritional and exercise behaviors, which are ultimately

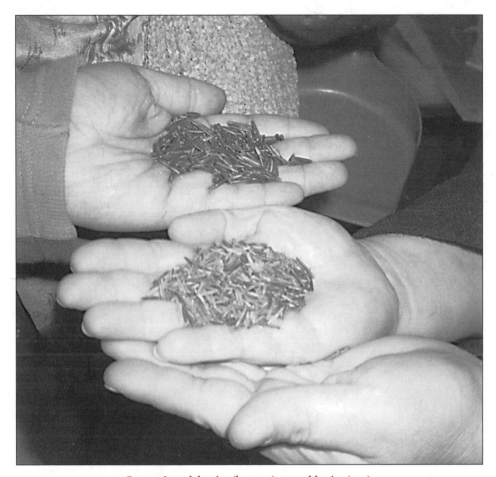

Comparison: lake rice (bottom) vs. paddy rice (top).

connected to individuals' genotypes. Such a narrow and dated conception of culture has prevented researchers from grasping the broader and deeper conceptions of self, identity, and the body which are at stake in determining the social and existential causes of degenerative diseases (Ferreira 2000: 4).

Ferreira echoes Farmer's concerns about the concentration on cultural behaviors obscuring underlying macro-social factors, including confinement on reservations, boarding schools, prisons and juvenile detention halls, poverty, and violence, which have shaped the difficult socio-economic situation and loss of resources impacting many Indigenous Peoples today (see Ferreira Ch. 3 and Ch. 14 in this volume).

The identification of a "diabetes lifestyle" implicitly places blame on affected individuals or communities and on specific cultural practices. Researchers such as Lang (2002; Ch. 2 & 9 in this volume) have remarked on the linkage of "native culture" and disease to the point where having diabetes becomes part of being Indian. Everywhere from physicians' guides to educational pamphlets, the mere status of being American Indian or Alaskan Native puts one at risk for diabetes (Eldeman et al. 2001: 11; Lee et al. 2000: 183). Indeed, the stigma that was previously attached to a poor living standard of an individual has now shifted to behavior attributed to cultural identity.

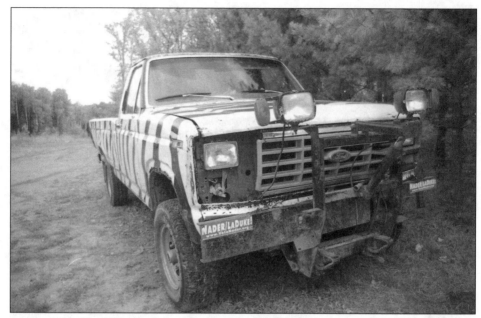

The White Earth Land Recovery Project (WELRP) two-toned truck.

> …the message that 'being Indian means to be diabetic' is widespread, and can lead to consequences such as those reported by Kozak as an attitude of 'surrender.' I suggest that such a notion can be considered another 'stereotype' that should be of great concern to those working with communities to achieve healthy lifestyles, and that efforts to concentrate—in future publications—on this point alone may be extremely important (Lang 2002).

The correlation between diabetes and Indianess is extremely detrimental to Indigenous communities in light of contemporary politics of ethnic identity. In addition, it perpetuates the notion of diabetes as a clinical disease rather than as a result of social inequality. Economic disparity and historical oppression fuel the conditions for the emergence of type 2 diabetes, as discussed in several chapters of this book.

To look beyond simplistic racial and ethnic correlations in the demographics of diabetes often made in the medical literature opens the door to looking at Indigenous Peoples as marginalized and disenfranchised communities who have been forced to be a part of foreign political and economic processes of "modernization" and "assimilation." Ethnic communities are often bound by shared histories, geographies, aspects of their cultural identities including food preferences and eating practices, and availability and accessibility of nutritional resources. These attributes, however, are not purely "cultural," that is, "different." The work of anthropologists like Lang, Ferreira, Farmer and others in this anthology encourages us to unpack the notion of diabetes solely as an Indigenous, that is, "cultural" disease.

Production of White Earth Traditional Food Packages

The components of each food package are brought together at the White Earth office, where some of the foods undergo final production. The importance of food is seen almost everywhere in White Earth. Wild rice is of much spiritual and culinary importance to many people on the reservation. It is native to northern Minnesota and highly integrated into the identity of the Anishinaabeg. Many people earn their living by ricing in the early fall and selling green rice to processors, such as the WELRP itself. The traditional food packages also include one-half pound of the mazon, or broken grains of wild rice. Wild rice is important spiritually and culturally within the community and it is important to the livelihood of many community members involved in its harvesting, processing and selling.

In addition to wild rice, Mino-Miijim packages contain maple syrup, coffee, buffalo meat, hominy and jam. The White Earth Project owns a large "sugar bush" on the reservation, a couple of miles outside of the village of White Earth. The maple syrup process starts with the collection of sap, which involves all of the able-bodied persons that WELRP can round up. The jam is made without sugar from local fruits and berries. The produce comes from local organic farms, the White Earth strawberry fields, or by the bucketful from the community in response to a call for chokecherries or wild plums. The buffalo meat usually comes from ranchers whose land borders the reservation. Coffee is one of the most popular items in the package, and the gourmet coffee is roasted in a local Indigenous owned business. Each Mino-Miijim package contains one pound of corn or hominy, which is usually purchased from a company in New Mexico. Although the White Earth Project has a small field of corn on the property, it is insufficient for the needs of Native Harvest and Mino-Miijim combined. The eventual goal of the WELRP is to locally produce all of the products it sells.

Traditional Food?

The concept of traditional food as preventive medicine for diabetes did not originate with Mino-Miijim. A study was conducted in 1991 on the Gila River Pima to watch the effect that a return to traditional foods (and a rejection of high fat and sugar foods) had on the rising incidence of diabetes (Higgins 1991: 94). The conclusion of the study found that behavioral changes that followed a rigorous nutritional education program at schools were very promising. While the purpose was to target what the medical community considered as a "genetically disadvantaged population," the study ended up using concepts of traditional food and culture to educate Native children and change their eating habits. What the Mino-Miijim program provides, however, is bringing the knowledge of the community to the forefront in managing chronic health conditions; it is a program based on traditional foods organized within the community by community members.

"Mino-Miijim provides alternatives to high-cholesterol and sugary foods by giving elders the makings of a traditional meal…the goal of Mino-Miijim is to replace a diet of poverty" (LaDuke 2002). The services that Mino-Miijim delivers reinforce the goals of the WELRP: to regain the resource of land and use sustainable methods to support healthy lifestyles for the community. Obviously, the content of these packages is not the strictly traditional pre-contact diet. Many of the foods are contestably not pre-contact. Both coffee and buffalo are not considered to have been staples in the Ojibwe diet before the creation of reservations. Ethnic identity as an Indigenous People plays a greater role in the promotion of this assortment of healthful foods than does the actuality of recreating past eating habits. The ideology of the White Earth Project, rather than founded on a past/present reality, is erected on the notion of tradition as based on the past but reinterpreted in terms of the present. In this respect, White Earth's selection of food items are marketed as traditional foods, resembling a complex process of "reinvention of tradition" (Hobsbawm and Ranger 1992). The manner in which food is produced and processed also promotes a cohesive community identity. The program makes sure that a medicine man is present for the buffalo kill and that there is support for Indigenous owned companies, such as the Muskrat Coffee. These are all important aspects of the relationship between Indigenous identity politics and food.

Some foods are readily available to people on the reservation. Hominy, for instance, is not difficult or expensive to buy, nor is jam. However, the Native Harvest jam is made with honey and the buffalo meat is not only expensive but also difficult to locate. The paradigm of ideals that were necessary to secure buffalo meat were complex and very confusing to me. It was clear, however, that the process of incorporating buffalo meat into traditional diet was deeply rooted in some aspect of Winona LaDuke's and the WELRP's ideology. Using locally raised buffalo meant supporting community agriculture and gaining the positive side effects that bison have on the environment, such as the preservation and restoration of prairie ecosystems (LaDuke 1998: 3).

The ways in which the Mino-Miijim program operates and produces traditional food it distributes are a steps towards the larger goal of lowering the incidence and severity of diabetes. For instance, production of food packages involves enhanced physical labor. Collecting sap, chopping the wood for the evaporator and bottling the syrup definitely burns more calories than picking a bottle off the supermarket shelves. Additionally, the traditional aspect of the food bundles implies that Mino-Miijim have control of the production process and regulate the methods that are used. Not adding sugar to the jam and having a medicine man present for the slaughter of the buffalo are ways of exercising this control. Mino-Miijim's efforts in the diabetes program illustrate WELRP's larger goal of the reclamation of production within the White Earth Community.

Food and Community Identity

The White Earth, Native Harvest and Mino-Miijim projects have ideals about the production and consumption of foods that are reflected in the programs' ideology. Among the programs' office staff, and presumably the greater community, there is somewhat of a division between "traditional food," "Indian food" and "good food." These distinctions were also found in research on Lakota diet and physical activity patterns. "For many American Indians, foods regarded as traditional have particular spiritual and social value and represent purity, healthfulness, and strength-symbols of pre-reservation (and pre-European) life and culture" (Harnack et al. 1999: 834). In discussing food preferences and foodways with Dakota people at Spirit Lake Reservation (formerly Devil's Lake Reservation), in North Dakota, Lang (1989: 310) found most residents invariably reflected upon traditional ("way back") foods as health promoting.

> Traditional foods and medicinal plants and wild game represent purity, healthfulness, and strength-symbols of pre-reservation (and pre-European) life and culture. Though today many traditional foods are generally in short supply, and had been consumed regularly by only a few people during their childhood as major components of the diet, the Dakota continue to hold these foods in very high regard and all spoke at length of their healthful properties in contrast to foods they find themselves eating today.

The ideological focus of the WELRP and Winona LaDuke cultivates the spirit of community empowerment and reclamation through publicized images of pre-European ideals. This approach is used by the WELRP to promote the program ideology within the community. Thus, the significance of giving out the food packages to elders at White Earth is not only to supplement meager pension checks. It also makes available foods that had vanished from the Anishinaabeg diet during many of the elders' lifetimes. These traditional foods are idealized symbols of identity cohesion and are associated with a past free of chronic illness conditions.

Indian identity has become a very complex issue, in light of highly polarized border towns of reservations, federal assistance, affirmative action, and other divisions along so-called racial and ethnic lines.

> American Indians have begun to become concerned about the possibility of people falsely identifying themselves as American Indian for personal gain. Further problems arise when the American Indian population will increasingly consist of mixed-blood Indians of less than 25% Indian blood quantum. This will make it necessary for both individuals and groups to reconsider definitions of ethnic identity (Gonzales 1998: 199).

Food has categorical distinctions that can be used to reaffirm "Indianness" and personal identity. Lang detailed the importance of this distinction between traditional foods and Indian" foods.

> Recipes and food preferences today at Devil's Lake reflect the major shift in subsistence that began when they were forcibly settled on the reservation in 1868 (Meyer 1967) and indicate an incorporation of "frontier" Euro-american cooking along with rations and commodity foodstuffs into a number of dishes regarded as "Indian" foods. An important distinction can be made between the wild plant and game foods that are associated with pre-European past or "way-back" history (Lang 1985) and the modified foods that are commonly referred to as "Indian" foods, such as fry bread or rich soups and stews that are often served at "Indian occasions" (Lang 1989: 312).

Obviously cultural identity is deeply invested with respect to these food categories, and it is interesting to note that the foods that people labeled as traditional were not part of the diet consumed prior to European contact. Rather, the idea of eating these foods, like buffalo and bannock, informed a sense of tradition and Indian identity, in-

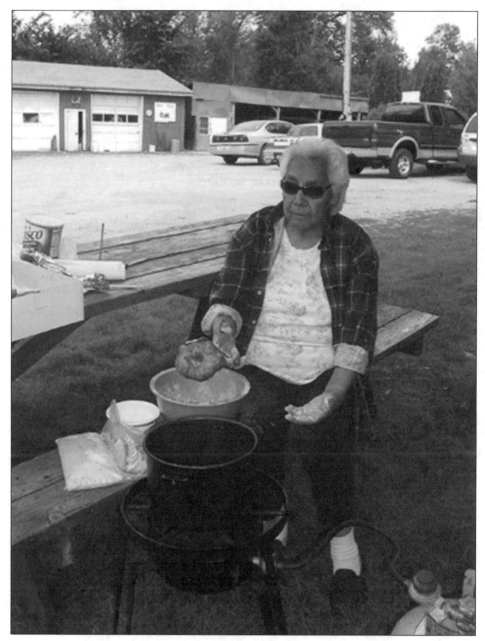

Margaret's special frybread.

dicating that traditions, too, are ever-changing—reinvented—over time (Hobsbawm and Ranger 1992).

> It just feels good to be sitting at the powwow, watching the veterans walk in and hearing the Drums, eating good food like fry bread and soup. Sometimes that opening ceremony almost makes me cry. It makes me really feel that part of myself. Proud and Indian (Personal Communication, Kandi McGregor, July 5, 2002).

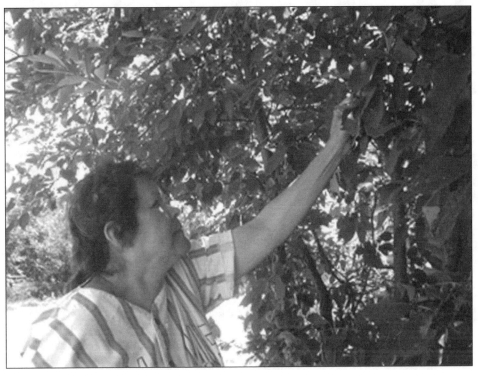

Florence picking chokecherries.

Personal identification with a particular ethnic or cultural group is very significant in the "lifestyle" of people suffering from diabetes, as the biomedical community often correlates Indian heritage with diabetes, however loosely defined "Indian heritage" is (cf. Ferreira Ch. 3 and Ch. 14 in this volume). Food can be an important symbol of cultural belonging and shared experiences of ethnic and cultural identity. "Like all culturally defined material substances used in the creation and maintenance of social relationships, food serves both to solidify group membership and to set groups apart" (Mintz and Du Bois 2002: 209).

History of Lifestyle Changes

The amalgam of many different Anishinaabeg bands in the area of northwestern Minnesota where the White Earth Reservation is located today is the result of a process that started over 1,000 years ago. Accounts of history are recounted in migration fables that begin long before the formation of the reservation. Conventional historical documentation and records are more plentiful after the 1858 installation of a U.S. government agency:

> Between 1874 and 1894 the U.S. government signed 371 treaties with Native people and made some 729 land-related seizures on Native territory... (LaDuke 116: 1999).

The formation of the White Earth Reservation created a fusion of different bands into a space of 1,300 square miles. The 1855 treaty established the first reservations for the Mississippi and Pillager bands, establishing concentrated areas around Leech Lake and Cass Lake. In 1867 a treaty finally established the White Earth Reservation to serve as a "model agrarian settlement for the Indians." (Brown et al. 1999: 1) Here, again, as Jo Scheder indicates for Hawaiian peoples also (in this volume), land and health are intimately connected.

Historian Melissa Meyer's book, *The White Earth Tragedy: Ethnicity and Dispossession at a Minnesota Anishinaabe Reservation, 1889-1920*, carefully details connections between the loss of sustaining seasonal migrations and the decline of community health (Meyer 1994: 203). While concentrating on the disenfranchisement of White Earth, Meyer identifies the end of seasonal migration as especially important to the subsequent manifestation of diabetes. A direct connection is drawn to the loss of seasonal migration, and the land and environmental rights implicit in the migration, and the disempowerment of the Anishinaabeg. The process links the lack of resources and economic fate of the community with the ability to sustain itself through the stewardship of the land. The control of resources and the outcomes of degenerative diseases, such as diabetes, are intertwined.

The title of Meyer's book, *White Earth Tragedy: Ethnicity and Dispossession* (1994), seems at first glance to be the indulgence of a historian railing against the crimes of dead politicians. Yet the repercussions of separating people from their resources and means of living is felt vividly today as in the impact of the diabetes epidemic. Meyer's documents have unveiled important current reservation figures, such as 50 percent unemployment and estimates of a lower general life expectancy (LaDuke 1999: 128). Both Meyer and LaDuke describe these circumstances as a "crisis between who lives on the land and who owns it." The importance of land accessibility and availability to the Anishinaabeg in terms of subsistence pattern, and nutritional patterns of sustenance, become clear in the next section of this chapter. Yet, even without a detailed knowledge of seasonal migration patterns and their disruption, the effect of environmental degradation, land dispossession, and U.S. mismanagement of resources and society can indeed be seen as a tragedy.

Frances Densmore, renowned for her detailed records of Ojibwe life, recorded valuable information on the seasonal movements of the Ojibwe and the ways in which this People used to gather and prepare food. A large section of the following relies on her book *Chippewa Customs*, published in 1929. Meyer also discusses seasonal migration in her account of the White Earth Reservation. The framework of a hunter/gather society fits insofar as the cyclical movements of people allowed them to return to a summer garden, their habitual ricing lakes, and winter camps, representing a mix of foraging and horticulture practices. The seasonal changes and movements are often referred to in literature from accounts of the early contact through the 1920s. However, the complexity of the seasonal migration in relationship to food availability and people's health demands more attention than a simple description of a harvesting pattern.

Densmore reports on many of the food practices and food availability in her 1929 publication of *Chippewa Customs*.

> The country of the Chippewa abounded in vegetable products, which the women prepared in a variety of ways and stored for winter use by drying. The principle vegetable foods were wild rice, corn and maple sugar. Rice was a sta-

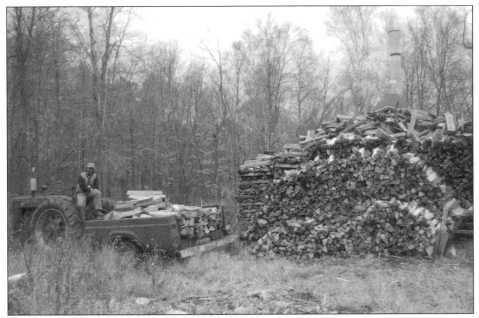

Ron's woodpile for maple sugaring.

ple article of food and was boiled in water or in broth as well as parched. Corn was roasted in the husk or parched in a hot kettle or dried and boiled. Pumpkins and squash were cultivated in gardens and either eaten fresh or dried for winter use. Maple sugar was prepared in the form of granulated sugar, "hard sugar," and "gum sugar." The grained sugar was used as a seasoning, and all forms of the sugar were extensively eaten as a delicacy. Wild potatoes were used, and the Chippewa obtained white potatoes at a fairly early date. Acorns were gathered and cooked in several ways. The Chippewa claim to have had both pumpkin and squash before the coming of the white man (Densmore 1929: 120).

The complexity of the seasonal migration pattern emerges from Densmore's description of everyday foodways. She describes systems of gathering, gardening, cultivating and hunting that were used to produce a dependable and well-rounded diet. This description of the Ojibwe food cultivation goes beyond the popular stereotyping of the simple hunter/gatherer category that many "feast/famine" theories of diabetes, in particular the "thrifty genotype" (Neel 1962, 1982), are based upon.

From the formation of the White Earth reservation to the present time, private property holdings of non-Ojibwe and hunting licenses heavily affected the White Earth community's ability to be self sufficient, and limited the options available to families during times of economic hardship. In the first part of the 20th Century while many continued to hunt deer and rabbits, the threat of action by local law enforcement and the added toll of boarding schools decreased the number of practicing hunters and fishermen.

Environmental degradation coupled with contemporary food preferences make fish fairly low on the list of foods commonly consumed on the reservation. The culmination of environmental degradation, enforced changes in diet, and loss of resources accounts for the poor nutritional value of foods consumed by the White Earth community today.

> According to a 1926–1927 Indian Affairs survey conducted in 55 of the 95 jurisdictions, the most important factor identified as affecting the health of American Indians was the food supply. Survey results indicated that both food quality and quantity was lacking and that many American Indian families never had enough to eat. Other families alternated between gourmandizing and starving. Ten years later in 1936, a report issued by the Public Health Service also identified diet as a major problem, particularly a lack of food availability (Story et al. 1998: 170).

The number of deaths directly and indirectly related to malnutrition during the early 1900s was very high. Many governmental investigations and BIA inspectors found the lack of adequate food to be the root of the health problems, so a number of supplemental food programs were put in place (Dillinger et al. 1999: 174). These programs, however, were never intended to provide a complete diet. Commodity foods, federal school lunch programs and elderly nutrition programs were all comprised of agricultural overstocks and high fat processed foods, such as cheese, purchased by the government. Reservations like Pine Ridge in South Dakota have successfully petitioned to have more traditional, healthful, and locally grown foods added to their commodities lists. On the White Earth Reservation commodities have been modified to include low-fat and low-sugar options as well as the possibility of bison during certain seasons. However, while this is an important step it is crucial not to reduce diabetes to a problem of nutritional intake.

This story of food availability and access is not unique to White Earth, or to Indigenous communities in the U.S. and worldwide. The Great Depression, World War II, and the following agricultural boom created extremely different historic patterns of food consumption and production all over the world. The change from what was considered insufficient food in light of seasonal fluctuations, to an abundance of food was seen by health professionals and government officials as a positive change. The consequences of such changes are now becoming apparent, and the ramifications of past actions and current resource control are being illuminated. Although erroneously claimed to be exclusively a "dietary" issue, the current situation of nutrition in Indigenous communities is obviously very complex, and any steps towards addressing its effects on Indigenous Peoples need to be fully cognizant of historical events and situational aspects of poverty.

In many political, environmental and economic analyses of diabetes anthropologists have used the concept of diabetes as a lingering symptom of colonialism (cf. Scheder and Ferreira in this volume). Mino-Miijim uses a similar understanding of the causation of diabetes in the structure of the project's goals. However, the "causation" of diabetes is most important to the founders of Mino-Miijim as it relates to possible solutions to the epidemic. In effect, Mino-Miijim and the White Earth Land Recovery Project treat diabetes as a devastating symptom of oppressive structures, starting with the perverse effects of colonization, including commodity foods delivered and made available on and around Indigenous reservations. Rather than proposing an idyllic "return" to the pre-European contact period or "traditional" diet which would indeed restore, if it were at all possible, community well-being, the WELRP proposes that restoring a healthy-lifestyle based on foods of historical and symbolic importance to the local community, address the larger problems of the historical disenfranchisement of the White Earth Anishinaabeg. It is this framework of diabetes as a product of colonialism that enables Winona LaDuke to say that her program moves beyond treating diabetes as a product of cultural behaviors, and instead, views diabetes as symptomatic of colonization. Understanding the path of nutritional change at White Earth is central to the current discourses about diabetes, both in the theoretical realm delineating the origin of diabetes, and more importantly, in the current actions that are being developed to reduce the prevalence and severity of diabetes among Indigenous Peoples.

Food Availability and Individual Choices

In general, American Indian communities are economically disadvantaged at two and a half times the U.S. all-races rate of 13%. Corresponding median family incomes in 1990 were $21,750 and $35,225 for American Indians and the total population, respectively. Thus, limited household resources, coupled with the limited availability of reasonably priced, high quality fresh foods at reservation stores in some sites, led to a diet high in total fat and low in fruits and vegetables, a finding that coincides with reports of other low-income groups (Gittelsohn et al. 2000: 10).

Food availability and dietary intake become a central concern of health workers when framed within the context of a disease like type 2 diabetes. Starchy foods, sugary foods and foods high in fat all have a metabolic impact on individuals suffering from diabetes or who are at risk for the ailment. Obesity is strongly linked to type 2 diabetes; approximately 90 percent of diagnosed patients are overweight (Edleman 2001: 26). In the medical literature, food and exercise contribute to the development and complications of diabetes, such as liver failure. However, the White Earth Project understands that underlying all of these contributing factors is the forced separation of people from their land. With the loss of traditional and pre-reservation food resources, the economic disenfranchisement of the community brought periods of starvation.

It might be pointed out that popular foods today are coincidentally composed of many of the foods found on commodity lists. Fry bread, macaroni and cheese, and hamburgers are all examples of tastes that developed from necessity. Foods that are frequently consumed at present in the community are accessible dishes that are high in fats, sugars, and carbohydrates. When examining the long-term effects on people who suffer from diabetes, it is crucial to understand the food politics of the community.

> "People always forget that we were hungry. I was happy to go to school so I would get three meals a day. My family always used what we got, and sometimes before the war, we really needed it. (Margaret Smith, Personal Communication, Summer, 2002)

Frequently Consumed Foods
Fried Chicken
Bacon
Sausage
Cheeseburger Casserole
Chicken and Dumplings
Wild Rice (w/bacon grease or Wild rice Hotdish)
Fry bread (Indian tacos, Indian hamburgers, or with maple syrup)
Lasagna
Pizza
Potato salad
Soup (Naboob)
Jell-O salad
Baked beans
Mountain Dew
Pepsi
Tater-tot Casserole
Macaroni and Cheese
Bacon
Ribs

Large governmental and industrial structures, like the U.S. Food Distribution Program, influence the availability of food, while community food practices may perpetuate detrimental food choices given the prevalence of diabetes in these communities. Numerous contemporary studies of American Indian diets come to the overwhelming conclusion that it has become a diet high in carbohydrates, fats and sugars (Casotacou et al. 2000: 833). However, such "incompatible" dietary patterns within the context of diabetes care were established after a well-documented history of colonization in the US, and across the globe. Changes in food practices are complex and frequently involve cultural and ethnic identity issues as well as situational factors that include dependence upon commodity foods and preferences for familiar food dishes that have been available over time. LaDuke (2004) has recently discussed the serious concerns of White Earth tribal leaders in her *Cultural Survival Quarterly* article, "Wild Rice and Ethics," setting forth arguments for protecting the genetic variants of wide rice (in light of research to genetically modify these strains) and the rights of Chippewa by treaty to this resource.

Current availability of certain foods and individuals' choices became apparent in the potlucks and lunches that the WELRP office staff frequently held for birthdays and to mark the coming and going of temporary staff members, like interns. Oftentimes these were the foods that the program sought to discourage. Interestingly, the food products that Native Harvest sells through catalogues are an example of tapping into food tastes of consumers elsewhere. The new line of freeze-dried wild rice soups and hot dishes are selling well to outside consumers, somewhat to the mystification of the WELRP staff, who find the soups "funny," "as having too much flavor," and "weird." Some staff members think they are "bland" and "a waste of wild rice," which would be better with bacon grease, a long-standing staple food during the past century. McIntosh (1996) discusses the complexity of understanding food in terms of both culture and in terms of socioeconomic factors as follows:

> Barriers at the individual level involve a host of factors including habit (or what Giddens describes as practical consciousness), strong cultural incompatibilities, or lack of resources (Ilmonen 1991). Food habits are part of practical consciousness, that part of individuals' everyday repertoire that cannot even be easily recognized and discussed. Part of the difficulty in making changes lies in the ease with which an individual can rely on habit versus the additional effort that must be undertaken if one chooses to change....Income and education also affect the adoption of new habits; generally those who have more of both of these resources are more willing and able to experiment with new crops, new cooking techniques, and new foods (McIntosh 1996: 55).

Buffalo and hominy are parts of the Mino-Miijim package that many people have difficulty preparing, even though these foods are appreciated and eagerly anticipated. However, due to the lack of familiarity with these foods many people are unsure about their preparation. Because buffalo is much leaner than beef, it needs to be cooked longer and at a lower temperature to remain tender. Hominy, or the dry, husked corn, is also a challenge to many people, as it must be slow simmered for over eight hours to be fully cooked. Many times when I entered a Mino-Miijim recipient's house to help put the food package away, I noticed that the previous months' worth of buffalo meat and the hominy were piling up, unused.

It is important to contextualize the list of "Food Categories" as foods that are not recommended for individuals with high blood sugars, yet many of these foods have become significant parts of family meals and community occasions. Another aspect of food choices to factor into individual diets is the high cost of "healthy" food. Economic status and situation are crucial determinants of nutritional health because they directly affect the types of foods that will be purchased and eaten (Sucher and Kittler 1991: 297).

Learning about food categories on the White Earth Reservation proved to be very useful in understanding local conceptions of food. "The Frybread Queen" by Annie Cecilia Smith (2002) defines categories and classifications of food within the larger American Indian or Pan-Indian community (Sister Nations 2002: 140). "The Frybread Queen" talks specifically about four categories of food in Pan-Indian culture: commodities, fry bread, traditional food and "the other stuff." The most noticeable difference between these categories and the WELRP food structure is that the White Earth Project stresses the separation of traditional food from other types of food rather than acknowledging the four equally weighted categories found in "Frybread Queen."

The categories below are compiled from many different conversations I had with people on the reservation, especially informed by Margaret Smith and other WELRP employees. During lunch I would ask people what their favorite foods and dishes were, and which commodities they remembered best. I organized the foods in Table 6.1 according to Annie Cecilia Smith's food categories (2002).

In White Earth, as in many local Indigenous communities, social relationships and cultural membership are heavily involved in food choices and practices. "Indian" foods

Table 6.1	Food Categories		
Commodities	Traditional Foods	Indian Foods	"Other Stuff"
Farina	Deer	Fry bread	Pepsi
Noodles	Moose	Indian tacos	Mountain Dew
Macaroni and	Wild Turkey	Hominy and buffalo	Chips
cheese	Beaver	Oatmeal w/ bacon	Donuts
Ground beef	Porcupine	grease	Pizza
Canned fruits	Squash	Wild rice	McDonalds
Canned vegetables	Onions	Wild rice w/bacon	Beer
Onions	Berries:	grease	Hotdogs
Carrots	*Blueberries*	Mac (macaroni and	Milk
Potatoes	*Chokecherries*	cheese)	Eggs
Canned	*Strawberries*	Wild rice hotdish	Lunch meat
Sweet Potatoes	*Highbush cranberries*	Wild rice soup	
Cheese	*Raspberries*		
Butter	Plums		
Vegetable oil	Fish		
Flour	Wild rice		
Dried milk	Rabbit		
Juice	Maple syrup/sugar		
Rice	Potatoes		
Raisins	Hominy/corn		
Evaporated milk	Soup		
	Bannock (made		
	with flour)		
	Buffalo*		

* Buffalo is included in the list of traditional foods because this is how the Ojibwe see it today. However, it is important to remember there is scanty documentation for its existence as a staple in the pre-reservation Ojibwe diet.

are not necessarily pre-European contact foods. They have changed with the availability of foodstuffs, and today include such foods as frybread, bacon grease, oatmeal and Indian tacos. These are distinguished from traditional foods, which are seen as more behavior-oriented foods—that is, as the outcome of an active pattern of subsistence, such as hunted deer, rabbit meat and fish, and gathered squash, berries and maple sugar.

Narratives of Diabetes

For individuals who worked for the White Earth Project, there was overriding consensus that White Earth is as an oppressed community which has integrated unhealthy foods into its diet. Both Florence Goodman and Margaret Smith spoke of the good diet that "traditional" food provided, and the "bad" foods like hamburgers, fries, chips, candy and pizza. Margaret would talk about the "sugary cereals" and "greasy food" which her grandkids would eat. "When they come over I give them oatmeal, they ask for things like oatmeal and pancakes. I like to feed them good food. Some of the kids are really big, our kids keep eating junk and get bigger" (Personal Communication, Margaret Smith, Aug. 12, 2002).

Florence Goodman is the production manager at WELRP, and an enrolled member of White Earth. She has lived on or around the White Earth Reservation for most of her life. Her sister died from kidney complications from diabetes. Florence herself does not have diabetes, and she believes it is due to her lack of a sweet tooth.

> My sister, even when she was sick, would eat all this sweet stuff, like candy and cookies and cake. Everyone in my family has diabetes, except me, I don't like sweet things, I like salty things. When I get home I like to make potatoes and gravy, but the boys like pizza so sometimes we eat that. Commods are bad. The people who eat only commods get fat, all that cheese and fat. Sometimes people sell the commods, but a lot eat it. I don't get commods, even though we could, I don't want it, it's not good food (Personal Communication, Florence Goodman, Sept 27, 2002).

It is important to point out that there are differences among community narratives and those of the WELRP staff.

> They have a lot of good food in commodities, like the juices and now they have vegetables. My neighbor she doesn't like farina, but I do so she'll save up that and the dried milk and give them to me (Personal Communication, Margaret Smith, Summer 2002).

A commonality throughout both Margaret and Florence's recollections is the understanding that traditional food was healthful, and that the means to acquire and collect this food has been eroded over time and through contact with non-Indians. This is a powerful statement which is also supported by Lang's work with the Dakota (Lang 1989 and in this volume). Lang has noted that in talking about diabetes, Dakota people often reflected upon "not only individual, but community identity" (Lang 1985: 305).

> While it may appear to be an ironic contradiction that there is reluctance to change food habits, given the commonly-expressed idea that 'white man's food made us sick,' foods and foodways constitute complex codes for social relations and symbols of cultural identity. Many contemporary preferred foods, while incorporated into a traditional foods system (as Powers and Powers 1984) are also recognized to have entered Dakota culture relatively recently, during a period recalled as one of great deprivation. Diabetes, especially as it affects food patterns, from an outsider's standpoint appears to have provided the Dakota with another means through which to reflect and comment upon matters of continual concern regarding their history and their place with respect to the majority society (Lang 1990: 309).

The implications of this knowledge are used to their full advantage by the WELRP and Mino-Miijim. Traditional food carries with it connotations of community identity, native pride, and healthfulness. The necessity of having traditional food being strictly pre-European contact is considered Eurocentric. It is therefore secondary to the importance of a sense of community which is expressed through the use of current traditional foods including buffalo, wild rice, and hominy, combined with the indigenously produced nature of the coffee and jam. In essence, this solution has somewhat compensated for the collective nature of the diabetes experience. The traditional foods

Mino-Miijim support today have more to do with Indigenous identity and the promotion of a healthy community, than with the idea of a pre-contact diet.

Conclusion

> We write today not about charity but about economic justice. With Native Harvest, the WELRP is building a strong marketing program through which White Earth tribal members can increase their income. For years, the marketing of locally grown foods and products has been an essential component of our overall economic improvement and social empowerment program (WELRP 2000: 2).

While many new diabetes programs have addressed the importance of "cultural appropriateness" in medical treatment, education and prevention, Mino-Miijim moves past a superficial handling of diabetes and addresses it as a disease of colonization. Mino-Miijim shows promise because it is based on a concept that promotes a sense of reclamation and possibilities for true socio-economic change, rather than simply raising an alarm about a community epidemic. This utilization of traditional foods harks back to an era before European contact and connotes positive images of Indigenous pride and identity, advocating a change in food practices that solidify community identity instead of preaching against "Indian foods," like fry bread. Within a political and economic context, the White Earth Project and Mino-Miijim are working toward reclamation of resources and control over food production and thus food accessibility. WELRP and Mino-Miijim are not simply creating a "culturally appropriate" prevention program; rather, they are attempting to alter the systems that create the impoverished conditions on which diabetes thrives, namely, socio-economic marginalization. Mino-Miijim is truly a movement for cultural restoration with the necessary tools for positive change, away from the historically repressive structures of the broader, non-Indian society in order to reclaim control over community resources and futures. The WELRP's ideology and implementation through the Mino-Miijim program are unique to the world of diabetes programs and an important position in the explanation of the social causes of the diabetes epidemic amidst Indigenous Peoples.

> Our work springs from our culture and history, and the need to control our destiny. Through our initiatives, we work to recover the land base of the reservation, while building a self-sustaining future for our People. We recognize that the root cause of the problems found on White Earth is the collective loss of culture and land. Diabetes is a symptom of the larger loss of our community, and needs to be redressed through the holistic approach of recovery of food production. This Initiative is about the process of sorting out what is valuable from both Anishinaabeg and European society, and restoring our community from this foundation (WERLP 2002).

Mino-Miijim is a new program, and it is a very small-scale operation. However, it provides an important, and even revolutionary model for diabetes programs. The ideology of the program leaders is expansive enough to address the deeper underlying contributors of poverty and oppression, viewing diabetes as a social ailment rather than exclusively as a biological disease.

Acknowledgments

My experience with the White Earth Land Recovery Project (WELRP) is due to the kindness and patience of Margaret Smith, Winona LaDuke, Ron Chilton and all of the WELRP community; who were very generous in sharing their histories and adventures with me, and who so kindly helped me learn about the workings of their program and the community. This chapter would never have been written without the help, advice, and guidance of Macalester College's Anthropology Department, especially Professors Sonia Patten, Jack Weatherford, Arjun Guneratne, Karen Nakamura, and Diana Shandy. My thanks also to the editors of this book for their encouragement in my efforts to write this chapter.

References

Brown, Marshall, Jerry Rawley, Georgia Wiemer, Edwin Goodwin and Kathy Roy Goodwin. 1999. White Earth, A History. Third Edition. Cass Lake, MN: The Minnesota Chippewa Tribe.

Casotacou, Tina, with Sarah Levin and Elizabeth J. Mayer-Davis. 2000. Dietary Patterns among Members of the Catawba Indian Nation. Journal of the American Dietetic Association 100(7): 833–39.

Centers for Disease Control. 2000. Diabetes in American Indians and Alaskan Natives. Electronic document, <www.cdc.gov/diabetes>, accessed March 19, 2003.

Densmore, Francis. 1929. Chippewa Customs. Fourth Edition. St. Paul, MN: Minnesota Historical Society.

Dillinger, Theresa L., Stephen C. Jett, Martha J. Macri, and Louis E. Grivetti. 1999. Feast or Famine? Supplemental Food Programs and their Impacts on Two American Indian Communities in California. International Journal of Food Sciences and Nutrition 50(3): 173–93.

Edleman, Stephan V. and Robert R. Henry. 1999. Diagnosis and Management of Type 2 Diabetes. Caddo, OK: Professional Communications, Inc.

Farmer, Paul. 1999. Infections and Inequalities: The Modern Plagues. Second Edition. Berkeley, CA: University of California Press.

Ferreira, Mariana L. 2000. Native Americans and Diabetes. New York Times Interview. Liz Neporent, ed. Sept. 11, 2000.

Gittelsohn, Joel, Elanah Toporoff, Mary Story, Marguerite Evans, Jean Anliker, Sally Davis, Anjali Sharma, and Jean White. 2000. Food Perceptions and Dietary Behaviour of American Indian Children, their Caregivers, and Educators: Formative Assessment Finding from Pathways. Journal of Nutritional Education 32(1): 2–13.

Gonzales, Angela. 1998. The Re(articulation) of American Indian Identity: Maintaining Boundaries and Regulating Access to Ethnically Tied Resources: American Indians and the Urban Experience. American Indian Culture and Research Journal 3: 199–201.

Harnack, Lisa, Mary Story and Bonnie Holy Rock. 1998. Diet and Physical Activity Patterns of Lakota Indian Adults. Journal of the American Dietetic Association 99(7): 829–35.

Higgins, Michael. 1989. Native People Take on Diabetes: Indigenous Peoples from America to Australia are Fighting Some of the Highest Rates of Diabetes in the World by Returning to Traditional Foods and Practices. East West 21(4): 94–100.

Eric Hobsbawm and Terence Ranger, Eds. 1992. Invention of Tradition. Cambridge U Press.

LaDuke, Winona. 1998. Pte Oyate: Buffalo Nations, Buffalo Peoples. Smart Set, Minneapolis, MN.

_____1999. All Our Relations: Native Struggles for Land and Life. Cambridge, MA: South End Press.

_____2002. Interview with the Associated Press, Oct. 16, 2002.

_____2004. Wild Rice and Ethics. Cultural Survival Quarterly 28(3): 15-17.

LaDuke, Winona with Sarah Alexander. 2004. Food is Medicine: Recovering Traditional Foods to Heal the People. Minneapolis, MN: Honor the Earth.

Lang, Gretchen Chesley. 1985. Diabetics and Health Care in a Sioux Community. Human Organization 44(3): 251–60.

_____1989. "Making Sense" about Diabetes: Dakota Narratives of Illness. Medical Anthropology 11(1): 305–27.

_____1990. Talking About a New Illness with the Dakota: Reflections on Diabetes, Food, and Culture. *In* Culture and the Anthropological Tradition, *Festschrift* for Robert F. Spencer. Robert Winthrop, ed. pp. 283–317. New York: University Press of America.

_____2002. Discussant Response, for Medical Anthropology Society Sponsored Session, entitled "Healthy Lifestyles and Communities: Future Scenarios to Reduce the Diabetes Epidemic, Chaired by Dennis Wiedman. American Anthropological Ass'n. Annual Meetings, November, 2002, New Orleans, LA.

Lee, Elisa T., Barbara V. Howard, Oscar Go, Peter J. Savage, Richard R. Fabsitz, David C. Robbins and Thomas K. Welty. 2000. Prevalence of Undiagnosed Diabetes in Three American Indian Populations. Diabetes Care 23(2): 181–91.

McGregor, Kandi. 2002. Personal Communication.

Meyer, Melissa. 1994. White Earth Tragedy: Ethnicity and Dispossession at a Minnesota Anishinaabe Reservation 1889–1920. Rev. Ed. 1984. Lincoln, NE: University of Nebraska Press.

Mintz, Sidney and Christine M. Du Bois. 2002. Anthropology of Food and Eating. Annual Review of Anthropology 34: 99–119.

Neel, James V. 1962. Diabetes mellitus: A "Thrifty" Genotype Rendered Detrimental by "Progress"? Amer. J. Human Genetics 14(4): 353–62.

_____1982. Thrifty Genotype Revisited: *In* The Genetics of Diabetes Mellitus. J. Kobberling and R. Tattersall, eds. pp. 283–93. NY: Academic Press.

Smith, Anne Cecilia. 2002. The FryBread Queen. *In* Sister Nations. Heidi E. Erdrich and Laura Tohe, eds. pp. 14–141. St. Paul, MN: Minnesota Historical Society.

Smith, Margaret. 2002. Personal Communication. 12 August 2002.

Story, Mary, Karen F. Strauss, Elenora Zephier, and Brenda A. Broussard. 1998. Nutritional Concerns in American Indian and Alaska Native Children: Transitions and Future Directions. Journal of the American Dietetic Association 98(2): 170–77.

Sucher, Kathryn P. and Pamela Goyan Kittler. 1991. Nutrition isn't Color Blind. Journal of the American Dietetic Association 91(3): 297–301.

The WELRP Wild Rice Brochure. 2001. Wild Rice Brochure. Unpublished Report. Detroit Lakes, MN.

The WELRP Report for the Year 2000. 2000. Report for the Year 2000. Unpublished Report. Ponsford, MN.

CHAPTER 7

DIABETES AND IDENTITY: CHANGES IN THE FOOD HABITS OF THE INNU

A Critical Look at Health Professionals' Interventions Regarding Diet

Bernard Roy

Eating habits fall within and reveal the social and, I insist, political dimension. Without any doubt, for the Innu, the act of eating is an act of recognition, of building solidarity, developing trust relations, differentiation and assertion of difference from the Other. Moreover, the analysis of the changes in the food habits and its contemporary and daily expression reveals the creative power of the social actors who, on a daily basis, build viable universes and moments of happiness with contemporary materials.

Bernard Roy, in this chapter

Summary of Chapter 7. The present chapter takes a critical look at classical approaches of the medical community, often constructed around the economic theory of rational choice. I attempt to illustrate that the emergence of the diabetes epidemic among the Innu people in Canada is directly related to the social, economic and political conditions in which the Innu evolve. To this end, rather than use the more popular concept of eating habits I prefer to use the "act of eating." This concept describes a social act through which one may create social contacts, define and construct boundaries, allowing us to identify those who will be accorded a place inside the boundary and those who will be excluded. The act of eating offers the possibility of a broader view of the social, economic and political dynamics at play in modern Innu society, shedding light onto the emergence and rapid increase of diabetes as a highly political phenomenon.

ও ও ও

The explanatory model of diabetes conveyed by biomedicine and public health professionals considers the disease to be closely related to nutrition. The public health view is that this disorder requires substantial modifications in many "lifestyle habits," notably in diet, regularity of mealtime and physical activity. This doctrine emphasizes that for most individuals, it is difficult to modify lifestyle habits and more particularly to maintain newly acquired habits. It is specified that lifestyle habits are often very resistant to change (<www.chbc.qc.ca\diabete>), and this resistance is often related to specific "cultural characteristics," especially when they occur among populations belonging to other "cultures." In associating themselves with the social sciences, public health professionals will then try to find, identify and understand cultural traits particular to the Other, as patient, in order to evaluate and by-pass what can act as obstacles (Fassin 2001).

For over a century, biomedicine has associated food with the onset of diabetes. Food-related factors suspected of playing a role in the evolution of diabetes include excessive calorie intake, unbalanced proportions of certain macro-nutrients (protein, fat, carbohydrate), excess of refined carbohydrates, lack of certain nutrients such as chrome and zinc, and low intake of dietary fibers. The medical community argues whether it is the quantity of ingested sugar that must be incriminated or the insulin response when sugar is ingested alone or with animal proteins. Alcohol is also suggested as a significant food-related risk factor (Colditz et al. 1991). Overall, inappropriate "food habits" are strongly associated with the onset of diabetes.

For the biomedical community, the rapid increase of the diabetes prevalence rate among Aboriginal Peoples since the end of World War II is attributed to far-reaching modifications that have changed the food habits of Aboriginal people following contact with Europeans. These changes, resulting from a fast process of "acculturation" along with particular "genetic characteristics," have driven Aboriginal people towards what biomedicine calls a diabetes epidemic (Harris et al. 1997; O'Dea 1991; Zimmet et al. 1990).

A Fight to the End Against "Bad Food Habits"

In 1996, the Pan American Health Organization (PAHO) approved the Declaration of the Americas on Diabetes. The Declaration proposed four basic objectives in order to help prevent and control the spread of diabetes, establish a national coordination center for the development of programs related to diabetes, implement a national monitoring system, develop a national strategic plan for prevention and control and establish immediate objectives nationally and locally. Consequently, at the end of the 1990s, the Canadian Government commissioned health institutions to make all necessary efforts to stamp out diabetes among Aboriginal Peoples. The selected strategies would have to ensure greater control by individuals and social groups affected by the disorder. Since it is considered that the occurrence of diabetes is primarily the result of inappropriate choices made by individuals, it was established that the epidemic could be stopped by increasing biomedical control and a broader dissemination of this kind of scientific knowledge in Aboriginal communities. From this perspective, it would be important to control the biological parameters of diabetic patients, detecting each new case as soon as possible, and finally, to successfully control the lifestyle habits of at-risk populations such as, for instance, their food habits.

Food Guide and "Culturization" of the Message

For the public health community, it appears that health-related behaviors are entities that can be modified by individuals. The latter would have the responsibility, the ability and the desire to modify their behavior and to do so "successfully." All individuals would have the responsibility to discipline themselves and to modify their behavior in order to live a healthy life (Becker 1993). To this end, the health community, adopting a fundamentally economic approach, developed programs based on the premise that human beings are fundamentally rational and systematically use the information at their disposal to make and carry out decisions that are in their best interest.

In this context, the initiatives of the health community and more particularly of the nutrition sector have been many. For example, in Québec, since the early 1990s, two culturally-sensitive food guides have been developed for the Innu[1] people (see Figures 1 and 2) by the Conseil Atikamekw Montagnais (CAM, created in 1991 by the Atikemakw and Montagnais Nations). The development of the food guides stems from the assumption, of the bio-medical school of thought among others, that it is crucial to put culture at the service of the health message that is being delivered. According to these approaches culture is considered an ally that can be profitably employed for developing promotional tools for a so-called "healthy lifestyle." Anthropological knowledge was thus called upon in the hope of finding the right formulas to identify the reasons for the Innu's cultural resistance to adapting a "healthy lifestyle." This culturalist approach aimed to identify "resistance factors" as well as the "cultural obstacles" faced by conventional prevention and health promotion programs. The health community's interest in the cultural dimension was supposed to allow for the identification of the "intractable differences" of the Innu culture that are responsible for the persistent misunderstanding, by the Innu, of the health education message. The admitted objective of these initiatives was, of course, to disseminate the scientific knowledge of the Canadian Food Guide in order to offer to the women and men of these populations the scientific information that would allow them to make clear and informed decisions regarding their health. These initiatives were consistent with the postulates of the economic theory of rational choice mentioned above and adapted by the culturalist approach.

In 1991, the first version of the Innu Food Guide developed by CAM was published and broadly distributed across all the Innu communities and training sessions were delivered to the health professionals and to Innu community workers. A few years later, a second version was developed by the Mamit Innuat Organization, an advisory organisation created in 1982 by the Innu Nation of the Lower North Shore. Since 1990, the Mamit Innuat Organisation is responsible for the management of the following economic development programs; health services, social development (social welfare) and social services. The distribution of the second version was limited to the member communities of this tribal council (Ekuanitshit, Nutakuan, Unamen Shipu and Pakua Shipi). A few years later, the three Atikamekw communities (Opitciwan, Wemotaci and

---

1. Throughout the essay the word Innu is used in the form favoured by the Innu themselves.

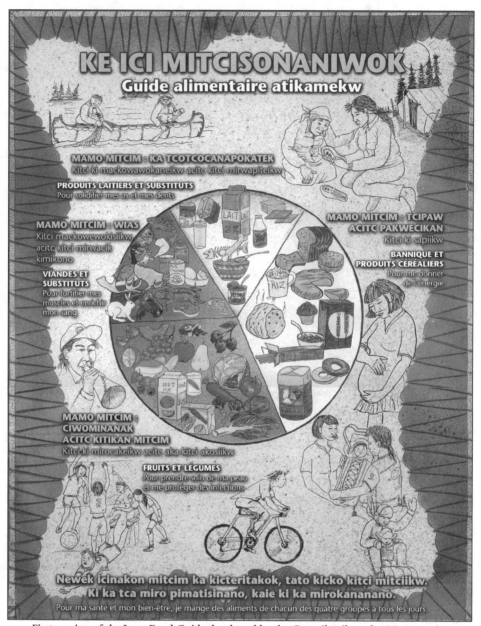

First version of the Innu Food Guide developed by the Conseil Atikamekw Montagnais.

Manawan), living in territories located in the Haute-Mauricie region in Québec, also developed their own food guide adapted to their cultural knowledge.

Mixed Results

Health programs usually have a strong assessment or evaluation component of "results." These evaluation processes are mainly aimed at verifying whether the estab-

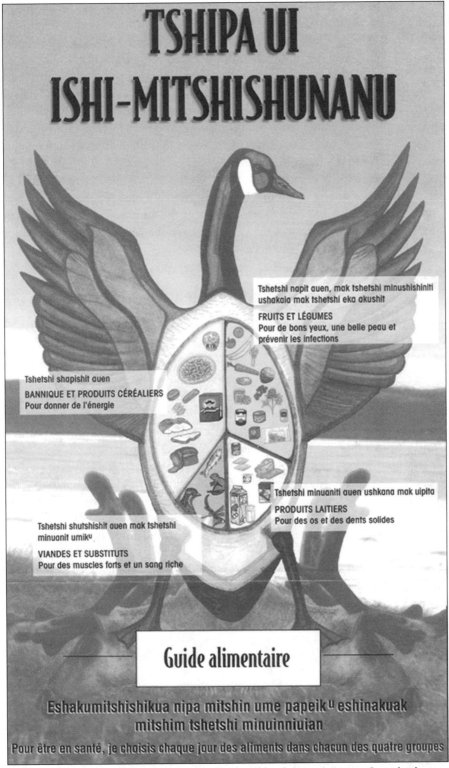

Second version of the Innu Food Guide developed by the Mamit Innuat Organization.

lished objectives were realistic and whether the established means and timeframe have
allowed to reach the said objectives. As an anthropologist I found it pertinent to take
a critical look at these initiatives which aim to bring substantial changes in the food
habits of the Innu. Did the health community's, and more particularly, the nutrition
sector's cultural approach, contribute to their reaching their objectives more quickly
and efficiently? As suggested by the rational choice theory, did the Innu, now having
access to relevant and scientifically proven knowledge delivered through "culturally appropriate symbolism," substantially modify their behavior and their so-called "lifestyle"?

Evaluative research conducted in several Innu communities where these food guides
have been distributed (Fecteau and Roy 1999, 2005; Fecteau 2000; Pouliot 2000; Roy 1999a;
Roy 2000; Valdebenito 2001) suggest that these efforts and investments have produced few
significant results, at least in terms of tangible results that show a significant slowdown in
the progression of the disease, a better control of the patients' biological parameters
(glycemia, weight, etc.) as well as significant changes in the said food habits of the Innu.[2]

Conscious and Knowledgeable Populations

The results obtained in the evaluative research mentioned above, which reached
large segments of the adult population, indicate that the Innu People have reached a
level of awareness and knowledge of diabetes that would make health professionals
green with envy. The Innu have a comprehensive and deep knowledge of the complications, symptoms and risk factors associated with the disorder. In all the concerned
villages, broad segments of the population identified diabetes as one of the most important threats—if not the most important threat—to their community's "health circle" and affirmed that it is important and urgent to take action.

From a biomedical point of view, the Innu are very knowledgeable on the subject of
diabetes. Large portions of the population can identify the risk factors (including food-
related factors), the symptoms as well as the adverse effects of the disorder. Indeed, in
all the concerned Innu villages, over 60 percent of the adult population (15 years and
older, including diabetics and non-diabetics) manage to identify a healthy person's normal blood sugar level. It should also be noted that another finding of the above research
was that Innu patients suffering from diabetes visited, on a regular basis, the different
health professionals (nurse, physician, nutritionist, etc.) available in their respective
communities. Indeed, a majority of patients suffering from diabetes in Innu communities covered by the evaluation, see health professionals more than once a month.

---

2. The Innu, formerly known as the Naskapi-Montagnais, are a First Nations people. The majority of the Innu live in the east of the Québec and Labrador peninsula and still primarily speak
Innu-aimun, an Algonquine language. In *innu-aimun*, the word *innu* means human being. Once no-
mads, today the Innu Nation, divided by the Canadian government into 11 separately administered
communities, is spread out through Québec to Labrador. Today the Innu (Nutshimiunnuat) constitute a group of distinct entities, who together through their territorial claims are redefining their
rights and living habits. The Innu's Aboriginal neighbours to the north are the Naskapi and the Cree,
the Atikamekw to the west and the Wendat to the south.

Despite this high level of awareness and knowledge and the regular visits to health professionals, the behavior and the eating habits of the Innu have obviously not changed significantly. On the contrary, it seems to have been strengthened and further developed.

If one of the ultimate objectives of the health community is to achieve optimal control of biological parameters, the results obtained by the evaluative research show that there is still a long way to go for the Innu. It appears that the main biological indicators such as weight and glycemia are out of control. Indeed, on a regular basis, the blood sugar level of a large majority of patients remain clearly above the desired standard, which is between 3.8 and 7 mmole per liter. As well, the average Body Mass Index[3] of the general Innu population is way above the "healthy zone" as the vast majority of individuals with high blood sugars cannot manage to substantially reduce their weight (Roy 1999b).

In addition, a significant number of new cases of type 2 diabetes are diagnosed each year among young people who, incidentally, become overweight at an increasingly younger age. All of this allows me to suggest that the lifestyle and particularly the eating habits targeted by these extensive and numerous prevention and promotion campaigns based on Innu cultural values have not significantly altered the eating behavior of the Innu, whose awareness and knowledge is remarkably high. It allows me to further suggest that the situation described above is contrary proof to the postulates of economic rational choice theory.

Why the Repeated Failures?

Despite important human and financial investments in diabetes prevention among the Innu, significant results have not been observed so far, even though, interventions specifically aimed at nutrition referred to in this essay, are made in addition to many other initiatives from health professionals and community workers.

The health community's repeated failures to prevent and treat diabetes using conventional approaches are partly due to the fact that the so-called hard sciences apply their methods and concepts in a certainly rigorous, but narrow manner. Bio-medicine and all scientific disciplines related to it, approach the Innu's eating habits as if they were mere cultural habits and behavior that need only be corrected by disseminating scientifically proven knowledge directly or indirectly pertaining to biomedicine. To maximize the understanding and effectiveness of the message, the health community increasingly calls upon the social sciences, and more particularly on anthropology, to culturally refine the message. But this culturalization of the message serves only, to bypass so-called cultural obstacles which are imprinted in a cultural frame deeply rooted in a mystical ancestrality. Biomedical science is trying to reduce two irreducible realities to a few quantifiable indicators or to a number of artifacts. First, biomedicine tries to reduce the act of eating to a simple physiological function and totally disregards the

---

3. The Body Mass Index (BMI) is a measurement obtained by dividing weight (kilograms) by the square of the height (meters). According to a report by a group of experts on weight standards and commissioned by the Health Promotion Directorate, the BMI is the only measurement likely to meet the eight criteria established to determine the best measurement to be used for the development of new guidelines associating weight and health (Canada, 1988: 21)

complexity of the act. However, complex and multidimensional phenomena such as the act of eating resist a strictly disciplinary approach, as noted by Fischler (1993).

The biomedical reductionism also affects the concept of culture used by health professionals, as seen in other chapters of this book (Ferreira, Kimberley). The health community is trying hard to understand and explain the persistence of the considered irrational behavior of the Other—Aboriginal people in this case—by attempting to identify and incriminate cultural motives. Ultimately health professionals identify what is missing for compliance and what acts as the obstacle. Culture is then reduced and reified into a number of "characteristics," "variables" and "behaviors" that can be isolated from reality and social dynamics (Fassin 2001). From this public health perspective, culture is a phenomenon that can be entirely circumscribed, a global entity, distinct and objectifiable, which can then be tracked down, evaluated and decoded (Gruzinski 1999).

The Complexity of Food Habits

Many anthropologists have shown to what extent the activity of eating transcends the biological function. Anthropologists understand eating as a deeply social act intimately associated with identity. Many anthropological studies show the profound relationship between food, and individual and group identities. (Beardsworth and Keil 1997; Counihan and Van Esterik 1997; Garine 1995; Giard 1994; Meigs 1997). Anthropologist Mary Douglas tries to show that foodways consist of more than simply feeding the body and that it is essential to explore its symbolism, meaning and social function (Douglas 1984).

Research conducted in a Dakota community by anthropologist Gretchen Chesley Lang (1989: 320; see also Chapters 2 and 9, this volume) pointed out that the discourse of individuals suffering from diabetes reveals "their collective identity and are creative enterprises in what Cohen calls 'symbolizing boundaries.'" This symbolizing of boundaries is expressed by referring to certain foods that appear to be included in the identity structure while others are totally excluded. What Lang and other researchers, including anthropologist Linda C. Garro, have explained is the fact that eating habits constitute phenomena with identity rules which allows the inclusion or exclusion of individuals in or from a given space (Garro 1987; Garro 1987; Lang 1985; Lang 1989). In their article, Garro and Lang (1993: 322) affirm that "Foods and foodways constitute complex codes for social relations and symbols of cultural identity and change, and as they are linked to aspects of health and illness, provide salient imagery in which to demarcate community and cultural boundaries."

If they don't want to feel "out of place," or even ostracized, those entering a space must meet the conditions tacitly imposed by its occupants (Bourdieu 1993). And suitable eating practices are precisely one of these essential conditions. Eating habits fall under the control of the local cultural order but cultures are dynamic. Changes in material conditions or the political organization can bring about substantial changes in eating habits as well as in the determination of the edible. Giard (1994: 214) wrote in this regard that food habits constitute a field where tradition and innovation are equally important, where the present and the past act interact in a current context to allow for the emergence and the construction of the "joys of a moment."

The Act of Eating—A Political Act

If it is true that humans feed on proteins, carbohydrates, vitamins and fat, they assimilate in their food, at the same time, a number of symbols, myths and dreams. The said "food habits" are all components of tiny crossroads of history (Giard 1994). The act of eating belongs to the social sphere. Anthropologist Richard R. Wilk (1999), addressing the issue of the *authentically national* cuisine in Belize, in the Caribbean, successfully demonstrates that food choices are used to express and show a sense of belonging to a people, a nation or to distinguish oneself from Others, from a personal, social and political perspective. Moreover, Wilk clearly shows that this cuisine albeit qualified as *authentic*, is in fact a construct. A construct that can be understood only when considering the current context, of course, but also the historical context with its social, economic and political dimensions. Wilk (1999: 249) then proposes that "to bring back the discussion to earth in Belize, we need to begin with the colonial regime of consumption and describe the way it set the stage and provided scenery for drama of local vs. global." By emphasizing the need to understand the local by not attempting to isolate it from the global, but rather by trying to identify the dynamics of that relationship, Wilk introduces a necessary and fundamental variable in the analysis of the act of eating. We are a long way from "food habits" that are only the result of simple individual decisions.

The Innu's discourse allows us to determine the far-reaching changes in their food habits over the past decades. It allows us to determine, from the micro-societal level, the dynamics that have inspired the local as well as the interrelations between the global and the local. It reveals that the act of eating creates a space within the community where members of the community who are deemed entitled to be associated with the Innu Nation and those who are excluded are strictly and clearly identified: the allies vs. the traitors. The act of eating creates a space for building and releasing the tensions that exist between the local and the global, as well as between the different interest groups making up and giving impetus to the local.

Recognition and Differentiation through Eating

It is fascinating to see how the attitudes of Innu women and men are paradoxically different towards food products from those promoted by the culturalist and traditionalist school which creates a mythical conception of the Other which does not reflect the history or reality of the subject under study. This school talks about Innu food by referring to game, fish, bannock and berries, but we have to admit that in the contemporary daily life of the Innu, the reality is utterly different. In fact, the food basket is made up, to a very large extent, of modern consumer products. Fast food, soft drinks such as Coca-Cola, chips of all kinds, French fries, pizza as well as all the other food products with low nutritional value and high refined sugar and fat content, make up the greater part of the food basket of a vast majority of Innu families. If the bioculturalist approach persists in interpreting these findings as a result of acculturation, we prefer to call upon the concept of *métissage* (a French term which may be roughly translated as "interactions or mixing of cultures") to characterize these new realities while building upon the concept of social stratification of foods and foodways developed and applied by Wilk in his work in Belize (1999).

Through *métissage*, Innu food habits went through profound changes in the second half of the 20th century, changes that were instrumental in building contemporary Innu identity. *Métissage* is not considered here as a strictly cultural phenomenon of solely aesthetic production but rather as an intersection of strategic assertion, of resistance to the hegemonic power by dominated minorities (Turgeon 2003).

The introduction of new products in their food code has allowed the Innu to symbolically integrate an outside westernized world from which they were excluded. This integration allows them to acquire, at least symbolically, the attributes of a condition or state deemed to be desirable and to take effective ownership of it. As mentioned by Fischler (1993: 80), food consumption has one essential characteristic: it is physically and literally incorporated. In this case, food consumption represents a territorial consumption to the extent that it expresses a geographical movement of foods, therefore allowing for the integration of this forbidden outside world, to internalize the outside from which the Innu is excluded (Turgeon 2002).

Innu discourse indicates that by the 1950s the Innu were systematically excluded from the industrial production process. Before the development of the large industrial towns of Baie-Comeau or Sept-Îles and the massive arrival of non-Aboriginal people from large urban centers, such as Montreal and Quebec City, relations between the Innu and the white population of the North Shore area had considerably, if not radically, changed. My research (Roy 1999b, 2002) shows that in this context, the food habits of the Innu were deeply and radically transformed.

The second half of the 20th century was a time of increasing exclusion of the Innu from the production process of Québec's market economy. In the previous decades, the Innu has been intimately associated with and involved in the production process of the North Shore region. Relations between Natives and non-Natives were, at that time, relatively close. With the end of World War II, economic activity increased in remote areas. Job opportunities in the new industrial towns of the North Shore region, such as Baie-Comeau and Sept-Îles attracted thousands of non-Aboriginal people to these areas. As a result, relations between the Innu and Quebecers changed considerably. In the early 20th century the Innu accounted for 23.7 percent of the North Shore population, but this percentage went down to only 7.4 percent at the beginning of the second half of the century. It continued to decline throughout the second half of the 20th century. It should be noted that this decline is solely due to the rapid growth of the non-Aboriginal population and not to a low birth rate among the Innu (Frenette 1996; see also Garneau 1997).

While paid employment was available to an important number of Innu prior to the 1950s, the situation changed drastically soon thereafter. A majority of Innu were then jobless and access to their territory became increasingly reduced as a result of growing forestry, hydro and mining activities. This period is characterized by the deep poverty faced with a large number of Innu families.

Sunday Meal

On the Innu reserve of Pessamit, the daily diet was limited to relatively few staple foods, "*Potatoes, carrots, turnip and bologna*"(Roy 2002: 90) in the second half of the 20th century and for many years thereafter. This is how many individuals described what their family's daily menu looked like during those years. However, these same respondents made reference to the Sunday meal menu of their childhood to describe the foods they would have liked to eat and of which they were generally deprived.

On Sunday, as Innu family members gathered for dinner, the mother would put those so much desired foods on the table. This kind of food was frequently eaten by white families of neighboring villages or by teachers, priests, nuns, nurses and physicians staying on the reserve for short or long periods of time. These foods included chicken or ham but more particularly "Jell-O", occasionally served with a thick layer of "Dreamwhip," "chocolate cake," "sugar pie" or "cookies" cooked by the mother or the grandmother, pizza, or French fries. Individuals remember these food products and refer to them as luxury foods that rarely found their way to their kitchen table. These foods symbolized pleasure, luxury, the inaccessible, wealth, success, and their availability was closely related to paid employment. An individual told me that when she was young, she would often do unpaid housekeeping work for her aunts who were employed by Hydro-Québec. The only benefit was that her aunts allowed her to eat anything she wanted. She longed for cakes, candies, soft drinks and similar foods that garnished her aunts' pantry and of which, in her view, she was painfully deprived.

These few observations are along the same lines as those made by Wilk (1999) in Belize and, to a lesser extent, by other anthropologists belonging to different schools of thought who have studied the mediatization of the act of eating in the cultural construct of reality, such as Roland Barthes (1961), Mary Douglas (1974), Marvin Harris (1985), Miriam Khan (1986), Carol Laderman (1983), Claude Lévi-Strauss (1966), and Lenore Manderson (1986).

The act of eating is an act of creation and of building social alliances. It evolves through time, adapts to circumstances and, from time to time, integrates innovation and reflects social dynamics (Fischler 1993: 179). Food may become a political tool contributing to the development of social solidarity, which serves to define "who is who." Guatemalan activist Rigoberta Menchù, 1992 Nobel Peace Prize Winner, says that her people "*only trust those who eat the same food as we do*" (Burgos 1983), a short and simple but highly significant phrase that allows us to appreciate the full extent of the political dimensions of eating habits.

The proponents of the culturalist doctrine will see the inclusion of new food products in the Innu cultural frame as a "loss of culture," as one more inevitable step towards total acculturation. We may see in this integrative phenomenon—which is part of a process of *métissage*—a phenomenon that allows individuals to acquire, at least symbolically, certain attributes of conditions or status deemed desirable at the local level. These consumable objects, with their meaning and imaginary content, are acquired partly for their status quo.

Eating as Differentiation

Food is central to the development of the collective sense of belonging. It allows to assert specificity, to trace the boundaries of alterity or difference from the Other (Fischler 1993). Distinguishing "who is" from "who is not" Aboriginal is central to the contemporary and daily discourse of the Innu. This sorting out process permeates all areas of Innu life and more particularly those aspects of life the French anthropologist Marcel Mauss (1950: 365) called the "*techniques du corps*": techniques or "ways by which man, in every society, traditionally uses his body." And the act of eating is one of these "body techniques" that allows individuals to acknowledge themselves as members of the same group.

When talking about diabetes, their relation to the body or food, the Innu actually talk about their identity, of who they are in comparison with Others and more specifically in comparison with white people. Garro and Lang (1993: 294) have also stressed this pervasive presence of the identity discourse. "It should also be noted that when Dakota and Anishinabeeg speak of diabetes—or about many other topics—they often make references to their cultural identity." Our work and research came to the same conclusions as shown below.

"*I would have never thought that my daughter would someday eat like the White man!*" This is how a woman in her early forties related her own mother's words the day her mother saw her eating lettuce. Obviously, this mother made a strong association between the simple fact of eating this type of food and the "White" man's world. Yet her daughter had been drinking all kinds of soft drinks and eating chips, pizza and other food products strongly associated with the "ready-to-eat" industry without ever being shown disapproval, or labeled as White. The association with the White world far from being a compliment, is an accusation and a disapproval. Associating her daughter with this food (considered as belonging to the White man) was sufficient for this mother to push off her own descendant to the borderline of the Aboriginal world.

An Innu woman from a Middle North Shore village told me that she preferred to travel five hours by car every two weeks to a grocery store located far from her community. The regular trips made by this women to buy her groceries have a direct impact on the amount of money she actually pays for her food. The price of gas, the vehicle depreciation and of course the time invested in traveling and shopping must all be added to the grocery bill.

What this story suggests is that this Innu woman prefers to be out of her community's sight in order to be out of its mind, away from the rules governing community life, from the place where each and everyone is under the practically inescapable rules of convenience. Out of her community's sight, she manages to act in accordance with her own choices and desires. She can choose the content of her food basket without the fear of seeing her food choices be disapproved of by her peers, of being repudiated as an Innu and marginalized by her own society. Because of this voluntary but occasional exile, she has been able to act according to her desires without feeling the burden of community control. To stop being watched, judged and ostracized, this respondent would rather go from time to time to a place where this difference is allowed, accepted, tolerated. But at what cost? Other Innu, and particularly women, will choose permanent exile and diaspora to be able to live their difference, which is often created and expressed by food habits that do not comply with the home community's rules of social acceptability.

A member of an Innu community located far away from any urban centers, told me it was very difficult for him to buy certain food products he wanted at the Northern store without being labeled as White. The simple fact of buying a tomato, he mentioned, would expose him to disapproving looks and to the excruciating accusation of belonging to the white world. In the collective memory of Aboriginal people, this is the world that has infringed on their rights and still segregates them today.

The manager of this small village's Northern store confirmed that the Innu very rarely bought certain fruits and vegetables. While these foods are literally rotting on the shelves, other products considered objectionable from a public health perspective are preferred by the Innu. These few observations suggest that certain modern food products did find their way into the Innu's identity frame while others simply did not make it to their table. What is particularly surprising is the fact that those foods strongly associated with the White man today, in other words, ignored by the Innu, belong to a large extent to the "health food" advocated by health authorities. But how is one to explain this selectivity, this cultural permeability to certain food products and impermeability to others?

Assertion and Withdrawal

If in the second half of the 20th century Innu food habits underwent considerable change through incorporation. Paradoxically as the Innu grew stronger, they closed in further and withdrew upon themselves. In this regard, taking into account the political context at a macro-societal level may shed new light and help find answers to the choices made by the Innu, including their food choices.

From a macro-societal perspective, the second half of the 20th century corresponds to the emergence of—or emphasis upon—an Aboriginal political discourse organized and structured on a Pan-American identity world wide. Broadly speaking, from the 1950s to the 1970s, in a context of emancipation and decolonisation, Aboriginal claims for self-determination and takeover of health, education and economic development increased significantly. At the same time, during this period and thereafter, there were many confrontations between Aboriginal peoples and State governments.

Examples of Aboriginal resistance are plentiful. At the local level, these struggles and power relations were also reflected in the Innu's daily actions. They penetrated and contributed, for example, to changes in Innu food habits and body. It should be no surprise that foods associated with modernity and part of the Innu's food habits correspond, in most cases, to foods that were highly valued in Québec society from the 1950s to the 1970s. White bread, candies, refined sugar and fat food did not, in those days, incur the frowns and contempt of public health rhetoric. On the contrary, these foods, just like cigarettes and alcohol, were strongly associated with social success and consequently, for the Innu, they were forbidden or difficult to obtain. It is during those same years that Aboriginal people included these foods in the "edible" category. Food was, and still is, as a cultural product, revealing the culture's mobility and polysemy. Incorporating these foreign foods associated with achievement, luxury and success has significantly contributed to the development of the Innu's modern identity. Integrating these foods in the edible order symbolically offered the Innu a part of this modernity from which they were increasingly and painfully excluded.

At the macro-societal level, this period also corresponds to the accentuating and hardening of the discourse surrounding identity. A discourse developed from the materials of a history built and interpreted in the present in order to serve the interests of Aboriginal peoples aspiring to territorial autonomy and self-government. This consolidation—not to say radicalization—of the Aboriginal discourse also occurred at the local level and particularly in the discourse concerning food habits and the relationship to the body. Through the assertion of their contemporary food specificity, the Innu added their voices from the local level, to that of their leaders who were advancing the official identity message at the macro level.

Eating as a Political Act

What I have attempted to demonstrate in the previous sections is that the act of eating, which is the focus of diabetes prevention, is more than a simple act which results from biological dictates. I have also tried to show that the Innu's persistent resistance to modify what the health establishment insists on calling "bad lifestyle" habits reveals and is embedded in political dimensions rather than in ignorance, failure to understand or inappropriate cultural traits.

For health professionals, it appears that the prescription and, of course, the diet elaborated from purely and essentially scientific criteria are clearly apolitical. Who could blame science in being involved in politics!? Didn't Michel Foucault's work unveil the strata of the doctrine that were used as raw material for the construction of what is known today as dietetics? According to Foucault, the Greek word for diet[4] refers to the manner in which one constitutes oneself as a subject who takes appropriate care of one's body and for whom life activities represent a health and moral issue (Foucault 1984: 143). Isn't dietetics at the origin of diets, which actually are prescribed conduct and rules to govern one's lifestyle? Aren't these diets, in a way, manifestations of this new form of governance that Foucault accurately called "bio-power"?

The Innu's resistance to change what is defined by the health community as "unhealthy food habits," is an eloquent demonstration that the health and dietetic community's teachings constitute, at the local level, a political offense. These teachings, clearly associated with the white society by the Innu, are construed as insults to the contemporary way of being Aboriginal by large segments of these populations. This creates a confrontational situation, opposing the "prescriptions" of the local community to those of public health and health practitioners. The Innu who, within their own community, adhere to the dietetic prescription, incur the risk of being marginalized by their own society and, consequently, of being doubly marginalized. If, in the eyes of the health establishment, non-acceptance of their diet and prescription creates risks for the Innu health condition, for the latter, accepting this "scientific prescription" incurs the risk of losing peer recognition.

---

4. In French, it is interesting to note that the etymology of the word "régime" (diet) is the same for the words "régiment" (regiment) and " régimentaire" (regimental). The Latin word *regimen* means to govern or the act of governing.

This is a space where symbolic power is asserted and exercised, and this power is exercised in subtle and sometimes violent ways. The act of eating is thus one of those forms of exercising power that Bourdieu (1979) associated with symbolic power. We are obviously not in the presence of so-called lifestyle habits, a concept regularly used by the health establishment and which is totally meaningless. Incidentally, it is hard to find in the biomedical and public health literature any statements that allows us to understand the theoretical support for the concept of "habits" so abundantly used by them. I am rather of the opinion that we are observing what Bourdieu called the *habitus*. This grammar that generates conforming practices, where the subjects adjust themselves between the objective structures and those structures internalized by them in a practical way that fosters their social existence (Pinto 1998: 51). In fact, long before Bourdieu, Marcel Mauss showed his preference for the Latin word *habitus* instead of *habit* which, for Aristotle, referred to the "exis", the "acquired" and the "faculty." For Mauss (1950: 369), the *habitus* varies within each community according to education, social convenience and fashion. *Habitus* means the "techniques et ouvrage de la raison pratique collective et individuelle" (techniques and work of the collective and individual practical reason).

It is evidently undeniable that human beings must ingest nutrients, proteins and vitamins on a daily basis to keep their biological body functional. But it is also true that as a social and political being, human beings must eat foods with symbolic meanings to successfully integrate into society. And this is particularly true for the Innu for whom the sense of belonging to the Aboriginal society is essential. As long as the Innu are at home, within their community and their village, which they often call their "country," they do not have, as Frantz Fanon said (1952), to prove themselves to others. If in the White world the Innu are regularly faced with the image people have of them, they can exist within their community without feeling like "savages," "lousy persons," "profiteers," "dealers," "non taxpayers." However, this sense of belonging to the Aboriginal world is governed by rules of social convenience providing access to Innu status but only if these rules are complied with.

Eating habits fall within and reveal the social and, I insist, political dimension. Without any doubt, for the Innu, the act of eating is an act of recognition, of building solidarity, developing trust relations, differentiation and assertion of difference from the Other. Moreover, the analysis of the changes in the food habits and its contemporary and daily expression reveals the creative power of the social actors who, on a daily basis, build viable universes and moments of happiness with contemporary materials. Like Giard (1994: 261), I believe that the foods that constitute the Innu's contemporary eating habits reveal the silent piling up of a stratification of orders and counter-orders, of an ethnohistory, a local economy, in sum, cultural creations resulting from the choices of individuals associated with or dissociated from interest groups. It is evident that we cannot deny the biological, the environmental and the climatic. But our understanding of food habits cannot be narrowed down to these sole components. We are far from the simple and sterile notion of "habits" that feeds the heart of the public health and biomedicine doctrine.

The near failure of numerous and recurring promotion and prevention initiatives are, from my point of view, an eloquent illustration of the inadequacy of the explanatory model developed by the health establishment. A model elaborated by people who, in my view, have an invested interest in refusing to recognize the political dimensions responsible for the origin of diabetes and its epidemic proportions, in Innu and other Aboriginal communities.

The contemporary Aboriginal identity feeds on the awareness of belonging to an ethnic group but also to a region and even to a country and to the international community (Hroch 1995). This identity has developed in a context of accelerated globalization of which the Innu have probably been the first victims, like all Aboriginal peoples in Canada and elsewhere in the world. Changes in food habits, gestural expressions and the relationship to the body, are all involved in the geneses of diabetes among Aboriginals in Canada and are closely associated with the process of identity development. This identity is, on one hand, the result of a legitimate resistance and, on the other hand, the exacerbated expression of an ethnocentrism resulting from the exclusion in which Aboriginal people are maintained.

Can we, like Amin Maalouf (1998) does, qualify certain aspects of Aboriginal identity as "killers"? We believe that some of the changes in the Innu identity in the past decades as well as certain views about identity that prevail today in Innu communities could probably be qualified as such. Undeniably, many aspects of the Innu's contemporary eating habits are, from a public health perspective, deeply pathological. The same goes for what we venture to call "Aboriginal fundamentalism" that compels all Innu to comply with the rules of social convenience which very often receive the sanction the defector. "*Les traditions ne méritent d'être respectées que dans la mesure où elles sont respectables, c'est-à dire dans l'exacte mesure où elles respectent les droits fondamentaux des hommes et des femmes.*" (Traditions deserve respect only to the extent that they are respectable, i.e. to the extent that they respect the fundamental rights of men and women. [Maalouf 1998: 124])

The development of this "killer identity" which is instrumental, though not solely, to the emergence and development of diseases like diabetes, is closely linked to the historical and current conditions of exclusion in which the Innu live. Today, we go as far as to say that as long as hostility towards Aboriginal people persists as well as their non-inclusion in all fields of social, economic and political activity, the personal identitfication that undeniably permeates eating habits as well as the relationship to the body, will remain as a rampart behind which the actors of the Aboriginal society will find comfort and security. There they experience, in their daily lives, "moments of joy" and a locally conceptualized and operationalized "health" condition through the actions of the social actors.

If the hostility of the non-Native society is to be considered, Aboriginal peoples' own intolerance towards members of their own group who stand out one way or another, is also to be noted and stressed. That this intolerance is the consequence of a history of colonialism, oppression and of a contemporary context where racism and intolerance occur daily in Innu society is indisputable. But withdrawal and retreat into a victim mentality is likely to be more detrimental than beneficial to Aboriginal people. As noted by Amin Maalouf (1998: 143), retreat into a victim and aggression mentality is likely to have a more devastating effect than aggression itself, as experienced as much by society as by its individual members.

Acknowledgments

As I crafted this chapter, there were hundreds of men and women from the Innu and Atikamekw nations at my side. In particular, Innus from the community of Pessamit have helped to direct my thinking in a more critical direction, a perspective that has taken me far beyond biomedicine's one-dimensional view of diabetes. Through their gaze and their science of the everyday, the Innu and the health care workers of Pessamit opened a door onto the social, economic and political dimensions underlying the emergence of the diabetes epidemic that affects First Nations communities today.

Ms. Sainte-Onge, an Innu woman and director of Innu health services in Pessamit, welcomed me into her circle, in spite of her distaste for anthropologists. In fact, she entitled her postscript to my book, *Sang sucré, pouvoirs codés et médecine amère*, "I hate anthropologists." Ms. Sainte-Onge trusted me, but she always kept me in clear view! She was determined that I not consider the Innu as "cultural objects," like so many other anthropologists in search of exoticism.

Many many thanks to you, Ms. Sainte-Onge and the Innu and Atikamekw who shared your words, your knowledge and your science of the everyday with me from 1986 to 2002.

References

Barthes, Roland. 1961. Pour une psychologie de l'alimentation. Annales ESC. 5: 977–86.

Beardsworth, Alan and Teresa Keil. 1997. Sociology on the Menu: An Invitation to the Study and Society. London: Routledge.

Becker, Marshall H. 1993. A Medical Sociologist Looks at Health Promotion. Journal of Health and Social Behavior 34: 1–6.

Bourdieu, Pierre. 1979. La Distinction—Critique sociale du jugement. Paris: Éditions de minuit.

_____1993. Effets de lieu: *In* La misère du monde. Pierre Bourdeau, *dir*. pp. 249–62. Paris: Éditions du Seuil.

_____1998. La domination masculine. Paris: Éditions du Seuil.

Burgos-Debray, Elisabeth. 1983. Moi, Rigoberta Menchú. Paris : Gallimard.

Canada. 1988. Niveaux de poids associés à la santé: lignes directrices canadiennes. Direction de la promotion de la santé, Direction générale des services et de la promotion de la santé, Santé et Bien-être social Canada.

Certeau, Michel De. 1990. L'invention du quotidien 1. Arts de faire. Paris: Gallimard.

Colditz, G.A., Giovannucci, E., et al.

_____1991. Alcohol Intake in relation to Diet and Obesity in Women and Men. Am .J Clin. Nutr. 54: 49–55.

Counihan, Carole M. and Penny Van Esterik. 1997. Food and Culture: A Reader. New York: Routledge.

Douglas, Mary. 1987. Food in the Social Order: Studies of Food and Festivities in Three American. Communities. New York: Russell Sage Foundation.

————1974. Food as an Art Form. Studio International 188 (969): 83–88.

Fanon Franz. 1995. Peau noire masques blancs. Paris: Éditions du Seuil.

Fassin, Didier. 2001. Le culturalisme pratique de la santé publique. *In* Critique de la santé publique. J.P. Dozon and D. Fassin, dirs. pp. 181–208. Paris: Balland.

Fecteau, Kathia (dir.). 2000. Évaluation de besoins, Centre de santé de Pakua Shipi. Québec. Groupe Recherche Focus.

Fischler, Claude. 1993. L'homnivore. Paris: Éditions Odile Jacob.

Foucault, Michael. 1984. Histoire de la sexualité II. L'usage des plaisirs. Pari: Gallimard.

Frenette, Pierre. 1996. Évolution démographique, développement institutionnel et vie culturelle. *In* Histoire de la Côte-Nord. P. Frenette, dir. pp. 389–422. Québec: Les Presses de l'Université Laval.

Garine, Igor de. 1995. Socio-cultural Aspects of the Male Fattening Sessions Among the Massa of Northern Cameroon. *In* Social Aspects of Obesity. I. De Garine, and N.J. Pollock, eds. pp. 45–70. Wellington: Gordon and Breach Publishers.

Garneau, Jean-Pierre. 1997. La population montagnaise. Données disponibles et évolution récente. Recherches amérindiennes au Québec XXVII (1): 7–18.

Garro, Linda C. 1987. Cultural Knowledge about Diabetes: *In* Diabetes in the Canadian Native Population: Biocultural Perspective. T. Kue Young, ed. pp. 97–109. Toronto: Canadian Diabetes Association.

_____1988. Explaining High Blood Pressure: Variation in Knowledge about Illness. American Ethnologist 15: 98–119.

Garro, Linda C. and Gretchen Chesley Lang. 1993. Explanations of Diabetes: Anishinaabeg and Dakota Deliberate upon a New Illness. *In* Diabetes as a Disease of Civilization: The Impact of Culture Change on Indigenous Peoples. Jenny Joe and Robert S. Young, eds. pp. 293–328. Berlin: Mouton de Gruyter.

Giard, Luce. 1994. Faire la cuisine. In L'invention du quotidien 2. Habiter, cuisiner. M. De Certeau, L. Giard and P. Mayol, dirs. pp. 213–352. Paris: Gallimard.

Gruzinski, Serge. 1999. La pensée métisse. Paris: Fayard.

Harris, Marvin. 1985. Good to Eat: Riddles of Food and Culture. New York: Simon and Schuster.

Harris, S.B., G. Helshn, A. Hanley, et al. 1997. The Prevalence of NIDDM and Associated Risk Factors in Native Canadians. Diabetes Care 20 (2): 185–87.

Hroch, Miroslav. 1995. De l'ethnicité à la nation. Un chemin oublié vers la modernité. Anthropologie et Sociétés 19(3): 71–86.

Khan, Miriam. 1986. Always Hungry, Never Greedy : Food and the Expression of Gender in a Melanesian Society. New York: Cambridge University.

Labbe M. 1936. Étiologie des maladies de la nutrition. *In* Maladies de la nutrition. Encyclopédie Médicochirurgicale, 1ere édition.

Laderman, Carol. 1983. Wives and Midwives: Childbirth and Nutrition in Rural Malaysia. Berkeley: University of California Press.

Lang, Gretchen Chesley. 1989. 'Making Sense' About Diabetes : Dakota Narratives of Illness. Medical Anthropology 11: 305–27.

_____1985. Diabetics and Health Care in a Sioux Community. Human Organization 44 (3): 251–60.

Levi-Strauss, Claude. 1966. The Culinary Triangle. Partisan Review 33: 586–95.

Maalouf, Amin. 1998. Les identités meurtrières. Paris: Éditions Grasset & Fasquelle.

Manderson, Lenore. 1986. Shared Wealth and Symbol : Food, Culture and Society in Oceania and Southeast Asia. New York: Cambridge University Press.

Mauss, Marcel. 1950. Sociologie et anthropologie. Paris: Presse Universitaires de France.

O'Dea, Kerin. 1991. Westernization, Insulin Resistance, and Diabetes in Australian Aborigines. Medical Journal of Australia 155(19): 258–63.

Pinto, Louis. 1998. Pierre Bourdieu et la théorie du monde social. Paris: Éditions Albin Michel.

Pouliot, Sophie (dir.). 2000. Étude de besoins, centre de santé d'Ékuanitshit. Québec: Groupe Recherche Focus.

Roy, Bernard. 2002. Sang, sucré, pouvoirs codés, médecine amère. Québec: Presses de l'Université Laval.

_____1999a. Évaluation quinquennale des services de santé montagnais de Natashquan. Québec. Groupe Recherche Focus.

_____1999b. Le diabète chez les Autochtones. Regard sur la situation à Betsiamites, Natasquan et La Romaine. Recherches amérindiennes au Québec XXIX, 3: 3–18.

Roy, Bernard (dir.). 2000. Études de besoins, Centre de santé de Matimékosh, pour la direction des services de santé Innu de Matimekosh, Québec. Québec. Groupe Recherche Focus.

Roy, Bernard and Kathia Fecteau (dir.). 1999. Étude de besoins, Centre de santé d'Unamen Shipu. Québec: Groupe Recherche Focus.

_____2005. Empowering Words of First Nations Women: Manual for Speaking Out about Life, Health and Diabetes. Quebec: University Presses, Laval University. (originally published in French, under the title Paroles et pouvoir de femmes des Premières Nations).

Szathmary, Emöke. 1987. Genetic and Environment Risk Factors. In Diabetes in the Canadian Native Population Bio-cultural Perspectives. T.K. Young, ed. pp. 29–55. Toronto: Canadian Diabetes Association.

Turgeon, Louis. 2002. Manger le monde. Rencontres postcoloniales dans les restaurants étrangers de la ville de Québec. In Regards croisés sur le métissage. L. Turgeon, dir. pp. 205–33. Québec: Les Presses de l'Université Laval.

_____2003. Patrimoines métissés. Contextes coloniaux et postcoloniaux. Paris: Éditions de la Maison des sciences de l'homme.

Valdebenito, Cécilia (dir.). 2001. Évaluation des programmes et des besoins en santé de Uashat mak Mani-Utenam. Québec. Groupe Recherche Focus.

Wilk, Richard R. 1999. "Real Belizean Food": Building Local Identity in the Trans-national Caribbean. American Anthropologist 101(2): 244–55.

Young, T. Kue. 1988. Health Care and Cultural Change: The Indian Experience in the Central Subarctic. Toronto: University of Toronto Press.

Zimmet, Paul, G. Dowse, C. Finch, et al. 1990. The Epidemiology and Natural History of NIDDM—Lessons from the South Pacific. Diabetes/Metabolism Review 6(2): 91–124. <www.chbc.qca\diabete\psychologie\habitudes.htm>, June 17, 2003.

CHAPTER 8

PRENATAL MYSTERIES AND SYMPTOMLESS DIABETES IN THE GILA RIVER INDIAN COMMUNITY

Carolyn Smith-Morris

At issue is how much information and autonomy will be allowed to groups of patients who can so clearly benefit from biomedical interventions. As in colonial settings, do we coerce and force our methods because of our conviction that we "know better", or allow Indigenous groups to understand and adopt those practices that are meaningful and useful within their lives? As women's discussions show, a medical pluralism exists in Pima society, which employs local notions of women's competence and a non-reliance on biomedicine.

Carolyn Smith-Morris in this chapter

Summary of Chapter 8. This chapter considers the importance placed on pregnancy in the struggle to prevent diabetes at the Gila River Indian Community, Arizona. It provides ethnographic data on Pima (Akimel O'odham) women's perspectives about this highly surveilled period in their lives. For many Pima women, the largely symptomless nature of gestational diabetes contributes to a sense of mystery about this disease. Pima women's narratives illustrate that their diabetes prevention behaviors during pregnancy are limited by their comprehension of and responsiveness to biomedical testing and surveillance data, even in contradiction of their own symptomless experience. Specific biomedical concepts such as "risk" and even the idea of a reliable diagnostic test are challenged by the economic and logistical problems of life in this community. Thus, while certain findings are generalizable to all women engaged with biomedical diabetes screening, pointed concerns about the political economy of health on Native American Reservations and the position of Indian women vis-à-vis biomedical praxis will be highlighted.

❦ ❦ ❦

(Jan. 5, 2000) Stephanie [age 22] has only been to one appointment in this pregnancy—she's now 31 weeks gestation. She told me she'd attend today because she knew they would do an ultrasound, and wanted me to give her a ride to the hospital.

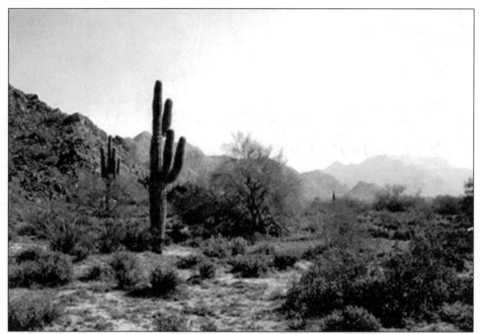

Landscape, Gila River Indian Community, Arizona.

She had a burrito for breakfast [2 eggs, 1 cup potatoes, one-quarter cup onions, one-half cup beef, 18-inch tortilla]. Her appointment was for 8:30. We arrived at 8:00 and sat with a friend she found in the waiting room. She had a Coke while she waited, and was called at 8:30 to update her record and give a urine sample. At 9:00, she was called back by the nurse for vitals and "all the questions". When she spoke to the nurse, she was reminded that she was supposed to have fasted, but Stephanie didn't admit to having had breakfast. She had blood drawn later that morning at the lab and would have to return in a couple of days for results. [This was for diabetes screening, but Stephanie didn't remember that.]

At home she talked about how getting back to the hospital this month would be a "pain" because it was winter and too cold to walk. Her mom had been getting sick a lot lately and wasn't able to watch the kids, so she'd have to take them with her. And whenever she did take her kids, the staff looked at her real "snotty" if they would make any noise or touch anything. And, of course, Sarah was into everything. And they would always give her a lecture about how Toby was too "chunky," and "you shouldn't be letting him drink that." These were the main reasons she didn't go to prenatal appointments. "They usually only have you pee in a cup and listen to the baby's heart beat. So if I feel fine, there wasn't much reason to go . . . except for that ultrasound picture."

(Jan. 12, 2000) Stephanie told me she wasn't going to go, but her mom had an appointment with podiatry the same day, so we all went together. Stephanie talked to the nurse, who said her sugars were high and she had to talk to the people over at Diabetes Education. Toby drew a couple of glares, I noticed, from a secretary for spilling his Coke on the floor. At Diabetes Education, they were telling her she had diabetes—230 sugars—and that it was going to hurt the baby if she didn't get it under control. Stephanie later told me, "the only reason it was so high is because of that breakfast burro, so I'm probably fine."

[Taken from fieldnotes. Postscript: Stephanie missed the education class scheduled for her at Diabetes Education at the end of October. Had baby boy February 25th, cesarean, 10 lbs., 1 oz. He had jaundice and a slight heart murmur.]

This scenario accentuates the everyday concerns that compete for pregnant Pima women's time and attention.[1] In particular, although a woman's general feelings about health care and health care providers might be good, there are logistic barriers that make attendance at appointments difficult and may distract her during those sometimes brief appointments. For a variety of reasons, screening tests for gestational diabetes (diabetes during pregnancy) have become a standard practice in the U.S. for all pregnant women. However, almost two-thirds of the Pima women with whom I spoke were, like Stephanie, reluctant to ask questions about what test results mean. The costs in time, effort, and mental anguish of finding out one's diabetes status outweigh the benefits of knowing, especially if this is a condition that one suspects will eventually crop up no matter what prevention efforts are made.

Introduction

Over half of Pima adults have diabetes. The Gila River Indian Community has borne a high disease prevalence since soon after World Ward II, to the extent that diabetes is now considered endemic to the Pima. According to the medical literature, three domains are claimed to influence Pima diabetes: genetics, culture, and political-economic factors (Smith-Morris 2004). The interaction of these factors has revealed a remarkably important linchpin in the perpetuation of high diabetes rates: the mother's womb.

The development of glucose intolerance during pregnancy (called gestational diabetes mellitus or GDM) is not unique to the Pima. GDM is a condition that occurs during 7% of pregnancies in the U.S. in which abnormally high amounts of glucose circulate in the blood of the pregnant woman. This creates an environment in the uterus that predisposes the fetus to the development of diabetes later in life. GDM also correlates with the mother's development of "outright" diabetes within 5-16 years (Carr 2001). Thus, pregnant women—in particular, pregnant Pima women—are monitored carefully for signs of gestational diabetes.

This chapter offers a perspective on diabetes as told by pregnant Pima women. Their narratives about this disease were informed by their own experiences of pregnancy and by their exposures to diabetes in friends and relatives. In many instances, women's talk was full of stories and anecdotes recounting the health dilemmas they or others had faced. Women used these stories to not only punctuate but to construct answers to my various probes into their knowledges and practices regarding diabetes.

---

1. Stephanie is a fictitious person; the scenario is compiled from field notes and various women's narratives to supply a snapshot or profile of pregnant participants in the study.

In the first section, I provide some detail on the ethnographic work and the women with whom I spoke. I then outline several biomedical and epidemiological facts about gestational diabetes in this community, in order to clarify the importance of gestational diabetes within the larger realm of "outright" diabetes, especially for Indigenous Peoples. Just before turning to focus on women's narratives, I offer further detail about the Gila River Indian Community and the health services available to persons with diabetes on this reservation. My discussion of women's understandings of GDM details three central themes that emerged from our interviews. I discuss each in turn then, in the summary and discussion, considering how women's forms of talk and learning might inform future diabetes prevention efforts.

An Ethnography of Pregnancy

Conversations with Pima women offer a window into the common, yet largely inscrutable, experience of diabetes in this community. Growing up in the context of an endemic disorder, pregnant women did not show a sense of urgency or trauma that might be associated with other prenatal ailments. Theirs was a seasoned view of diabetes and its impact, not simply on individual lives, but on the life and identify of a community. In efforts to find a common ground, I could neither rely on biomedical explanations of this disease nor upon western or Anglo norms surrounding patient attitude and responsibility. What I did rely on was my own first experience of pregnancy, as it unfolded simultaneously with these women's. My ethnographic method was the embodiment of participation observation: an ethnography of pregnancy conducted while I was pregnant.

The methods for this ethnography were otherwise very traditional: open-ended, lengthy interviews with Pimas on the topics of diabetes, its causes and consequences, health care, pregnancy, and the meanings they attached to their illness experiences. I conducted 63 tape-recorded interviews with Pimas age 18–67; interviews lasted from 40 minutes to over 4 hours. Thirty-six of these were non-pregnant adults and the remaining twenty-seven were pregnant women who provided multiple interviews over the course of their pregnancy. I tested my list of interview questions carefully, using key contributors to evaluate the appropriateness and clarity of each question. The average age of participants was 28.5 years old. Most of the pregnant women were in the twenties or early thirties, although a majority of women had been pregnant with their first child in their teen years. Seventeen (27% of tape-recorded) adults reported they have diabetes. I recruited participants primarily from the waiting rooms at the prenatal clinics, WIC and Well Baby (Public Health) clinics, and through word-of-mouth. Most (43 out of 63) of the interviews were conducted in the participant's home and I conducted interviews in all seven districts of the Reservation as well as off-Reservation in parks and restaurants.

Talk about illness has always been a subject of medical anthropology. These narratives, including the Pima narratives in this chapter, are not only talk about one's own illness but also situated, limited, and socially strategic accounts. Medical anthropologists (e.g., Garro 1994; Good 1994; Lang 1989; Mattingly 1998), as various chapters in this book illustrate, consider illness narratives more than a simple story—they are a way for speakers to manage new information or experiences, and to prepare accounts that are appropriate for a specific audience or context. The essence of illness narratives is the story-telling efforts of speakers to explain and, some argue, impact what is going on in an illness experience. In studying illness narratives, I aim to answer the questions, "What is the relationship between story and experience?" (Good 1994) and how do women use narratives to understand, cope with, and act upon diabetes in their lives?

Gestational Diabetes

Gestational Diabetes mellitus is carbohydrate intolerance with onset or first diagnosis during pregnancy. Glucose intolerance that existed prior to pregnancy but was unrecognized, therefore, falls into this diagnostic category. Roughly 8-9% of Pima pregnancies are complicated by GDM (Association 2000; Pettitt et al. 1996). The American Diabetes Association (ADA) recommends that all pregnant women receive a risk assessment for this disease at their first prenatal visit. For Pima women, this assessment—which checks for marked obesity, personal history of GDM, glycosuria (glucose in the urine), or a strong family history of diabetes—is considered unnecessary based on the strong family history of diabetes for almost all Pimas. The ADA does not recommend further glucose testing for no-risk or low-risk status women; that is, women who are "less than 25 years old, normal weight before pregnancy, member of an ethnic group with a low prevalence of GDM, no known diabetes in first-degree relatives, no history of abnormal glucose tolerance and no history of poor obstetric outcome" (American Diabetes Association 2000). Thus, as members of a high risk ethnic group, *all* Pima women undergo diabetes testing.

Although Pima women are at high risk for diabetes, they are no different from other diabetes patients who struggle with the often symptomless nature of this disorder and the lifestyle changes necessary to avoid health problems. The few symptoms that might be present in early diabetes can easily be confused with symptoms related to any pregnancy in the Sonoran Desert of Arizona—fatigue, excessive thirst, and swelling in lower extremities. The lack of symptoms indicative of diabetes not only creates a technology-bound diagnosis, but exacerbates the competition between professional, authoritative knowledge and women's lay, experiential knowledge. In short, where Pima women experience a symptomless pregnancy, biomedical surveillance provides evidence of disease or its imminence. Providers trying to make accurate diagnoses can likewise be frustrated with the necessity for multiple glucose readings over time and the lack of symptoms upon which to base a diagnosis or because of which to urge patients in behavioral changes. The screening process is therefore an essential tool in diabetes prevention and screening, but is also one that requires both patients and professionals to attend to non-experience-based markers of health.

At Gila River's Huhukam Memorial Hospital, all pregnant women between 24 and 26 weeks gestation are first screened for diabetes. This screening involves a 50-gram glucose load with a 1-hour (non-fasting) waiting period before blood is drawn. If this screen yields a positive result, the pregnant woman is referred for the 3-hour 100-gram glucose test. If that test yields a positive result, then a diagnosis of gestational diabetes is made. If the test result is negative, the test is repeated at 32 weeks gestation. The testing process therefore means that some women may undergo testing several times during a pregnancy. These follow-up tests, of course, require additional trips to the hospital and added worry about the results.

As with type 2 diabetes, the form of diabetes that is predominant in the Gila River Indian Community, GDM is treated through a combination of daily self-monitoring of blood glucose, nutritional counseling, and in some cases pharmacologic therapy. Additional considerations for diabetes management during pregnancy include: the measurement of fetal abdominal circumference to predict macrosomia (high birth weight); maternal surveillance for hyperglycemia high enough to pose increased risks to the fetus; maternal surveillance for blood pressure and protein in the urine, to detect hypertensive disorders; counseling on exercise and lifestyle factors; and ultrasonography to measure asymmetric fetal growth and fetal stress. GDM is not an indication for cesarean delivery or for delivery before 38 weeks gestation, although it makes a cesarean more likely. Maternal morbidity associated with GDM includes hypertensive disorders, specifically preeclampsia, and increased maternal length of stay (Carr 2001). Neonatal morbidity can include macrosomia, birth trauma, fetal demise, hypoglycemia, and hyperbilirubinemia (ibid.).

Healing Practices on the Reservation

While I learned of one traditional Pima healer (training under a man from the neighboring Tohono O'odham nation), many Pimas know of one or several healing practices and medicinal plants. This knowledge is not codified to my knowledge, but passed down through the generations. Thus, for a fallen fontanel, many Pima women would take their infants to an elderly relative for healing, rather than to a healer. And several Pima women told me that "doctors don't know about" fallen fontanel, although providers assured me they had indeed treated Pima children for dehydration—one symptom of which may be a fallen fontanel. The prescribed treatment for this condition, however, differs between the two healing traditions: traditional Pima practices require the mechanical "lifting" or "pushing up" of the fontanel through pressure on the roof of the child's mouth; biomedical practitioners prescribe liquids for re-hydration.

Pimas, however, are principally engaged in biomedical forms of healing. The Huhukam Memorial Hospital houses an inpatient, surgical, and many specialty clinics. A smaller satellite clinic also exists near the far western end of the reservation. A shuttle service is available to both sites, although some women report this service can be unreliable. The Huhukam Memorial Hospital is tribally-owned and houses the Diabetes Education Center (DEC). Public health nursing, environmental health services, and other Indian Health Service (IHS) programs are active on the reservation. The IHS trains Community Health Representatives, about 21 of whom work on the Reservation—most in the Public Health services. There are also offices for Tobacco Tax funding, Women, Infant and Children (WIC) services, Head Start, and various Tribal services. There is a Wellness Center gymnasium and weight room in Sacaton, as well as an additional fitness center and program in the hospital. There are also District Service Centers in each District where public health clinics (e.g., "Well Baby Clinics" for immunizations) are held and where I held the focus groups for the project. Additional programs, including ones run by the National Institutes of Health specifically aimed at diabetes reduction, also exist on the reservation.

In Sacaton, a woman might travel two miles from home to the hospital. From the nearest settlement outside of Sacaton, in Sacaton Flats or Stotonic, a patient would travel at least 5 miles and up to 12 miles to the hospital. The westernmost areas of the Reservation are a 40–60 minute drive away by car. Vehicle transportation is thus essential, especially due to the extreme high temperatures in this part of the Sonoran Desert (110–115 degrees F. each day of the summer). And many women who skip or miss medical appointments do so because of a lack of transportation. In these scenarios, women develop strong(er) family and social supports to help answer questions about prenatal health and symptoms, thereby strengthening the non-professional arena of knowledge.

Women, however, make great efforts to attend prenatal and other scheduled appointments. Eighty-three percent of the women I interviewed had generally good things to say about the biomedical care services available on the reservation. "Positive" comments were made by women who felt the care was good or fairly good, or that "I get what I need to know." Only 6 participants had an overall negative response, including statements such as, "[The care's] not good cause they really don't know that much." And five participants were neutral or replied, "I don't know" concerning their overall feeling about health care on the reservation. This generally positive view reflects that health care is responsive to the needs of these women, and that providers are generally attentive and skilled.

However, as the interviews continued and questions began to probe more deeply into issues and scenarios, women also expressed several concerns. In short, there were often both positive and negative feelings about health care expressed within a single interview. From the many factors influencing women's decisions about prenatal care and diabetes management, I will focus on three: lay understandings of GDM and its screening process; women's ideas about risk; and women's reactions to the co-morbid problems in diabetes.

Pima Women's Understandings of GDM

CSM: Why do pregnant women get diabetes?

Alice: The body doesn't break down the sugar. The insulin doesn't work, so it makes all your food turn to sugar.

Vina: The baby probably takes a lot of your sugar.

Eileen: Like when you drink too much sugar—and you don't drink enough water and stuff.

Mary: Probably most people that eat a lot of sweets when they're pregnant can get it.

Pima women's discussions of gestational diabetes are influenced by biomedical, traditional, and popular notions. Their ideas also change over time and in response to experience and exposures. I focus here on those features of GDM upon which women

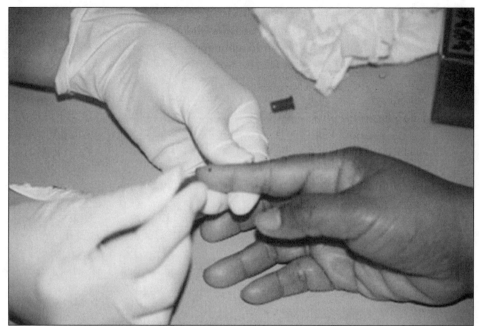

Regular monitoring of blood sugar, sometimes through several of these finger pricks each day, is an important part of controlling diabetes.

hinge their understandings; those traits that are most salient to women: the fluctuation in diabetes screening test results; women's lack of symptoms with GDM—especially in comparison to the outright diabetes they have witnessed in others; and the complex of health problems that often occur with uncontrolled or late-stage diabetes.

Fluctuating Test Results

Screening tests for symptomless or pre-symptomatic diseases are a hallmark of epidemiology and biomedicine. The ability to identify disease or it precursors before any bodily symptoms are present is seen as an important advantage in biomedicine, and is largely attributable to the population-based research conducted on disease events by epidemiologists. Through epidemiology, characteristics of a disease, as well as of the diseased population after and before disease onset, are tentatively identified. This research would greatly enhance our ability to identify, prevent, and provide early treatment for disease. But the benefits of screening tests are complicated in gestational diabetes by the fact that all indications of disease usually disappear after the birth of the baby. This disappearance seems to indicate good health when, in fact, the infant may be overweight, hypoglycemic, and at higher risk for diabetes; the mother may also be recovering from Cesarean section delivery and is also at higher risk for developing "outright" diabetes later on.

I began this chapter with a scenario from field notes detailing Stephanie's experience and perceptions of prenatal screening tests for gestational diabetes. Stephanie and other pregnant Pima women are like other women in being unsure of how to interpret the results of GDM screenings. To understand the reason for multiple tests over the course of the pregnancy, women must be aware of the cumulative effect of glucose intolerance.

> Kelly: It's like…you do these two hours [of tests]. You do the one hour, you
> do a three hour. Ok, your sugars are up and then it's like, now, *now* I'm clas-
> sified GCI [gestational carbohydrate intolerance—a precursor to diabetes].
> And then they do them again six months later and I'm classified 'gestational
> diabetes.' I'm, like, wait a minute. So what comes next? That's all I have to
> say…is "what comes next?" But as far as it happening [what causes it], that
> just blows my mind…I really couldn't answer that question. I just don't know.

Kelly had not yet learned about either the biological or the social processes behind
her changing glucose readings. In the absence of that perspective, she (1) felt frustration and lack of control over her glucose—"what comes next?"; and (2) was not likely
to have participated in blood sugar control behaviors between tests. At Gila River,
women are referred to the Diabetes Education Center as soon as they receive a diagnosis of GCI, in an attempt to prevent their progression to diabetes through behavioral change (e.g., diet and exercise). But these referrals are not always followed up,
and women do not always complete the day-long class in diabetes education. The end
result, for Kelly and many other Pima women, is no change in behavior and, subsequently, an earlier diagnosis of gestational diabetes in each pregnancy.

> Kelly: I can catch it, I mean I had it with my first daughter at 28 weeks, my
> second daughter at 27 weeks, but with this pregnancy, I had it at 7 to 8 weeks.
> And that part of it, I just don't understand. I could never [understand that]
> because afterwards, I'm fine. After the deliveries and the six weeks [post par-
> tum] glucose testing, yet I'm fine.

Unfortunately, Kelly's six-week post-partum blood glucose might not be "fine".

Symptomless Diabetes

Illness bodily clues undergo cognitive screening and cultural interpretation quickly
and pre-consciously. "Whether or not a particular behavior or experience is viewed by
members of a society as a sign or symptom of illness depends on cultural values, social norms, and culturally shared rules of interpretation" (Mishler 1981: 141). For
many pregnant Pima women, no bodily clues to diabetes exist; they have no experience of illness. The pregnant women with whom I spoke were relatively young (average age=25) and, therefore, had less hypertension, less use of insulin, and fewer co-
morbid diabetes conditions than older Pimas. For biomedicine, risk information
attempts to "fill in" information where experience stops. Risk is treated as disease and
not just as its potential—risk becomes *symptom*. *"And because symptoms and bodily
signs are "malleable," risk lurks in every twitch, ever-present"* (Gifford 1992).

For Pima women—and many women with GDM—a lived experience of health is
redefined as symptomless disease and unhealthy pregnancy. Further, biomedicine tends
to conceptualize pregnancy and diabetes as antagonistic states, the combination of
which creates a *life-long* period of vulnerability to diabetes for both the mother and
child. Women are taught, contrary to their physical experience, that their pregnancy is
potentially harmful to their bodies, that a diabetic pregnancy will harm them and their
baby, and that such a pregnancy will continue to affect them both throughout their lives.

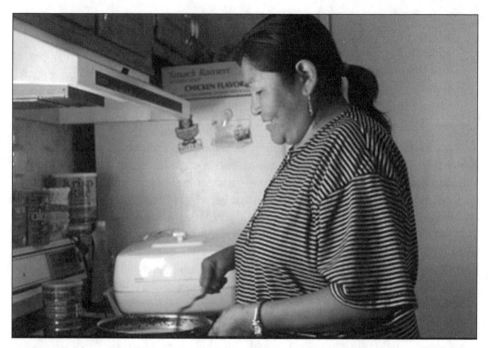

To Pima women, health is not about "avoiding risk" but about "taking care" of yourself.

Not surprisingly, this unhealthy and risk-laden view of pregnancy is unpopular and confusing, especially when presented by persons from a "dominant" ethnic category, socioeconomic status, and power position (as is quite often the case in biomedical institutions on American Indian reservations). Yet, clinicians use prenatal tests as teaching tools that reveal symptomless processes in the body and expect patients to undergo examinations and treatments in an understanding and cooperative way.

How, then, is this risk information interpreted by Pima women? Within biomedical paradigms, risk data are considered objective, scientific knowledge to which patients have the right and through which patients can become 'empowered' to prevent disease. From the patient's point of view, however, his or her sense of vulnerability to disease is typically informed by professional and lay information as well as personal experience, and intuition about the likelihood of developing disease in a given context, time, and circumstance.[2] Comparative risks and optimism also factor into individuals' considerations (van der Pligt 1998). Thus, a broad combination of subjective and objective information blends with Pima explanatory models to produce health-seeking behaviors: "taking care" of oneself involves more than avoiding "risky" behaviors. As Florence understands it,

> I think it all depends on your body, on yourself, on your own thinking. That
> [you're more likely to get it if] you're gonna be down and out or all negative.

---

2. Several things may contribute to a person's sense of vulnerability including emotional states (e.g., Hammer 1995 on fear) or culturally-determined periods of vulnerability (see, for example, Frazer 1922). Likewise, people will have periods of resiliency, during which they may feel able to engage in risky behaviors with relative safety (see Nichter 1998).

Local interpretations of risk are especially important in communities with endemic disease and long-standing prevention programs. The rise in diabetes prevalence coupled with a falling age of initial diagnosis, means that young Pima women are considered closer in years to a diagnosis of diabetes than ever before. However, after their first child, some of the pregnant women I interviewed were more willing to skip prenatal appointments based on how they were feeling. They expressed greater knowledge of pregnancy and what their bodies were going through, and a greater confidence that they would know if something were wrong. For these women, prenatal visits are seen a superfluous and inconvenient. Therefore, because of its symptomless nature, gestational diabetes can easily go undiagnosed. Patricia said she normally attends appointments at the Reservation hospital, but hasn't gone much during her current pregnancy because, as she explained, "I think I know what's going on with me". The subjective experience thus continues to drive much of women's decisions about health care, despite ample objective risk data.

Therefore, I sought specifically to understand women's ideas about risk and how these informed knowledge of diabetes. In general, women agreed that risk for disease did not equate with disease itself.

> Angela: Risk means that you're gonna…get diabetes, and if you don't control the way you're eating, you could get it. But if you do control, you won't get it.

Angela highlights the importance of dietary control in the prevention of diabetes. But she also implies that a controlled diet is a guarantee for avoiding diabetes, which it is not. In response to the same question—"What do you think it means to be 'at risk' for diabetes?"—other women employed the term 'borderline':

> CMS: What do you think it means to be at risk for diabetes?
> Priscilla: That they were borderline.

> CMS: What do you think it means to be at risk for diabetes?
> Denise: Just, is that like another term for borderline?

Sarah's use of the term 'borderline' reveals its ambiguity—although she says she was diagnosed with diabetes four years ago, the fact that the term "borderline" was used leaves her uncertain as to whether she has it now or not.

> [I think I'll get it] when I get older.…About 4 years ago I was diagnosed with diabetes—I have borderline diabetes. [But] someone told me, you either are or you're not, there is no borderline."

Many providers at Gila River agree that use of the term "borderline" misleads patients. Yet, since diabetes is diagnosed with the use of a numerical scale (indicating a blood glucose level), then numbers close to the diagnostic cut-off are often described as "borderline" by both patients and a few care givers. Further, these numbers fluctuate all the time. So a reading one day might be well within diabetic range, while the next day may be normal. And "borderline" can soften the psychological impact of a diagnostic lab report by implying "you're not too sick…yet." Also, some Pimas who are tested over a period of time show a progressive rise in their glucose readings, furthering the cultural meaningfulness of the *linear* progress and the idea of "borderline diabetes."

What happens when 'borderline' is used as a synonym for 'being at risk for' diabetes? For most women, it meant that you were close to having diabetes, and that behavioral change or medication was needed immediately. For others like Sarah above, it is a slippery slope, such that becoming "borderline" was essentially the same as receiving the diagnosis.

> Maureen: I don't know because…you know people that had been told they were a borderline candidate—here, you know, because…I've talked to different people and they have different reactions. So what does that mean, borderline? Either you are or you aren't!

In these women's comments resounded a frustration, if not pessimism, with providers and biomedical knowledge for not being more precise or more reliable. They also reflect a desire to develop a linear sense of diabetes—its closeness or inevitability—so that the urgency and/or futility of the situation could be gauged. In sum, risk information is flexible and imprecise for these women, and therefore open to interpretation based not only on biomedical perspectives but on Pima knowledge and experience.

Related Problems in Diabetes

The distinction between health problems that often develop with advanced diabetes, and diabetes itself is often blurred. While differences between causal factors and disease symptomatology may not be relevant in patients' lived experiences, the distinction between diabetes and its consequences does have relevance for prevention messages. Associating the disorder with its related (or co-morbid) conditions may influence young, pregnant women's willingness or ability to recognize symptomless GDM as part of the same process. In this section, I will explore how co-morbid conditions are included in Pima definitions of diabetes, and consider how the combination of these problems impact women's disease management efforts.

Because the biomedical etiology of diabetes includes a complex set of genetic and environmental factors (see, for example, Smith-Morris 2003), it is often co-morbid with a range of neural, heart, eye, and kidney problems. Diabetes-related conditions account for 19.5% of all Pima deaths which is four times that of whites and two times that of blacks (age adjusted) (Newman et al. 1993; Sievers et al. 1992). Pimas' fears of a slow, painful, and withering death to diabetes are, therefore, warranted. In this section, I wish to demonstrate the knowledge participants have about the complications of diabetes, even when their understanding of the disease itself is not always accurate in biomedical terms. Women's horror with amputations and the pain suffered by relatives undergoing dialysis were profoundly distressing. These emotions are strong motivations for women. Laura talks about her father:

> Laura: Talking about it, this hurts me, you know. His body started shutting down and he got on dialysis. And then he had an ulcer or something…and they found out that he was getting an infection under his foot. And he had, I don't remember what else. So they sent him to Tucson and they amputated up to his knee. And so then he had to get a prosthesis. And, you know, he couldn't ever,

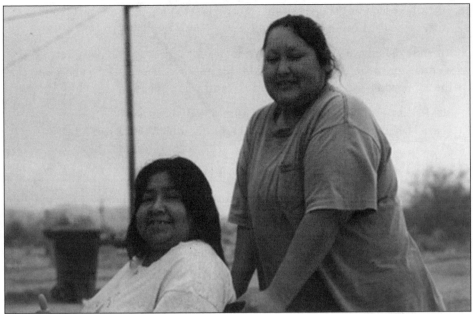

Pimas often know diabetes more by its outward signs in the late stages of disease, like amputations and dialysis, than by a number on a glucose meter. But such complications are now affecting Pimas at a younger age than for previous generations.

he never gained the strength to get back. I think he gave up from that point. He gave up.

Observations of diabetes' physical impact on the body's organs and extremities provoke a more visceral awareness of disease than does information from a glucose meter. Complications of diabetes, such as blindness, nerve and circulatory damage, and the need for dialysis, are the outward signs of diabetes, and these signs draw upon the fears and disgust of all Pimas from an early age.

> Maureen: I have been diabetic for quite some time....I know infection has a lot to do with your blood sugar and other things. And my amputation came because, that other complex I lived in, the neighbor didn't want to...get involved. And my mother didn't live too near at the time, and she was on vacation. And I had to wait until she came....And so by the time I got to the doctor, you know, I didn't have a choice. [They had to amputate.] That's why I don't like to put things off because I know if you put it off too long, something like that can happen.

The co-morbid conditions of diabetes are recognized as signs of impending death. But Pimas speak somewhat metaphysically about death by diabetes, explaining that patients grow tired of fighting the disease and "give up," rather than being overtaken by the disease.

> Caroline: My best friend's grandmother, I was real close to her, she died because of her diabetes. She had to take insulin shots. She took them every day and she got one blister on her foot and they amputated and amputated until

the whole leg was gone. Then they were going to amputate the next one and that's when she gave up and just died.

Patients, thus, have some agency even in death by diabetes complications.

A crucial theme in women's discussions for improved diabetes education is to clarify the confusion between diabetes, and its causes and consequences.

CMS: In your own words, what do you think diabetes is?
Fay: They can't control their, I don't know, their high blood pressure?

CMS: What do you think diabetes is?
Nancy: High blood pressure and that's all I know about it.

The association between high blood pressure and diabetes indicates that the Pima incorporate other signs and symptoms into their own diagnosis of diabetes. High blood pressure is a frequent problem for persons with type 2 diabetes and can be a problem for pregnant Pima women, leading to complications during childbirth including c-section deliveries.

Summary and Discussion

Three main issues contribute to Pima women's difficulty to understand and undergo diabetes testing during pregnancy. Biomedical multi-stage screenings and the assignment of numerical indicators of health is the first issue. In the second place stands the clinical use of risk information that contradicts women's experiences and first-hand knowledge about incidence and prevalence of diabetes among family and friends. This leads to the third issue, which encompasses co-morbid disorders and diabetes complicating factors identified by biomedicine that further blur the distinction between diabetes and a variety of other illnesses. The implications of these perceptions for GDM are profound. Since diabetes is now endemic at Gila River, the long-term effectiveness of prevention efforts are frequently questioned because they seem to be ineffective in the long run.

In talking with Pima women about their pregnancies, I was repeatedly struck by the importance they placed on their own and others' experiences. Rather than driven by biomedical knowledge, it was the women's experiences of health events that informed their decisions about healthy behaviors and the meanings of signs and symptoms. The centrality of experience is an important feature of Pima knowledge and the ways in which they structure their actions in everyday life. Life experiences and perceptions are particularly relevant in attempts to control symptomless disorders like gestational diabetes.

It also became clear that in the context of women's talk about pregnancy, oral tradition as a mode of communication and reliance on kin networks for social support remain central to Pima life. The help of health professionals and information acquired during hospital visits is certainly important, but it is not accepted uncritically by the Pima. Biomedical perspectives are evaluated by family and friends, who compare their experiences with those of others. And while atypical experiences are not entirely ignored, the most common experiences become truisms—for example, the inability of hospital employees to treat a fallen fontanel, or the sense that diabetes is, in some cases, unavoidable.

By paying close attention to Indigenous forms of producing knowledge, health professionals can help improve diabetes programs. Diabetes during pregnancy already is the critical focus of prevention efforts among American Indians and Indigenous Peoples all over the world, broadly speaking. Pregnant women thus emerge as an important group to consult and understand (Smith-Morris 2003). O'Neil and Kaufert (1995: 70) describe an effort in community-based healing in which a birthing center recruited and trained local Inuit women as midwives:

> [T]his case was a unique attempt to take the sometimes disparate ideological frameworks that surround the childbirth issue in northern Canada and merge these to create a unified challenge to the hegemony of obstetrical ideology. Probably most remarkably, the decisions to pursue this type of program were made in response to practical needs...

The principal challenge in such community-based planning is arriving at agreements on conceptions of health, what is considered reasonable treatment, and what are sound and realistic expectations for outcome. Indigenous understandings of the meanings of "risk" are instrumental to develop effective prevention and treatment plans for gestational diabetes.

Acknowledgments

I am most grateful to the women of Gila River who shared their lives and pregnancies with me. Their warm and enthusiastic welcome made this a wholly gratifying experience and I value their friendships. I also thank the elders and leaders at Gila River, particularly the Gila River Community Council and its Health and Social Committee, for their guidance, constructive criticism, and encouragement. The work would not have been possible without the financial support of the National Science Foundation (#9910441), the Wenner-Gren Foundation (#6502), and the Agency for Health Care Quality and Research (#R03HS10802). I also remain gratefully indebted to my advisors at the University of Arizona: Ana Ortiz, Mark Nichter, Susan Philips, Jennie Joe, and Tom Weaver. Finally, thanks to my family and friends who were simultaneously support, critics, editors, and assistants.

References

American Diabetes Association. 2000. Gestational Diabetes mellitus. Diabetes Care 23(Suppl. 1): 577–79.

Carr, S. R. 2001. Evidence-Based Diabetes Screening for Pregnancy. Journal of Midwifery and Women's Health 46(3): 152–58.

Farmer, Paul. 1994. AIDS-Talk and the Constitution of Cultural Models. Social Science and Medicine 38(6): 801–9.

Garro, Linda C. 1994. Narrative Representations of Chronic Illness Experience: Cultural Models of Illness, Mind, and Body in Stories Concerning the Temporomandibular Joint (TMJ). Social Science and Medicine 18(6): 775–88.

Gifford, Sandra M. 1992. Pathologies of Risk: Managing the New Social Morbidity. *In* Annual Meetings of the American Anthropology Association, San Francisco, California, Dec 4, 1992. pp. 1–20.

Good, Byron J. 1994. The Narrative Representation of Illness. *In* Medicine, Rationality, and Experience: An Anthropological Perspective. New York: Cambridge University Press.

Good, Byron J., and Mary-Jo Delvecchio Good. 1994. In the Subjunctive Mode: Epilepsy Narratives in Turkey. Social Science and Medicine 38(6): 835–42.

Lang, Gretchen Chesley. 1989. Making Sense" About Diabetes: Dakota Narratives of Illness. Medical Anthropology 11: 305–27.

Mattingly, Cheryl. 1998. Healing Dramas and Clinical Plots: The Narrative Structure of Experience. Cambridge: Cambridge University Press.

Mishler, Elliot. 1981. Social Contexts of Health, Illness and Patient Care. Cambridge, UK: Cambridge University Press.

Newman, Jeffrey M., et al. 1993. Diabetes-associated Mortality in Native Americans. Diabetes Care 16(1): 297–99.

O'Neil, John D., and Patricia Leyland Kaufert. 1995. *Irniktakpunga!* Sex Determination and the Inuit Struggle for Birthing Rights in Northern Canada. *In* Conceiving the New World Order: The Global Politics of Reproduction. F.D. Ginsburg and R. Rapp, eds. Los Angeles: University of California Press.

Pettitt, David J., et al. 1996. Incidence of Diabetes mellitus in Women Following Impaired Glucose Tolerance in Pregnancy is Lower than Following Impaired Glucose Tolerance in the Non-Pregnant State. Diabetologia 39: 1334–37.

Sievers, Maurice L., et al. 1992. Impact of NIDDM on Mortality and Causes of Death in Pima Indians. Diabetes Care 15(11): 1541–49.

Smith-Morris, Carolyn M. 2004. Reducing Diabetes in Indian Country: Lessons Learned from Gila River. Human Organization 63(1): 34–46.

_____2003. (*unpublished manuscript*) Native American Revival of Community Participation Models: Old and New Lessons for Diabetes Prevention and Treatment.

van der Pligt, Joop. 1998. Perceived Risk and Vulnerability as Predictors of Precautionary Behaviour. British Journal of Health Psychology 3: 1–14.

CHAPTER 9

TALKING ABOUT A NEW ILLNESS WITH THE DAKOTA: REFLECTIONS ON DIABETES, FOODS, AND CULTURE[1]

Gretchen Chesley Lang

In the old days, we had more people, more elders, there were lots of old couples, and on this reservation nearly everybody lived in log cabins, very few frame houses. They were spread out on this reservation, and people used to pay visits to each other, that's what I was saying. They didn't have jobs, see. And if they knew someone had a problem they would go and look them up. And on a visit, these people who were going to visit, they'd cook up their own meal, and take it along and share it with their neighbor. This is the way we visited a long time ago. And in our Sioux tradition, my grandma used to say, "If anyone comes to visit, even if you just have water and bread, serve it to them. This is the first thing we were taught to do—to feed the people that visit...And this is what we had in those days...We were so poor from the time I was born. I had a hard time with my family, I struggled, I was on my own most of my life. And where we lived when I was young, out south where they call it Jackson Hole, we all lived in log cabins, we all got along..."

> Ignatius Jackson, 1985

Summary of Chapter 9. Dakota people of the Devil's Lake Sioux Tribe have been concerned about the diabetes 'epidemic' that emerged in the 1970s. To some, it is one more trial in a series of hardships that have occurred over a century and more of disjunction from their pre-European lifeways in the eastern Plains. In talking with residents during the 1980s who had experience with diabetes, I found that conversations invariably turned to changes in the community during the late 19th century and for most of the 20th century, including decades of food scarcity, unemployment, dependence on government rations, and later, commodity foods. Some elders harked back, often with nostalgia, recounting stories from the earlier time of reliance on wild game and prairie plant foods. Their autobiographical accounts were interwoven with commentaries on changes in Dakota lifeways, housing, family relations, and present-day efforts to retain "tradition." Talking about a "new" affliction with the Dakota brings up "old" issues—evoking

---

1. Reprinted, with permission, from Lanham/University Press of America. Originally published in *Culture and the Anthropological Tradition: Essays in Honor of Robert F. Spencer*, Robert H. Winthrop, Ed. NY: Lanham, 1990, pp. 283–317.

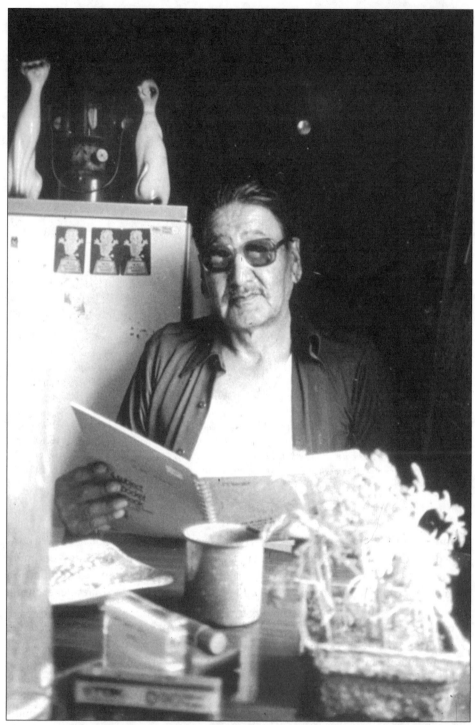

This chapter is dedicated in remembrance of Ignatius Jackson (1920–1986), traditional singer and drummer, St. Michael, ND.

strongly felt reflections on an on-going relationship between Dakota people and the "outside" non-Native American society and culture. Dakota narratives about illness and health reflect what Williams (1984) described, as peoples' "attempts to establish points of reference between body, self, and society…narrative reconstruction(s) of their changing relationship to the world in which they live and the genesis of illness within it." This chapter explores perspectives on foodways, health, and Dakota culture within the past and present, in keeping with themes voiced by community residents as they considered a new health condition and larger issues of wellness.

ཟ   ཟ   ཟ

Introduction

Two years ago at a university conference on health issues sponsored by Native American medical students, in between speakers' citing new health statistics and presenting profiles of health care delivery in remote reservation settings, a slight and somewhat frail-appearing Dakota woman in her 70s moved forward to present a community perspective on health care. In characteristic Dakota fashion, Mrs. Peters (pseudonym) began in a soft voice to tell what became a long account of her childhood recollections during a much earlier time on the reservation, around 1910 and 1915. Her description was extremely detailed, telling of specific wild plants and game that they were able to procure, and of the frequent periods of hardship in their log house when she recalled that their diet at times primarily consisted of potatoes and somewhat erratic government hand-outs of flour, sugar, lard and coffee. She continued, eloquently, to describe the challenges in later years of raising her own seven children, of whom four survive as adults in their 30's and 40's today. She then referred back to a longer time ago in the pre-reservation days before 1867, portraying a lifestyle centered upon the buffalo and prairie plants and when people were actively engaged in traditional methods of making a living:

> "We once ate the right foods and lived the right way as *Wakan Tanka* intended us to do. People used to live to a very old age, before we were put onto reservations. Today we have these diseases like cancer and heart disease and now we all seem to be coming down with diabetes. I remember when my father was told that he had "sugar"—it was about 1952. There was little that they could do at the clinic. They couldn't stop the sugar from building up in him. He was the first person at Devil's Lake to get diabetes. It is all the foods we eat now—they make us sick—all the sugar in these junk foods that everyone is eating around here that doesn't agree with us. For me, I think it also is the stress from living all bunched together in these new housing projects that I think keeps my sugar up. Some days I just know it is high when I am worried about things. Everyone seems to have it. It used to be tuberculosis and other diseases that were brought to us, and now it is diabetes."

Mrs. Peters' speech, as one might ascertain, seems to be more than nostalgia. At the same conference a medicine man from another reservation community in western South Dakota spoke of the beneficial "holistic" aspects of traditional Dakota medicine

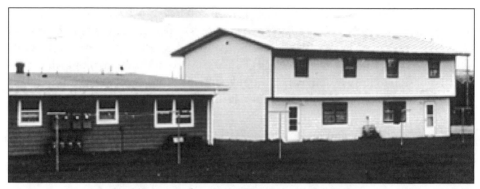

Government housing at Ft. Totten, N.D. (1982).

as opposed to the mind-body dualism of Euro-American medicine.[2] His perspective, as well, represented the growing number of often quite diverse commentaries on health and illness that extend to a wider social critique, currently voiced by Native Americans healers in mainstream settings. For me, Mrs. Peters' speech was interesting in a number of ways. Having talked with many Dakota about diabetes as a new health condition during the past 3 years, I had heard similar etiological explanations and commentaries on treatment in varied individualized contexts. When I asked about why people thought they had diabetes, conversations inevitably turned to the diabetic diet, then to traditional foods, and to reflections on their history. In 1981, diabetes was an increasingly prevalent chronic illness that was just starting to concern Dakota people. At this time, most people who had "sugar" (which is how Dakota have referred to diabetes) did not want others to know about it, perhaps because it was unclear as to its origins, and perhaps because standard diabetic dietary therapy posed a dilemma at the numerous Dakota social occasions that almost always involve major meals and feasts and it has been considered rude to not eat heartily and with appreciation. What interested me here was that Mrs. Peters was now publicly drawing upon diabetes as a way to talk about larger issues, including the on-going difficulties of the Dakota as she continually reflects upon them.

This paper is an attempt to examine ways in which Dakota women and men talk about and personally deal with an illness that is new for them—diabetes, and represents an effort to look at the conversations that I had with people at Devil's Lake Sioux Reservation[3] regarding their beliefs about its origins (etiology) and their experience in living with this chronic condition and its prescribed treatments. I suggest that as a "new" illness, diabetes and its treatment is interpreted and talked about in ways that reveal sym-

---

2. The terms "biomedicine" or "mainstream" medicine used here refer to current Euro-American medical concepts and practices. Alternative medical practices occur in the West as in other pluralistic societies (cf. Helman 1984). To use these broad terms is to imply that there is a shared agreement between researchers, clinicians, and other health professionals, which is not necessarily the case; furthermore, the "state of the art" regarding any particular condition is constantly changing, and gradually diffuses through the health professional hierarchy. It should be noted that Native American beliefs and practices have been in a long interaction with mainstream medicine.

3. Devil's Lake Sioux Reservation changed its name to Spirit Lake Nation in the 1990s; the earlier name is retained in this chapter, as a reprint of the original publication (cited in footnote 1).

bolic boundaries of Dakota culture within a larger society. Almost all the Dakota with whom I talked took these occasions to interweave extensive autobiographical accounts of their illness experience with what I see as revealing commentaries on their reflections on the relationship between a Dakota and a non-Dakota world, in the past and in the present.

The work on which this paper is based stems from a larger study of community perspectives on health and illness and on existing health care resources in the Devil's Lake Sioux Reservation community located in eastern North Dakota, reported on elsewhere (Lang 1985). This was a self-initiated project carried out between 1981 and 1983 in cooperation with the Tribal Health Committee of the Devil's Lake Sioux Tribe and the newly-instituted Diabetes Program Office located in the Indian Health Service Clinic.[4] Devil's Lake is about 120 miles west of the University of North Dakota, and for two years I made weekly visits with people in all walks of life, patients and their families, community people and Dakota and non-Dakota health workers. During the summers I have had the opportunity to spend longer periods of participant-observation time in the community with two families in particular and have attended a number of celebrations such as powwows, community dances, school and tribal events,and several funerals and memorial feasts held one year after a death. In 1982, I carried out a series of lengthy, unstructured interviews with people who have diabetes, in which we discussed how they thought that they had developed this condition, their experience in following the standard mainstream medical treatments, and if they had sought other forms of treatment. At the outset, it may be pointed out that despite the focus upon diabetes here, it is important to emphasize that diabetes is not *the* major life concern for most people; on the other hand, for a number of persons affected, diabetes has created significant personal incapacitation and suffering due to complications.

Theoretical Considerations

The critical distinction between the concept of *illnesses* ("experiences of disvalued changes in states of being and in social function") as distinguished from *diseases* ("in the scientific paradigm of modern medicine,...abnormalities in the structure and function of body organs and systems") (Eisenberg 1977: 11), recognizes that illness is strongly influenced by culture, and is part of a social system of shared meanings and rules for behavior (cf. Kleinman 1978). Thus, cultural orientation influences/shapes ways in which illness is presented, how care is evaluated by the patient, and how one cares for oneself (Kleinman et al. 1978: 252; Foster 1978: 251). Most medical anthropological approaches to the study of illness rest on W.H.R. River's early recognition that "...medical practices follow from and make sense in terms of underlying medical beliefs, and...that both are best conceived not as quaint folklorisms but as integral parts of culture" (Wellin 1977: 49). Studies of illness gen-

---

4. The Indian Health Service Five-Sites Diabetes Project is headed by Dorothy Gohdes, M.D., Indian Health Service Hospital, Albuquerque, NM. ; this program to develop models for diabetes education and treatment in Native American communities was initiated in l979, and included the Ft. Totten Indian Health Service Clinic on the Devil's Lake Sioux Reservation, Ft. Totten, ND.

erally have attempted to elucidate and explore the rationale underlying health beliefs and behaviors to assist health professionals to provide more culturally-sensitive and culturally-appropriate care.

In his critique of theoretical approaches taken by (medical) anthropologists and sociologists in their studies of health and illness, in particular their emphasis upon patients' explanatory models ("EM's"), Allan Young (1982) proposed an additional focus on what he calls the "anthropology of sickness." By this definition, *sickness* is conceptualized as "the process through which worrisome behavioral and biological signs, particularly ones originating in disease, are given socially recognizable meanings" (1982: 270). According to Young (1982: 272), researchers have neglected the "social relations of sickness" that tend to sustain and perpetuate larger social relations within the society as a whole (cf. also Frankenberg 1980 and Taussig 1980, who have similar concerns). In Taussig's (1980) case study of a chronically-ill, hospitalized woman who intermittently cooperated and rebelled against what appeared to be a "constructed" role of dependency and helplessness as a patient, Taussig uncovers an ideology of bio(medicine) that reveals the relations of power in the wider society. This woman's reflections on her illness and role as patient are formulated in an autobiographical, and thus idiosyncratic, framework. Young points out that patients' statements regarding their illness experience are basically of a different order from those of mainstream clinicians who operate in a dyadic doctor-patient framework. Laypeople's explanations involve different *kinds* of medical knowledge, combining "strings of events and circumstances recalled from the past" that he calls "prototypes," and the individual's associations of various events and circumstances that are likely to be highly idiosyncratic that he calls "chain complexes" (1982: 274). In a similar vein, Williams and Wood (1986) refer to patients' beliefs about their condition as "common sense" beliefs with a different *purpose* from that of clinician. Both patient and clinician strive to make sense of a particular disorder, but the patient's explanation—often presented as an autobiographical narrative or story—is to "find meaning or sense of coherence in the midst of the disruption which the illness has caused" (Williams and Wood 1986: 1437). In his in-depth study of beliefs of British arthritis patients, Williams (1984: 177) conceptualizes patients' etiological explanations for their condition as part of a larger interpretive process" that he calls "narrative reconstruction." Such narratives, as Young's prototypes and chain complexes, may be deceptively congruent, in parts, with clinician's etiological models for particular diseases; however, such narratives spring from a significantly different matrix of thinking, one which for patients is an attempt to integrate and find meaning in their "changing relationship to the world and the genesis of illness within it" (Williams 1984: 175).

In presenting this material I have two objectives: first, is to examine how a new illness and treatments for it are deliberated upon and interpreted by Dakota, as diabetes is increasingly recognized as a new affliction by them, and secondly, I have also tried to consider etiological explanations and descriptions of illness experience as narratives that are also a form of social commentary. The Dakota, as Native Americans in other reservation and urban communities, have combined many elements of their traditional culture with aspects of contemporary American life (Grobsmith 1981: ix) in styles that often express a good deal of individual variation, yet retain distinctly Dakota ways of interpreting and doing things. The Dakota, as M. Powers (1986) has pointed out with respect to the Oglala Sioux, are very clear about what is "traditional" and what is "modern"; individuals move easily between such categories in their roles in daily life. Like-wise, such eclecticism occurs with respect to health; a number of studies of medical choices in pluralistic societies (cf. Leslie 1976; Kleinman 1980; Helman 1984) show complex ways in which people draw upon or combine quite distinct bodies of med-ical/religious knowledge and practice for the relief of illness and disorder. In discussing either present-day Dakota culture or specific medical beliefs and practices it would be somewhat misleading to categorize individuals from an analytic outsider viewpoint that would suggest individuals' exclusively drawing upon "traditional" or "modern" mainstream medicine, or various forms of alternative medicine. Furthermore, clini-cal medicine does not precisely replace or substitute for other kinds of medical knowl-edge and treatment, that, as will be described shortly for Dakota patients, may be in-terwoven with religious prescriptions and proscriptions, and that reflects the long interactions between Dakota and Euro-American.

When Dakota patients speak of diabetes—its possible origins, their considerations in seeking treatment, and following prescribed treatments—their statements were often presented and phrased in terms of "our people" or what emerged from individual's ac-counts to me as an instructive commentary on how the Dakota people view their col-lective traditions and their history. It is recognized here that, as Williams (1984) points out, narratives that occur in the context of interviews, no matter how open-ended and lengthy, are co-authored enterprises. Thus, Dakota people speak of illness experience to a non-Dakota or non-Indian (in this instance) in terms that make commentary on what can be called their ethnic boundaries, an "ethnic autobiographical" narrative that implies a collective experience despite individual differences. Though "factionalism" at all levels is pronounced at Devil's Lake, and consensus is rarely attained outside of the household, there is an on-going dialogue between individuals regarding this new chronic condition that affects increasing numbers of the community (and currently, as will be seen below, is directly or indirectly experienced by nearly everyone). While interpretations vary be-tween individuals, diabetes is a symbol that can be used to convey meaning (and agree-ment) at many levels. That diabetes treatment impinges on customary foodways makes imagery of diabetes perhaps more salient. Thus, Dakota culture incorporates and trans-forms events and circumstances surrounding one health condition in a manner that may be understood as part of a Dakota narrative vis-à-vis the larger majority society.

Diabetes from a Biomedical Perspective

The Dakota would agree with epidemiologists that diabetes mellitus (type II, or ma-turity-onset) is a new disease for them as it appears to be for other Native Americans. Examinations of existing clinic and hospital records reveal that diabetes was virtually non-existent among Native American populations until about 45 years ago (West 1974, 1978). Current biomedical explanations for this dramatic increase consider a number of etiological factors in attempts to explain prevalence rates for many American Indian groups that are currently 5–8 times higher with respect to the total population (West 1978; Neel 1982; Knowler 1984). During the past two decades, the Dakota as other Na-tive Americans of the Plains region have shown an increasing prevalence; in 1983 approximately 24% of people 35 years and older were receiving treatment for diabetes.[5] (This increase of diabetes among Native Americans reflects a larger trend that has been documented for many non-Western populations in diverse parts of the world, in particular, indigenous populations in Oceania, Australia, Africa and parts of Asia (cf. West 1978; Eaton 1977; Hagey 1984, for partial bibliographies). Diabetes, along with cancer, hypertension, and coronary heart disease are commonly referred to as "diseases of modernization" or "diseases of civilization" (Foster 1978: 124) in that they are associated with major lifestyle changes including a greater life expectancy. Generally, the health profile for Native American populations parallels trends in the total U.S. population, despite differing prevalence rates of specific conditions, which has been an increase in chronic conditions, and a lessening of a number of communicable diseases. However, diseases associated with poverty are disproportionately higher (with respect to the total population) in many Native American communities (cf. Harwood 1981; Kosa 1969); and a majority of tribal leaders and health workers agree that alcohol-related problems remain the most serious health and social problem in most Native American communities.

The factors identified as playing a role in the occurrence of diabetes, while not fully understood, include obesity, not enough exercise, and a genetic predisposition for an impairment in the transport of glucose from the blood to body cells (cf. West 1978; Keen, et al. 1979; Neel 1982). For clinicians, the primary aim of treatment is to regulate blood sugar levels so that they fall within a norm established for the non-diabetic population. Diagnostic testing for diabetes involves standardized blood tests to determine blood sugar levels, and it is customary practice for diabetic patients to make regular visits to a clinic for blood sugar determinations to ascertain whether their condition is "in control." Biomedical research on efficacious medication and dietary treatments modifies clinical practice over time. Basically, conventional methods of treatment for type II diabetes may be dietary regulation and weight control, dietary regulation in conjunction with hypoglycemic oral medication, or diet along with insulin injections. Diabetes is a complex condition, with marked diversity in its interpretation and treatment choice by clinicians (cf. Posner 1974), and indeed, experts recognize their incomplete understanding of the underlying physiological and genetic processes (Neel 1982). The primary task from the health professional's standpoint is to explain the basic characteristics and "causes" of diabetes and the prescribed treatment to patients through personal consultation and educational materials such as brochures, dietary plans, medication schedules, etc..The central message of physicians, nurses and dietitians to patients most generally rests upon concepts such as "compliance," "adherence," "management," and "control" of dietary intake,

---

5. To date [1990], comprehensive epidemiological studies of diabetes have not been carried out among Plains Indian peoples; it is estimated that more than 20% of adults 35 years and over have diabetes (cf. Brosseau 1979 for Mandan, Hidatsa and Arikara; Diabetes Program, IHS 1983). Diabetes occurs increasingly frequently in the under-35 age group; at Devil's Lake, 163 of the 167 diabetics are 35 and older. Of residents at Devil's Lake, 644 of the total 2800 who are 35 years or older; the percentage of diabetics (163/644) in this age category is therefore approximately 24%. This may be an underestimation because of those currently undiagnosed. Devil's Lake Sioux, as the Dakota at Standing Rock (Bass and Wakefield 1974), concomitantly have a high prevalence of obesity. A survey carried out in the clinic revealed 60% of all clinic patients to be 20% or more overweight (Butts 1981).

body weight, and exercise to eliminate symptoms and to avoid serious complications that primarily involve the vascular system. It is generally recognized by health workers that for all diabetics compliance with daily dietary regimens is a more difficult challenge than with medication schedules (cf. Eckerling and Kohrs 1985; Haynes et al. 1979).

Health workers at the Devil's Lake Public Health Service Clinic are predominantly non-Indian at the higher echelons, and despite their efforts to encourage "compliance" have been discouraged with what they perceived as a lack of success in patient control and/or reduction of body weight and their following the diabetic diets. Informally, their explanations for why this was occurring fall into two categories: 1) patients don't understand the instructions, and 2) people don't really seem to be concerned about their condition. On another level, either the Dakota culture or low socioeconomic status were seen as the underlying causes of low compliance. The Diabetes Program described elsewhere in cooperation with the Tribal Health Office (Lang 1985) has provided patients and their families, as well as the community at large, with more information and supportive assistance than clinics that do not have such a program.

Surprisingly little attention has been focused on ways in which diabetes is experienced by patients and prescribed treatments carried out in the home setting, or how such chronic illness is perceived by diabetics and their families. For Native American groups there are only a few studies at present: Joos (1984) work with the Seminole explores food preferences and dietary patterns; Judkins' (1974, 1978) papers situate perceptions of diabetes with respect to traditional Seneca concepts of disease causation and healing; Hagey (1984) describes a cooperative Native-health worker effort in Toronto in diabetes education in which a traditional story "Nanabush and the Stranger" is reworked to include diabetes. Her paper provides insightful considerations of metaphorical aspects of both Native and biomedical concepts of illness and disease, respectively, and the reconstruction of meanings for a shared purpose in health education.

Background: Devil's Lake Sioux Community

Historically, reservations in the Northern Plains were created by the U.S. government in the late 1860's with most Native Americans settled in allotted land areas by the 1890's. At present, the Devil's Lake Sioux community numbers about 2800 residents, with an official enrolled membership in the Devil's Lake Sioux Tribe of 3100. The Eastern Dakota at Devil's Lake trace their origins to several bands of the Eastern and Middle Divisions of the larger Dakota people (cf. Albers and James 1984) extensive discussion of subjective and objective tribal designation, with special attention to this community). The extensive ethnographic and historical literature on the Dakota primarily focused upon the more well-known Western Division or Teton Dakota, whose descendants today live at Pine Ridge and Rosebud Reservations in western South Dakota. Accounts of traditional Dakota religious beliefs and practices, including healing, have likewise primarily centered on the Teton Dakota, most notably in the recently published Walker (1980) papers. Scholars generally agree that there is less formal organization and elaboration of religious practices among the Eastern Dakota, noted first by Lowie (1913).

Two striking characteristics of the Devil's Lake Sioux community are both the strong extended family ties and intense community involvement of most reservation residents and, secondly, a rural poverty associated with a number of social problems that are frequently expressed in the all too-familiar statistics for many Native American communities. On one hand, many aspects of traditional Dakota cultural patterns—such as the high value placed on reciprocity and generosity—can be viewed as effective strategies for coping with aspects of poverty. On the other hand, in this small community, problems related to poverty and unemployment affect almost every family and have resulted in personal and family crises disproportionately higher than for most other ethnic groups in the U.S., including urban Indian populations.

Diabetes occurs most frequently among the middle-aged and older people, those who are often the mainstay of extended families. Very elderly people frequently care for their grandchildren during the day or on a semi-permanent basis while the parents are at work or away from the community sometimes for extended periods of a year or more. In many households, it is common for 8–12 people to share one or more meals together each day, and many households generally include one or more grown children and their children. Grandparents often mediate between younger family members, their spouses or ex-spouses, and provide an important source of emotional and economic support in times of difficulty. Alber's (1974) study of personal and social networks at Devil's Lake documents the strong and continuously reinforced ties between "blood" relatives, fictive kin ("the formalized 'taking' or 'adoption' of someone as brother, sister, father, or mother"), and friends that reflect sharing and support between individuals and families throughout the Plains communities, often extending into the large Native American community in Minneapolis-St. Paul.

Frequent school, church, and other community functions draw people together at Devil's Lake at all times of the year. Food plays a central role in each level of interaction, and is one of the most important elements of hospitality in the family and community context. Along with items such as star quilts, beadwork, and blankets, food in the form of a side of beef, prepared dishes, and assorted canned or boxed grocery items in a basket may be auctioned off at a school fund-raiser, presented in a give-away in honor of someone, or awarded as prizes for raffles or bingo games. When available, as I will discuss shortly, special "traditional" or "Indian" dishes are featured in the shared meals for such occasions, as well as having a significant place in wakes and memorial feasts held one year after a death.

Devil's Lake Reservation is beset by economic difficulties. Unemployment in 1983 was estimated to be approximately 62% (B.I.A. 1983) and nearly one-third of those employed had annual incomes less than $5000. Numerous statistics could be marshaled to illustrate the many facets of poverty. Here it may suffice to indicate a few of the small "realities" of daily life by mentioning such factors as unpredictable or no available transport in a harsh climate, not having a telephone, numerous breakdowns in appliances such as electric pumps for wells, plumbing, hot water heaters and other technology, and long waits at government and tribal offices, including the clinic. Tribal leaders and the Tribal Health Committee are especially concerned with recent cutbacks in government and tribal positions at all levels; the high prevalence of alcohol-related problems, often in association with car accidents; and increasing financial problems of maintaining or improving social programs started during the late sixties and early seventies that include elderly housing, the nursing home, the half-way house, and a family counseling center.

Traditional Medicine and Religion

Albers (1974) describes the extensive contemporary social systems that cross-cut reservation boundaries, original band or tribal division, and link Devil's Lake residents with other Dakota. Today, it is common for many families from Devil's Lake to travel hundreds of miles almost every weekend in the summer to participate in powwows, *Yuwipi* healing rituals, the vision quest, the Sun Dance, and other celebrations or ritual occasions in communities in South and North Dakota, Manitoba, Saskatchewan and Minnesota. Those at Devil's Lake who draw upon traditional healing practices today and the smaller minority who are Native American Church followers of the "Peyote Road" are in continual contact with people in communities to the west. Currently, at Devil's Lake there are no practicing medicine men or women, respectively, *wakan wicasa* or *winyan wicasa* (who employ supernatural power in healing). These sacred persons are distinguished from *pejuta wicasa* and *pejuta winyan*, medicine men and women who are recognized as having extensive secular knowledge of herbal medicines and a knowledge of specific medical techniques for common ailments and injuries. Several elderly women at Devil's Lake are considered to possess such knowledge, but are distinguished from those in the past who are remembered as having a more complete repertoire of healing techniques.

Individuals may consult both types of traditional practitioners for diagnosis of their affliction.[6] Persons seeking assistance may be referred to the mainstream clinic, or may be advised by sacred persons to take part in the *Yuwipi* healing ritual which is common in the Western Dakota communities; it is on rare occasions if a medicine man visits Devil's Lake that such healing rituals would be carried out in the community. *Yuwipi* ceremonies are primarily used for dealing with what is considered "Indian sickness," those conditions that existed " prior to the white man's arrival and that are caused by disharmony between common man and the supernatural beings and powers" (Powers 1975: 130). Such sicknesses are brought on by the breaking of "spirit-imposed taboos" (Kemnitzer 1980: 274). Older people say that sickness may result along with other misfortune, as a result of not keeping "a promise" (for example, neglecting to hold a memorial ceremony for one who is deceased after stating that one would do this or by not following obligations understood in a vision, such as taking up a spiritual calling). In a related sense, illness is understood to result from not carrying out obligations and duties with respect to others who are living—friends, relatives, neighbors, thus leading a "bad life," morally and spiritually. Sometimes sickness or disability is interpreted as the result of a deliberate action against someone by means of "magic" or "power." It would be difficult to ascertain how often sorcery is perceived as a specific cause of particular illnesses, though older people enjoy recounting instances in which "power" was used to determine the outcome in gambling, romantic pursuits and sex-

---

6. An initial gift of tobacco is presented to a medicine man whom one wishes to consult; later "gratuities" may take the form of goods or money as deemed appropriate for the particular circumstances and ritual expenses.

ual manipulation, and at times in causing a person to be susceptible to illness, failing in energy, or "wasting" which refers to unexplained weight loss. The effects of such "bad medicine" must be reversed with the intervention of a ritual specialist.

Nearly everyone at Devil's Lake claims a church affiliation (the majority of people are either Episcopalians or Catholics), though participation in church activities may be limited to attending funerals or weddings. Contrary to what some church officials may suggest, few individuals consider their dual participation in Christian religion and traditional religious practices a contradiction. In his study of Oglala religion, Powers puts it this way: that individuals today are born into or join Christian churches, but participation in traditional religion (which includes healing) occurs as individual needs arise"(Power 1975: 129). Traditional healers as well as Dakota "patients" consider by what means particular ailments should be treated, as will be seen in statements below, and despite statements that diabetes is a "white man's disease" and the fact that virtually everyone is a regular user of the mainstream Indian Health Service Clinic, consideration is given, or at least verbalized, to a range of possible forms of treatment and relief of symptoms.

Foods, Eating and the "Diabetic Diet"

Before the nineteenth century, the Eastern Dakota hunted, fished, collected wild rice, and grew corn in the woodlands along the river systems of Minnesota, along with involvement in buffalo hunts and trade with western bands of Lakota Sioux. By the 1800s, however, wars with the Ojibway and encroachments by white settlers reinforced a growing reliance upon buffalo hunting and a subsistence pattern focused upon other animal and plants resources of the prairie. The first residents of the Devil's Lake Sioux Reservation, settled there by treaty in 1867, were primarily Santee Sioux from Minnesota, and Cuthead bands of the Yanktonais Sioux living in the eastern Plains region. Early reports by reservation superintendents sent back to the U.S. Commission of Indian Affairs portrayed those early years at Devil's Lake as ones of hardship and near starvation, with poorly-administered attempts to introduce unfamiliar forms of "modern" agriculture (Meyer 1967: 233). By the end of the 1800s, more than half of the original reservation holding was lost through sales of individual allotments as allowed by the Dawes Act of 1887. Today older people recount stories they heard about the early decades of the present century, and recall personally the Depression years in particular. A constant theme in these recollections is an ever-present threat of food shortage—summers when the weather was bad and gardens failed, a lack of basic staples and meat, and the toll of tuberculosis, pneumonia, and alcohol-related problems.

Government rations were distributed from the first years of reservation administration, and included flour, salt pork, meat (sometimes "on the hoof" and often low-grade beef and pork that was frequently spoiled), salt, sugar, dried tea leaves, and green coffee. The government agents distributed these rations, deciding who should receive them and how much, so that allotments varied according to an individual agent's estimation of conditions and needs. Nurge (1970) depicted subsistence during these years as involving an on-going collection of prairie plant foods, a dependence upon hunting, and a continuing reliance upon rations and store-bought foods.

Today a few older people still have large vegetable gardens, primarily raising items that can be dried or stored in cellars for the winter: potatoes, onions, and the "Indian" corn. Ethnobotanical reports and compendia of native plants and their uses illustrate the broad range of plants that were once used for food and/or had a place in the pharmacopoeia (Densmore 1928; Vogel 1970; Gilmore 1977; Rogers 1980). Nurge (1970) has reconstructed the history of the Dakota diet, detailing the development of contemporary dietary patterns of the Lakota at Rosebud Reservation in South Dakota.

At Devil's Lake, several elderly women and men are respected for their knowledge of plants and their uses; in checking Nurge's (1970) lists of traditional plants (in English and Dakota) with them it appeared that they had only heard of some of them from their parents; they now find it difficult to obtain the fewer plants that are used today. The items most frequently mentioned that that are used in dishes when available include: prairie turnips (*tipsina*), chokecherries (*cham pah*), buffalo berries (*mastincha-pute*), wild onion (*pshin*), June berries or Saskatoons (*wipazuka*), red plums (*cauntah*), wild artichokes (*panghai*), wild rice (*psin*) brought in from northern Minnesota, venison, and occasionally rabbit. Some families raise what they call "Indian" corn (*wamnaheza*), parching the kernals for later use in soups and stews. Food dishes would include prairie turnips added to stews and soups, corn soup, fruit pudding (*wojapi*), the ritually-important chokecherry balls, or pemmican, (*wasna*) served at memorial feasts, made by pounding meat , berries, lard and sugar. (see photos, below). Other traditional dishes include plum jam, berry soup, buffalo stew (today buffalo meat and "beefalo" (hybrid buffalo/cattle cross) are available from commercial sources and are not considered as healthful as the wild buffalo of the past), rabbit stew, and boiled venison.

Many people employ home remedies for fever, headache, colds, aching, and gastrointestinal ailments, the most common being sweet flag (*sinke ta wote*) obtained today from friends or relatives from communities to the west. Certain older women are considered knowledgeable about the uses of other plants (often prepared as an herbal tea) for particular ailments, but most people agreed that much of this knowledge is disappearing. Taken together, these traditional foods and medicinal plants and wild game represent purity, healthfulness and strength that is central to present-day concepts of a pre-reservation (and pre-European influence) life and culture. Though these foods are generally in short supply, and had been eaten regularly by only a few people during their childhood as major components of the diet, the Dakota hold these foods in very high regard and all spoke at length of their healthful properties in contrast to foods they find themselves eating today.

A distinction can be made between the wild plant and game foods that are associated with the pre-European past or "way-back" history (Lang 1982) and the modified foods that are commonly referred to as "Indian" foods, such as fry bread[7] or rich soups and stews that are often served at "Indian occasions." Powers and Powers (1984: 64–65) suggest that the introduced ration foods (e.g. beef, flour, crackers, bacon, and coffee)

---

7. "Fry bread" is the hallmark of contemporary Native American gatherings through out much of North America. Common ingredients consist of white flour, sugar, lard, salt, and baking soda, and it is fried in an inch or so of shortening. Fry bread is a component of meals in many homes, and is frequently modified into a sandwich bun with chili, taco, or other rich meat fillings.

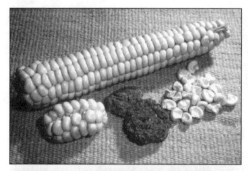

Traditional corn, *wamnaheza*, grown by a few families dried and stored for special meals, and pemmican, *wasna*.

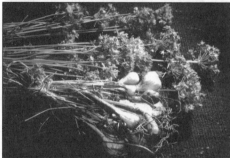

Wild onion, *pshin*.

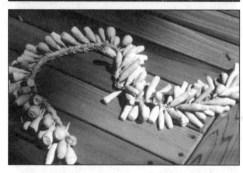

Prairie turnips, *tipsina*, dried and braided, worn by traditional dancers.

were "transformed at the same time as a system" (around 1870) into the Oglala food system , and thus have "status as traditional foods," with buffalo retaining a privileged sacred status as the main ritual food. I found that at Devil's Lake, people made a distinction between the indigenous foods, endowed with qualities of freshness, non-domesticated, a sacred endowment of the Great Spirit, and the more recent introductions. Both the "way back" traditional foods and the more recent "Indian" dishes are served at occasions that involve (and often promote) community and distinctly Native American identity such as powwows, social gathering at the school or tribal office building, or at the University of North Dakota Native American Center. Food dishes that may be advertised for such occasions as "Indian" and that must be prepared in large quantities would include soups and stews that contain meat rich in fat along with corn, potatoes, macaroni, tomatoes and onions, along with fry bread. If venison or buffalo are available, this will be a highlighted feature of the meal, almost as an additional "marker" of authenticity.

Older people are very clear about individual and family preferences in foods and cooking, however, and at Devil's Lake a more "traditional" method of cooking is boiling and simmering, as opposed to frying. Today, it would be rare to find a meal consisting en-

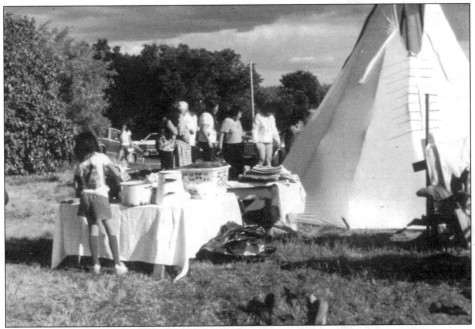

A memorial feast held one year after a death, in this instance, of an elder (1983).

tirely of the "way back" traditional foods at Devil's Lake. (One exception that approached this end of the continuum was the recent Dakota Women's Conference at which sample dishes were prepared by older women to demonstrate the art of traditional cookery.) Some individuals and families, however, strive to serve a traditional meal illustrated by a recent memorial feast held for an elderly man one year after his death.

The family of the deceased in this instance identify themselves as following tradition, and planned a "traditional" meal for the approximately 90 invited guests. The meal followed the memorial service in which the medicine man made a last food offering to the deceased. Guests at the ceremony were seated outside in a large circle around the yard, on lawn chairs placed in front of their cars and pick-up trucks. The two middle-aged daughters of the deceased with the assistance of relatives served portions clockwise around this circle from large kettles of beef soup, quantities of fry bread, and as a special dish, a soup made from dried prairie turnips and "Indian" corn that had been raised by the deceased man in his large garden, and parched and saved by his wife. In addition, coffee carried in large pots and cigarettes (placed on a platter) were offered to all the guests. Each guest was offered several helpings of the main dishes, and were encouraged to take additional food home with them. The large kettles of soup and the large cardboard boxes of fry bread had been prepared by relatives, while the special prairie turnip and corn soup was prepared by the immediate family. Though this meal did not consist strictly of indigenous traditional foods, the context and the interpretation by hosts and guests was that it was carried out in the "old way." Canned or bottled soft drinks, snack foods or other commercially prepared store-foods were noticeably absent. At this memorial feast the "give-away" of the large accumulation of star quilts, blankets, and dry goods such as sheets, towels, and pillows with embroidered pillowcases, was carried out immediately after the meal. A number of older residents at Devil's

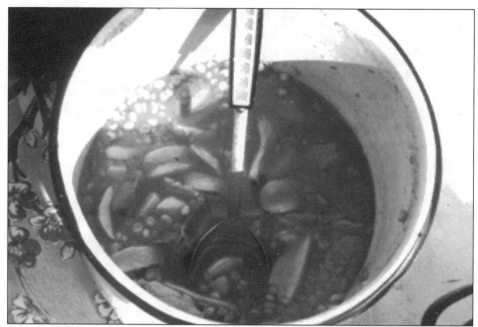

A traditional corn soup (*wamnaheza*), with prairie turnips.

Lake who had been present spoke highly, later, of the manner in which this occasion had been conducted, with particular reference to the traditional meal.

On an even larger scale, at the yearly summer celebration "Ft. Totten Days," the pow-wow committee serves a meal to all "visitors" from other reservations and communities. Kettles of soup (generally beef and macaroni or buffalo stew), wild rice dishes and fry bread are served to upwards of 300–400 people as an important gesture of hospitality by the host reservation. Reminiscences by older people about the quality and quantity of foods at such meals in times past held by other communities indicate the significance of a generous and complete repast. An older man who has attended many ceremonial occasions and powwows recalled the generosity of the hosts at a Montana powwow in the 1960s:

> In the summer meat is dried right away so it won't spoil. They hang it out in the sun. At celebrations they give out rations and a lot of beef—great big chunks. You can see meat hanging between the tents and from the tent poles. Families may donate a beef to whomever is sponsoring the event. Sometimes they might have a dozen beefs that are eaten during a three-day celebration. This time they passed out a lot to my wife and me—so much that we had to go uptown to get bags of ice to keep it from spoiling on the long drive back. They wanted to give extra portions to those of us who were from out-of-state.

The same man also spoke of food preferences in various communities, and in his family:

> Each reservation has its own favorite food. Like those people out west—New Town, White Shield, Twin Buttes, Mandarie—all they like is beef. They eat a lot out there. You go over to Red Lake (in Minnesota) and they mostly eat fish.

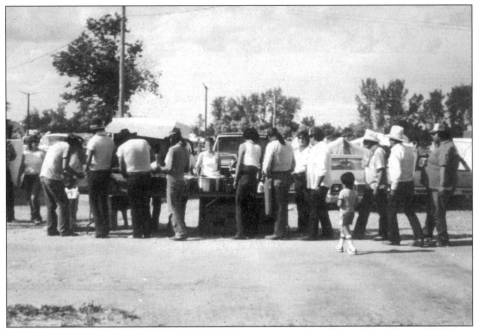

Meal hosted by community for out-of-town attendees, Ft. Totten Days Pow-wow, July, 1983).

And you go south, around Roosevelt and down that way—their main food is pork. We've mixed here, and eat anything, mainly chicken and beef....Now me, I've eaten everything there is, I think, except mink. One of my aunts did—she was the only one in the family who used to eat mink. When I was young, I used to like skunk, but in my family nobody ate this but me and my grandpa and grandma. Porcupine is good. I've eaten raccoon, muskrat, beaver, badger, deer, elk, bear and moose. These foods are good for you. I don't know why. They taste better, I know that.

During the past 50 years, the Dakota diet has greatly diminished in the amount of wild and home-grown foods, and a significantly greater proportion of store-bought foods supplements the government commodity foodstuffs. Today at Devil's Lake, the great majority of households rely upon government commodity foods, with a small number of families raising foods in gardens. The commodity foods are more variable than in the past, and are canned or storable shelf products not intended to provide a balanced diet. The basic elements are fruits packed in syrup, canned meats, peanut butter, canned vegetables, rice, macaroni, dried potatoes, flour, sugar, dried milk and shortening. Store-bought meat, preferably inexpensive cuts of beef and chicken, a small amount of fresh fruit and vegetables, and beverages—often soft drinks—are incorporated into the menu. Those who have gardens raise items that can be dried or stored in cellars for the winter: potatoes, onions, and occasionally "Indian" corn though this is in short supply and always in demand from certain elderly people known to raise and parch it. The food groups that dietitians consider under represented in Dakota diets today are green vegetables and fresh fruits. People on diabetic diets complained that they didn't like many of the suggested selections in the diet pamphlets, saying that they were expensive, or foods that Indian people didn't like , citing in particular broc-coli, spinach, asparagus, celery, and lettuce. The main components of large family meals include rich stews (preferably beef) and soups, fried potatoes, bacon and eggs, pan bread, oven-baked bread, sweet rolls, cakes, cookies and fry bread. In criticizing diabetic diets, a number of people emphasized strongly that "Indian people like to feel full" because as children they often had gone hungry.

Recipes and food preferences today at Devil's Lake reflect the major shift in subsis-tence, and reflect an incorporation of "frontier" Euro-American cooking" along with ra-tions and commodity foodstuffs into a number of dishes regarded as "Indian" foods. Powers and Powers (1984: 64) illustrate the "transformation of foreign foods into tradi-tional Oglala foods" in showing how particular foods were classified into Oglala food cat-egories and processed, cooked and eaten within the larger symbolic food system. Many of these foods bear a striking similarity on the surface to the traditional Euro-American farmer's diet in this region, yet are distinguished from these recipes by the addition of a traditional ingredient when possible, or by not adding an ingredient that would be found in a non-Indian household. Certain foods are highlighted within the community as " markers" of Indian identity, such as tripe soup. At a recent powwow, the announcer jok-ingly referred to the food stand selling tripe soup as a good meal for the "real Indians." Yet, interestingly at the same occasion, a food stand serving "genuine Buffalo-burgers" run by college-age whites was virtually ignored, though there was no antagonism dis-played towards their entrepreneurship. As Powers and Powers (1984: 86) point out:

> "Food is capable of symbolizing the manner in which people view themselves with respect to insiders and outsiders of society...gastronomic categories and culinary practices have meanings far beyond their biological and historical contexts. Food systems may be treated as codes, bearing messages relative to everyday social interactions."

The "shape, color, taste, odor, or special preparation of food" (Powers and Powers 1984: 92) all carry information about social relationships. Thus, dietary modification in treatment is inherently laden with potential meanings that are not immediately ap-parent to an outsider unfamiliar with the social and cultural context in which food-ways have developed.

Etiological Explanations, Experience of Illness and Efficacy of Treatments

When individuals talked with me about why they thought that they had gotten di-abetes, their statements often covered and combined what could be called etiological explanations, experience of illness, and efficacy of treatments as the following accounts will illustrate. In the open-ended and loosely structured interviews, people frequently started out with standard biomedical explanations, and developed their more personal narratives as time went on. As Mrs. Peters' statement at the beginning of this paper, most people make a connection between this new "epidemic" as the most recent de-velopment in a chronicle of other afflictions that have been brought by the Europeans.

These afflictions include smallpox, measles, influenza, tuberculosis[8] and more recently, alcohol-related problems. The majority of people, as Mrs. Peters, commented on a distant past without these "sicknesses." Another woman put it this way: "Long ago, people died of old age, not from all these diseases we hear so much about now. Many people used to live to be 100."

One of the first persons I talked with recalled her fear in the late 1960's when she was told at the clinic that she had diabetes:

> I went to the clinic because I was feeling very weak and tired all the time. I was very frightened when they told me I had "diabetes" because I had never heard of this disease before. They seemed to almost blame me for having something—I remember the nurse saying you've got a high sugar and will have to lose about 35 pounds. Now I know that others have it on this reservation, but at first I didn't dare tell anyone. My sisters have it now and my niece. I might have to change from pills to insulin soon, the doctor said, but I am afraid of giving myself a shot.

This woman now in her mid-sixties is aware of potential complications of diabetes that for some at Devil's Lake have resulted in the amputation of lower extremities. To her the shift from oral medication to insulin represents a step along a linear course towards such severe complications. She attributes her diabetes to "stress" caused by family crises.

> I think that I have gotten diabetes because I have been under so much stress with problems at home. My daughter died in a car accident the year that I came down with diabetes, I worry all the time about my son and two other daughters, and I think it makes my blood sugar go up. One daughter lives in Texas but I haven't heard from her for a long time. She has two children but I have never seen them. I made beadwork medallions for them, but I haven't gotten a letter back now, and I keep waiting.

Another woman speaks of her weight gain as a causal factor in developing diabetes, but also sees her need to work very hard as instrumental in "bringing it on." She is very precise about the weight that the doctor has told her to lose, yet does not attempt to follow the dietary plan. A woman in her late 40s, she put it this way:

> To tell you the truth I don't ever look at the literature that they send home with you from the clinic. I have had diabetes now for 9 years. When I got it the first time I was working in Wyoming as a cleaning woman at a school. I had to work hard every day, but I started to notice that I was so tired and weak all the time, and dizzy. They gave me some pills for "sugar," and it seemed to go away for several years. I think that it was the work I did that brought it on, because I had my 3 small children at the time and I had gone out there to live near my sister. When I came back here I was dizzy a lot, and they told me at the clinic that I should lose weight. They said that I was too heavy. I know I

---

8. People at Devil's Lake view tuberculosis as having been introduced by Europeans to Native Americans. A consensus of medical opinion at present is that tuberculosis was present in the New World prior to European contact; the epidemics of infectious tuberculosis among virtually all North American reservation populations are seen as primarily exacerbated by environmental conditions of reservation life (Buikstra 1981).

should lose 17 pounds, that's what the doctor said. But once when I did lose some weight everyone at my house thought I looked sick. I now take pills again but I can't seem to find time to follow the diet—it is hard when you are cooking for a lot of people to eat a separate meal. The medicine has made me feel a lot better, but I haven't done anything about the weight. I am worried about my children getting diabetes because they say it runs in families. In fact, I think that all the young people are much heavier than they used to be. My mother and father both had it; my mother found out just about the time that I did that she had sugar. It does worry me a lot.

Such a series of misfortunes, as in the first example, suggests to another man that supernatural forces are at work. Though he does not attribute such causes to the origin of his own diabetes and speaks of it as a "new disease" for Dakota, he referred to such instances of illnesses and accidents as the one recorded above as "people who aren't living their life the right way." Such difficulties can arise, he pointed out, when someone doesn't carry out their responsibilities, such as following the one-year restrictions on a mourner for a deceased relative, or taking up a calling when "one has been told something" (in a vision). It may affect the whole family into the future, not just the individual who has taken the wrong path. He extends his analysis to the whole community, referring to lots of "disturbances" at night and people seeing faces at their windows, which he interprets as ghosts of deceased who are restless when things aren't being done the right way (by the living).

This man now 70, who is considered to be one of the most knowledgeable regarding "tradition," is highly respected as an "informal" spokesperson, just as Mrs. Peters (p. 1) is. Though he is not a medicine man, his considerations and pronouncements are taken seriously by others. He is primarily concerned that younger people will not know their own traditions, and talks of diabetes as another sign that things aren't right in the way people are living their lives, that with the loss of knowledge of tradition conditions will continue to decline. With regard to his own health, he has never attributed his own diabetes to a particular source, but as someone afflicted with many complications, primarily circulation in his extremities and numbness in his hands and feet he often speaks at length of what his disability has kept him from doing. As a well-known singer and member of a drum group, he still travels to many celebrations but is finding it increasingly difficult to walk and to stand for long periods of time. To him, his illness keeps him from attending ceremonies and occasions that are of the greatest importance to him, and that are for him obligations to keep tradition and pass it on to young people and occasions when he reciprocates for such activities by others for his family and community. He has invitations to perform naming ceremonies, to be an announcer at a powwows, to sing at memorial services on a number of reservations that he cannot always keep. The experience of illness is one that prevents his participation in the activities that for him have primary meaning.

I was a lot heavier then, which may be why I got diabetes, that was about 19 years ago now. These days I have been losing weight. and the doctor says my vision is going. This is a new disease for us Indian people you know; we didn't have this in the old days, and I think that it has to be treated by white man's medicine—I don't think traditional medicine will work for this condition, but I have been considering trying something besides the clinic. I've known many medicine men over the years, and many are charlatans. Now they say that there is a medicine man out at Ft. Smith that can cure diabetes, but I'm not so sure. I used to know this man when we were young. But then lately I've heard that he's lost his " power." I know about *Yuwipi* and I have been to ceremonies. Once I went to help my voice because suddenly at a celebration I was hoarse and it was getting worse so that I couldn't sing; something was sent through the air at me over at Red Lake (a Chippewa community to the east). I think nowadays this *Yuwipi* business is full of trickery, and they carry it out in the dark, not like it was when my grandfather practiced medicine. My grandfather was a "Traditional Holy Man" whose knowledge was brought to him by the Great Spirit *(Wakan Tanka)*. My grandmother helped my grandfather and people came from all around. She knew all the roots and plants, she didn't have "power' but she knew the medicines. But I don't think that diabetes can be cured in a *Yuwipi* ceremony.

Almost all medicine men seem to eventually lose their reputation and their power as they become older, and many considerations of seeking a medicine man for treatment involve lengthy deliberations about the current "status" of a particular individual's " power". For example, drinking and carousing and other inappropriate behaviors such as "misuse" of such power can mark the end of a ritual specialist's following. A medicine men who claims to be able to cure diabetics in a *Yuwipi* healing ceremony requires that the sufferer is to give up other medications, and to purify oneself beforehand by eating traditional foods. Nevertheless, no one with whom I talked had actually gone through a *Yuwipi* ceremony for their diabetic condition, nor had any been under treatment with a medicine man.

George, a man in his early 60's, speaks of his "coming down with" diabetes as resulting from a buildup of sugar throughout his body. Until recently he has been taking pills (oral hypoglycemics) for his condition and apparently does not have serious complications. At present, he lives in a small apartment in a senior citizen housing complex and often has friends in who sit and talk around the kitchen table. For many years he was away from Devil's Lake, living in a community in Washington state, where he worked as a farmhand and casual laborer; he has never been married. George attributes his diabetes the kinds of foods that he has eaten and to an earlier history of heavy drinking. He spoke at length about food and possible "cures":

> No one used to have diabetes; if they had, the real medicine men in those days would have found a cure for it. My grandfather was one of the last medicine men here at Devil's Lake. There is one here sometimes from farther west, but I don't have confidence in him..I am a member of the Native American Church, but I don't think of peyote as being a *cure* for diabetes. It can suppress it, but not cure it. Recently I've changed from taking pills to giving myself insulin shots, but I still don't feel good a lot of the time. These pills are much too small to have any effect on all that sugar in my body. I think a medicine is needed to take after meals to "cut the grease" and balance the sugar that one has just eaten. I used to drink a lot of soft drinks, and I think the sugar built up in me. I've heard that there is a man down in Texas who can cure diabetes with a liquid that will get the sugar out of the

blood. It costs a lot, and you have to drink a great big jar of it—about a gal-lon—but it is made with herbs and can cure you, so that you can eat the kinds of food that you want to without having to worry. A lot of the foods that we eat these days aren't fresh— store-bought meat is often spoiled. It seems to be the foods we eat now, especially the canned foods that are slowly poisoning us. If we had more fresh foods we would be healthy. When I was a young man, we used to do a lot of hunting here on the reservation, for deer, rabbits, and pheasants, but now there aren't many of these animals left around here.

Many others also referred to foods and the manner in which modern foods were processed and prepared as a pathway through which they developed diabetes[9]. All of the diabetics and those family members who helped care for them (e.g. the wife or husband) were well informed about the medication doses, the prescribed weight program, and the basic elements of their suggested diet. Many were complementary about the dietitian, nurse, and visiting physician at the Diabetic Program office. Following medication schedules (including self-administered insulin injections) was not perceived as unduly difficult, However, many people were candid and outspoken that they had not modified their dietary intake and methods of food preparation as they had been instructed at the clinic.

Discussion and Conclusion

In a review of studies of health and healing among Native American societies in the Plains region, Kemnitzer (1980: 272) points to a lack of information on ways in which Native American beliefs and practices interact with mainstream health concepts and practices in the context of clinical health care. The Dakota, as most Native Americans, are regular "users" of mainstream health facilities (generally the IHS Clinic) for most disorders and illnesses. Individuals, in the interactive context of family and larger Dakota community, as in all societies, continually weigh the benefit or efficacy of a va-riety of possible treatment for their afflictions, as the accounts of Dakota patients pre-sented here suggest. Diabetes for residents of Devil's Lake appeared to emerge suddenly, and this phenomenon has been perceived as a kind of "epidemic" (a term employed by epidemiologists as well, with different connotations). Clinically the disease is "created" as often rather "diffuse" symptoms (such as fatigue, weakness, dizziness) are interpreted by the doctor or nurse as a cluster and related to blood sugar determinations. As the

---

9. In her 1966 study of perspectives on "modern" medical care by Rosebud Reservation (Lakota) Sioux, Ford reported that traditionalists who used *Yuwipi* healing rituals and those who relied pri-marily on herbal remedies attributed many of the present- day diseases of Indian people to modern processed and/or canned foods. Likewise, these groups as Devil's Lake residents, felt that their gen-eral state of health had greatly declined in the recent century or more of contact with Europeans (1966: 99). Ford also noted that *Yuwipi* followers (more than users of peyote, herbal remedies, or "modern" medicine sometimes refused both injections and surgery; while injections per se did not appear to be an issue for diabetics at Devil's Lake, there was great antipathy towards surgery that would involve removal of any part of the body.

Diabetes Program at Ft. Totten has provided information about diabetes, and carried out screening and treatment on a community-wide basis, the awareness of an illness that seemed to have materialized rapidly in the community has been heightened. For example, in a number of families middle-aged people were diagnosed at approximately the same time or shortly after their aged parents were found to be diabetic.

Additionally, the prescribed treatment generally included a dietary format that (no matter how flexible) restricts intake of preferred foods. Such regimens are capable of, and are, being seen as another "imposition" on Indian people by a non-Indian world (cf. Hagey 1984: 270). While it may appear to be an ironic contradiction that there is reluctance to change food habits given the commonly-expressed idea that "white man's foods have made us sick," foods and foodways are seen to be complex codes for social relations and symbols of cultural meanings. Many contemporary preferred foods while understood as having come in recent history (and during a period recalled as one of great deprivation) from the outside, were also "incorporated" into the traditional food system (as Powers and Powers (1984) have pointed out). Diabetes, especially as it impacts food patterns, from an outsider's viewpoint appears to have provided Dakota with another means through which to reflect upon and make commentary on matters of continual concern to them regarding their history and on their place with respect to the majority society.

Anthony Cohen (1987: 9) points out that "It is in the symbolic that we now look for people's sense of difference, and in symbolism...that we seek the boundaries of their worlds of identity and diversity." Diabetes as a new illness, and foods and foodways, lend themselves to symbolic usefulness for on-going Dakota concerns with their distinctiveness in the past and in the present. Recognition of this dimension is not to underplay the personal experience of this chronic illness and the challenges of its day-to-day and often lifelong treatment, but rather to see such experience in a wider context.

When people were asked about why they thought that they had diabetes, and about the efficacy of their current treatments, most individuals turned the conversation to the discussion of foods and eating, a recalled traditional lifestyle, and at times to a commentary upon their political history. Herzlich (1973: vii) observed in her analysis of French lay beliefs that "When an individual talks about health and illness, he also talks about something else: the nature of his links with his environment, physical and social, as well as aspects of social organization." Foods—as they are linked to aspects of health and illness—provide a rich imagery in which to demarcate boundaries. At Devil's Lake , for example, food preferences and styles of cooking, for example, mark family (and individual) orientation, community solidarity (vis-à-vis other Dakota communities of the region), Dakota identity (vis-à-vis other Native American groups, such as the Chippewa to the east), and with respect to "white" society), and likewise provide a means by which Dakota make connections with an idealized past.

It appears obvious that underlying many Dakota narratives about illness—its origin, experience and treatment— is a quite different set of *purposes*, as Williams and Wood (1986: 1437) have suggested, than those of the health professional. The mainstream health worker operates from what Young (1982: 260) calls a "desocializing" framework in which the objective is to create a positive and constructive dyadic relationship with a patient; a "successful" diabetic is one who complies with prescribed regimens and is able to reduce diabetic symptoms and complications. Clinical medicine as experienced by the Dakota is part of what they frequently consider the "outside" white or majority society; their considerations not surprisingly center less on themselves as diverse individuals, but rather result in narratives with symbols that represent for them, in that context, an "Indian," a "Dakota" or a Devil's Lake resident's orientation. Though Williams and Wood's (1986) focus is the *individual's* " making sense" through common sense statements (or "narrative reconstructions") of the disruption caused by illness, the Dakota produce narratives (to an outsider) that reflect more on their collective identity and that are creative enterprises in what Cohen (1987) calls "symbolizing boundaries."

The material presented here regarding reflections on a new illness and its treatment is bounded by a time frame as well as by the particular position of the writer with respect to those who conversed with me. Some of the applied implications of my work with the Dakota are described elsewhere (1985, 1986). If there is a "usefulness" here, it is not to portray of Dakota beliefs and ideas regarding diabetes as a static "reality", but hopefully to convey some aspects of the complexity of cultural process as it relates to health beliefs in an ever-shifting context. Nurse-anthropologist Hagey's (1984: 271) description of her cooperative efforts with Native educators to draw upon metaphors and meanings held by Cree and Ojibway is perhaps instructive:

> Seldom did key participants in the Native Diabetes Program assume that there was any such thing as information pure and simple. All utterances, facts, ideas were taken to be coming from a professional way of understanding or a Native way of understanding. Value was placed on the discussion of meanings, and interpretation. Mutual recognition was held of some topics being better left not discussed. Integral to the process of cooperation between Natives and professionals, was a basic recognition of the metaphors each other was using to order perceptions.

Such recognition of "constructions of meanings" that occur in the sphere of biomedicine as well as within communities from which patients come is central, it would appear, to bridging—rather than futilely attempting to mask or blend—the basic counterpoints of cultural distinctiveness in a pluralistic society.

Acknowledgments

I wish to thank the many residents of the Devil's Lake Sioux Reservation who talked with me about diabetes, diet and foods; the Diabetes Program staff at the Ft. Totten Indian Health Service Clinic; and members of the Tribal Health Committee of the Devil's Lake Sioux Tribe. Permission to do this project was received from the Devil's Lake Sioux Tribe and IHS Diabetes Program (1982); this research was partially supported by a Faculty Research Grant, University of North Dakota.

References

Albers, Patricia C. 1974. The Regional System of the Devil's Lake Sioux: Its Structure, Composition, Development, and Functions. Ph.D. Dissertation, Univ. of Wisconsin.

_____1983. Sioux Women in Transition: A Study of Their Changing Status in Domestic and Capitalist Sectors of Production. *In* The Hidden Half: Studies of Plains Indian Women. Patricia Albers and Beatrice Medicine, eds. pp. 175–236. University Press of America.

Albers, Patricia C. and William R. James. 1984. On the Dialectics of Ethnicity: To Be or Not to be Santee Sioux. Journal of Ethnic Studies 14: 1–27.

Bass, Mary and Lucille Wakefield. 1974. Nutrient Intake and Food Patterning of Indians in Standing Rock Reservation. J. of the Amer. Dietetic Assoc. 64: 36–41.

Brosseau, J., R.C. Eelkema, C. Crawford and T.A. Abe. 1979. Diabetes Among the Three Affiliated Tribes: Correlation with Degree of Indian Inheritance. Am. J. Public Health 69(12): 1277–78.

Brown, Linda and Kay Mussell, Eds. 1984. Ethnic and Regional Foodways in the United States: The Performance of Group Identity. Knoxville: University of Tennessee Press.

Buikstra, J.E. 1981. Introduction. *In* Prehistoric Tuberculosis in the Americas. J.Buikstra, ed. pp. 1–24. Evanston, Ill: Northwestern University Archaeology Program.

Bureau of Indian Affairs. 1983. Indian Service Population and Labor Force Estimates (Jan. l983). Mimeo, Aberdeen, S.D.

Butts, Jeanette. 1981. Diabetes Program, St. Totten Indian Health Service Clinic. Mimeo.

Cohen, Anthony P. 1986. Of Symbols and Boundaries. *In* Symbolising Boundaries: Identity and Diversity in British Cultures. Anthony. P. Cohen, ed. pp. 1–19. Manchester, England: University of Manchester Press.

Densmore, Frances. 1928. Uses of Plants by the Chippewa Indians. *In* 44th Annual Report of the Bureau of American Ethnology, 1926–1927. Washington, D.C.: U.S. Gov't. Printing Office.

Diabetes Program. 1983. Mimeo and personal communication. Ft. Totten Indian Health Service Clinic, N.D.

Eaton, Cynthia. 1977. Diabetes, Culture Change, and Acculturation: A Biocultural Analysis. Medical Anthropology 1(2): 41–63.

Eckerling, L. and M.B. Kohrs. 1984. Research on Compliance with Diabetic Regimens: Applications to Practice. J. Am. Dietetics Assoc. 84(7): 805–9.

Ford, Virginia. 1966. Cultural Criteria and Determinants for Acceptance of Modern Medical Theory and Practice among the Teton Dakota. Ph.D. Dissertation, Catholic University of America.

Foster, George and B.G. Anderson. 1978. Medical Anthropology. New York: John Wiley and Sons.

Frankenberg, Ronald. 1980. Medical Anthropology and Development: A Theoretical Perspective. Social Science and Medicine B 14: 197–207.

Gilmore, M. R. 1977. Uses of Plants by the Indians of the Missouri River Region. Lincoln: University of Nebraska Press.

Hagey, Rebecca. 1984. The Phenomenon, the Explanations and the Responses: Metaphors Surrounding Diabetes in Urban Canadian Indians. Social Science and Medicine 18(3): 265–72.

Harwood, Alan. 1981. Ethnicity and Medical Care. Cambridge: Harvard University Press.

Haynes, R.B., D.W. Taylor and D. L. Sackett. 1979. Compliance in Health Care. Baltimore: Johns Hopkins Univ. Press.

Helman, Cecil. 1984. Culture, Health and Illness. Bristol, Boston: Wright-PSG Publ. Co.

Joos, Sandra. 1984. Economic, Social, and Cultural Factors in the Analysis of Disease: Dietary Change and Diabetes Mellitus among the Florida Seminole Indians. In Ethnic and Regional Foodways in the United States: The Performance of Group Identity. L. Brown and K. Mussels, eds. pp. 217–37. Knoxville: University of Tennessee Press.

Judkins, Russell A. 1976. Diet and Diabetes among the Iroquois—An Integrative Approach. Actas Del XLI Congreso Internacional de Americanistas III: 313–22.

_____1978. American Indian Medicine and Contemporary Health Problems IV.Diabetes and Perception of Diabetes among Seneca Indians. N.Y. State J. Med. 1978(7): 1137–41.

Keen, H., R.J. Harrett, B.J. Thomas, and J.H. Fuller. 1979. Diabetes, Obesity, and Nutrition: Epidemiological Areas. In Diabetes and Obesity. J. Vague and Ph. Vague, eds. pp. 91–103. Amsterdam-Oxford: Exerpta Medica,

Kemnitzer, Luis S. 1976. Structure, Content, and Cultural Meaning of Yuwipi: A Modern Lakota Healing Ritual. American Ethnologist 3: 261–80.

_____1980. Research in Health and Healing on the Plains. In Anthropology on the Great Plains, Raymond Wood and Margot Liberty, eds. pp. 272–83. Lincoln: University of Nebraska Press.

Kleinman, A. L. 1980. Patients and Healers in the Context of Culture. Berkeley: University of California Press.

Kleinman, A., L. Eisenberg and B. Good. 1978. Culture, Illness and Care: Clinical Lessons from Anthropologic and Cross-Cultural Research. Annals of Int. Med. 88: 251–58.

Knowler, William D. 1983. Diabetes Mellitus in the Pima Indians: Genetic and Evolutionary Considerations. Am. J. Phys. Anthropol. 62: 107–14.

Kosa, J., A. Antonovsky and I.K. Zola. 1969. Poverty and Health: A Sociological Analysis. Cambridge: Harvard U. Press.

Lang, Gretchen Chesley. 1985. Diabetics and Health Care in a Sioux Community. Human Organization 44(3): 251–60.

_____1986. Contemporary Native American Health Issues: How Can Anthropologists Contribute? High Plains Applied Anthropologist 6(1): 1–7.

Leslie, Charles. 1974. Role Adaptation: Traditional Curers Under the Impact of Western Medicine. American Ethnologist 1: 103–27.

Lowie, Robert. 1913. Dance Associations of the Eastern Dakota. Anthropological Papers of the American Museum of Natural History 11(2).

Maurer, A. C. 1979. The Therapy of Diabetes. American Scientist 67: 422–31.

Metropolitan Life Insurance Tables. 1983. Ideal Body Weight Chart.

Meyer, Roy W. 1967. History of the Santee Sioux: United States Indian Policy on Trial. Lincoln: University of Nebraska Press.

Mirsky, R. M. 1981. Perspectives in the Study of Food Habits. *In* Foodways and Eating Habits: Directions for Research, Special Issue, M. Jones, ed. Western Folklore XL(1): 125–33.

Neel, James V. 1982. The Thrifty Genotype Revisited. *In* The Genetics of Diabetes Mellitus. J. Kobberling and R. Tattersall, eds. pp. 283–93. New York: Academic Press.

Nurge, Ethel. 1970. Dakota Diet: Traditional and Contemporary. *In* The Modern Sioux: Social Systems and Reservation Culture. Ethel Nurge, ed. pp. 35–91. Lincoln: University of Nebraska Press.

Posner, Tina. 1977. Magical Elements in Orthodox Medicine: Diabetes as a Medical Thought System. *In* Health Care and Health Knowledge. R. Dingwall, et al., eds. Pp. 142–58. London: Croom Helm.

Powers, Marla. 1986. Oglala Women. New Brunswick: Rutgers University Press.

Powers, William. 1975. Oglala Religion. Lincoln: University of Nebraska Press.

Powers, William and Marla Powers. 1984. Metaphysical Aspects of an Oglala Food System. *In* Food in the Social Order: Studies of Food and Festivities in Three American Communities. Mary Douglas, ed. pp. 40–96. New York: Russell Sage Foundation.

Rogers, Dilwyn J. 1980. Lakota Names and Traditional Uses of Native Plants by Sicangu People in the Rosebud Area, South Dakota (Fa. Buechel's Collection of Plants of Rosebud, 1920). St. Frances, S.D.: Rosebud Educational Society, Inc.

Taussig, Michael T. 1980. Reification and the Consciousness of the Patient. Social Science and Medicine B 14: 3–13.

Toma, R.B. and M. L. Curry. 1980. North Dakota Indians' Traditional Foods. J. Am. Dietet. Assoc. 76(6): 589–90.

U.S. Dept. of Health, Education, and Welfare. 1978. Indian Health Trends and Services. Washington, D.C.: Gov't. Printing Office.

Vogel, V. J. 1970. American Indian Medicine. Norman: Univ. of Oklahoma Press.

Walker, James R. 1980. Lakota Belief and Ritual. R.J. Demaille and Elaine A. Jahner, eds. Lincoln: University of Nebraska Press.

Wellin, Edward. 1977. Theoretical Orientations in Medical Anthropology: Continuity and Change Over the Past Half-Century. *In* Culture, Disease and Healing: Studies in Medical Anthropology. David Landy, ed. pp. 47–58. New York: Macmillan Publ. Co.

West, Kelly M. 1974. Diabetes in American Indians and Other Native Populations in the New World. Diabetes 23(10): 841–55.

_____1978. Diabetes in American Indians. Adv. Metab. Disord. 9: 29–48.

Williams, Gareth. 1984. The Genesis of Chronic Illness: Narrative Reconstruction. Sociology of Health and Illness 6(2): 175–200.

Williams, Gareth and Phillip Wood. 1986. Common-Sense Beliefs about Illness: A Mediating Role for the Doctor. The Lancet, Dec. 20/27, 1986: 1435–37.

Young, Allan. 1982. The Anthropologies of Illness and Sickness. Annual Review Anthropology 11: 257–85.

BURYING THE UMBILICUS: NUTRITION TRAUMA, DIABETES AND TRADITIONAL MEDICINE IN RURAL WEST MEXICO

Leslie E. Korn and Rudolph C. Ryser

If you do not care where your umbilical cord is buried, it is as if you had no mother.

Luisa Lorenzo, Community leader

Summary of Chapter 10. This chapter explores the intersections of traditional medicine, nutrition trauma and diabetes in a small Indigenous community on the west coast of Mexico based on 27 years of Leslie Korn's direct experience and research. Beginning with the philosophy and practices of the Center for Traditional Medicine, a rural grassroots, natural medicine and public health center, the chapter discusses the current and historical use of traditional medicines in west Mexico, and locates them in the context of the emerging movement of integrative methods in health care. A detailed exploration of the cultures and peoples of the region and the effects of "defective development" leads to an examination of development, tourism and community trauma on health in the area. A definition of nutrition trauma provides a basis from which to explore an innovative women-directed community-determined program designed to address diabetes with an intergenerational focus. Intercultural exchanges, clinical health change strategies, authentic nutrition and culinary arts, detoxification, the creative arts and medicinal plants provide the methods by which the community defines its priorities and enacts self-determination to regain control over its health.

&a. &a. &a.

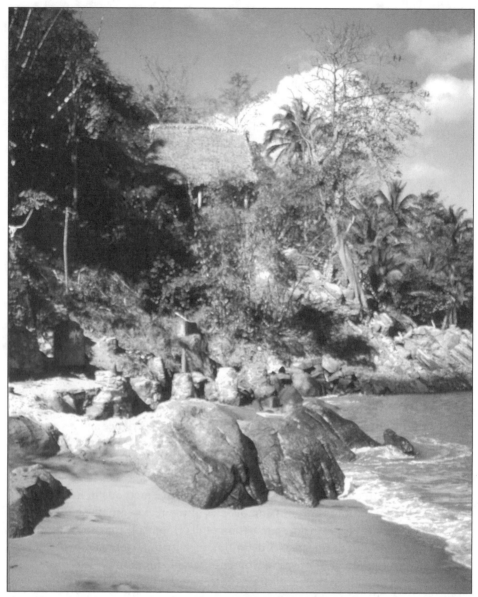

The Center for Traditional Medicine (1977–1997).

Part 1. Center for Traditional Medicine— Philosophy and Practice

I founded the Center for Traditional Medicine (CTM) in 1977 as a small natural medicine public health clinic set in a traditional dwelling on the edge of a precipice overlooking the Pacific Ocean in the *Comunidad Indigena de Chacala* in *Cabo Corrientes*, Mexico.

I had been living in the village of Yelapa for three years, where I taught schoolchildren in a one-room schoolhouse organized at the request of local Chacalans. I arrived when I was 20 years old having left Washington University, I was in search of my

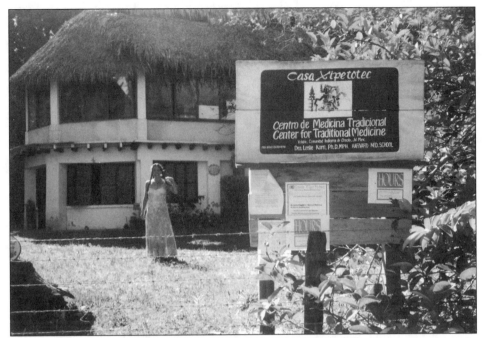

The Center for Traditional Medicine (1997–2002).

life-purpose. In my first years in Yelapa I became ill with many of the infectious mal-adies endemic to the sub-tropics. Since there was no doctor in the village I turned to my new friends and neighbors to teach me about staying healthy using nature's reme-dies. My knowledge of local medicinal flora and fauna grew from my friendship with the women and from the spontaneous exchanges that arose in daily life. I had been in-volved in the feminist movement of the early 1970s and shared my knowledge of con-traception in a village where the pill had not yet arrived and vasectomies were not yet whispered about. More than once this brought the village priest to my door. The small, ocean front clinic, was equipped with a treatment table, herbs and a few donated books and art supplies for the children to play with while their *madres* came for treatment.

Over the years the activities of the center evolved organically to include additional volunteer staff members, and the provision of educational programs and internships for visiting health professionals who sought ways of incorporating traditional healing approaches into their work. Along with our barter in the village, these programs pro-vided us with the subsistence required to operate year round and provide free services to people of the *comunidad*.

Our focus on diabetes grew from the Center for Traditional Medicine's work and my own clinical observations during more than 25 years in Mexico and over the last 10 years with First Nations and Indigenous Peoples in the Pacific Northwest and the Northeast Atlantic region. In addition to the diabetes programs in Mexico with the Chacalan com-munity described here, we now conduct research and training in traditional approaches to diabetes as practiced in Anishinabek culture, and in Salish and Sahaptin cultures.

From its inception, the Center's work in Mexico was intercultural in nature. Women and men in the village contributed their knowledge and skills and in turn shared and re-ceived from the visiting students and health professionals, many of whom donated their

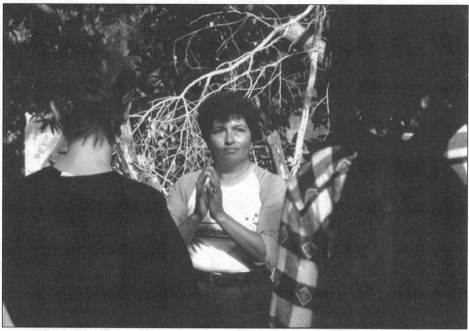

Local faculty teaching visiting students to about medicinal plants.

services while in residence. Our philosophy of health care promotes the healing arts and sciences, in which culture (cult: worship / ure: earth) is understood as the fulcrum for nature, the central element underlying health and illness in the personal and social domains.

Every society conceptualizes what wellness and health is, and ways of maintaining health, curing illness, or addressing disability. Indigenous Peoples exchange and trade their medicinal knowledge with other peoples. Traditional healing systems are taught inter-generationally among families and are based on Indigenous empirical sciences, borne of observation and experience in the healing arts and sciences. Distinctive cultures develop within the environments that shape them (Kuhnlein et al. 1996; Wadsworth and Robson 1977) and thus nature in its myriad forms shapes the foundation from which traditional medicine and food choices evolve. As access to the land is impeded, or as medicines are destroyed as a result of neo-colonial practices, the practice of medicine itself and community health is undermined.

The Indigenous and non-Indigenous staff and faculty emphasize the personal role of *indigeneity* as a primary source of identity linked to the promotion of health. The staff undertakes intensive pursuit of their own Indigenous origins and medical traditions whether they derive from the Americas, Europe Africa or Asia. We place women and children at the front and center of our work and apply a feminist analysis of health in the context of power, cultures and societies. In addition to members of the *comunidad,* who serve as staff, educators and the recipients of our services, the center has received Indigenous academics, healers and researchers from urban and rural centers around Mexico including Oaxaca and Puebla and from around the world, including Aboriginal Peoples from Australia and New Zealand, First Nation Peoples from Canada, and European Indigenous representatives, such as the Sapmelas (Sami) of Finland and Sierra Leone, Africa.

The Center for Traditional Medicine affiliated with Center for World Indigenous Studies, an independent non- profit research and education organization in 1994, thereby expanding our reach beyond rural Mexico, and facilitating linkages with reservation and urban Indigenous People in the USA and Canada. Dr. Rudolph Ryser (Taidnapum-Cowlitz) formed the Center for World Indigenous Studies (CWIS) in 1979 in response to a call from Northwest Pacific tribal governments. In 1983 Chief George Manuel (Sushwap) who was then President of the World Council of Indigenous Peoples called on the Center for World Indigenous Studies to serve as a documentation and education center on a global scale addressing Indigenous Peoples. It now houses one of the largest digital and hard copy library collections on Indigenous Peoples and conducts research and policy deliberations for tribal communities worldwide. In 2000, the Center for Traditional Medicine opened an office in Olympia, Washington, where CWIS is located and incorporated under state law to provide clinical care, research and education opportunities directly to peoples in the Pacific Northwest in the U.S. and Canada. We also conduct a program entitled *Nutrients for Natives*, which provides *pro bono* clinical care and nutrient support to Indigenous Peoples with diabetes and other chronic diseases.

As the Director of the Center for Traditional Medicine, I also oversee the only certificate and graduate degree program in Traditional Medicine and Fourth World Studies in the western hemisphere in collaboration with Lesley University in Cambridge, Massachusetts. This two-year training program relies upon Indigenous epistemologies (Ryser 1998) as the foundation which equips students with clinical and research skills from Indigenous perspectives. The program is unique in that it facilitates training in multi-vocality within and across the social science and humanities disciplines. Our goal is to enable students and professionals to traverse the diverse worlds they choose with ease, to integrate and translate ideas and practices that all too often are compartmentalized as separate disciplines in the academy and, perhaps most importantly, to envision and enact change through an Indigenous, not a *colonized* mind.

A basic principle of our work at the Center is as follows: Food and medicine are intimately tied to personal identity and personal health. Our approach also requires a commitment to personal integration of new learning and health seeking behaviors. We have observed and experienced first-hand that most often, meetings and conventions on diabetes, attended by activists, academics and policy makers serve coffee and sweets while discussing diabetes and "Indian health." The failure of individuals and groups to recognize and act on these lingering disjunctions precludes their ability to directly effect the necessary change of consciousness that ensures systematic, societal-wide change. Our work uses a heuristic and phenomenological approach to address what we consider the social and somatic dissociation that underlies diabetes and other chronic diseases. Thus, each staff member, faculty and patient engages in a process of "personal detoxification" and authentic health-building that is bio-culturally isomorphic with achieving his or her health goals.

Detoxification involves activities that support liver function and metabolic balance, including eliminating refined foods such as white flour and sugars, soft drinks and (excessive use of) alcohol. For Indigenous Peoples this means eliminating "introduced" or "colonial" substances that act like poisons. This call for the rejection of colonial nutrition may be located historically with other nodal moments when leaders, such as Shirley Palmer, a Colville Confederated Tribes council woman, stood before the meeting of the

Affiliated tribes of Northwest Indians in 1977 and implored every leader there to take responsibility for the alcohol abuse that is "killing our people" (Ryser, personal communication). This call to action was a turning point leading to the elimination of alcohol at leaders' meetings and a turn to sobriety by many in the sovereignty movement.

Every culture that we have looked into includes detoxification strategies in their traditional medicine repertoire. Indigenous societies use alterative (blood-purifying) plants, bitter, digestive-stimulating plants and foods, and substances that absorb toxins. Many peoples use purge-and-cleanse systems such as clays, various plant and animal-derived oils and enemas to detoxify the body and reestablish metabolic balance. In west Mexico, Indigenous Peoples use practices derived from *curanderismo* and incorporate the use of particular herbal teas, herbal enemas, *temazcales* (sweatbaths) and bathing rituals (Goldwater 1983; Korn 1983). At the clinic we have applied detoxification methods that include the use of castor oil packs, and coffee enemas, which serve as "dialysis of the blood across the gut wall" (Walker 2001: 49). Coffee enemas are theorized to dilute bile and dilate blood vessels countering inflammation of the gut and to enhance *Gluthianone S Transferase*, facilitating the phase-two liver detoxification pathway so integral to health in people with diabetes. While often ridiculed by the uninformed, coffee enemas were until recently included in the "bible of medicine," the *Merck Manual* (Gonzalez and Issacs 1999). In our patient population in Mexico and in the northwest USA patients readily embrace the coffee enemas in part because they promote a sense of relaxation and well being and because enemas are a tradition for many. Among the people who resist using coffee enemas are those who have experienced sexual abuse and offer the abuse as a reason for their refusal.

Authentic health building derives from the dynamic discovery and use of foods and practices that are Indigenous to a region or, if resulting from syncretic practices, nonetheless provide nutritive or medicinal sustenance and balance. This contrasts with foods that are exotic or introduced into an environment that contribute to or cause addictions and illness, acting like poison. Authentic foods and foodways always support a balanced approach to glucose levels. Even where peoples cultivate authentic sweet foods such as sugar cane, tree sap like maple syrup, honey, or wines, (or sweet wild plants such as Stevia, *stevia rebaudiana*, found primarily in Paraguay) these foods retain nutrients that add nutrition and are consumed in ratios conducive to psychophysiological balance.

Drugless Medicine in the Tropical Forest

During the early years in Mexico, the Center focused on addressing women and children's health: infectious diseases, malnutrition and women's reproductive health. There was no doctor in the village. Our texts were *Our Bodies Ourselves* (Boston Women's Health Book Collective 1998, the early newspaper print version) and *Where There is No Doctor* (Werner 1996). Women gathered weekly to cook together and share healing strategies, exchange knowledge, and integrate new knowledge about what kinds of sanitary practices would promote health, and how nutrition could improve or prove detrimental to health. The main health problems faced by the people in this region of Mexico included infectious diseases such as typhoid, dysentery, hepatitis, helminthiasis and amoebiasis. Concurrent with the socioeconomic changes during the 1980s the incidence of infectious disease decreased while chronic diseases increased.

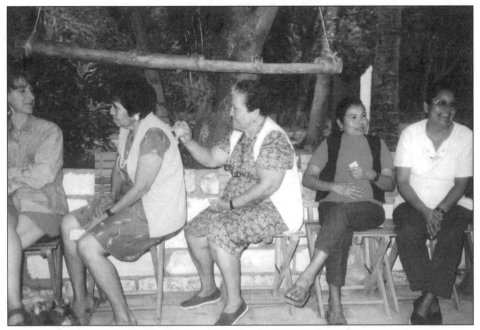

Sharing polarity therapy and massage techniques.

During these early years I trained in and practiced Naturopathic modalities such as polarity therapy, massage, hydrotherapy, nutrition and fasting, meditation, rehabilitative exercise and the internal and external application of medicinal foods and plants. Polarity therapy is a syncretic system of healing derived from Ayurvedic medical traditions from India and the cranial Osteopathy from early 20th century "drugless" medicine practitioners (Korn 2000). It is an art and science of healing, which brings balance to the human energy field by hands-on manipulation of bones, soft tissue and energy points; nutritional and attitudinal counseling; and specific stretching exercises using sound and movement. Polarity therapy and other massage modalities proved harmonizing with *curanderismo* (Goldwater 1983), known to the villagers and practiced under the radar of the physicians with whom the few wealthier, Catholic church-going community members traveled to the city to consult. These methods link to traditions dating back to Greco-Roman natural medicine, which is a major arm of the syncretic tradition of *curanderismo* (Davidow 1999; Trotter et al. 1997), which is active in its many forms throughout Mexico and by various Indigenous Peoples in the southwest USA.

As the Center for Traditional Medicine grew we offered traditional (local) and natural medicine services for chronic and primary health needs as well as for emergencies, such as bee and scorpion stings, burns and wounds. We applied high-dose vitamin therapies such as ascorbic acid to counteract scorpion and snake venoms, and acupuncture for dysentery. We offered polarity therapy and massage therapies for all types of physical and emotional distress and designed a specific protocol for the sequelae of decompression illness, which afflicts divers along the coast and leads to severe disability. We incorporated homeopathy and hydrotherapy for the growing number of cases of asthma and allergies and conducted post trauma counseling for men and women and domestic violence support (and often a safe house) to women.

The Center provided the only sustained health care in the village, in addition to the local *hueseros* (bone-setters) and *parteras* (midwives). During the early years of our work the public health nurses occasionally visited, traveling by boat from Puerto Vallarta, carrying out vaccination programs. Since it took a day's wages for a round trip fare by boat, many people who could not afford to travel to the city for health care instead used our clinic. We attended to many, many people who suffered from what we identified as *iatrogenic* (*Iatros*: Greek for physician and *genic*, meaning induced by) problems following their visits to doctors in the city, and to people who simply had not been helped at all. I observed only rarely the success of the medical interventions and pharmacotherapy ordered by the biomedical doctors, and as a result, I grew increasingly skeptical of the efficacy of allopathic medicine except in acute physical emergencies.

We focused our health education outreach from the early 1970s to mid 1980s on the use and abuse of pharmaceutical drugs that were (and still are) piped into the villages and are available at the *tienda* counter, used only on the advice of the store owner. Entero-Vioform (clioquinol) an over-the-counter pharmaceutical widely used for amoebic dysentery, was withdrawn from the pharmacies of industrialized countries following the decision of the Japanese government in 1970 due to its putative role in subacute myelo-optico-neuropathy (Silverman et al. 1982). During these years, Enterovioform, or as it was known, Mexaform, was used like candy by adults and children for episodes of diarrhea in the village. The *comunidad*'s village *tiendas* stocked the drug and *farmacias* in the cities as late as the mid 1980s stocked the drug on front shelves when it was supposed to have been withdrawn from the worldwide markets by Ciba Geigy, the manufacturer.

Our researchers found more pharmaceuticals with dubious value when we again renewed our store surveys in 1998. This time we identified 12 different pharmaceuticals, primarily steroids, painkillers, parasiticides and antibiotics. The indiscriminate use of antibiotics and other pharmaceuticals continues to remain high. Community members purchase injections of an antibiotic merely by contacting a person on the beach for 60 pesos to 100 pesos (about 5 to 10 dollars). Nearly any kind of drug remains accessible on the beach by simply paying for it. If a person has a cold, penicillin may be available and injected even though there is no relationship between the drug and the condition. Steroids, antibiotics and assorted other pharmaceuticals are consumed, without diagnosis in the same manner one would buy a *taco* to eat.

Meaning and Success

The Center for Traditional Medicine's health and healing programs achieved popularity throughout the *comunidad*. Word spread throughout the villages and people traveled by boat and over land to our clinic door. We believe that a complex interaction of forces contributed to our success. First, we supported the body's natural ability to heal while avoiding secondary side effects: The gentle, non-toxic effect is generally a hallmark of natural medicines. The use of these natural, traditional medicines draws from a deep wellspring of somatically-encoded (Ferreira 1998) familial histories that when tapped, reinforce a healing response.

Because we interpret most of the disease states within a holistic model, we are able to treat and respond to the whole person. Thus where chronic pain or somatization is at best generally understood by allopathic physicians as merely physical or emotional symptoms, and therefore to be medicated psychotropically, or where people with diabetes deteriorate in spite of the multiplicity of medications, we respond to these calls of distress by addressing each individual's situation as a reality whose symptoms, when listened to, tell a whole narrative that contains the answers (Korn 1987). We take time to learn the language of each person, listening and treating with our hands, eyes, ears and heart as well as with nutrition, herbs and all the other modalities within our repertoire.

The Center for Traditional Medicine serves as a cross-roads of medicine, and people feel validated when they are invited to discuss their knowledges and practices about the causes of their illness in an historical and cultural context. We listen openly and actively engage narratives that reveal the symptoms of *susto* (loss of spirit, extreme fright), *mal de ojo* (evil eye), *empacho* (indigestion with multiple etiologies) and *mal aire* (technically, bad air or wind, but can be associated with supernatural forces).

We believe that efficacy also arises from the added effect that I was an outsider, who had weathered many seasons in the village and had sought help myself for my own illnesses, thereby validating local knowledge systems through relationships. Each of these acts of validation, both private and public alike, make meaning, that in turn creates trust and reinforces self-agency that, for all of us lead to healing at many levels. We had also witnessed healing episodes that we could not easily explain. The 84-year old woman with crippling arthritis in her knees was able to walk after a week of receiving care at the clinic. The 35-year old woman, who suffered the humiliation of 15 years of infertility in a culture where her mother had birthed twelve children and her friends were birthing six, became pregnant after three weeks of care. The 15-year-old girl with Bell's Palsy whose face had been frozen for a year, returned to normal with a full bright smile after 4 weeks of care. The 56-year-old woman whose blood glucose hovered around 400 and who normalized her level to 110 and continued to maintain this level with diet, herbs and nutrients. These and many others demonstrated the value and success of our holistic approach to healing.

A. Traditional Medicine Practices in Western Mexico

The use of medicinal plants, animals, foods, touch and massage, the elements and spirit ways are all methods of healing that continue to evolve in rural western Mexico. Beginning in the 1970s, I compiled oral histories with local herbalists and healers to document the use of plants and their categories of knowledge and practices (Korn 1983).

The purpose of this action research was to affirm and sustain knowledge in the community and to support its practice inside and outside of my clinic. I have continued this process for 25 years with the assistance of interns and graduate students enrolled in the Center's two-year certificate program in Traditional Medicine, and Ethnonutrition and Ethnobotany.

During the 1980s, the social movement towards natural or holistic medicine grew in metropolitan areas in Mexico as well as in the United States of America. We identified the *lacunae* of cultural context that normally inform and give rise to these syncretized practices in traditional societies. We theorized that denuded of a cultural context, these practices, though effective for many, also reinforced the cultural homogenization of medicine and contributed to the theft of cultural property.

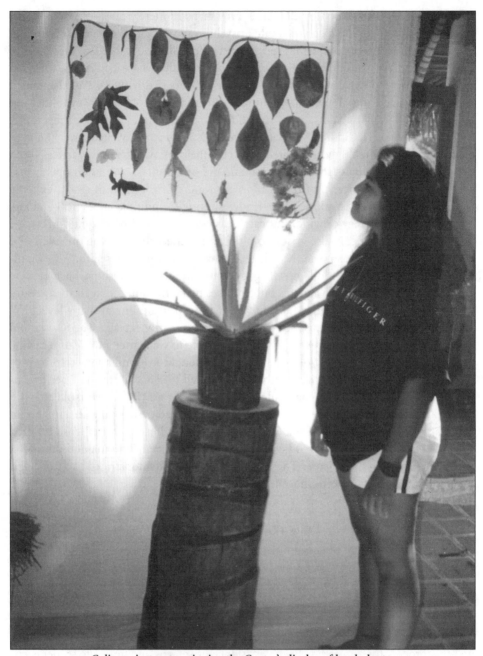

Culinary instructor viewing the Center's display of local plants.

At the Center, we also observed and experienced the effects of the unspoken internalized shame that Indigenous Peoples in the western hemisphere experience. Many peoples express shame over generations from the time of colonization, following the imposed criminalization of various cultural and medical healing practices by colonizing powers. As a consequence many healing and spiritual traditions are practiced secretly. The fear of punishment is the legacy of this trauma.

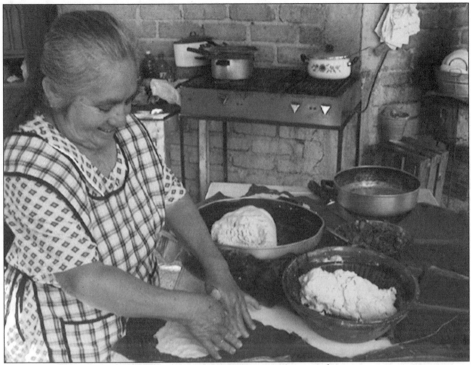

Elder culinary instructor preparing tamales.

By the late 1980s several socioeconomic classes emerged in this western Mexican *comunidad*. Twenty years earlier, class distinctions were not as severely demarcated. During these same years, the introduction and consumption of sugar, flour and hydrogenated oils became new staples in the daily diet. Introduced foods progressively replaced the use of authentic foods. Authentic foods native to the environment of west Mexico include zapote, chayote, the Mexican sweet potato called *camote*, beans, amaranth, maize, fish from the sea, deer, avocado, turkey (guacalote), chilies (Andrews 1984) chocolate (Coe and Coe 1996) and the ubiquitous coconuts (*coco nucifera*; Duke 1983).

Several changes contributed to shifts in food quality and security. A major Mexican national policy initiative that reached the *comunidad* was the CONASUPO. Established in 1965 to maintain price supports for introduced foods, the *Compañia Nacional de Subsistencias Populares* (CONASUPO) delivered large quantities of cheap foodstuffs like flour, refined sugar, canned fruit juices, honey and packaged ground corn. However, this attempt by a parastatal organization (subsequently implicated in massive corruption and illicit drug trade) to deliver food to the rural poor only served to further displace the role of traditional food gathering activities of Indigenous Peoples of both the west and east coast alike.

The *comunidad* members who were acquiring wealth were also, we observed, among the first to become ill with the chronic diseases. They sought help in the city while the poor continued their visits to the Center for Traditional Medicine's clinic. It was common that following dissatisfaction with the medicine in the city, the wealthier members then returned to our clinic, not for traditional medicine *per se*, but for the latest "alternative" or "complementary medicine" that was commanding attention in the

media. Thus, my task was to respond not only to the illness at hand but also to the belief systems that influenced people to reject various Indigenous traditional healing
methods, only to accept these same treatments known by different names in the lexicon of "complementary medicine."

B. "Defective Modernization"

If we had known then what we know now, I don't think we would have let in the tourists.

      Epifanio Solario

Throughout our time in Mexico, we have witnessed a persistent trend of socioeconomic and cultural changes resulting from modernization, which in turn severely affected the overall health of the community. Economic and social forces introduced into
the *Comunidad* from the rapid growth of Puerto Vallarta in the last thirty years had a
significant effect on the level of self-sufficiency, self-esteem, absenteeism, and the growing use and abuse of alcohol and drugs. As the economy, external development and
political influences became apparent by the late 1970s, Puerto Vallarta became an economic focal point for developers and investors.

One Chacalan, Lupita Ramos C., explained that increasing housing construction
along the Rio Tuito (one of two major water sources serving the *comunidad* and the
ancient link to the mountain town of El Tuito) and other rivers increased levels of water
contamination and radically reduced the water availability in the *Comunidad*. According to Cruz Ramos (1999):

> The rivers are no longer as beautiful as before. Before, they were cleaner; they
> did not dry up; one could swim all the time. Now, there are many houses,
> and the water is wasted all over the place, and it does not rain like before.

When I arrived at the *comunidad* in 1973, the use of pharmaceuticals and refined
foods were growing at an accelerated pace. Denatured oils and refined wheat and sugar
products, including white flour, corn oils, powdered and on-the-shelf milks and candies, were flooding the market. Yet most people also continued to grow coffee, beans
and squash and grind corn, make fresh fish soups, slaughter pigs and pick fruits from
family plots. Yet the pace of change accelerated and put pressure on the attempts to balance these influences. By 1982 we witnessed the smoke rising from the beach as the *Fed-
erales* stormed the small village of *Mismaloya* 10 miles north and burned down the
palapa homes and restaurants, chasing the villagers back into the mountains in order
to clear the beach for the development of a "five star resort." That resort stands where
the village had been located, now limiting access to the beach to all but registered guests.

Rapid change from development imposed by expansion of Puerto Vallarta, the role
of drug trafficking, now considered to be the driving economic power in the city and
increasingly a significant factor in the *comunidad* (Cruz 1999), and the growing influence of economic and social pressures flowing from the North American Free Trade
Agreement have paralleled changes in health patterns.

Jalisco is the largest corn growing state in Mexico, but the value of corn is low compared with the export value of soybeans. Growing investments in tourism and agricultural changes portend even more rapid and larger-scale economic—and thus social

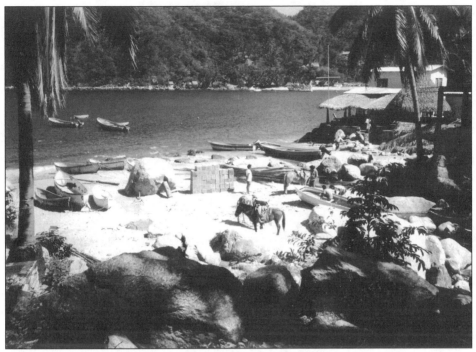

The little beach receiving cargo, 1975.

and cultural changes—in western Mexico. Such rapid externally-induced change appears to have given little time for members of the *comunidad* to understand these changes within their own cultural background. A serious consequence is the increasing levels of cultural stress coupled with social, health and economic dislocation and imbalance (Zimmet 2000), as discussed by the authors of this book.

Externally imposed and internally adopted dietary and health transitions also reduced access to wild foods and medicines by altering communal knowledge systems. The migration from the villages by young adults began in the late 1980s. The increase in diabetes along with other chronic diseases rose side-by-side with these changes. The pace of life increased along with stress-related disorders. White bread sandwiches with cut-off crusts replaced corn tortillas. Children and young adults came in to the clinic with high blood pressure, high blood sugar, insomnia (often due to over-consumption of Coca Cola and other commercially produced sugar water products), allergies and diabetes. An epidemic of chronic diseases was unfolding.

Additional influence emerged with the arrival of the Protestant evangelical ministers who brought a new wave of colonization. The message of these ministries to their "brown flocks" is to focus on the "blond savior," then rise above poverty (and by implication your Indian-ness) aided by the promise of NAFTA, consumption of commercially made products, and rejection of "primitive" use of plants and natural healing. These new ministries focused on recruiting young adults in the *comunidad*. By the late 1990s the children of these young adults were struggling themselves with increasing use of alcohol and drugs and growing addiction to sugar—whether alcohol-based or through Coca Cola. Smoking, which was not seen in the village among women or teen boys and girls, became increasingly evident. Alcoholism and recreational drug consumption in these age groups and among women increased as well. The Women's Traditional Medicine Group held several months of meetings to consider what could be done with the growing use of drugs like crack cocaine among school children. Because everyone knows who does what in a small village, the women expressed fear for their lives if they took action by going to the authorities.

C. Imposed Development and Chronic Disease

…the pressures from a dominant society intensify precisely when the presence of a group with distinct identity constitute an obstacle to practical objectives.

Bonfil (1996: 46)

The gestation period of "defective modernization" (Simonelli 1987: 23) that we began observing in the early 1970s had resulted by the 1990s in a village-wide diabetes epidemic and the related triad of cardiovascular disease, stroke and high blood pressure. There was a palpable shift from infectious to chronic disease. Whereas people in the rural subtropics are subject to sanitation-based disorders such as intestinal parasites, typhoid fever, dengue, hepatitis A and non-A and the usual forms of influenza, colds and pneumonias the prevalence of chronic disease rose in the *comunidad*. Heart disease, stroke, cancer, high blood pressure, diabetes (adult onset), chronic pain and stress became the primary health maladies. Villagers developed huge and multiple lipomas (benign fatty tissue tumors) on their bodies and reported high rates of insomnia. At the same time, there were growing rates of drug and alcohol abuse. Traditional healers using healing remedies from the tropical forest's pharmacopoeia would each typically have detailed knowledge of more than 1000 plants and their multiple uses. By the late 1970s modernization had severely affected access and use of traditional medicines, in particular medicinal and authentic foods and plants. By the 1990s community knowledge and use of these systems were severely diminished.

Iatrogenic symptom rates grew as most villagers now traveled by boat to the city an hour away to obtain health care at the Social Security Clinic. We identified and catalogued iatrogenic symptoms including severe allergic reactions to pharmaceuticals, dermatitis, antibiotic resistance, over-use of cortisone, vertigo, and secondary digestive problems all resulting from inaccurate diagnoses or over-medication. All of these problems were exacerbated by the (undiagnosed) chronic dehydration experienced by most of the patients seen at our clinic. The commonly practiced proscription against drinking quantities of water appears to have arisen out of the history of sanitation problems. However traditional *agua frescas*, drinks made from fresh water, local fruits and berries, and anthelmintic herbs teas that traditionally took the place of plain water were replaced by Coca Cola and other commercially produced sugared juices. Not only were the benefits of water, fresh fruits and teas substantially reduced, but also adverse affects of refined sugar consumption became the norm.

Together with some of the village women, I organized a gathering to evaluate the role the social security clinic doctor might play in our effort to document community stress and community healing strategies. This gathering produced a rather eye-opening realization that the Social Security doctor herself was identified as an important stressor. A young woman of 23 years from Guadalajara, the doctor expressed intensely negative views toward the men of Yelapa. She also felt free to express her belief that the people are "lazy, prone to drunkenness and heavily dependent on illicit drugs." These remarks got a quick and firm retort from Doña Maya. This presumption of superiority of status, methods and of the inevitability of development and progress (cf. Bodley 1982) undermined our work. Conventional medical practitioners in the city and in the village had a disastrous affect in the community both in terms of general health and community confidence. The only exception was in the practice of homeopathy, which is practiced by many physicians in Mexico.

Homeopathy arrived in Mexico around 1850 shortly after it was introduced in the USA from Germany.[1] In 1910, after decades of internecine battles between competing medical groups seeking hegemonic right-to-practice, the Carnegie Foundation in alignment with newly formed American Medical Association issued the Flexner Report. This document led to the demise of Homeopathy in the USA for nearly a century by making it impossible for homeopathic medical school graduates to obtain a license to practice medicine (Ullman 1991). However, homeopathic medicine remained accessible in Mexico, popular especially among many poor segments of the population and Indigenous Peoples. When we introduced homeopathic medicine at the clinic our patients embraced it and responded exceptionally well.

D. Community Trauma

For the first 20 years of operation, the Center for Traditional Medicine was supported through volunteerism, small donations and educational training programs that brought community health practitioners to the clinic for study for one-month periods. Barter was an important form of exchange. People brought fresh eggs and fish to the clinic and our training programs brought health professionals from around the world to learn about rural health to train with us and local healers, in exchange for tuition and for donating their services. In the nearby cities of Puerto Vallarta and Guadalajara interest in complementary medicine grew slowly toward the middle of the 1990s.

In 1998, we received major outside financial support for our work, and this allowed us to design and undertake the Women's Traditional Medicine Community Trauma Study, in which the diabetes-healing project became a major component. The purpose of the community trauma study in Yelapa was to determine the role of culture in the healing of community stress and to develop a replicable template for restoring balance in a community that was modifiable according to each community's needs. The approach used in our study relied on a proven participatory action research model. The methods of community-determined research are designed so that the community can control the decision making process from inception in order to allow culturally sensitive programs to be carefully crafted. In this project, which we discuss in detail below,

---

1. Homoeopathy is an alternative method of treatment, based on the nature's Law of Cure, namely 'Like Cures Like'. The truth of this law was discovered by a German scientist Dr. Samuel Hahnemann in 1796, and has been verified experimentally and clinically for 200 years. The remedies are prepared from natural substances to precise standards and work by stimulating the body's own healing power.

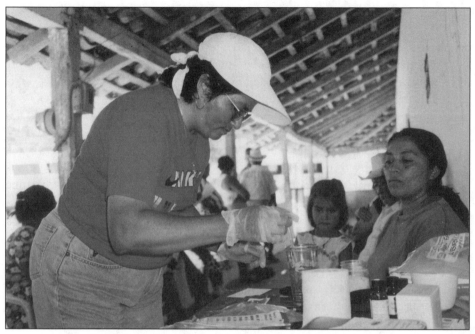

Health promoters visit mountain villages to test blood glucose.

we emphasized community-determined research to elaborate the desired goals of the community with respect to resolving emerging community health problems and the validation of cultural knowledges.

The study was developed with the Women's Traditional Medicine Group whose members were volunteers from the *comunidad*. The Women's group included members with extensive knowledge of healing plant and animal medicines and techniques. They chose this as an important area of knowledge to encourage throughout the *comunidad*. In addition members encouraged designing and implementing a community natural medicine health promoter program for local women throughout three villages in the *comunidad*.

A women's sewing circle was organized on a weekly basis. The project also coordinated intergenerational sharing opportunities to collect and recycle community knowledge through *comunidad* school-wide creative arts classes. *Comunidad* youngsters were involved in traditional healing plant identification by our encouraging them to draw colorful pictures of plants from the tropical forest.

The knowledge of healers and pictures drawn by the children were combined into a unique Spanish and English booklet designed for use in the *comunidad*. The clinic became the focal point for practicing traditional medicine as well as documenting evidence of community stress and trauma in an effort to identify the role of culture as a healing factor for community trauma. Cultural practices as represented in traditional healing approaches were to be identified for the prevention and management of infectious disease and chronic disease.

While prevention and the management of infectious diseases remained a strong component of the clinic's work, the results of modernization and the social influences of encroaching development brought many adults and children to the clinic suffering with symptoms of (traumatic) stress. Where family and community cohesion had pre-

viously served as a deterrent to stress, the growing migration of the younger generation out of the villages and the intense pressures of market economy *commodification*
overwhelmed many. Children came to the clinic with high blood pressure; women were
gaining weight, experiencing sleepless nights and increasingly reporting rapes. More
men were drinking beer and *Raiclla* (a local cactus-based brew) excessively and using
hard drugs We collected the case reports of women who came to the clinic for treatment for a range of problems, which were as we began to learn, associated with the
sequelae of the growing stress and violence domestically.

One woman whom we attended at the clinic reported:

> My husband rapes me whenever he wants. I try to tell him that I cannot have
> relations because of my health condition. My family tells me that I have to live
> with him and that my children need a father. But I am the one who works and
> I am the one who raises him.

Another mother who also was the victim of domestic violence and her alcoholic
husband's rage was one of the few women who left her husband, much to the opprobrium of others. She told us:

> The woman needs more support. She is always working inside and outside the
> house to get things for her family but it is never enough. There are a lot of
> lazy men and egotistical men that don't like to help.

And yet another woman with diabetes whom we interviewed at the clinic said:

> The majority of the women are oppressed. There is a lot of family abuse gen-
> erally because men are drunk. Alcoholism is the biggest problem in the family.

To assign these experiences solely to the stress of development would be inaccurate.
Machismo and the rigid formation of gender roles and gender identity arrived with the
Europeans and slowly influenced Indigenous Peoples, for whom gender and hence
power relations are more fluid concepts (Joyce 2000). *Machismo* remains strong
throughout Indigenous Mesoamerica today.

Through our everyday conversations and more formal interviews in the community and at the clinic we identified both the subtle and overt ways that externally imposed economic development was increasingly stressful and contributed to the increase of physical and emotional violence that in turn is causal of traumatic or
extreme stress (Herman 1992). Historically the Chacalans are a strong, resourceful,
and resilient people. Individuals, families and a whole community increasingly (as
our data began to demonstrate) suffered a decrement in mental and physical health
patterns particularly the chronic diseases such as diabetes and psychosomatic distress.
We named these phenomena community trauma. This process clearly began to develop over a 15 to 25 year period, but began to show marked and accelerated changes
in community health in the final 5 years of that period. We believed it was not only
the types of changes that were occurring but the pace at which they occurred. To better understand the exponential increase in the pace of life we examined the speed of
travel, by boat between the coastal villages and the nearest city, Puerto Vallarta. In
1950 people traveled in a canoe with a small sail, taking 12 hours when the wind was
favorable. By 1970, a larger boat with a 40 horsepower outboard motor, called a

panga, required 2 to 3 hours to navigate the seas. Between 1970 and 1990 the boat and motors grew in power so that by 1990 the boats carried a 75 horsepower. By 2000, boats carried 175 horsepower or more and bounced along the wake, arriving in the city in 35 minutes.

We define development that is imposed from outside the community as traumatogenic and we define community trauma as "events that overwhelm communities' capacities to function in stable and generative ways" (Korn 2003). Habitat destruction, economic dislocation, food security interruption, social order disruption, physical relocation, educational colonization, religious conversion, natural resource piracy, distortion of decision-making, and externally imposed priority-making are all together and individually characteristics of community trauma. Externally-induced development is defined as choices made by others ostensibly for the benefit of the group being changed, when in reality those choices are primarily beneficial to the promoters of development (Ryser 2001). We were in contact and exchanging ideas and practices with our colleagues working in East Papua and among the Bhil in West India who also identified similar patterns of community trauma. Clearly we were systematically identifying a phenomenon, a community disorder that has profound significance in other regions of the world as well. Helena Norberg-Hodge (*Ancient Futures* 1991) working in Ladakh also mirrored our observations of the destructive effects of externally-induced development and globalization among Indigenous Peoples.

As one of our collaborators, Tonio Lopez, said of the disintegration of community cohesion:

> Before people were more united. It was truly a community. Everyone helped everyone and they gave more value to the natural resources than money. There were abundant fruits and vegetables that grew easily, plants that cured and finally resources that satisfied the demand of the people. When Puerto Vallarta began to grow, a lot of people began to arrive here and many people in the community began to compete and to want to make money and it was precisely at this time the divisions and envy began to develop. People became dependent on tourism and life here changed enormously. Before we were self-sufficient and living with what we had here. Everyone lived without problems and the guarantee of subsistence.

Many people in the community were suffering from some form of traumatic experience, and we observed how these experiences passed among family members inter-generationally. We observed various degrees of breakdown among families experiencing mental and physical health illnesses that originated in or were exacerbated by consumption of alcohol and refined foods. A complex relationship between access to local food, development and the cash economy and diabetes and hyperglycemia became evident. We carefully monitored buying patterns, *tienda* stocks of commercially produced and refined foods and locations of peoples suffering from chronic conditions over several years. Rates of insomnia increased dramatically—our community screenings and clinic records documented stress and the high rates of Coca-Cola and other sugared soft drinks. The relationship between consumption rates, stress and chronic conditions appeared palpable. Sugar and caffeine addiction appeared to contribute significantly to the inability to sleep. Our community screenings indicate that 13% of 243 surveyed (nearly 9% overall of *co-*

munidad residents) in the community at random indicated they consumed at least 3 to 5 cans of Coca Cola or other sugared beverage daily. Our clinic records further indicated that the majority of primary complaints between 1996 and 1999 were chronic pain disorders (40%) and chronic, preventable diseases (31%) that arose out of a "nexus of stress."

We include diabetes and other autonomically mediated dysfunction in the nervous, digestive, circulatory systems, as well as lifestyle or development-related changes in nutrition as conditions that have been initiated or exacerbated by this stress (Evans 1985; Surwit 1993). Diabetes, heart disease, and obesity form the trinity of community trauma resulting from induced development. In order to address diabetes by focusing on prevention and treatment, we had no choice but to respond to the persistent and mutable influences of colonial trauma and the resulting nutrition trauma that affected the villagers.

E. Nutrition Trauma

Now if you have money you eat, if you don't have money you don't eat. Everything is more difficult. Now the people are maintained only by tourism. The beach is very small and everyone wants a business there and everyone is competing. There is a lot of envy and a lot of gossip all over.

      Lucio Rodriguez, elder Comunero, 1999

Community trauma includes a subset concept we call "nutrition trauma." We define this type of trauma as a disruption in access to endemic natural food resources due to overwhelming forces that make inaccessible foodstuffs that are bio-culturally and biochemically suited to healthy digestion and nutrient utilization. Such outside forces include externally introduced economy, cultural genocide or ethnocide in the form of *Mestizoization* policies (Salvador 1996), the *melting pot* theory in the United States and *Russification* in the Union of Soviet Socialist Republics; all are examples of state integration policies that are imposed on culturally distinct peoples (Fallon 1985). Agrarian reform policies like the Mexican constitutional revision of Article 24 that disbanded *ejiido* land rights were originally the heart of the Mexican constitution designed to protect Indian lands from sale or confiscation. The repeal of the *ejido* provision in 1994 led to the immediate sale of 25% of all *ejidos* transferring that land to corporate farmers seeking to consolidate land for the production and export of soybeans. An even more drastic result was the massive migration of Indigenous men primarily from rural to urban areas mainly in the north of Mexico along the border with the United States where manufacturing companies were quickly built by US companies after the adoption of the North American Free Trade Agreement. Self-sufficient and collective reliance practices among rural Indigenous Peoples were replaced by landless peoples now dependent on unseen economic forces and dependence on commercial foods not suitable for Indigenous metabolisms. Dependence and food scarcity replaced self-sufficiency and plentiful and appropriate foods.

Nutrition trauma occurs when introduced foods overwhelm the capacity of the local Indigenous Peoples to digest and metabolize these new foods, which often cause conditions that were unknown or rare before the colonial process. A 1946 study of the Otomi people (who live in Puebla) found that they suffered no malnutrition, despite difficult conditions, relied on traditional foods such as *quelites* (greens) and ate no refined or processed foods, no wheat, and little dairy (Anderson 1946). A 1996 study found a prevalence of hypertriglyceridemia in 26% of the Otomi population (Alvarado-

Osuna, Milian-Suazo and Valles-Sanchez 2001). Larsen (2000: 167) asserts that bioarcheological evidence from the America suggests "most settings involving pro-longed interactions between Europeans and Indians led to a decline in the quality of life and changes in activities for the latter."

Introduction of single-species agriculture or mono-culture in the Americas dra-matically altered the ecology as well as the health of the Indigenous Peoples. Such a change in quality of life and dramatically-altered health affects can also result from changes slowly introduced into a society from outside trade.

Instead of leading active physical lives, many Indigenous Peoples have become seden-tary as a direct consequence of decades of land appropriation and relocation, and forced models of development. The association between sedentism, and the prevalence of dia-betes is well-defined (Larson 2000; Murray and Pizzorno 1998; Nabhan 1997; Jackson 1994; Lang 1989; cf. Wiedman, this volume). Even where people are active, as many are in the *comunidad*, the balance has tipped in favor of a process of "dis-ease" that has over-whelmed the body's capacity to adjust to change. In *Cabo Corrientes*, nutrition trauma includes a sharp reduction in available arable land; reduction in fish supply in the bay (the seventh largest in the world) due to over fishing in response to tourism and devel-opment; pesticide poisoning; media propaganda; and by a greater dependence on com-mercially produced foods in the 1990s. Electricity and hence television arrived in 2002 in Yelapa, later than most of the other *comunidad* villages. The images and storylines portrayed through the television clearly associated certain foods with being "Indian," poor and disenfranchised, and, thus, undesirable. Commercially-produced foods loaded with wheat, sugar, corn syrup, and preservatives are promoted as desirable and "modern."

Reductions in arable land and fish supply caused an out-pricing of certain traditional foods by highly processed, less healthy foods that were mass-produced by corporate con-glomerates. Our food surveys of the village *tiendas* revealed over 100 food and toxic cleaning items with nearly all supplied by transnational corporations such as Kraft, (Phillip Morris) Pronto Unilever, Coca Cola, Quaker, Colgate, Palmolive, McCormick, Kimberley Clark and del Valle (Hirch 2003). Not surprisingly, people in the villages want to be "modern" so they work to acquire currency in order to buy the new products. "In-dian foods" that have sustained members of the community, require physical labor and are sometimes unavailable, appear destined to be replaced by convenient products.

F. Intergenerational Traumatic Stress

To be an "Indian" in Mexico is to be called lazy, stupid and shifty. To be an Indian in Mexico is to be in danger. This is so well understood that, given the opportunity, what has been forgotten or is rarely said, is that one is "Indian" or *indigenista*. This is also seen in the apparent obsession of many who ask if someone is really an Indian or how **much** Indian they are. Rarely are Europeans asked how English they are or how French they are. What has become well understood, though, is passivity and submission in the face of other authority. To be an Indian often requires the need to "pass" as non-Indian, and Indians on the west coast of Mexico don't "pass" by using traditional medicines.

This newly desired behavior spans multiple generations and speaks to the inter-gen-erational stresses (Duran et al. 1998) that pass for normalcy in the *comunidad*. This behavior may explain, in part, the chronic health disease patterns related to stresses that are increasing in rural Mexico and in the *Comunidad de Chacala* in particular. Socio- political changes have resulted in the rescinding of many edicts outlawing traditional medical practices, even as new ones are constructed in the name of "Public Health" (Friedland 2000: 1995). Elders retain the active memory of both threat and shame and these observations lead us naturally to integrate clinical care with social activism and conclude that most of the chronic health problems we observe are due to the legacy of colonization trauma and intergenerational transmission of traumatic stress. In the 1980s many clinicians came to believe that diagnostic categories of post-traumatic stress failed to reflect the profound personality changes in victims of prolonged totalitarian rule—such as in prisoners of war, cult survivors and battered wives. Thus a new category, called Complex Traumatic Stress or Disorders of Extreme Stress Not Otherwise Specified (DESNOS) was proposed. Just as we observe similar responses to nutrition trauma among Indigenous Peoples in North and Mesoamerica, there are similarities in the responses to experiences of colonization among Indigenous Peoples in the U.S. and Mexico. Referring to members of a study on trauma among tribal members in the Southwest U.S., Manson et al. (1996: 262) stated:

> How does one recognize and identify psychic numbing? In the presence of cultural disintegration and high levels of cultural demoralization, how does one accurately assess loss of interest, feelings of detachment or estrangement or a sense of a foreshortened future?...Perhaps the degree of trauma itself is sufficiently greater in many native communities so that the individual threshold for clinical response has been reset at higher levels, as trauma has become more the norm than the exception.

Stress and traumatic stress are intergenerational experiences for colonized Indigenous Peoples all over the world (Gagne 1998; Duran et al. 1998), as discussed in most chapters of this volume. Trauma alters the eco-system of the body, mind, and spirit, like oil pollutes water. Stress and trauma negatively affect the autonomic nervous system and endocrine function (Kiecolt-Glaser et al. 1994) and this chronic decrement in function is correlated with Syndrome X, a precursor to diabetes (Reaven 1992) and to diabetes itself (Cordain 2001). Cultural and historical traumas precipitate the disruption of communal psychobiological rhythms resulting in adrenal stress and dysglycemia. Community trauma affects individuals, families and whole communities' capacity to exercise self-determination and generate community well being. Stress and trauma affect the metabolism of a community; the ability to find, absorb and use both edible and interpersonal nourishment. Elsewhere we have referred to the digestion of trauma in the context of undigested traumatic experiences as a psychological correlate of autonomically mediated digestive dysfunctions (Korn 1996). Stress causes anxiety and depression and leads to self-medication with drugs, alcohol, carbohydrates and sugar; in turn these substances exacerbate stress.

Recent history suggests native coping strategies were reinforced by alcohol early in the colonial process. Distilled alcohol was introduced into native societies in Mexico in the 1520s. The Spaniards traded alcohol along with the Russians, English and French with Indigenous Peoples in western North America at the beginning of the 19th century. Of course societies in these regions had fermented beverages, and for those societies there were strict regulations for consumption. The intensity of distilled alcohols and fortified beverages proved poisonous to local peoples.

All pre-contact societies used a variety of psychoactive substances in highly regulated and customary rituals (French 2000). The Nahuatl in Mexico employed strict taboos against alcohol consumption—only high priests could consume the authentic fermented *tequino,* a corn beer with a very low alcohol content. The higher alcohol and sugar content of introduced beverages from Europe quickly replaced the domestic variety, and taboos proscribing alcohol broke down alongside the rest of the fabric of pre-European contact mores. In societies where alcoholic beverages were first consumed as a controlled ritual alcohol beverage, alcohol now became a commodity used as self-medication (Khantzian 1985) against dislocation, stress and trauma (Robin et al. 1996).

G. Stress and Diabetes

Stress is a trigger for hyperglycemia and the development of adult onset diabetes (Surwit 1999; Scheder 1988 and in this volume). The hypersecretion of stress hormones called glucocorticoids are antagonists to the production of insulin (Roman 1980). Emotional, psychological and spiritual stressors combine with nutrition trauma to contribute to the dramatic breakdown of Indigenous societies—manifestations of neo-colonial induced cultural and historical trauma.

When the stress response is called into action again and again, without the ability to affect the outcome, then despondency, despair and rage will set in (Rossi 1986). These conditions result in biochemical changes: lactic acid builds up in the muscles, and leads to rigidity, pain, and anxiety. The nervous system is dysregulated and the immune system weakens, along with digestion and heart function. Individual reactions alternate between depression and helplessness to anxiety and irritability and self blame (van der Kolk 1987). People hurt themselves and others and abuse drugs and alcohol to not feel the collective rage and pain. Self-harming behavior, physical pain and self-medication, like the extensive abuse of pharmaceuticals, drugs and alcohol, only reinforce a sense of being out of control. Helpless to change the present, the individual believes there is no future (Korn 1996). This loss of self-efficacy and ability to mobilize change spreads throughout members of a community. Our experience suggests that if this loss is not addressed at the individual and community level, trauma often leads to the reenactment of behaviors that in turn traumatize others (Korn 2003; van der Kolk 1987).

Once diabetes becomes apparent in a community it is already a signifier of a long process of metabolic imbalance that began years earlier. The stress that underlies and contributes to metabolic dysfunction often prevents the individual from mobilizing the extraordinary effort required to stabilize or reverse the disease. It is not uncommon for health providers working in Indigenous communities to express their frustration with the apparent failure of people with diabetes to undertake self-care or to comply or adhere to their assigned health protocols. But what if (even when interventions are culturally isomorphic) people are suffering from learned helplessness (Garber and Seligman 1980; Seligman 1972), depression, and cultural demoralization of which diabetes is yet the latest symptom?

Part 2. Metabolizing Trauma: The Case of the *Comunidad Indigena de Chacala*

The *Comunidad Indigena de Chacala* is one of the few remaining *Comunidades Indigenas* in Mexico whose political sovereignty dates back to a writ by the King of Spain in 1525. Its population reflects the confluence of multiethnic and multicultural peoples who have flourished on the west coast for 3000 years and more (Townsend 1998). Because no great archaeological discoveries had been made in the region, the general attitude of government, scholars and tourists has been that there is no "culture" in Western Mexico and research in this region has grown slowly. To our knowledge, only a few researchers have in the last 100 years looked at the culture of Western Mexico. Adela Breton, a British artist, arrived in Guadalajara in 1895 with an interest in antiquities and became the first serious scholar to inquire into the substance of western Mexico's ancient cultures (Townsend 1998). Little public acknowledgment of this research was granted until the late 1990s.

Peoples of Western Mexico (generally including the states of Nayarit, Jalisco, Michoacan and Colima) have experienced intense externally initiated and motivated demands to impose a Hispanic ethos on the Indigenous Peoples. The culture of the *Comunidad* has its roots in the 2300-year influence of what modern scholars now refer to as the Teuchitlán tradition and the 400-year dominance of the Purépecha (Tarascans as they are known by outsiders) in the eastern part of west Mexico. The Teuchitlán tradition is recognized to have begun in approximately 1500 BC in the lakebeds area to the west of what is now Guadalajara. Mountjoy has conducted radiocarbon determinations in the region dating to the archaic period identifying markers ranging from 2200 BC to 1730 BC (Mountjoy 2000).

The region was apparently defined by the direct influence of the Olmec culture from southeastern Mexico. Constructing a centralized chieftain in round *palapas* and circular cities on the lakeshores (unlike the rectangular cities of the Valley of the Moon), the culture emphasized civic ritual and ceremony, ancestor worship and organization of personal power around the practice of accumulation and ceremonial give-away (Townsend 1998). The region appears to be further influenced by a 3500-year trading relationship with what is now the coast of Ecuador and Peru. The trade centered on acquisition of the beautiful *Spondylus* oyster shell a "large spiny, tropical bivalve, its exterior and lips are scarlet, its interior cavity with color of white porcelain" (Anawalt 1998: 246) off the coast of present-day Colima, the state immediately south of Jalisco. The shell of this oyster was so prized by the peoples of the Andes in Peru that great effort was expended to acquire large quantities. The trade also involved textiles, pottery, dried beans, and technological knowledge including smelting of copper and silver (Townsend 1998). The relationship continued until the 16th century when the invading Spanish disrupted the Toltec-based and Mayan based civilizations in Mexico, and later the civilizations along the Andean mountain spine. The devastation brought on by the advance of small pox, influenza, typhoid, cowpox, mumps, and other bacterial and viral epidemics combined with military actions made easy by such diseases, to bring about economic, cultural and social collapse in 1521.

The militaristic Purépecha Empire (dubbed by the Spanish the "Tarasacan Empire") emerged after the collapse of the Teuchitlán tradition in the high valleys of what is now the state of Michoacan—south of Guadalajara. The Purépecha Empire ruled much of western Mexico before and contemporaneously with the Aztec Empire. By virtue of its intense military culture, and the forbidding mountains, the Mexica of the Aztec Empire in the Valley of the Moon had little influence in western Mexico.

The Spanish slowly subdued the Purépecha though the people and their culture remains a strong influence in Michoacan to this day. Around the time when complex societies all over the Americas were experiencing stress and collapse, the Teuchitlán tradition came to an end about 700 AD. In a relatively short time, the Teuchitlán tradition was transformed into the Purépecha State located in the high valley of what is now the state of Michoacan just south of the city of Guadalajara. The Empire came to an end in 1525 when Spanish invaders arrived (Carmack et al. 1996).

The government of the United States of Mexico in Mexico City, Federal District, recognizes the *Comunidad Indigena de Chacala* as a semi-legal entity with a standing that predates the formation of the Mexican state in 1821. In 1940 there were 10 small houses in Yelapa (Diaz 2000). While the political seat remains the mountain village—now nearly deserted as a result of an outflow of the younger people—power has shifted with an economic focus now on the tourism burgeoning in three ocean villages.

Early 20th century small-scale agriculture included activities such as the collection of *chicle* gum from the sub-deciduous, medium size height canopy tropical forest, and later coconut oil extraction, followed by post- subsistence fishing in the Pacific Ocean. Subsistence crops include corn, squash, bean, chili, tomato, sesame seed, cartamo, copra, sunflower, barley, tobacco, peanut, cantaloupe, watermelon, sweet potato, papaya, *guamuchil, ilama, anona, mamey, chico zapote,* lime, orange, avocado, guava, coconut, banana, pineapple, peach, pear, sugar cane and mango. Today, tourism, drugs and the migration of the younger family members to find employment in the U.S. form the backbone of the current cash economy.

The region where Chacala is located is considered to host some of the richest endemic species of vertebrates and plants in the world (Alejandra Valero et al. 2001). The coast road, which opened the region to intense natural resource exploitation beginning in 1972, remains inaccessible to Yelapa and all but one of the villages in the *comunidad.* Temperatures range from 60° to 85° F. The dry rain forest has cycles of rain between May and October and a dry period of five months between November and April. Every May, when the heat parches and the waterfalls are nearly dry, the women continue the ancient tradition of calling to Tlaloc, the rain god, the memory of which is inscribed in petroglyphs on boulders in the hills (Mountjoy 2000), by traveling up river and singing their way back to town.

The *Comunidad Indigena de Chacala,* and indeed the whole region, is at its root steeped in a rich culture quite distinct from other parts of Mexico. The culture of the *Communidad Indigena de Chacala* is characterized by self-reliance, militant protection of access to land, community property ownership, and individual identity associated with community identity. These people do not identify, nor have they ever generally identified themselves according to "tribal affiliations." Instead of thinking of themselves as "Indians," "Nahua," "Zapoteca," or some other linguistic, ethnic, or tribal group, the Indigenous Peoples of western Mexico think of themselves as *Chacalan.* Alisia Rodriguez is the only person we have heard say the word "Indigena" in relation to herself and that was said as though a secret was proudly pronounced to people whose ears were listening without fear. Pizota, Yelapa and other communities in the southern re-

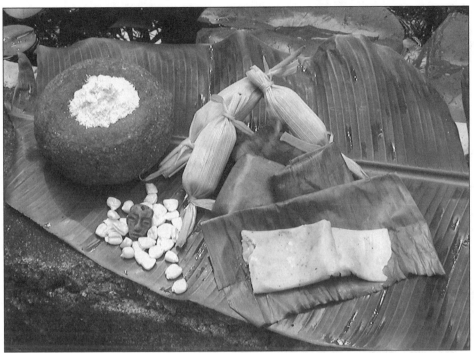

Tamales prepared traditionally with banana leaves and no fat (Cole Photography).

gion of the Bahía de Banderas where the *comunidad* sits have many Puré-influenced names in their populations (Romo 2000).

Our studies over the years of culinary practices include the recording of over 100 food and medicinal recipes. One of our favorites and now rarely prepared in the mountains are *Los Corundos*, a Purépecha traditional tamale from Michoacan (Romo 2000), reddened by the bark of the Brasil tree .

Like their ancestors, the Caxcanes and the Pures, peoples of the central Pacific coast of Mexico are intensely independent, and resist identification with state and federal jurisdictions (Romo 2000). As of 1995, only nine inhabitants spoke the *Indigenous* language for it was virtually forgotten by the time of the revolution of 1910 (Romo 2000). Like their cousins the Nayari (Cora) across the bay and to the north (Coyle 2001), the peoples of Chacala have a strong sense of ancestor worship, social ceremony, and ritual associated with maintaining civil unity and enacting rituals informed by stellar, lunar, solar and planetary events. Individuals and their communities have traditionally balanced the use of domesticated and wild plants and animals, and shared wealth in a distributive manner, connected with feasts (Butterwick 1998), similar to the Potlach economies (Kinley 1989) of the Pacific Northwest peoples and Indigenous communities worldwide (Lévi-Strauss 1965; Mauss 1990).

Despite metropolitan efforts to proclaim western Mexico and the *Comunidad Indigena de Chacala* culturally dead and *terra nullias* in terms of an Indigenous population, Indigenous Peoples' knowledges and practices are part of daily life albeit suffering from intense exploitation and pressure to change.

Part 3. History of Nutrition Trauma in Mexico

We are living in a gold mine. If we looked for the properties of medicinal plants, we would leave more valuable things for the future of the people…also the medicinal animals because they eat medicinal plants. We are losing the iguana and armadillo whose fat helps cure bronchitis. The animals feel the vibration of the people. Now there is a lot of cancer and diabetes in Yelapa. The Nopale helps arthritis, the kidneys and diabetes.

> Santiago Cruz, age 73

In Mexico, nutrition trauma arises out of the effects of uneven trade dynamics, confiscation of land and natural resources, and the current wave of globalization, in which large-scale mechanized agriculture controls access to food. Nutrition trauma also occurs under government subsidy programs that supply food that is not bio-culturally nourishing for a local population. Mexico is the largest consumer in the world of the carbonated sugar water consuming 16 billion crates per year, via 900 thousand sales sites and 87 bottling plants. Indeed, the former director of Coca Cola-Mexico, Vincente Fox, became the president of Mexico.

As the Hispanics colonized various regions of Mexico they reorganized the local and then the regional economy to siphon wealth away from Indigenous Peoples into Hispanic hands (Carmack 1996). To effectively transfer wealth to themselves the Hispanic leaders defined the Indigenous population out of existence by declaring their status as *mestizo*. The *mestizo* is a Mexican "melting pot" identity that effectively eliminates the so-called Indian. The "mestizocization" of Indigenous Peoples in Central Mexico was widely practiced throughout Mexico. By redefining Indians as *mestizos* it became possible to eliminate what few rights they had as Indigenous Peoples—particularly their collective control over land—legally protected under the Mexican Constitution for perpetual use by Indians. The result has been a direct outflow of wealth from Indigenous communities into the Hispanic society and a net inflow of Hispanic control over Indigenous lands and resources. This process has resulted in cultural dislocation within the Indigenous populations. While legally recognized as "Indigenous," but popularly identified by Mexico as neither Hispanic nor as an Indigenous society, the people of the *Comunidad Indigena de Chacala* nevertheless retain a deep sense of group identity. Accelerations of development and external intrusions have recently divided the population along economic lines. Its begins with the educational system and use of television in the schools to separate the younger population from the older. Social policies of "deIndianization" have driven Mexico's agricultural policies (Bonfil 1996) and hence nutrition since the 16th century.

Pre-Colonial Diet

Before European contact in the 16th century, wheat was not available in the diet of Indigenous Peoples of Mexico (Joe and Young 1994), nor were fried foods, bovine or porcine animal fats. European settlers introduced monocropping (the practice of single crop planting usually enhanced with fertilizers, herbicides and pesticides) into a previously efficient and abundant culture of Indigenous intercropping farming system. European introduction of wheat and the near destruction of amaranth as an important food led to an agricultural dominance of corn. Amaranth was a major ceremonial grain for the peoples of west Mexico out of which deity icons were made for the thirteen three-week celebration periods each year praising different gods (Butterwick 1998). Not only is the seed a major source of protein (seeds contain 16–18% compared to 12–14% for corn or wheat), but the flower, the leaves and the roots provide rich nutritional benefits that rival and exceed all other plants in Mexico. Amaranth is very rich in the amino acid lysine (Karasch 2000), richer in iron than spinach but, unlike corn, it has hypoglycemic qualities.

Today in west Mexico honey is added to the amaranth seed and is now sold as the candy *alegrias*, meaning happiness—the name the Spanish gave to amaranth. Yet one need only travel today a few hours from Mexico City to discover that amaranth as a seed or plant is virtually unheard of. The Spanish prohibited amaranth cultivation because of its use as a ceremonial food (Karasch 2000) and this caused its near complete disappearance as a major grain (seed) in Mexico.

However, like the ceremonial sacred mushrooms used by the Mazatecs and Maya, some peoples continued cultivation in secret or outside the boundaries of colonial rule. And even as amaranth was outlawed in Mexico by the Spanish crown, it was exported to Europe as late as the 1700s (Centéotl 2002; López 2003). There is a renewal of cultivation and use of amaranth by various community-based groups in Mexico and its value as a source of authentic nutrition is highly regarded by the National Academy of Sciences, agronomists, and food enthusiasts promoting healthy and exotic foods.

In spite of millennia of exchange and trade among Indigenous Peoples, the introduction of different foods did not contribute significantly to diabetes and other chronic disease patterns until recently. For many years, refined sugar and white flour were products for the very few and very rich (Erasmus 1993). We can trace the parallel course of sugar production with diabetes development. By 1930 worldwide production of sugar catapulted sales to 16 million tons and by 1950 it was approximately 19 million tons. By 2000 more than 120 million tons of refined sugar were produced worldwide in one year (Galloway 2000).

Not long after his arrival in Mexico, Hernando Córtez developed large sugar plantations to support export back to Europe where it became widely available by the 18th century (Mintz 1995). It was not until the centrifugal or highly-refined sugar was mass produced with new industrial methods in the early part of the 20th century that a shift in consumption occurred. Just as white flour was a rich man's food and hence rich men developed diseases related to these foods so did sugar slowly become a "consumer product." Mintz (1995) asserts that market capitalism developed on the backs of slaves who produced the sugar. Slaves had no access to sugar until the advent of machines and mass production. The new method of processing produced such large quantities that the descendents of slaves and Indigenous Peoples of the North America became consumers themselves (Mintz 1995).

Even where certain foods were introduced that may have caused adaptive difficulties, the overwhelming diet of rural Indigenous Peoples of Mexico remained dependent on wild foods and intercrop agriculture (the practice of planting and encouraging plants of various kinds to grow together in much the same way they might grow in the wild). The link between diversity of foods and the physical expenditure of energy to hunt, gather and prepare those foods created a metabolically stimulating and reciprocal dynamic of energy exchange that is absent among most peoples in metropolitan societies today.

NAFTA-Cized Mexico: The Global Soybean, Defective Modernization and Diabetes

We used to fish for a few nights and make enough for the week. Now a few nights won't even cover our expenses.

        Emilio Sanchez R., 35-year-old fisherman

Economic forces of globalization are shifting the staple of Indigenous diets in Mexico from maize (corn) to corn flour, wheat flour and soybeans. The 1998 government decided to eliminate corn production and replace it with soybeans for export. Jalisco is the largest corn producing state in Mexico. Replacement of corn production with soy was not for the benefit of local consumption, but for export as animal feed. The corn market is a four-billion dollar market: The lighter, more efficient and nutritionally poorer source for tortillas, *Maseca*, is replacing ground corn (fresh masa) tortillas. Flour producers increased their share of the market from 20% in 1990 to 40% by 1996. It is estimated that by 2005 corn flour production will comprise 85% of the market (Donnelly 1999).

Additionally, soybeans are invading the diet in Mexico, as elsewhere in the Americas. The craze for soybeans that began among urban health food advocates has spread to rural populations. Soy is a anti-nutrient, a substance that while not necessarily toxic per se, is detrimental because it either inhibits digestion of certain nutrients or binds with them during digestion to prevent uptake. Soy contains the most powerful digestive enzyme inhibitors of any food known—it has also been shown to depress thyroid function contributing to weight gain (Fallon and Enig 2003). Soy textured protein, the most potent anti-nutrient (Fallon 2003) known has been a staple in the surplus food programs on Indigenous reservations in the U.S. and reserves in Canada for more than 40 years (USDA 2003). In rural west Mexico textured soy protein is now often used to replace fish in *ceviche*, the traditional dish made from raw marinated fish.

Before colonization of the Americas there was virtually no diabetes among Indigenous Peoples. Diabetes was rare before the 1930s in North America (Schacht et al. 1999) and in Mexico the estimated prevalence currently is 14.2% of the population, ranking it fourth worldwide in prevalence (Federation 2000).

The Center's approach to diabetes focused on using blood and metabolic type for different peoples. This approach is different than much of the current scientific research focus on genetic theories of Indigenous "difference" that attempt to account for Indigenous Peoples' susceptibility to diabetes. Commercial producers of foods and medicines imply that there is something wrong with Indigenous Peoples because they cannot digest processed and genetically altered foods without becoming fat, instead of recognizing that there is something wrong with the foods and medicines that the commercial producers manufacture (Zimmet 2001, 2000).

Authentic foods have historically nourished the community. Following years of work with individuals and small groups we chose the opportunity to organize more extensively within the community by undertaking a community-wide project to validate local knowledge of medicinal foods and medicines and to support their vigorous sustenance in the community.

Part 4. The Pedagogy of the Nourished

...healing must be sought in the blood of the wound itself. It is of another of the old alchemical truths that no solution should be made except in its own blood.

Nor Hall (1976)

As discussed throughout this book, diabetes mellitus is a symptom of community illness and we believe the answer is to be found in the community. Our work leads us to conclude that the failure of conventional diabetes prevention and treatment programs is due in large part to the onus placed on the individual to change instead of recognizing culture and the community's role in the healing process. The failure to act from an integrated analysis of causality, in turn precludes appropriate prevention. Treatment then remains dissociated from cultural identity and reinforces separation from authentic systems of support. In response to our conclusions we developed a community-wide intergenerational project to assess if the support of traditional medicine could mitigate the effects of community trauma. We received funding for this project between 1997 and 2000.

The Center for Traditional Medicine began by gathering women and teens throughout the community to share healthy meals and to discuss their concerns and interests. Participants were invited by their friends or chose themselves and represented a cross section of the community; rich and poor, catholic and protestant, married and unmarried, living in town and up river. Over time, some members engaged the cooperation of the Catholic and Protestant churches and their priests and ministers. We traveled into the mountain towns several hours away and by boat to neighboring villages. As plans for the project evolved we educated the influential community actors—the doctors and clergy—to prevent them from doing harm to the project and to also assess and engage their support for the value of traditional medicines.

The role of the facilitator in a community-determined action project is to collaborate in processes that validate community knowledge that is beneficial to the community (Minugh 1989), define questions to be answered, the methods to use, the action to take and in this project, to define the health problems to be addressed. The principal emphasis is to encourage an exchange of knowledge and then present the knowledge as visible information—to mirror the information back to the source. Our role was to offer conditions under which the *Comunidad's* knowledge base could be viewed, examined and recognized as a valid way to understand the community's cultural reality. Our work proceeded from the protocols defined by the Center for World Indigenous Studies for the conduct of community-determined research:

Community-determined Research (Center for World Indigenous Studies)

1. The project must be community-based, that is, the knowledge of the community must have a primary role determining the shape and direction of the project with

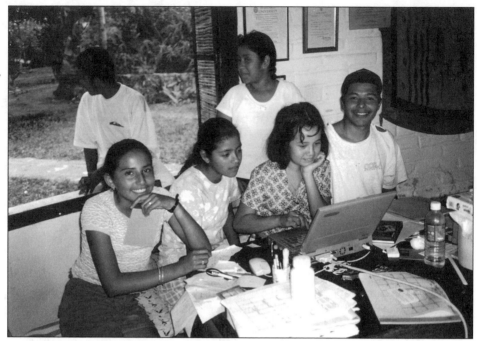

Village teens designing the medicinal plants book.

outside researchers, activists and educators serving as collaborators and cohorts engaged in a process of the free exchange of knowledge.

2. The project must be bi-technological, that is, outside practitioners and researchers and community researchers and practitioners must be able to do some of each other's work.

3. The project and its outcome must be economically and technologically appropriate, that is, affordable, doable, teachable and accessible.

4. The project must be accurate, that is, cultural information, the research, the organization, the learning and teaching and the final report must be the very best possible.

5. The dissemination of the project knowledge and format must meet with agreement by the participants.

During our initial meetings we listed priorities, designed activities, and developed a plan of action that addressed each area of the group's interest. These activities and interest areas included a priority stated by the teen girls to learn the use of medicinal plants from their mothers and *abuelas*, sewing classes for the women, art classes for the children, and classes to train women in natural medicine health promotion and to conduct community screenings for diabetes, high blood pressure and stress.

We knew that from the earliest years of our work, when we shared food over the book *Our Bodies Ourselves* (Boston Women's Health Book Collective 1998), gathering and preparing food together provides a common ground that simultaneously elevates mood and community spirit, initiates sharing, and dispels community tension. During our meetings about diabetes we focused attention on traditional foods and health, and generated the following questions to explore:

- What foods nourished our families and communities prior to diabetes?
- What of this knowledge do we know or have recorded?
- What of this knowledge have we lost?
- What can we recover and how can we go about it?
- What foods and medicines did we use?
- How do we nourish our health?
- How do we prepare healthy foods?
- How do we work with the health service doctors and nurses when they don't want to hear about our healings?
- How much will it cost to take vitamins?

Within the smaller planning circle we discussed how to engage the support of the men, which was essential for the activities to occur unobstructed and for the successes to be sustained. Occasionally, drunken men came by the Center, keeping a safe distance while half-seated upon a horse, railed at the project and left. A number of women either had to sneak out of their homes or had to stop attending the sewing group because their husbands would not allow them to participate. It was essential to allay their fears that women were planning and acting "without them."

With rare exception, the men were not interested in nutrition or cooking, but when they joined us for group meals we discussed plants used for healing, or initiated discussion about their mothers' health. Several of the men expressed concerns about the agricultural changes occurring in the mountains and in particular, the loss of certain plant species. Concurrently the teens were interviewing the elders about medicinal plant use for diabetes and during these interviews some men discussed their concerns over the growing resource exploitation (Hurtado 1999) from Guadalajara businesses seeking access to the Maguey (*agave*) plants in the mountains. So central is the Maguey and its fermented fluids to the life of this region that the Nahua named a female deity, Mayahuel, for the Maguey. In a tradition dating back thousands of years, women oversee the production of the mescal or *raicilla* made from the fermented juice of baked Maguey hearts.

The practice of traditional and integrative medicine must include satisfying the requirement that actions protect the cultural property rights of Indigenous Peoples—the products of each distinctive culture, including the knowledge of healing practices. This led to discussions with the *comunidad* men using this approach arising from the work of Center for World Indigenous Studies Chair, Dr. Rudolph Ryser (1997), and Rodney Bobbiwash (2001), Director of the Forum for Global Exchange. Their work focuses on the definition of laws protecting Indigenous Peoples' rights, which develop from the requirements of Indigenous nations themselves, not subject to definition or modification by state-level governments. In the forum Ryser (1997) noted:

> Only through new mutually agreed and enforceable treaties and the maintenance of existing treaties can Indians hope to preserve the diversity of tribal cultures and ensure the diversity of fish wildlife plants and their habitats for seven generations unborn.

Yet even where traditional medicine is integrated at the policy level (WHO 2002), there remains a wide gap between rural peoples with respect to NGO's and university-educated policy makers. Community members are rarely privy to the ongoing mechanisms promoting or countering the effects of development. While rural peoples are often the subjects of policy deliberations, they are most often excluded from the discussion table. Thus, our work in this project included facilitating network links within Mexico that would inform the *comunidad* members about policy development in other communities. With the men feeling satisfied with their roles we were proceeding smoothly with training women and teens as natural medicine health promoters.

Natural Medicine Health Promoter Training

We designed a natural medicine health promotion curriculum that combined conventional public health screening methods, with the traditional medicine services provided at the clinic. One challenge was to design training materials that addressed the diverse literacy capacities of the participants. We focused on experiential learning and limited the writing and reading required. People worked together in teams of two, some measuring and interviewing, and others writing. Together we designed a community survey that was designed to assess blood pressure, blood glucose and stress levels. The women suggested that we avoid asking directly about stress, which they believed people, especially men, would not readily admit to. So instead we asked about insomnia. From there, we were able to explore the possible causes of insomnia, which we found was a good marker for stress.

When the natural medicine health promoters were trained they offered post-lunch daily glucose screenings at the clinic and in the community. These lunches provided an opportunity for people to observe the effects of food intake on blood glucose. They also provided daily "pep" talks followed by lymphatic massage to reduce edema and alleviate neuropathic pain. We designed specialized manual therapy protocols to include lymphatic drainage (Chikly 2001) for edema and neuropathies and recently produced a training video (Korn 2004), which is designed to teach this specialized touch therapy for health practitioners and diabetes family members. The sense of well being generated by these lunches and massages in turn supported adherence to a challenging regimen. People with diabetes who sustained their food, supplement and local plant remedies protocols reduced their glucose levels from a consistent 400 to 125–150 without the use of insulin.

A. Exotic Food Preparation Using Local Foods

Discussions of ancestral foods and nutrition led naturally to sharing foods. During one group session, the community members suggested making "Chinese food". A few young men joined in the cooking, by sneaking through the back door, as their interest in cooking challenged the strict gender role assignments that normally prevailed. Since one of the male team members from the north was a chef, he undertook the task of food preparation of exotic dishes. Together we gathered and prepared a feast of different Chinese (Han) dishes, using the often neglected local foods such as Chaya

(Chayamansa cnidoscolus), Capomo *(Brosimum alicastrum)*, and Jicama *(Pachyrhizus erosu)*. These ingredients became "Huevos Foo Yung" and Chaya Chow Mein.

Group food gathering and preparation also provided opportunities to discuss Chinese medicine and its similarities with *curanderismo* and its principles of Hot and Cold disease familiar to the group. In turn, the discussion about the ancient trade in chilies, indigenous to Mexico and finding their way east, gave breadth to the discussion about cultural continuity, change, and the value of local indigenous foods. We discussed the speculations that the that the Chinese traveled to the Mexico 2000 years earlier (Crossley), perhaps accounting for the local pottery known as the *Chinesco* tradition. (Xu). These dialogues over healthy food provided an opportunity to explore feelings about changes in the community and to link these feelings to action, choice and empowerment.

B. Intergenerational Activities

The children joined in the feasts and also attended arts classes at the center where we emphasized themes of nature and respect for the environment. We engaged the schoolteachers to provide time for the young ones to make art of local (anti-diabetic) plants and provided the supplies; the teenage girls interviewed their grandmothers, adult women gathered plants, and made herbal tinctures and formed sewing circles. Some women sewed clothing for their daughters; still others embroidered dresses, aprons and potholders with local food theme designs: *Nopales* (Cactus), *Obelisko* (Hibiscus), and *Pinas* (pineapples).

The project sparked conversation between villages as well, as people traveled to collect items from around the community and exchanged plants for the gardens. More than once an elder would appear with an ancient herbal recipe and recite the utility of its application.

Otherwise uninterested teen boys joined the project by participating in sports medicine classes where they learned how nutrition (not sugar) would enhance their soccer performance. The boys also learned to use computers and along with teen girls, scanned the botanical art of their younger siblings. Together we all designed the medicinal plant book, mapping out the dialogue that would be used to share community knowledge.

We validated community knowledge as we encouraged the use of the edible cactus nopale *(Opuntia sp.;* Ramos 1980), aloe vera (Bunyapraphatsara et al. 1996; Yongchaiyudha et al. 1996), cundeamor *(Momordica Charantia L.;* Raman 1996), garlic *(allium sativum)*, onion *(Allium Cepa)*, tamarindo *(Tamarindus indica)* and papaya *(Carica papaya)*. Among the dozens of plants we catalogued, the group chose 11 plants to highlight for the book, which was annotated with edited dialogues that occurred between the teens and their *abuelas*.

C. Herbal Validation

Plants have been used extensively for medicinal purposes throughout Mexico and North America (Moerman 1998). Mexico is one of the most biologically diverse regions in the world, with over 30,000 species of plants, an estimated 5000 of which have some medicinal value (Toledo 1995). Many of these are hypoglycemic in action and also support metabolic (Davidow 1999), cardio-vascular, lymphatic and kidney function for a person with blood glucose dysfunction (IBIS 1999; Marles and Fransworth 1996).

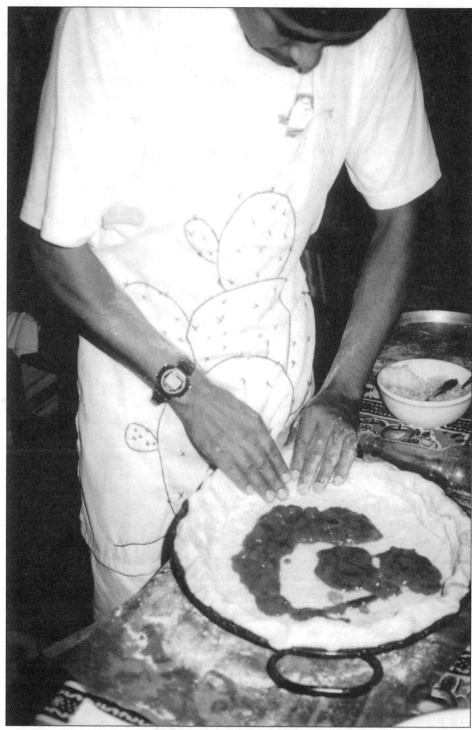

Aaron preparing "wheatless" pizza.

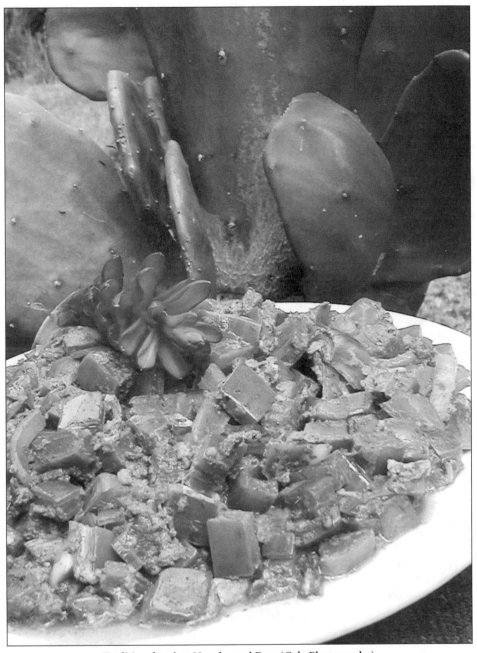

Traditional recipe: Nopales and Eggs (Cole Photography).

The *Comunidad* is rich in natural anti-diabetic plants, and there is a history of using these plants medicinally and particularly as food. The most common of these plants include cundeamor *(Mormordica charantia L.;* Sarcar et al. 1995), zabila (*Aloe vera*; Bunyapraphatsara and Yongchaiyudha 1996; Yongchaiyudha 1996; Ghannam et al. 1986), ajo *(Allium sativum;* Day 1998), canela *(Cinnamomum verum)*, capomo *(Brosimum alicastrum)* and linaza (Enig 2000; Fallon 1995; Michael and Pizzorno 1997; Erasmus 1993).

There are ongoing challenges to overcoming the dependency cultivated by (post) colonial medical systems. The *comunidad*, like much of the Indigenous world is currently caught between the degradation of local habitat containing Indigenous medicines and the resultant loss of traditional knowledges. Many of these plants, like *Mormordica charantia L (Cucurbitacae)*, which grew abundantly alongside the dirt paths, were all but gone from the village by the 1990s. Others, such as *nopale* or prickly pear cactus (*Opuntia sp.*), while still cultivated, are used less frequently now. Still other plants, like breadnut *(Brosimum alicastrum)*, which along with chaya were a diet staple for centuries, are poised to become the next "designer food" for import into the U.S. The breadnut or *capomo*, as it is known in the *comunidad* is rich in amino acids (Brucher 1969). It is used traditionally as a beverage and food for human nourishment to increase lactation in humans and animals alike. *Capomo* is one of the main plants we focused on for renewal especially for people with diabetes. We spent countless hours with the elders gathering the capomo seeds and preparing and eating them in all the ways the elders said their mothers did.

In addition we focused on the renewal of traditional food uses that had medicinal value. We found that the local practice of drinking tea made from cinnamon every morning is all but gone except among some elders and people living in the small ranches of the *comunidad* and coconut—whose value as a source of essential fatty acids cannot be overestimated (Enig 1999)—are increasingly left on the trees and are ignored except for their value to tourists.

Nutritional Protocols for the Treatment of Diabetes

Diabetes is often referred to as a "disease of civilization" (Joe and Young 1994) and occurs in response to the complex synergy between the use of refined foods, chronic stress, and sedentary lifestyle. By mobilizing communities to research, renew and reinvent uses of traditional and authentic nutrition and preparation methods we engage community involvement in a process of construction of historical continuity.

Indigenous Peoples are in different stages of capacity to self-sufficiently supply all the nutrition necessary to fully sustain their members. The Center's clinic provides a range of treatment and educational approaches that are isomorphic to our clients' needs and beliefs. Our approach emphasizes the Indigenous sciences with a minimal influence from the biomedical model. In response to demand from people in the village and, in particular, suggestions from the traditional medicine advisors, we refined our approaches to integrate traditional approaches Indigenous to the community, with natural medicine and complementary medicine approaches from around the world. This satisfied the need to feel that people were getting the "latest" medicine and also affirmed their own knowledge base. Community members often asked for pills in bottles, expressed interest in the remedios caseros, or home remedies packaged and sold in the *farmacias*. We responded by including high quality nutrients and exotic herbs to reply to this need.

The Center provides options through the integration of behavioral interventions with individuals, families and whole communities and the use of vitamins, minerals, and standardized botanical substances that people can take as pills or capsules. We have observed that a combination of natural and traditional medicine modalities are required to effect the potent changes necessary for metabolic function to return to normal or to stabilize.

Nonetheless, people are often confused by their options for healing from diabetes for a variety of reasons; one elder spent her hard earned money because she thought that the packaged, dehydrated *Nopale* she saw in the city was better than the fresh plants growing in her yard. Others cited the difficulty of addressing the jealousy of others as they made positive choices that caused imagined or actual emotional separation. Whether it is diabetes and "sugar sobriety" or alcohol sobriety often the men's friends would pressure and jeer at them and call them *maricones* (pejorative for male homosexual). Thus, our work was not always smooth. At times some men with uncontrolled diabetes, suffering from painful neuropathy, made substantial improvement only to receive the opprobrium by their peer group, upset that they were refusing the sweets offered by the women.

A. Nutritional Supplementation

There is a substantial body of scientific and clinical evidence to support the use of nutritional supplementation to prevent and treat diabetes and its sequelae. We have worked successfully to help people reduce or eliminate their pharmaceutical medications and to stabilize their symptoms. We teach the philosophy and these protocols periodically in Indigenous communities throughout North America. What follows below is a brief introduction to some options and directions that communities may explore based on empirical and laboratory research. What follows is not designed to provide a specific protocol for individuals but rather to provide information on what we (and others) have used successfully with many people who suffer from diabetes.

B. Essential Fatty Acids

Essential fatty acids deficiency result from the loss of authentic foods and the introduction of hydrogenated fats has, along with sugar and refined flour, contributed significantly to the development of type 2 diabetes. Essential fatty acids are nutrients that must be obtained in the diet because humans do not produce them endogenously (McColl 2003) and must be in appropriate ratios.

These essential fats are found in Mexico in tropical nuts, seafood and plant food such as coconuts. Coconuts and coconut fat are especially significant since they have served as major sources of high quality fats, rich in lauric and capric acid (Enig 1999) for Indigenous Peoples of coastal Mexico. Two types of Coconut trees, the Cohune Palm (*Orbygnia guacuyule*) and the *Coco nucifera*, are distributed throughout Mexico and Central America. Traditionally the people of Chacala use coconuts as a source of protein and energy and medicinally for the treatment of protozoal infections. The efficacy has been confirmed empirically though traditional use and in laboratory research, which demonstrates that coconut fat normalizes blood lipids (Enig 1999). The use of coconuts by Indigenous Peoples over the millennia has been protective against high blood lipids and cardiovascular inflammation leading us to wonder how the decline in its use contributes to diabetes and cardiovascular disease (Enig 1993; Fallon 1995). Lipid abnormalities are common in individuals with type 2 diabetes, and a number of randomized controlled trials have found that fish oil supplementation significantly lowers serum triglyceride levels in diabetic individuals (Montori et al. 2000). These fats also serve to

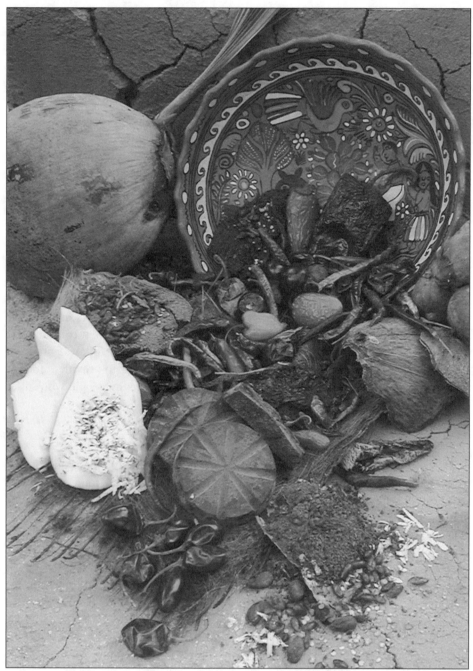

Still Life: "Chocolate, Chilies and Coconuts," a seminar designed to support traditional foods use (Cole Photography).

reduce inflammation, a common result of an inauthentic diet high in trans-fatty acids, and to decrease neuropathic pain (Jamal 1990; Jamal and Carmichael 1990).

For diabetes and cardiovascular disease we emphasize the nutritional and medicinal use of coconut as well as locale-specific sources of essential fats, like the *ooligan (Thaleichthys pacificus)* oil among the Pacific Northwest peoples (Ryser 2004; Kuhnlein

1996b). Fats and their plant and animal sources always prove to be intimately connected with cultural identity and the use of these food sources is an excellent starting point for culinary research in diabetes and as a culinary pedagogical method. Oftentimes, however, it is difficult or impossible for the diabetic patient to obtain a medicinal dose of essential fatty acids and thus supplementation of dietary sources is required. The suggested dosage is from 4000 to 6000 grams of fish or plant oils daily (Erasmus 1993).

C. Vitamin & Mineral Supplementation

Mineral deficiencies are common in diabetes. Minerals are cofactors that signal intermediary actions for metabolic function (Day 1998). Studies have shown that magnesium deficiency is frequently observed in patients with diabetes, and plasma magnesium levels are inversely related to occurrence or progression of diabetic retinopathy. Magnesium supplementation has improved insulin sensitivity and metabolic control (Moran and Guerrero-Romero 2003) and demonstrated reduction in insulin requirements without changing glycemic control (deValk 1999). We supplement with a high quality vitamin mineral complex (Ali 2002), high in chromium (Meletis 2001) and magnesium. Vitamin B6 and B12 have shown utility for prevention and mitigation of both nerve damage and diabetic neuropathy. Antioxidants, such as Vitamin E, protect blood vessel integrity, improve glucose tolerance, normalize retinal flow (deValk 1999; deValk 2000; Jain 1999) and significantly improve nerve conduction velocity in neuropathy (Weintraub 2001). Alpha Lipoic Acid improves blood flow to peripheral nerves and stimulates regeneration of nerve fiber, improving blood flow to nerves. It also reduces pain associated with nerve damage (Konrad et al. 1999; Packer et al. 1995; Weintraub 2001; Ziegler and Gries 1997).

Project Significance

Authentic foods and medicines (those foods and medicines that naturally evolved over time within a specific human culture) bring balance to the body, mind and spirit. Health practitioners and Indigenous Peoples living in *comunidades*, on reservations, reserves and in urban communities, however, do not generally turn to authentic foods and medicines because of access and cost. Furthermore, with the passing of elders, these individuals do not necessarily possess the traditional knowledge required to make appropriate dietary changes. Foods introduced into a culture often serve as substitutes for natural foods that are readily available, but their consumption can produce disastrous dietary and health results, as shown throughout this book.

Our study of culture and community as healing for chronic illness is the first major effort to document the relationship between imposed development, community trauma and diabetes in Indigenous Mexico. We have demonstrated the efficacy of culture and the validated knowledge of an Indigenous community as important elements in the process of promoting public health in Indigenous communities and reversing the trend toward greater prevalence of chronic diseases like diabetes. The role of a culturally distinct community in the process of self-healing is palpable. Individual incidence of chronic disease can be reversed through cultural validation, reintroduction of local wild and cultivated foods and employment of traditional healing techniques.

Acknowledgments

We wish to thank the people of the Comunidad Indigena de Chacala, in particular our friends Alisia, Jose Garcia, Chamba and Aaron, who contributed immeasurably through their trust and friendship to this important work. We also express our gratitude to Dr. Peter D'Adamo and Pharmacal, Inc. who generously contributed supplies we used in this study and at our clinic. We give our thanks to Medora Woods, whose generous financial support allowed us to set our sights high and to many others who contributed funds and time. We had the benefit of many student interns who worked with us for periods of a month, three months and in a few instances for years without pay. Among these gifted people were LizAnn Pastore, Christian Ryser, Mirjam Hirch, Emily Horowitz, Dr. Karen Frangos, Joyce Arafeh, Christine Labriola and the many others too numerous to list.

References

Ali, Majiid. 2002. Beyond Insulin Resistance and Syndrome X. Townsend Letter for Doctor and Patients (232): 114–18.

Alvarado-Osuna, F. Milian-Suazo, V. Valles-Sanchez. 2001. Prevalence of Diabetes mellitus and Hyperlipemias in Otomi Indians. Salud Public Mex 43: 459–63.

Anawalt, Patricia Rieff. 1998. They Came to Trade Exquisite Things: Ancient West Mexican-Ecuadorian Contacts. *In* Ancient West Mexico: Art and Archeology of the Unknown Past. R.F. Townsend, ed. pp. 233–50. New York: Thames and Hudson.

Anderson, R.K., J. Calvo and G. Serrano. 1946. A Study of the Nutritional Status and Food Habits of Otomi Indians in the Mezquital Valley of Mexico. American Journal of Public Health 36: 883–903.

Andrews, J. 1984. Peppers: The Domesticated Capsicums. Austin: University of Texas Press.

Bobbiwash, A. Rodney. 2001. The Fourth World: Site of Struggle and Resistance in the Fight against Global Capital. World Social Forum, Port Alegre, Brazil.

Bodley, John H. 1982. Victims of Progress. Menlo Park, CA: Benjamin-Cummings Publishing Co.

Bonfil, Guillermo Batalla. 1996. Mexico Profundo: Reclaiming a Civilization. P.A. Dennis, Transl. Austin: University of Texas Press.

Boston Women's Health Book Collective. 1998. Our Bodies Our Selves for the New Century: A Book by and for Women. New York: Touchstone, Simon & Schuster Inc.

Brucher, Heinz. 1969. Useful Plants of Neotropical Origin and Their Wild Relatives. Berlin: Springer-Verlag.

Bunyapraphatsara, N., V. Rungpitarangsi, S.Yongchaiyudha and O. Chokechai-jaroenporn. 1996. Antidiabetic Activitiy of Aloe Vera L. Juice II. Clinical Trial in Diabetes Mellitus Patients in Combination with Glibenclamide. Phytomedicine 3(3): 241–43.

Butterwick, Kristi. 1998. Food for the Dead: The West Mexican Art of Feasting. *In* Ancient West Mexico: Art and Archeology of the Unknown Past. R.E. Townsend, ed. pp. 89–105. New York: Thames and Hudson.

Carmack, Robert M, Janine Casco and Gary H. Gossen. 1996. The Legacy of Mesoamerica. Upper Saddle River, NJ: Prentice Hall.

Carter, George F. <www.epigraphy.org/ancient_scripts.htm> (The Epigraphic Society).

Centéotl, Centro de Desarollo Comunitario. 2002. El Amaranto: Alimento por los dioses para los hombres y mujeres de hoy.

Chikly, Bruno. 2001. Silent Waves: The Theory and Practice of Lymph Drainage Therapy. Scottsdale, AZ: I.H.H. Publishing.

Coe, Sophie D. and Michael D Coe. 1996. The True History of Chocolate. New York: Thames and Hudson.

Cordain, Loren. 2001. Syndrome X: Just the Tip of the Hyperinsulinemia Iceberg. Medikament (6): 46–51.

Coyle, Phillip E. 2001. From Flowers to Ash: Nayari History, Politics and Violence. Tuscon: University of Arizona Press.

Crossley, Mimi. <www.humanities-interactive.org/unknown/unknowntext.htm> ("Unknown Mexico").

Cruz, Maya. 1999. Interview, Oral History. L. Korn. Yelapa, Jalisco, Mexico.

Cruz Ramos, Lupita. 1999. Personal Communication, Interview. L. Korn, ed. Yelapa, Jalisco, Mexico.

D'Ádamo, P. and C. Whitney. 1996. Eat Right for Your Type: The Individualized Diet Solution to Staying Healthy, Living Longer & Achieving your Ideal Weight. New York: G.P. Putnam's Sons.

_____1998. Cook Right for Your Blood Type: The Practical Kitchen Companion to Eat Right for Your Type. New York: G. P. Putnam's Sons.

Davidow, Joie. 1999. Infusions of Healing: A Treasury of Mexican American Remedies. New York: Simom and Schuster.

Day, Caroline. 1998. Invited Commentary: Traditional Plant Treatments for Diabetes Mellitus: Pharmaceutical Foods. British Journal of Nutrition 80: 5–6.

deValk, H.W. 1999. Magnesium in Diabetes. Netherland J Med 54: 139–46.

_____2000. With Moderate Pharmacologic Doses of Vitamin E Are Saturable and Reversible in Patients with Type 1 Diabetes. Am J Clin Nutr 72: 1142–49.

Diaz, Bella. 2000. Interview-Oral History. L. Korn, ed. Yelapa: Center for Traditional Medicine.

Donnelly, Robert. 1999. Tortilla Riddle. *In* Business Mexico. Vol. 9-10: 26–36.

Duke, James A. 1983. Handbook of Energy Crops: Handbook of Energy Crops.

Duran, Eduardo, et al. 1998. Healing the American Indian Soul Wound. *In* International Handbook of Multigenerational Legacies of Trauma: Group Project for Holocaust Survivors and Their Children. New York: Plenum.

Enig, Mary G. 1993. Diet, Serum Cholesterol and Coronary Heart Disease. *In* Coronary Heart Disease: The Dietary Sense and Nonsense. G. Mann, ed. pp. 36–60. London: Janus Publishing.

———1999. Coconut: In Support of Good Health in the 21st Century. 36th Session of Asian Pacific Coconut Community, Singapore. pp. 1–26. APCC.

———2000. Know Your Fats: The Complete Primer for Understanding the Nutrition of Fats, Oils and Cholesterol. Silver Spring: Bethesda Press.

Erasmus, Udo. 1993. Fats that Heal, Fats that Kill. Burnaby, Canada: Alive Books.

Evans, Michael B. 1985. Emotional Stress and Diabetic Control: A Postulated Model for the Effect of Emotional Distress upon Intermediary Metabolism in the Diabetic. Biofeedback and Self-Regulation 10(3): 240.

Fallon, Joseph E. 1985. Soviet Union or Soviet Russia. Fourth World Journal 1(1): 11–32.

Fallon, Sally. 1995. Nourishing Traditions. San Diego, CA: ProMotion Publishing.

Fallon, Sally and Mary G. Enig. 2003. Cinderella's Dark Side: Newest Research on Why You Should Avoid Soy. Dr. Joseph Mercola's Newsletter. <www.mercola.com/article/ soy/avoid_soy.htm>.

Ferreira, Mariana K. Leal. 1998. Slipping through Sky Holes: Yurok Body Imagery in Northern California. Culture, Medicine and Psychiatry 22: 171–202.

French, Armand Laurence. 2000. Addictions and Native Americans. Westport, CT: Praeger Publishers.

Friedland, Jonathan. 2000. Labor Conflict: An American in Mexico Champions Midwifery as a Worthy Profession. *In* The Wall Street Journal, Feb. 15, New York.

Furst, Stacey and Peter Shaefer, eds. 1998. People of the Peyote: Huichol Indian History, Ritual and Survival. Albuquerque: University of New Mexico Press.

Gagne, Marie-Anik. 1998. The Role of Dependency and Colonialism in Generating Trauma in First Nations Citizens: The James Bay Cree. *In* International Handbook of Multigenerational Legacies of Trauma: Group Project for Holocaust Survivors and their Children. Y. Danieli, ed. The Plenum Series on Stress and Coping. New York: Plenum Press.

Galloway, J. H. 2000. Sugar. *In* The Cambridge World History of Food. K. Kiple and K.C. Ornelas, eds. pp. 437–50. New York: Cambridge University Press.

Garber, J. and M.E.P. Seligman, eds. 1980. Human Helplessness: Theory and Applications. New York: Academic Press.

Ghannam, Nadia, Michael Kingston, Ibrahim A. Meshaal, Tariq Al Meshaal, Parmar Mohamed, S. Narayan and Nicholas Woodhouse. 1986. The Antidiabetic Activity of Aloes: Preliminary Clinical and Experimental Observations. Hormone Research 24: 288–94.

Goldwater, Carmel. 1983. Traditional Medicine in Latin America. *In* Traditional Medicine and Health Care Coverage. R.H. Bannerman, J. Burton and C. Wen-Chieh, C., eds. pp. 37–49. Geneva: WHO.

Gonzalez, Nicholas J. and Linda Issacs. 1999. Evaluation of Pancreatic Proteolytic Enzyme Treatment of Adenocarcinoma of the Pancreas, with Nutrition and Detoxification Support. Nutrition and Cancer 33(2): 117–24.

Hall, Nor. 1976. Mothers and Daughters. Minneapolis, MN: Rusoff Books.

Harris, Bruce. 2003. American Accused of Sexual Abuse of Mexican Boys Arrested in Thailand. *In* Alianza Newsletter, 14 Feb. Bangkok.

Herman, Judith. 1992. Trauma and Recovery. New York: Basic Books.

Hirch, Mirjam. 2003. Store Surveys: Quantities and Sources of Dry Goods Pharmaceuticals and Fresh Produce in Yelapa. Olympia, WA: Center for Traditional Medicine.

Hurtado, Lorenzo Muelas. 1999. Access to the Resources and Biodiversity and Indigenous Peoples. *In* The Edmonds Institute Occasional Papers. p. 17. Edmonds, WA: Edmonds Institute.

Integrative BodyMind Information System (IBIS). 1999. Natural Medicine Database: Integrated Medical Arts Group, Beaverton, *or* <www.ibismedical.com>.

International Diabetes Federation (IDF). 2000. Diabetes Atlas. Brussels: International Diabetes Federation.

Jackson, Yvonne M. 1994. Diet, Culture and Diabetes. *In* Diabetes As a Disease of Civilization: The Impact of Culture Change on Indigenous Peoples. Jennie R. Joe and Robert S. Young, eds. Vol. 50. pp. 381–406. New York: Mouton de Gruyter.

Jain, SK. 1999. Should High Doses of Vitamin E Supplementation be Recommended to Diabetic Patients? Diabetes Care 22(8): 1242–44.

Jamal, G.A. 1990. Panthogenesis of Diabetic Neuropathy: The Role of the N-6 Essential Fatty Acids and Their Eicosanoid Derivatives. Diabetic Medicine 7: 574–79.

Jamal, G.A. and H. Carmichael. 1990. The Effect of Gamma Linolenic Acid on Human Diabetic Peripheral Neuropathy. Diabetic Medicine 7(4): 319–23.

Joe, Jennie R. and Robert S. Young, eds. 1994. Diabetes As a Disease of Civilization: The Impact of Culture Change on Indigenous Peoples. Vol. 50. New York: Mouton de Gruyter.

Joyce, Rosemary A. 2000. Gender and Power in Prehispanic Mesoamerica. Austin: University of Texas Press.

Karasch, Mary. 2000. Amaranth. *In* The Cambridge World History of Food. K.F. Kipple and K.C. Ormelas, eds. pp. 75–81. New York: Cambridge University Press.

Khantzian, Edward. 1985. The Self-Medication Hypothesis of Addictive Disorders: Focus on Heroin and Cocaine Dependence. Am J Psychiatry 142: 1259–64.

Kiecolt-Glaser, J.K., W.B. Malarkey, J.T. Cacioppo and R. Glaser. 1994. Stressful Personal Relationships: Immune and Endocrine Function. *In* Handbook of Human Stress and Immunity. J.K. Kiecolt-Glaser and R. Glaser, eds. pp. 321–339. San Diego: Academic Press.

Kinley, Larry. 1989. Potlatch Economics and Governing Ourselves Fully. *In* Indian Self-Governance: Perspectives on the Political Status of Indian Nations in the United States. R. Ryser, ed. Olympia: Center for World Indigenous Studies.

Konrad, T., P. Vicini, K. Kusterer, A. Hoflich, A.Assadkhanni, H.J. Bohles, A. Sewell, H.J. Tritschler and C. Cobelli. 1999. Alpha-Lipoic Acid Treatment Decreases Serum Lactate and Pyruvate Concentrations and Improves Glucose Effectiveness in Lean and Obese Patients with Type 2 Diabetes. Diabetes Care 22(2): 280–87.

Korn, Leslie. 1983. Oral History in Rural Mexico. pp. 46: Lesley University.

_____1987. Polarity Therapy: To Touch the Heart of (the) Matter. Somatics Magazine-Journal of the Bodily Arts and Sciences VI(2): 30–34.

_____1996. Somatic Empathy. Olympia, Center for World Indigenous Studies, DayKeeper Press. p. 56.

_____2000. Polarity Therapy. In Clinician's Complete Reference to Complementary and Alternative Medicine. D.W. Novey, ed. St. Louis: Mosby.

_____2003. Community Trauma and Development. Fourth World Journal 5(1): 1–9.

Kuhnlein, Harriet V. and Olivier Receveur

1996   Dietary Change and Traditional Food Systems of Indigenous Peoples. Annual Review of Nutrition 16: 417–42.

Kuhnlein, Harriet V., Faustinius Yeboah, Maggie Sedgemore, Scotty Sedgemore and Hing Man Chan. 1996. Nutritional Qualities of Ooligan Grease: A Traditional Food Fat of British Columbia First Nations. Journal of Food Composition and Analysis 9: 18–31.

Lang, Gretchen Chesley. 1989. "Making Sense" about Diabetes: Dakota Narratives of Illness. Medical Anthropology 11: 305–27.

Larson, Clark Spencer. 2000. Skeletons in Our Closet: Revealing Our Past Through Bioarchaeology. Princeton, NJ: Princeton University Press.

Levi-Strauss, C. 1965. The Principle of Reciprocity. In Sociological Theory. L.A.C.L. Rosenberg, ed. New York: Macmillan.

López, Juan and Manuel Vargas. 2003. Amaranto: Cultivo de los Aztecas prohibido por los conquistadores Españoles, Vol. 2003: Horizantes Revista.

Manson, Spero, Janette Beals, Theresa Nell, Joan Piasecki, Donald Bechtold, Ellen Keane and Monica Jones. 1996. Wounded Spirits, Ailing Hearts: PTSD and Related Disorders Among American Indians. In Ethnocultural Aspects of Post Traumatic Stress Disorder: Issues, Research, and Clinical Application. A.J. Marsella, Mathew J. Friedman, Ellen T. Gerrity and Raymond M. Scurfield, eds. Washington, DC: American Psychological Association.

Marles, R.J. and N.R. Fransworth. 1996. Antidiabetic Plants and Their Active Constituents. The Protocol Journal of Botanical Medicine 1(3): 85–137.

Mauss, Marcel. 1990. The Gift: The Form and Reason for Exchange in Archaic Societies. W.D. Halls, transl. New York: W. W Norton and Company.

McColl, Janice. 2003. Essential Fatty Acids and Their Interaction with Other Nutrients and Drugs. Integrative Medicine 2(3): 36–41.

Meletis, Chris D. 2001. Natural Approaches to the Prevention and Management of Diabetes. Alternative and Complementary Therapies, June, 7(3): 132–37.

Michael, M. and J. Pizzorno. 1997. Encyclopedia of Natural Medicine. Rocklin, CA: Prima Publ.

Mintz, Sidney. 1995. Sweetness and Power: The Place of Sugar in Modern History. New York: Viking Press.

Minugh, Carol and Russell Fox. 1989. Community-determined Liberal Arts Education. International Encounter on Participatory Research, Managua, Nicaragua, 1989. Olympia, WA: Center for World Indigenous Studies.

Moerman, Daniel. 1998. Native American Ethnobotany. Oregon: Timber Press.

Montori, V.M., et al. 2000. Fish Oil Supplementation in type 2 Diabetes: A Quantitative Systematic Review. Diabetes Care 9(23): 1407–15.

Moran, Martha Rodriguez and Fernando Guerrero-Romero. 2003. Oral Magnesium Supplementation Improves Insulin Sensitivity and Metabolic Control in type 2 Diabetic Subjects. Diabetes Care 26(4): 1147–51.

Mountjoy, Joseph B. 2000. Pre-Hispanic Cultural Development Along the Southern Coast of West Mexico. In Greater Mesoamerica: The Archaeology of West and Northwest Mexico. M.S. Foster, and Shirley Gorenstein, eds. pp. 81–106. Salt Lake City, UT: The University of Utah Press.

Murray, Michael and Joseph Pizzorno. 1998. Encyclopedia of Natural Medicine. Rocklin, CA: Prima Publishing.

Nabhan, Gary Paul. 1997. Cultures of Habitat. Washington, D.C.: Counterpoint.

Norberg-Hodge, Helena. 1991. Ancient Futures: Learning from Ladakh. San Francisco: Sierra Club Books.

Packer, L., E.H. Witt and H.J. Trtschler. 1995. Alpha-Lipoic Acid as a Biological Antioxidant. Free Radical Biological Medicine 19(2): 227–50.

Page, J.T. 1995. Health policy and Legislation Concerning Traditional Indigenous Medicine in Mexico. Cad Saude Publica. Jun 11(2): 202–11.

Raman, A. and C. Lau. 1996. Anti-diabetic Properties and Phytochemistry of Momordica charantia L. (Cucurbitaceae). Phytomedicine 2: 349–62.

Ramos, Ruben Roman. 1980. Una observacion clinica sobre el efecto hipoglucamiante del nopal (Opuntia sp). Medicina Tradicional 3(10): 71.

Robin, Robert, Barbara Chester and David Goldman. 1996. Cumulative Trauma and PTSD in American Indian Communities. In Ethnocultural Aspects of Postraumatic Stress Disorder: Issues, Research and Clinical Applications. A.J. Marsella, Mathew J. Friedman, Ellen T. Gerrity and Raymond M. Scurfield, eds. p. 576. Washington, DC: American Psychological Association.

Roman, Ramos Ruben. 1980. Investigacion y Clinica de la Diabetes. Medicina Tradicional 3(10): 71.

Romo, L. FyL. Edmundo Andrade. 2000. Characterization of the Municipality of Cabo Corrientes, Jalisco, Mexico, University of Guadalajara.

Rossi, Ernest. 1986. Psychobiology of Mind-Body Healing: New Concepts of Therapeutic Hypnosis. New York: W.W Norton and Company.

Ryser, Rudolph. 1997. New Treaties Need to Protect Native Peoples' Biological and Cultural Diversity. National Congress of American Indians Annual Convention, Santa Fe, New Mexico.

_____1998. Observations on 'Self' and 'Knowing.'" *In* Tribal Epistemologies: Essays in the Philosophy of Anthropology. Helmut Wautischer, ed. pp. 3–14. Aldershot, UK: Ashgate.

_____2001. Definitions of Development from a Fourth World Perspective. Olympia, WA: Center for World Indigenous Studies.

_____2004. Romancing the Oil. Nutritional Therapy Association Newsletter: Nutritional Therapy Association.

Salvador, Ricardo J. 1996 (Oct.4). Ulterior Motives for Indigenous Language Broadcast in Mexico? <www.bris.ac.uk/Depts/Philosophy/CTLL/FEL/i4/iat4.rtf>.

Sarcar, Shubhashish, Maddali Pranava and Rosalind A. Marita. 1995. Demonstration of the Hypoglycemic Action of Momordica Charantia in a Validated Animal Model of Diabetes. Pharmalogical Research 33(1).

Schacht, Robert M., et al. 1999. Emerging Disabilities: American Indian Issues. p. 106. Flagstaff: American Indian Rehabilitation Research and Training Center.

Scheder, Jo C. 1988. A Sickly-Sweet Harvest: Farmworker Diabetes and Social Equality. Medical Anthropology Quarterly 2: 251–77.

Seligman, M.E.P. 1972. Learned Helplessness. Annual Review of Medicine 23: 407–12.

Silverman, Milton, Phillip Lee and Mia Lydecker. 1982. Prescriptions for Death: The Drugging of the Third World. Berkeley, CA: University of California Press.

Simonelli, Jeane Marie. 1987. Defective Modernization and Health in Mexico. Social Science and Medicine 21(1): 23–26.

Streuver, Stuart and Felicia Antonelli Holton: New York. 1979. KOSTER, Americans in Search of their Prehistoric Past: The New American Library.

Surwit, Richard S. 1993. Role of Stress in the Etiology and Treatment of Diabetes Mellitus. Psychosomatic Medicine 55: 380–93.

Toledo, Victor Manuel. 1995. New Paradigms for a New Ethnobotany: Reflections on the Case of Mexico. *In* Ethnobotany: Evolution of a Discipline. R.E. Schultes, von Reis, Siri, ed. pp. 75-85. Portland, OR: Dioscorides Press.

Townsend, Richard F., ed. 1998. Ancient West Mexico, Art and Archaeology of the Unknown Past: Thames and Hudson.

Trotter, Robert T., Luis D Leon and Juan Chavira. 1997. Curanderismo: Mexican American Folk Healing. Athens: University of Georgia Press.

Ullman, Dana. 1991. Discovering Homeopathy: Medicine for the 21st Century. Berkeley: North Atlantic Books.

USDA United States Department of Agriculture. 2003. Food Distribution Programs.

Valero, Alejandra, Jan Schipper and Tom Allnutt. 2001. Jalisco Dry Forests: World Wildlife Fund.

van der Kolk, Bessel. 1987. Psychological Trauma. Washington, D.C.: American Psychiatric Press.

Wadsworth, J.R. K. and G.R. Robson. 1977. The Health and Nutritional Status of Native Populations. Ecology of Food and Nutrition 6: 187–202.

Walker, Morton. 2001. Liver Detoxification with Coffee Enemas as Employed in the Gerson Therapy. Townsend Letter 2001: 46–50.

Weintraub, Michael I. 2001. Alternative and Complementary Treatment in Neurologic Illness. Philadelphia: Churchill Livingston.

Werner, David. 1996. Where There is No Doctor. Berkeley, CA: Hesperian Foundation Press.

WHO (World Health Organization). 2002. WHO Policy and Strategy on Traditional Medicine. Geneva: World Health Organization.

Wilkinson, Clive, ed. 2002. Status of Coral Reefs of the World: 2002. Perth: Australian Institute of Marine Science.

Xu, Mike. <www.chinese.tcu.edu/www chinese3 tcu edu.htm> ("Artifact comparisons between ancient Mesoamerica and China").

Yongchaiyudha, S., V. Rungpitarangsi, N. Bunyapraphatsara and O. Chokechai-jaroenporn. 1996. Antidiabetic Activity of Aloe Vera Juice I. Clinical Trial in New Cases of Diabetes Mellitus. Phytomedicine 3(3): 245–48.

Ziegler, D. and F.A. Gries. 1997. A-Lipoic Acid in the Treatment of Diabetic Peripheral and Cardiac Autonomic Neuropathy. Diabetes (46): S62–S66.

Zimmet, Paul. 2000. Globalization, Coca-colonization and the Chronic Disease Epidemic: Can the Doomsday Scenario be Averted? Journal of Internal Medicine 247(3): 301–10.

_____2001. Global and Societal Implications of the Diabetes Epidemic. Nature 414(6865): 782–87.

CHAPTER 11

A SICKLY-SWEET HARVEST: FARMWORKER DIABETES AND SOCIAL (IN)EQUALITY[1]

Jo C. Scheder

Yesterday at the Mujer Latina Conference

Gloria Anzaldua told the packed auditorium that she has 'really bad hyperglycemia.' The crowd nod-
ded and sighed. Hyperglycemia. Instant understanding. Anzaldua had just been diagnosed, telling us
that her blood sugars were 'in the 300s-to-400s.' Collective moan. Whoa. This crowd knows. This is
common, this is shared. In what other collection of conferees—students and community people from
outside of the health professions—would this information have such salience, be met with such collec-
tive compassion, such shared emotion? In this community everyone's life is touched by this disease. I
mention to a Chicana student that my work was with diabetes; she tells me her mother has it. And so
do the other students' families. She tells me that the Chicano students are very concerned about it.
They are concerned for their families and for the raza. Is this generation to follow their parents and
grandparents in this epidemiology? Gloria Anzaldua taught the audience a customized healing mantra,
based on a Nahuatl word. She understands the links to oppression. And yet in a week from now on this
campus there will be another assemblage of conferees, this time prominent researchers in emotion and
health, who will not mention diabetes and who will convene in a political vacuum and who will chat
informally and somewhat collusively about the unscholarly stigma that attaches to academics who
study the health fringe, like massage and, by implication, mantras and meditation.

Diabetes prevalence is not the sum effect of individual units of lifestyle or diet. We see the falsity of this
reification in the audience reaction to Anzaldua. Diabetes is an emergent social phenomenon, tied to
the relations of individuals within their social and economic circumstances. The issue is with the collec-
tive antecedent to onset, the sociopolitical etiology of exposure and risk, and the continuum of collective
mediation of symptoms, course, and cosmological incorporation of the disease.

[Gloria Anzaldua died May 15, 2004, from complications due to diabetes.]

written by Jo Scheder 4.27.97, Madison, WI

---

1. Reprinted with permission, from the American Anthropological Association. Originally published in *Medical Anthropology Quarterly* 2:3 (NS): 251–77. September 1988. At the time of the initial research in 1979–80, and the writing and publication of this article in the mid-1980s, "NIDDM"
was standard usage for what is currently named "type 2 diabetes." The terms "diabetic" and "non-diabetic" were the accepted clinical descriptors for people with, and without, diabetes. The epigraph,
Yesterday at the Mujer Latina Conference, was added for this volume.

Summary of Chapter 11. Type II diabetes mellitus (NIDDM) is used as a model in examining neuroendocrine and experiential linkages between social inequality and health outcome. Ethnographic, psychosocial, and biochemical data collected among Mexican-American migrant farmworkers reveal that diabetic workers spent more years in migrant labor (p < .01), and reported a greater number of stressful life events (p < .001), than nondiabetics. Body mass index (BMI) did not differ significantly between the two groups. Dopamine-beta-hydroxylase, a regulating enzyme in the stress-responsive catecholamine system, may contribute to diabetes risk for some individuals; other pathways for neuroendocrine mediation of psychosocial stress are discussed. It is proposed that the oppressive life conditions of migrant farmworkers contribute to adverse health outcomes through specific physiological responses to life experiences.

ᵛ   ᵛ   ᵛ

The emerging critical perspective in medical anthropology is increasingly focusing attention on the inescapable influence of the political economy on health (e.g., Baer 1982; Baer, Singer, and Johnsen 1986; Elling 1981; Morsy 1979; M. Singer 1986; P. Singer 1977). However, specific analyses connecting macro-level economic and political phenomena with micro-level social contexts lag behind. The work described in this article is just such an attempt to analyze the interweaving of macro- and micro-levels.

Initially undertaken in 1978, the analysis grew out of my observations as a community health worker and clinical interpreter at a multiservice clinic for migrant farmworkers (Scheder 1981). Drawing on neuroendocrinology as well as anthropology and social psychology, the study is an exploration specifically of the relationships between diabetes, a common and intractable health problem in the farmworker population, and psychosocial stress.[2] More generally, my purpose is to suggest how a specific health outcome (Type II diabetes mellitus) relates to macro-level politics and economics as they affect and shape the mediating micro-level experiences of migrant farmworkers. I also contend that the prevailing research focus on obesity, nutrition, and individual health behaviors—although undeniably contributors to health outcome—obscures the social issues more fundamental to the etiology of the disease.

Background: Social Conditions, Stress, and Diabetes

In recent decades stress research has concentrated on psychosocial correlates of illness (e.g., Marmot, Kogevinas, and Elston 1987). Although methodological issues remain in this field (see reviews by Barglow et al. 1984; Rabkin and Struening 1976), various tools have been developed to examine psychosocial stress objectively and quantitatively. Two of the main areas of research, social support and stressful life events (Berkman and Syme 1979; Cassel 1974; Cobb 1976), have dealt specifically with the

---

2. "Stress" is defined in accordance with Lipowski (1977: 237): "psychosocial stress refers to external and internal stimuli that are perceived by and are meaningful to the person, activate emotions, and elicit physiological changes that threaten health and survival."

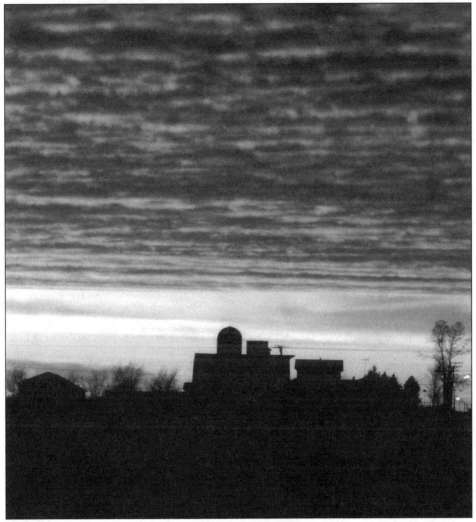

Wisconsin sunrise, 1980.

effects of social inequality. An early community survey by Dohrenwend (1970), for example, indicates that lower-income respondents are more exposed to stressful life events than higher-income respondents. A later study (Dohrenwend 1973) finds social class to be inversely related to life change scores (readjustment required by life events). Dohrenwend's interpretation is that members of the lower class are exposed to a relatively high degree of instability in their lives, requiring frequent social or psychological adjustment. It is this requirement for readjustment that is thought to act as a key stressor, leading to adverse psychological or health outcomes (Holmes and Rahe 1967).

The theoretical framework that underlies the research presented in this article is consonant with the views of these stress researchers. Basically the framework is psychosomatic and sees physical disorders as engendered by psychological and/or social factors that have physiological consequences involving the neuroendocrine and immune systems (Frankenhaeuser 1980; Locke and Hornig-Rohan 1983). The psychosomatic framework thus incorporates as environmental contributors to morbidity the various psychosocial elements of stress theorists and includes individual biopsychological responses in the physiological diathesis. This psychosomatic approach provides the following explanation for the etiology of Type II or non-insulin-dependent diabetes mellitus (NIDDM) among migrant farmworkers: fostered by the larger political and economic system that benefits from cheap labor, the migrant lifestyle fosters social and psychological stresses that place the individual at risk for disorders that are mediated at least in part by the neuroendocrine system. To explicate and support this theory of the etiology of NIDDM, in the following sections I review the evidence both for psychological and social contributions to diabetes risk and course and for biological evidence that links stress to hyperglycemia (diabetes).

Psychological and Social Correlates of Diabetes

Worldwide the overall pattern of increased diabetes prevalence in migrating, modernizing, or socioeconomically disadvantaged groups (Bennett, Burch, and Miller 1971; Fatani, Mira, and El-Zubier 1987; O'Dea, Spargo, and Ackerman 1980; West 1974; Zimmet et al. 1977) implies some underlying commonality behind their shared glucose intolerance. In the United States diabetes mellitus is generally more common among low-income Americans, particularly non-white females (U.S. Department of Health, Education and Welfare 1978). The 1973 National Health Interview Surveys (HIS), conducted by the National Center for Health Statistics, found that diabetes prevalence was 1.4% for those whose annual family income was greater than $10,000; 2% for the $5,000-10,000 income bracket; and 4% for those with less than $5,000 annual family income.

It has also been suggested that Type II diabetes mellitus may be precipitated by stress (Cobb and Rose 1973; Danowski 1963; Weiner 1981, Williams and Porte 1974), by loss and separation (Bruhn 1974; Slawson, Flynn, and Kollar 1963), or by disordered physiological and psychological adaptation to acculturation (Eaton 1977; Neel 1962).[3] From the 17th-century writings of Willis (1679) to the current elucidation of neuroendocrine mechanisms (Waldhausl et al. 1987) and the efficacy of relaxation training in improving glucose tolerance (Surwit and Feinglos 1983), interest in diabetes and behavior has been scattered throughout the literature.

Claude Bernard first formulated the notion of a neural role in the development of diabetes. Subsequent investigators have demonstrated links between metabolic control and psychosocial variables such as life events (Bradley 1979, Grant et al. 1974), family environment (Anderson et al. 1981), and anxiety, depression, and quality of life (Mazze, Lucido, and Shamoon 1984). Emotional and psychosocial factors have been related to onset or exacerbation of diabetes (Baker and Barcai 1970; Hauser and Pollets 1979; Kimball 1971; Schade and Eaton 1980). On the basis of the extant literature, there is thus reason to believe that a connection exists between NIDDM and psychological stress and social status.

---

3. This notion smacks of manifest destiny and of blaming the victim, but analysis on this level must await another occasion.

The Neurophysiological Link Between
Stress and Glucose Intolerance

Changes in circulating hormones that are part of the stress response system are also known to affect glucose metabolism (Cryer 1980; Porte and Robertson 1973). Cortisol, glucagon, growth hormone, and the catecholamines epinephrine and norepinephrine are of primary importance. These counter-regulatory hormones are under neural control, and are responsive to psychological stress, and function to increase blood glucose (Curtis et al. 1978; Schade and Eaton 1980; Shamoon, Hendler, and Sherwin 1980; Surwit et al. 1982). Cortisol elevates blood glucose and impairs glucose tolerance through increased gluconeogenesis and inhibition of glucose uptake in peripheral tissues (Felig et al. 1979; Rizza, Mandarino, and Gerich 1982). The secretion of insulin, a hormone essential to the transport of blood glucose into the cells, is inhibited by sympathetic nervous system activation of alpha-adrenergic receptors in the pancreas. Pancreatic beta-adrenergic receptors stimulate insulin secretion, but are inhibited by epinephrine and norepinephrine (Gerich and Lorenzi 1978; Williams and Porte 1981). Small increments in epinephrine, comparable to those seen during minor stress, can adversely affect glucose tolerance (Hamberg, Hendler, and Sherwin 1980). Catecholamines in particular have been studied in relation to psychosocial stress (Brown 1981; Usdin, Kvetnansky, and Kopin 1976) and to diabetes (Christensen 1974; Lebovitz and Feldman 1973). The rate-limiting enzyme in the synthesis of norepinephrine, dopamine-beta-hydroxylase (DBH), has been studied in relation to diabetes (Berkowitz et al. 1980; Schmidt, Geller, and Johnson 1981) and psychosocial stress (Mathew et al. 1981). Increases in catecholamine levels and DBH activity accompany physical and psychological stress. Finally, endogenous opiates have been shown to affect pancreatic islet function and may be pertinent to insulin response to glucose (Giugliano 1984).

A population exposed to stressors that tax the physiological system may be at greater risk for stress-related disorders. Best described as a threshold effect, the physiological responses to psychological stress would push the individual who is at risk (by virtue of family history and genetic background) closer to a threshold for actually manifesting the disorder. Relative degrees of psychological stress and biological risk vary among individuals. Therefore individual biopsychological responses to the environment are of interest, and part of the interest must focus on social conditions, like migrant farmwork, that might present a greater challenge to those responses, and provide the setting and exposure for individuals to express physiological symptoms.

The Mexican-American Migrant
Lifestyle, Stress, and Diabetes

The general paradigm of psychosomatic causality of NIDDM, outlined above, will be applied in this article to a sample of Mexican-American migrant farmworkers in Wisconsin. Two considerations underlie the selection of this group for study: (1) Mexican-American farmworkers' marginal status as an ethnic minority further exacerbates their marginality as migrants, and thus the effects of social stress on this group may

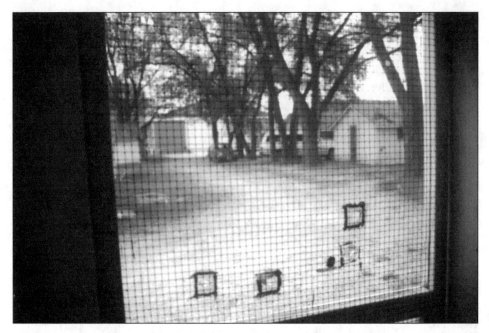

Migrant camp viewed thru laundry room screen door, 1998.

be expected to be heightened over those of other migrant groups; and (2) Mexican-Americans are reported as having higher rates of diabetes than other disadvantaged groups in this country (Fonner 1975). Before describing the research itself, it is therefore necessary to review these special characteristics of the sampled population.

Stressors Among Mexican-American Migrants

The historical link between Mexican-Americans and migrant labor officially dates to 1942, when the *bracero* program was initiated to alleviate U.S. labor shortages during World War II. Although the program ended in 1964, the well-established seasonal migration pattern has persisted. The Texas-Mexico border area, home base for more than 90% of Wisconsin's seasonal agricultural workers, is devoid of its own defining political boundary but remains culturally distinct, structured in a "social form known as border culture" (Nolasco 1978: 55). Contact with *el otro lado*, the other side, is a way of life and bears witness to border life as a "living and organic union of the two cultures" (McWilliams 1968: 62). For migrants, leaving this home base involves a radical departure from a milieu in which their cultural norms are preeminent and recognized, to a setting in which they are treated as unwelcome intruders. Social and family supports are disrupted, roles are obscured, and seemingly routine matters, such as grocery shopping and church attendance, are obstructed by geographic and cultural distances.

Texas-based migrants follow the Midwest "migrant stream" from May to November or for some portion of that time. Some people work a circuit each year, moving from state to state within an established network. Others migrate directly between Texas and

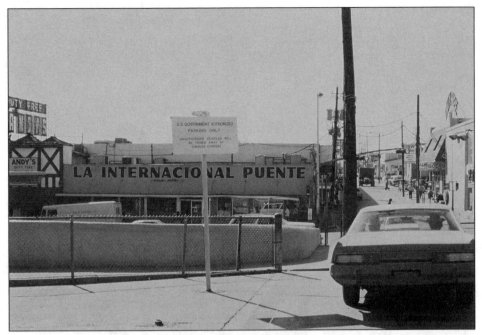

Laredo border crossing, 1980.

a target state such as Wisconsin, traveling in family units, buses, or quasi-caravans. Most families live in trailers, barracks, or shacks, usually on the grounds of the employing farm or cannery. "Singles," workers who travel without families, live in dormitory-style housing or occasionally in trailers, and include adults of any age, married or unmarried, and often widowed. Conditions vary from camp to camp, and can differ widely within camps (cf. Friedland and Nelkin 1971 for a description of migrant labor camps, comparable to Wisconsin, in the northeast).

Work schedules run from 10 to 16 hours per day, although most contracts guarantee only 20 hours of work per week. The weather dictates the availability of work for cannery and field workers alike, and rain can unexpectedly cause a loss of work time and income. Local transportation is difficult, as people are dependent upon service agencies or overworked relatives and friends to take them to the clinic, the grocery, the social service office, or the church. People are reluctant to ask others to sacrifice time from work, or to lose time themselves, in order to take care of personal needs.

The average 1977 family income for migrant farmworkers in Wisconsin was near $6,000. However, in 1978 an estimated 50% of farmworker households in Wisconsin earned less than $3,000, and some 45% of households had one or more disabled members. Yet fewer than 10% of migrant families receive public assistance. Infant mortality among migrants is two to three times higher than the national rate, and average adult life expectancy is 49 years, a full generation shorter than the U.S. population at large (La Clínica de Los Campesinos 1979).

Statistics and demographics cannot capture the flavor of ethnic discrimination and outright harassment the migrants receive, however. In Wisconsin local people resent

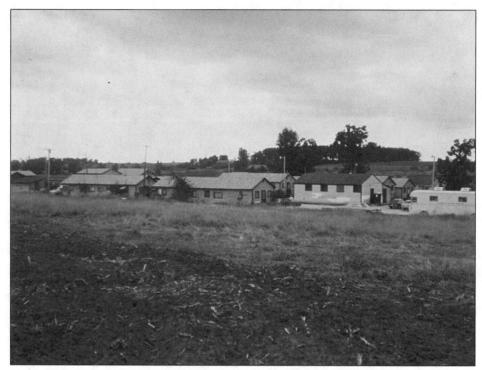

Housing for cannery workers in Wisconsin, 1978. The migrant health clinic's rented van is at right; funding cuts in the 1980s ended the mobile clinic program.

migrants as outsiders who take jobs away from them. Yet these jobs in fact go begging among locals, who are unwilling to accept the low wages and arduous work. The few townspeople who are friendly to migrants are met with ostracism from their peers. One of the rare instances of public documentation of hostility was reported in the October 18, 1980, *Milwaukee Journal*. In an article captioned, "Migrant Center Gets Quiet Start," it was reported that local residents protested the building of a migrant housing complex, saying "it posed a threat to the community." The article went on to cite "promises by residents...to block any construction attempts."

Social marginality is amplified by continued migration. Every season there is talk that "next year will be the last year up north," "the cannery won't hire migrants next year," I am going to school next year." Inevitably, some of these things occur. Just as inevitably, people return again and again, in a cycle that is for many impossible to break. For some, age and family responsibilities overpower their chances of developing alternatives. Others believe that it is "too late" for them, and there is an undercurrent of hopelessness and powerlessness. What masquerades as resignation, however, may be a way of dealing with frustration, not simply a surrender to the system. Poet Tomás Rivera (1975: 154) describes the cycle of frustration: "I'm tired of always arriving someplace. Arriving is the same as leaving....Maybe I should say when we don't arrive, because that's the plain truth. We never really arrive anywhere." Additional stress on the Mexican-American migrants results from pressures at home in Texas. These may include separation from family, obligations

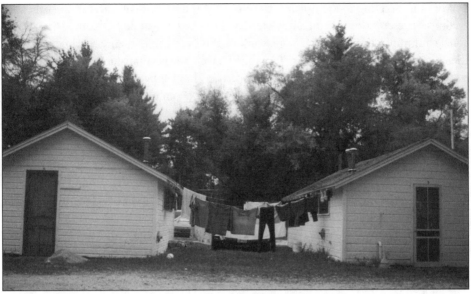

Laundry line at Wisconsin migrant camp, 1998.

to send money to relatives, expectation of an improved life position, and burglarizing of homes while the migrants are working in the north (cf. Dunbar and Kravitz 1976 and Thomas-Lycklama á Nijeholt 1980 for more detailed descriptions of migratory labor).

Mortality and Morbidity from Diabetes Mellitus Among Mexican-Americans

In South Texas overall death rates attributable to diabetes mellitus were three to four times higher for Mexican-Americans than for other Caucasians (Mexican-American Policy Research Project 1979; Stern 1985). An analysis of deaths from diabetes in this same population by age, sex, and ethnicity revealed a greater proportion among Mexican-Americans for both sexes and across all age groups (Fonner 1975; Mexican-American Policy Research Report 1979).

The Mexican-American Policy study (1979) also reports morbidity from diabetes to be four times higher for Mexican-Americans than for other Caucasians. The rates of diabetes among clinic patients at a San Antonio hospital are also reported as higher among low-income Mexican-Americans than low-income Anglos, regardless of sex (Fonner 1975).[4]

---

4. Differences in population genetic characteristics, such as degree of American Indian ancestry, could underlie differences in clinical expression of diabetes in different groups (Rotter and Rimoin 1979), and American Indian ancestry among Mexican-Americans is often suggested as a factor in their high diabetes rates. The highest known diabetes prevalence in the world occurs among the Pima of Arizona (50% of adults over age 35), and American Indian groups in general suffer from high rates of diabetes (Bennett, Burch, and Miller 1971; West 1974). Stern (1985) suggests that just such genetic heterogeneity might explain a portion of the differences in diabetes prevalence across neighborhoods in San Antonio. He reports a 15% prevalence of diabetes among Mexican-Americans liv-

Migrants arriving in the north for the start of their labor contracts frequently have a clinical presentation of uncontrolled diabetes (La Clínica de los Campesinos, personal communication, 1987). The reasons for this have been obscure, particularly since their pre-travel diabetes status in Texas may have appeared satisfactory. However, the pre-travel status for many migrants is uncertain, having been inferred from a lack of interstate clinic referrals. The lack of referral may be an outcome of limited access to health care, preferential utilization of selected clinics, breakdown in the referral system, or use of alternative healers not involved in the referral system.

It is unlikely, furthermore, that this clinical presentation is merely a transitory glucose intolerance related to a diet of truck-stop candy and soda during travel. Most migrants make the journey in one long 40-hour trip, alternating drivers and taking only brief rest stops along the way. Upon arrival in the north there is a delay of days or weeks before seeking health services, during which time the people begin to work and have reestablished their households and dietary patterns. The migrants' diet in Wisconsin is similar to the diet in Texas, and local supermarkets have begun to stock specialty items, such as *fajitas* (beef skirts). Staples, such as pinto beans and rice, are readily available, and homemade tortillas, tamales, and soups are common fare. In addition, fluctuations in glucose tolerance persist throughout the labor season and are not confined to initial presentation. Other aspects of the migrant lifestyle, which I have discussed earlier, thus take on clinical importance.

Research Design

This pilot study involved a biochemical analysis of a stress-related catecholamine system enzyme in matched diabetic and nondiabetic Mexican-American farmworkers. These physiological data were compared with assessments of subjects' life stresses, as

---

ing in the barrio, decreasing progressively to 5% in the suburbs. Using skin reflectance as a measure of American Indian ancestry, he finds that Mexican-Americans in the barrio have darker skin color (in a sun-protected skin region), those in transitional neighborhoods are intermediate, and those in the suburbs are lighter. Stern postulates that the relative rates of diabetes across neighborhoods are related to the degree of American Indian ancestry and are thereby a matter of genetic heterogeneity. These findings, however, are confounded by socioeconomic factors. The degree of American Indian ancestry may be related to diabetes by virtue of discrimination and the experience of inequality of opportunity rather than because of an ill-defined genetic factor. Darker-skinned (i.e., "more Indian") individuals may remain in the barrio for the same overall social and political reasons that concomitantly tender them more stress-exposed, and that stress exposure may be a causal trigger for the development of diabetes. Conversely, lighter-skinned ("less Indian") individuals may escape the social restraints and attain all that is implied by residence in the suburbs, and in so doing escape the chronic frustration of barrio dwellers. A more recent report by Stern's research group (Chakraborty et al. 1986) revealed a pattern of decreasing NIDDM prevalence with decreasing American Indian admixture and increasing SES, leaving questions regarding causality still unanswered. Within neighborhood categories, though, the diversity of American Indian admixture did not support a pattern of greater admixture among diabetic persons. This suggests that SES as indicated by neighborhood residence is more influential than American Indian ancestry in determining NIDDM prevalence, at least in this population.

measured by interviews concerning psychological stress variables, a life events protocol, and life history data.

Diabetic clients ($N = 28$) were identified through the Wisconsin migrant clinic's patient rolls and subsequently contacted in Texas. Nondiabetic clients ($N = 11$) were
drawn from the same clinic population of Texas-based migrants who worked in Wisconsin and were chosen on the basis of the diabetic clients' demographics for age, sex,
number of pregnancies, and place of residence in Texas. Diagnosis of diabetic subjects
was made according to clinical standards of fasting plasma glucose concentrations equal
to or greater than 140 mg/dl on at least two occasions (American Diabetes Association
1974; National Diabetes Data Group 1979). All subjects' identities were coded by assigning numbers from a table of random numbers, to disguise their status as diabetic
or nondiabetic.

Portions of the interview concerning life stresses had been used in previous studies
of similar populations (Nall and Spielberg 1967; Slesinger 1979). A modification of the
Social Readjustment Rating Scale (SRRS) (Holmes and Rahe 1967) and the Scale of
Life Events (SLE) (Paykel, Guiness, and Gomez 1976) were used. The SRRS was developed under the assumption that social events require life adjustment and that clustering of such events is significant in illness etiology. The SRRS attempts to measure
the magnitude of frequency of these events. The SLE is similar to the SRRS in content,
and like the SRRS, has been tested among Spanish-speaking people (Paykel, Guiness,
and Gomez 1976).

Although life event studies have provided insights and tools for use in stress research,
there are methodological issues concerning the validity and interpretation of these data,
including the ambiguity of items and the comparative significance of varying types of life
changes (Mechanic 1975). The interpretive experience of a stressful event may also be influenced by social support, and event scales in themselves do not account for other mediating factors. In addition, major illnesses, or illnesses that demand daily attention, may
alter the individual's perception of events or may make the sufferer more aware of events
(Rabkin and Struening 1976). Reporting on these instruments is affected by the social appropriateness of a response (e.g., being detained by police), and by distortions introduced
through recall (Jenkins, Hurst, and Rose 1979). Yet, despite these shortcomings, life event
data remain useful in conjunction with other types of data, when applied with caution.

A further issue that had to be considered in this research was the content validity of
these tests. Many event checklists emphasize events that are common to some groups
but are irrelevant to others. In light of this problem, I modified the event lists by introducing events characteristic of the migrant lifestyle: travel for work, separation from
family, loss or theft of property during the migrant season. These additions account
for 10% of the events used in the protocol; the remaining events were drawn directly
from the SRRS and SLE. The new events were chosen because they were mentioned repeatedly by migrants in nondirective discussions during two seasons of outreach/com-
munity health work prior to design of the protocols. Certain items from the SRRS were
not used because they were either inappropriate for the adult farmworker population
(e.g., take important exam) or for the time period (e.g., son drafted).

Subjects were asked to rate each event according to the degree of disruption presented by the event, regardless of whether the subject had experienced any of the

events, and the dates of the experienced events were recorded. Subjects were scored on the "number of events" reported and on "perceived stress" (each subject's overall rating of the "distress" assigned to the entire list of events, with scores ranging from 0 to a maximum of 20). Migration histories included data on the number of years in migrant labor, the number of states worked, and type of work (field or cannery).

The enzyme measured in the research was dopamine-beta-hydroxylase (DBH) (Weinshilboum 1979), which is involved in the synthesis of the hormone norepinephrine (a catecholamine), which in turn suppresses release of insulin by cells in the pancreas. When insulin levels are insufficient, the entry of glucose into the body's cells is impaired and the glucose accumulates in the bloodstream. An elevated level of glucose in the circulation, or hyperglycemia, is a hallmark of diabetes.

It was predicted that diabetic subjects would have altered DBH activity relative to the nondiabetics, with the catecholamine system acting as a physiological link between social stress and diabetes. Plasma samples were obtained for analysis of DBH activity, and all assays were performed "blind" so that the investigator did not know which samples belonged to diabetic subjects. Upon completion of the assays, a histogram of enzyme activity was constructed. Individuals on the extremes of the distributions were predicted to have diabetes, since high enzyme activity related to catecholamine synthesis and low DBH activity has been reported as being associated with diabetic neuropathy (Noth and Mulrow 1976). After removal of the extremes, 75% of the subjects remained in the middle range for enzyme activity. These were selected for special study to see whether their resemblance with regard to the biological variable—that is, mid-range DBH level—was countered by difference in one or more of the stress variables as well.

The relatively small sample sizes placed limitations both on the types of statistical tests appropriate for the data and on the strength of inferences to be drawn from them. Because of these limitations, statistical analyses were confined to nonparametric procedures.

Results

The study population, although small, reflected the demographic characteristics of Slesinger's (1979) larger sample (a 10% stratified random sample of migrants working in Wisconsin during the 1978 season), and may be considered representative of the Wisconsin migrant population at large with respect to ethnic heritage, place of birth, primary language, religious affiliation, and education (Table 1).

Upon completion of the blind predictions of diabetes status, each subject's health status was compared to predicted status. Of those predictions based on DBH activity alone, 86% were correct. Of those predictions based on "perceived stress" scores in mid-DBH-range subjects, 63% were correct. For those mid-range DBH subjects predicted as diabetic on the basis of the number of life events reported, 94% of the predictions were correct. By means of Fisher's Exact Test, only the association with life events was significant ($p = .0007$; $N = 16$). "Perceived stress" ($p = .30$; $N = 15$) and DBH ($p = .70$; $N = 10$) were not statistically significant. For comparison with these variables, a fourth set of predictions was made using body weight to height ratio (the Body Mass Index, weight/height). Only 62% of these predictions were correct, nearly

Table 1   Demographic characteristics of 1978 migrant population
in Wisconsin and of the pilot study sample.

	Mexican ethnic heritage	Born in Mexico	Spanish spoken most often	Religious preference: Catholic / None	x years education
Migrant Study (1978)[a] (N = 979)	91%	47%	86%	80% / 4%	4.5[b]
Pilot study (N = 39)	100%	49%	90%	85% / 3%	4.0

a. See Slesinger 1979.
b. Subjects over age 25 only.

the same rate of accuracy as the "perceived stress" predictions.[5] This relationship was not significant, again by means of Fisher's Exact Test ($p = .18$, $N = 13$).

After the analysis of the predictions was completed, subjects were grouped according to health status (presence or absence of diabetes) for further analysis (Table 2). The primary stress-related finding was that of a significantly greater number of stressful life events for diabetics by a nonparametric t-test (Siegel 1956; $p < .001$). This more frequent reporting of life events held for diabetic subjects as a group, for diabetic women over nondiabetic women, and for mid-DBH activity diabetics over mid-DBH nondiabetics. It is important to note that the kinds of stressful life events reported by diabetics were unrelated to their medical condition (e.g., miscarriages or diabetes-related hospitalizations) and were no different from the kinds of events listed by nondiabetics.

Correlations between the biochemical and stress data supported an association between stress and diabetes (Table 3). For diabetic subjects there was a positive correlation between "perceived stress" scores and fasting blood glucose ($p < .05$, Spearman's rank correlation coefficient). DBH activity was positively correlated with the number of life events for diabetics, but not for nondiabetics ($p < .05$).

In a further examination of physiological responses to life events, graphs of blood pressure and glucose data were constructed from medical records of diabetic and nondiabetic subjects. These graphs were then juxtaposed with the reported time of occurrence of life events to analyze whether subjects might be physiological "responders" to those events, in terms of blood pressure or glucose elevations. The word "response" is used loosely here, as the physiological measures are chronologically coincident with the reported events and not necessarily results of the events. Of the possible "responders," all were diabetic subjects. No nondiabetics were responders to life events by these criteria. The events that were associated with physiological responses were related to

5. These percentages are rounded to the nearest full percent. The precise values are 85.7, 62.5, 93.8, and 61.5, respectively.

Table 2   Summary Characteristics of diabetic and nondiabetic subjects (mean values).

	N	Age in years	Number of years migrating	DBH activity (mol/min/l)	Fasting glucose (mg/dl)	Insulin level (units/ml)	Body mass index	Number of life events[a]	Perceived stress score
Nondiabetic	11	47.7	11.7	4.05 (N = 9)	112	25	0.038	1.2	10.97
Males	4	54.8	12.0	3.84 (N = 2)	101	b	0.041	1.3	10.73
Females	7	43.8	11.6	4.11 (N = 7)	115	25	0.037	1.1	11.12
Diabetic	28	52.4	19.6[e]	4.03 (N = 15)	282	27	0.044	4.7[c]	10.38
Males	8	53.8	25.6	3.96 (N = 4)	216	b	0.042	3.1	9.65
Females	20	47.1	17.2	4.09 (N = 11)	307	28	0.045	5.4[d]	10.64

a. Mean number of life events for mid-DBH activity subjects:
Diabetic 5.9 (N = 8)
Nondiabetic 1.2 (N = 11)
    $p < .0001$ Student's t-test
b. Insufficient data.
c. $p < .0001$ Student's t-test.
d. $p < .001$ Student's t-test.
e. $p < .01$ Student's t-test.

Table 3   Spearman rank correlation coefficients for stress variables, fasting plasma glucose, and DBH activity.

	Fasting glucose		DBH activity	
	Perceived stress	No. of events	Perceived stress	No. of events
Nondiabetic	-0.3	-0.1	0.4	0.0
Diabetic	0.6[a]	0.3	0.3	0.5[a]

a. p<.05.

the migrant lifestyle: travel for work, loss or theft of belongings while in the north, and (less specific to migration) personal illness.

The only statistically significant difference between diabetics and nondiabetics with respect to social background was a greater number of years in migrant labor for diabetics ($p < .01$). One might suspect this difference to be due to age, but the two groups were not significantly different on this variable (see Table 2). Although the mean age for diabetics was 52.4 years and for nondiabetics 47.7 years (median ages were approximately the same—53 and 46 years, respectively), these differences were not found to be significant ($p > .4$, Mann-Whitney U Test).

For diabetics and nondiabetics alike there was a positive correlation between the number of years in the migration stream and the number of states in which individuals had worked. The latter variable was in turn related to educational experience. Roughly equal proportions of diabetics and nondiabetics had attended school for less than five years (64% and 67%, respectively), but more than half (56%) of the diabetics and a third (33%) of the nondiabetics had one or fewer years of school. Among those individuals with one or fewer years of school, the diabetics had worked in an average of four different states, while the nondiabetics had worked in only one state. Indeed, almost one-half (46%) of the nondiabetics had worked in only one state (Table 4).

Putting this another way, the entire subject sample can be categorized according to variables such as education and stability of worksites, and the relative proportions of diabetics and nondiabetics within each category can be calculated (Table 5). Because there were more diabetics than nondiabetics in the sample, the relative proportion of diabetics comprising any given category of subjects should reflect the original proportion of diabetics in the entire sample. After correcting for the skewed proportion of diabetics,[6]

---

6. The correction for skewed sample proportions is as follows:

$$\frac{N_D}{N_D + N_3} = \text{% of entire sample, per variable, who had diabetes,}$$

where N_D is the number of diabetics having the trait in question, and N_3 is the corrected number of diabetics having the trait.

Table 4   Education and migration history within diagnostic groups.

| | Within-group proportions: | |
Trait	% of diabetics (N = 25)	% of nondiabetics (N = 11)
Fewer than 5 years' education	64	67
Worked in more than one state	88	55
Worked in only one state	12	46
More than 20 years' migrating	52	9
Began migrating as:		
Children (11 years)	16	0
Adolescents (12-17)	8	0
Adults (20–29)	20	46
(30–39)	8	18
(40–49)	36	9
(50–59)	12	27
Adults (18 and older)	76	100

the following differences emerged: of the entire group of subjects who had worked in only one state, 18% had diabetes and 82% did not have diabetes. Of the entire group of subjects who had worked in more than one state, 58% had diabetes and 42% did not.

Duration of exposure to the migrant system also appeared to affect health outcome: 52% of the diabetics and only 9% of the nondiabetics had been migrating for more than 20 years (see Table 4). Seen across diagnostic categories, 82% of the subjects who had been migrants for more than 20 years had diabetes (see Table 5). There appeared to be a further difference in diabetes risk based on the age at which one entered the migrant stream. Virtually all of the migrants in this study who en-

---

N_3 is calculated as follows: $N_1 + N_2 = N_3$, where:

    N_1 = the original number of diabetics;

    N_2 = the correction factor = $X\%$ of 20, or the number of nondiabetic individuals expected to have the trait among 20 nondiabetics hypothetically added to the sample to equalize the number of diabetic and nondiabetic subjects. $X\%$ is the proportion of actual nondiabetic subjects who had the trait in question.

Table 5   Breakdown of education and migration histories by health status.

| Trait | N | Corrected[a] proportions of subjects positive for the trait who are also: | |
		Diabetic	Nondiabetic
Fewer than 5 years' education	22	45%	55%
Worked in more than one state	29	58%	42%
Worked in only one state	8	18%	82%
More than 20 years' migrating	14	82%	18%
Began migrating as:	4	100%[b]	0%
Children (11 years)			
Adolescents (12-17)	2	100%[b]	0%
Adults (20-29)	10	26%	74%
(30-39)	4	26%	74%
(40-49)	10	76%	24%
(50-59)	6	26%	74%
Adults(18 and older)	30	38%	62%

a. See Note 5.
b. Unable to correct for sampling due to absence of nondiabetics in this category.

tered the system during childhood and adolescence later developed diabetes. Of the migrants who entered the system in their 40s, 76% later developed diabetes. Equal numbers of diabetic and nondiabetic individuals were seen in the remaining entry-age groups.

A closer look at the diabetics according to age at initial migration revealed several group characteristics (Table 6).[7] Beginning with the relatively low-risk group of initial migration at age 20-29 years, the diabetics and nondiabetics differed on several dimensions, although the number of subjects in each category was too small for statistical analysis. Descriptively 80% of the diabetics were born in Texas and 20% were born in Mexico; all began migration in the 1950s, had less education as a group than the nondiabetics, worked predominantly in field labor rather than in canneries, and re-

7. Data on people who began migrant labor from age 30 to 50 are included in Table 6 but not discussed because of the small sample size.

Table 6   Mean values for migration and stress data, by age at initial migration (N = 36a).

Place of birth[c]	Decade of initial migration[b]	Number of years migrating	Age at initial migration	Number of years migrating prior to diabetes onset	Age at diabetes onset	Current age	Number of years education	Cannery or field labor[c]	Number of states worked	Number of stressful life events	Perceived stress	Fasting plasma glucose (mg/dl)
Initial migration:												
Childhood/adolescence (Diabetics, N = 6)												
TX	1940s	38	10	33	43	48	5	F	6	5	11	220
Age 20–29 (Diabetics, N = 5)												
TX	1950s	25	25	15	40	50	3	F	5	4	11	377
Age 20–29 (Nondiabetics, N = 5)												
b	1960s	15	24	d	d	39	6	C	4	1	14	113
Age 30–39 (Diabetics, N = 2)												
MX	1960s	18	38	13	51	56	4	b	3	13	14	182
Age 30–39 (Nondiabetics, N = 2)												
MX	1970s	9	37	d	d	46	4	b	5	1	14	104
Age 40–49 (Diabetics, N = 9)												
MX	1970s	11	44	5	49	55	3	b	3	4	8	213
Age 40–49 (Nondiabetics, N = 1)												
TX	1967	13	45	d	d	58	0	C	1	1	4	112
Age 50–59 (Diabetics, N = 3)												
b	1970s	3	52	8	44	55	3	b	1	5	14	410
Age 50–59 (Nondiabetics, N = 3)												
TX	1970s	7	53	d	d	61	0	C	1	1	7	119

a. Three subjects were removed from this tabulation, as their ages at initial migration were unknown.
b. Mode or mean inappropriate because no clear predominance of place of birth or type of labor exists.
c. These values are modes rather than means.
d. Variables not applicable to nondiabetic subjects.

ported a greater number of stressful life events. Of the nondiabetics 40% were born in Texas, and 60% in Mexico; all entered migrant labor in the 1960s, worked predominantly in canneries, and had more education and fewer stressful life events than the diabetics. In sum, a young adult entering migrant labor in the 1950s was likely to work in the fields and have less formal education than a young adult entering migrant labor in the 1960s, when cannery work began to replace field labor.

Subjects who entered migrant labor in childhood/adolescence began migration in the 1940s, worked predominantly in the fields, worked in the greatest number of states, had the highest number of stressful life events, and all developed diabetes (see Table 6). Those who began migration in their 40s worked in fewer states, but also had less education than most of the younger entrants, and had a large number of stressful life events. Age at diabetes onset for those who began migration in their 40s was older than the mean age at onset for the total diabetic sample, whereas age at diabetes onset for those who began migrating in childhood or their 20s was younger than the average for the total diabetic sample.

Discussion

I shall here explore patterns and relationships underlying NIDDM with respect to social inequality and psychosocial stress. This is a broader, yet more substantively precise analysis than most efforts at defining behavioral elements in diabetes (cf. Fisher et al. 1982; Skyler 1981; Surwit, Feinglos, and Scovern 1983) in its attempted weaving of experiential and social contributors and in its questioning of prevailing clinical notions of cause and course. Initial support for this perspective is evident in the predictions of diabetes status. The most reliable predictors of diabetes status were DBH activity and the number of stressful life events experienced. Predictions based on "perceived stress" or body weight (BMI) were essentially equivalent in accuracy, and neither was particularly discriminating with regard to diabetes status.

The similarity in outcome of the latter predictions can be interpreted in several ways. First, obesity (defined as 120% of recommended body weight for height, Society of Actuaries 1978) is generally considered to be a major etiologic factor in Type II diabetes mellitus; yet 67% of the nondiabetic subjects were obese, and 23% of the diabetic subjects were not obese. Second, the obesity-based (BMI) predictions were correct no more often than the perceived stress-based predictions, implying that perceived stress is equally important etiologically. Conversely, if perceived stress is not a major factor in distinguishing diabetics from nondiabetics, then in this context obesity is not a primary factor either. Third, the BMI for diabetics was not statistically different from the BMI for nondiabetics. Thus although accepted as an important contributor, obesity cannot be seen as the only contributor to diabetes risk.

At the time of the pilot study, little interest in non-obesity-related etiologies was evident in the literature. Only recently have reports begun to acknowledge that obesity is an inadequate explanation in NIDDM (cf. Knowler et al. 1981; Stern et al. 1983; Szathmary and Holt 1983). For example, Stern (1985), after finding a statistically significant four-fold excess of diabetes among Mexican-Americans even after adjusting

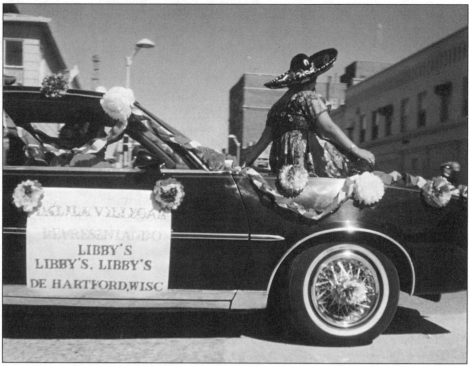

Cannery workers in Wisconsin hold a parade on Mexican Independence Day, 1979.

for obesity, rejected obesity as the sole contributor to the marked differences in diabetes prevalence. Similarly, though central body obesity has become popular as a correlate of NIDDM, Haffner et al. (1986) found that the increased risk of NIDDM in
Mexican-Americans cannot be explained by trunk fat deposition alone.

Vague et al. (1979) have considered the role of cortisol in centripetal obesity, suggesting that minor but long-term elevations in glucocorticoids may contribute to diabetes risk by way of the pituitary-adrenal axis. Cortisol and its regulatory hormone
from the anterior pituitary, ACTH, are secreted in response to a variety of stressful
stimuli (Eaton and Schade 1978), and in addition to its established action in stress
physiology, cortisol promotes central body fat deposition (most notably in Cushing's
Syndrome). Szathmary and Holt (1983) have proposed that the psychological stress of
acculturation may influence glucocorticoid secretion. It is plausible that centripetal
obesity may in some cases be an artifact of stress, arising from recurrent or chronic
stress-induced elevation of cortisol. Obesity might then become a tertiary factor, trail-
ing cortisol and the triggering/facilitation of social stressors.

Let me describe alternatives to a strict biomedical etiology of diabetes that are suggested by the data. In the present study, the importance of life events emerged in several contexts. Although the meaning of events to the individual cannot be dismissed,[8]

8. Cultural conceptions of health and illness among Mexican-Americans have become stereotyped, but what appear valid for at least some members of the migrant population are the associa-

the relatively greater usefulness of the number of events rather than the perceived stress variable in predicting health status supports the idea that it is the frequent experience of events, and not the generalized perception of stress, that is involved in glucose tolerance.

Since the life event data are drawn from self-reports, we must ask how reliable the memory of past events is. Might the nondiabetics be underreporting their experience of events? Do diabetics remember more events than nondiabetics? If so, is that an artifact of being aware of one's chronic disorder in a culture that associates emotion with health outcomes? Or is the awareness of and responsiveness to events contributory to diabetes onset and course? Whatever the ultimate answers to these questions, the people with diabetes in this sample have a different set of life events from the nondiabetics. For example, the theme of loss can be seen throughout the data on "perceived stress" and frequency of events: loss through death, loss of social/emotional support (i.e., marital separation), or loss/theft of property were perceived by both diagnostic groups as highly stressful. However, it was the diabetics who reported the frequent experience of such loss, particularly through death and loss of property. Nondiabetics reported the experience of personal illness. This pattern suggests not only a qualitative difference in event experiences, but also that the events reported by diabetics are not a consequence of their focus on their own health experience.

The correlations between life events, perceived stress, fasting blood glucose, and DBH invite further thought. Since the events and the physiological measures in this study were correlated but not temporally associated, the question remains as to whether the diabetics might in fact have different physiological response patterns from the nondiabetics, such as vigilance or hyperarousal (Kuhn et al. 1987), rather than having had different life experiences that engendered long-term changes in DBH or other neuroendocrine parameters. Evidence supporting the former idea is seen by examining physiological responses to life events among subjects in this study by using the graphs of blood pressure and glucose data from their health charts in juxtaposition with events. Changes in fasting blood glucose and blood pressures coincident with the occurrences of events in diabetic "responders" support the finding of Grant et al. (1974) and Baker and Barcai (1970) on subgroups of diabetics who were life-event responsive and others who were not. The findings here are similar: some diabetics are responders to life events, other are not; and none of the nondiabetics is event responsive.

The importance of the number of events is again seen with regard to subjects who were similar for DBH activity. The mid-DBH-activity diabetics and nondiabetics, sim-

---

tion between illness in the individual and in the social body (cf. Scheper-Hughes and Lock 1987), and the association between strong emotions and adverse health outcome. How may we interpret these beliefs in light of our data? Do they indicate that Mexican-American adherents to these beliefs are more "susceptible" to notions of sociogenic illness? Does that then affect neuroendocrine responses and illness liability? Is this yet another form of blaming the victim? Perhaps, on the other hand, these people are implicitly more aware of a fundamental union between social and individual health. The high rates of illness can then be a result of sensitivity to the sickness of the encompassing society. If so, illness is not a poetic metaphor, but a painful reality, a symbol only in the same way that a scream of agony is a symbol of distress.

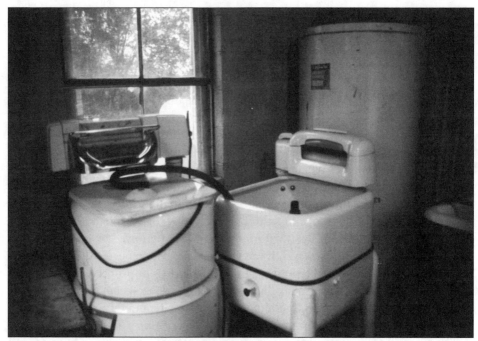

Wringer laundry at Wisconsin migrant housing camp, 1998.

ilar for the physiological stress system variable, were significantly different for the number of life events. This supports the idea of a greater stress requirement for the expression of diabetes when the relative biological risk is absent.

For comprehending the social context of stressful events, the positive correlation between the number of years migrating and number of worksites is intriguing, although
the data do not reveal the possible sources of this correlation. For example, several underlying patterns are possible; migrants may work in an increasing number of states over
time, long-term migrants may currently work in more than one state but began by working in only one, or long-term migrants may have begun their migrant careers by working in many states and later reduced that number. These distinctions are important with
respect to life change, because these different migration patterns imply either long-term
exposure to life change or life change clustered at certain times in the life cycle, and we
wish to know whether these two patterns contribute differently to diabetes risk.

The data on age at initial migration suggest that exposure to migrant labor may contribute to diabetes risk in different ways, depending upon the stage in one's life cycle
when migration begins. Marmot, Shipley, and Rose (1984) and Forsdahl (1977) speculate that poverty and social class-related factors operating in childhood might be important in risk for adult coronary heart disease. A developmental effect on diabetes
risk might also operate in this way. Those individuals with early life exposure to migrant labor had earlier onset of diabetes; those with later life exposure to migrancy had
later onset, but it occurred shortly after entering the migrant system. Migrancy for
older entrants, particularly those in their 40s, may have served as a "last resort" in the

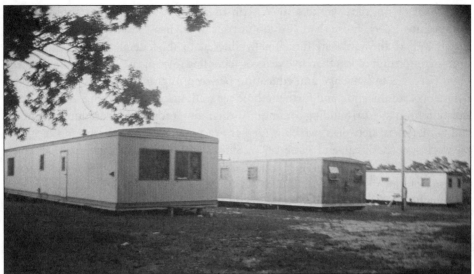

The three trailers of "Hidden Camp," Wisconsin, 1998.

effort to provide subsistence for themselves and their families, and the adjustments required by this major life change may have acted as final environmental triggers for the
clinical expression of diabetes. Nearly half of this age group (44%) developed the disorder within one year of initial migration, and the rest of them did so within five years.
Yet it is difficult to identify specific factors in their lives that may have contributed to
their current health status or to their decision to migrate.

These data introduce the idea of individual difference in propensity to develop the
disease, as well as the relative contribution of different stressors within the threshold
model. For example, the 40-year-old entrants to migration who reported few stressful
life events had a longer period of migration prior to diabetes onset than did 40-year-
old entrants who reported many stressful life events. Those at low risk on the basis of
life events were at higher risk on the basis of migrancy, and vice versa. By extension,
those individuals with many stressful life events would require less exposure to a cat-
alyst like migrant labor before crossing a threshold for expression of diabetes.

The social data suggest that migration to more than one state and having one or
fewer years of education also place one at greater risk for diabetes. What might there
be about emotional level or the number of work sites that places one at risk for diabetes? It may be that these variables reflect a single variable: access to coping resources.
Persons with more assets, resources, skills, and broader experience (equals educational
level?) tend to fare better in mediating stressful events (Rabkin and Struening 1976).

A related factor, ethnic group density, is also pertinent to risk. The assumption is
that the smaller the ethnic community, the less social support is available to any one
member (Rabkin and Struening 1976). Migrants in Wisconsin, as in many states, are
cloistered in labor camps, surrounded by a generally unsympathetic population of non-
Hispanic nonmigrants, and socially separated from surrounding communities. As one
moves from state to state, these conditions are repeated. Furthermore, although more

than 90% of migrant workers in Wisconsin are U.S. citizens (La Clínica de los Campesinos 1979), more than 40% do not speak English (Slesinger 1979). Approximately 29% of the adults are functionally illiterate by the federal government's definition—completion of less than five years of schooling (Slesinger 1979). In combination, the differences in language and education between migrants and host communities hamper communication and further ethnic separation and stereotyping. Added to this isolation from the surrounding community, migration promotes separation from home and family social networks, which is further exacerbated by moving around to multiple work sites (Berkman and Syme 1979). Since social networks are generally acknowledged as serving as buffers for life events (Cobb 1976; Sarason et al. 1985), seasonal migration not only disrupts these buffers but also affects the meanings of social support, marginality, and ostracism, and limits access to coping resources.

Education and migration histories might also have an indirect effect on health through their influence on biopsychological processes, such as adaptation to change and unpredictability. Situations analogous to those inherent in the migrant lifestyle have been shown to exacerbate physiological reactions to stressful stimuli. These include laboratory studies of novelty, unpredictability, and lack of control over situations (Frankenhaeuser 1971, 1975; Frankenhaeuser and Rissler 1970; Glass and Singer 1972). The distinguishing factor between diabetics and nondiabetics with less than one year of education was that the nondiabetics had stable worksites, and by extension more predictability in their surroundings. The effect of working in more than one state can be explained in terms of the life change model. Each state represents a new set of circumstances that demand at least some amount of adjustment. The more states worked, the more one accumulates exposure to novelty or recurrent stimuli associated with novelty. The more years spent in migration, the greater the possibility of a cumulative effect on physiological functioning. For life events as well, if the sheer experience of change evokes a physiological response, with repeated events the potential risk of metabolic decompensation might increase.

Models of Social Conditions and Diabetes

Glucose intolerance, hyperglycemia, and diabetes are terms that now appear to reflect symptom complexes and abnormalities detected in the laboratory, which can result from a number of distinct etiologic factors (Rotter and Rimoin 1979). It is likely that a number of individual disorders comprise the diabetes complex, each with its particular set of contributory factors. These disorders are yet to be clearly distinguished, but certainly the contributors include genetics, nutrition, obesity, physical activity, and psychosocial stress. The latter is the most difficult to define, measure, and interpret (Barglow et al. 1986), but it may offer potential suggestions or solutions to the problem of increased diabetes prevalence among migrating, modernizing, or socioeconomically disadvantaged populations.

Certainly, one physiological system is not enough to explain a complex metabolic imbalance. The contribution of other systems and other aspects of the catecholamine system is critical to a mature understanding of the mechanisms involved in such a transmutation of experience into health outcome. At minimum, corticosteroids, endorphins, free fatty acids, and gluconeogenesis are involved in this rich psychoneuroendocrine complex (Axelrod and Reisine 1984).

In the years since this study was undertaken, Surwit and Feinglos have explored the influence of behavioral variables on central and autonomic nervous system control of glucose metabolism (Surwit and Feinglos 1987, 1988). The findings of this study are consistent with their work: diabetics appear to be reacting physiologically to stressors, whereas nondiabetics do not show such reactions. DBH activity was positively correlated with the number of stressful life events for diabetics only; fasting plasma glucose was positively correlated with perceived stress for diabetics only. This pattern is consistent with laboratory evidence of a stress-induced hyperglycemic response in diabetic but not in control animals (Surwit 1983).

In conjunction with the life event results, the greater exposure of diabetics to the migrant lifestyle complements laboratory work on recurrent environmental stress and catecholamines (Cassens et al. 1980; McCarty et al. 1978) and glucose levels (Surwit, McCubbin, and Livingston 1985). Environmental stimuli associated with stressful events are sufficient to increase peripheral catecholamine and glucose levels in experimental animals. Stress-induced increases in norepinephrine metabolism and turnover are not diminished after repeated sessions with various intermittent stressors. Similarly, in diabetic humans blood glucose levels have been shown to decline steadily within sessions of a cognitive task experiment, but not across sessions (Edwards and Yates 1985), indicating a lack of metabolic habituation to the repeated stressor over time. Small physiologic increases of epinephrine, equivalent to those observed in mild stress, produce a significant impairment in glucose tolerance in nondiabetic humans (Hamberg, Hendler, and Sherwin 1980). Taken together, these findings suggest that catecholamine-mediated or cognitively generated impairments in glucose tolerance may persist despite repeated exposure to the stressors. In terms of the present study, psychological habituation to the quality of the event ("perceived stress") does not imply physiological habituation to the actual experience of the event. Continued or periodic exposure to event-associated cues (e.g., incidents of discrimination) over years of migrant labor could trigger intermittent elevations of catecholamine levels and fluctuations in blood glucose.

Analogous to the repeated stressor is the migrants' seasonal travel for work. Some individuals would be expected to exhibit a physiological response to such travel or to the circumstances surrounding travel. In this light it is not surprising that "uncontrolled" hyperglycemia is seen upon the migrants' arrival in the north. This observation also informs an interpretation of the "pathogenicity" of multiple worksites for some individuals.

Conclusion

As Peyrot and McMurray (1985) warn, complex relationships exist among the psychosocial factors influencing glucose tolerance, and these factors cannot be fully appreciated when studied separately. That fact sets a difficult task. In untangling the migrant experience, however, profiles of the diabetic and nondiabetic groups clarify the experiential differences. The number of life events and the number of years migrating were the discriminating variables. Nondiabetics presented a profile of relative stability. They were newer to the migrant lifestyle and lacked the developmental exposure

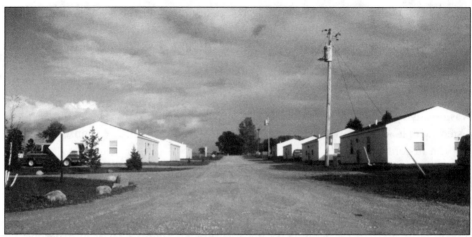

Temporary housing camp, Wisconsin, 1998.

to migrancy that was seen for many of the diabetics. Nondiabetics also lacked the frequent experience of stressful life events seen among the diabetics.

One might argue that the patterns seen here are an exaggerated effect of limited sampling. One must also consider alternative explanations of the patterns. Specifically, is it the number of years migrating that is important, or age at initial migration? Is it the length of exposure to the migrant lifestyle that increases diabetes risk, or is it a developmental effect of the lifestyle? Is it the lifestyle itself, or is it the circumstances that cause one to enter or remain in the lifestyle?

These questions lead to further questions of coping and adaptation, which must be carefully framed with an awareness of their political meanings. Ideas of inadequate coping or disordered adaptation might be regarded as the latest incarnations of a blame-the-victim schema in which responsibility for illness is implicitly assigned to the person whose health has been damaged by acculturation or by repeated exposure to events beyond personal control. These notions persist in diabetes, despite the fact that is has been clear for some time that hormonal consequences of stress are important to metabolic equilibrium.

The results of the pilot study suggest, in sum, that the frequent adjustment to stressful life events and life change, compounded by social inequality and psychosocial stress inherent in the migrant lifestyle, act via a series of physiological responses to culminate in hyperglycemia. Given such a scheme, preventive interventions are more appropriate at the social than at the individual level. The tenets of health promotion imply that individuals have power and autonomy over their choices and behaviors. Given the proper information and opportunity, individuals will choose behavior patterns that lead to good health. Even if this were true, can we further assume that these individual efforts can override continual political, economic, and social pressures that do not disappear on the wings of exercise and "proper" nutrition?

Medical relief of stress pathology is not enough. While such effort may provide transient (or even illusory) relief to the individual sufferer, it also provides a diversion from the remedy of underlying causes. Reductionistic treatment of symptoms is in itself an exploitation, as it encourages the perpetuation of an exploitative system (cf. P. Singer

1977). The possibility of treatment cannot permit a passive legitimation of the social contributors. Palliative measures then become forms of political control, offering no useful, long-term way out.

Dependency theorists have been criticized for evading or deemphasizing the biological factors in disease etiology (Morgan 1987). It is an unfortunate evasion because it leaves unexplored an unnecessarily forbidden territory in the cartography of sociopolitics and health. We must build bridges to this territory or risk never having the tools or access or knowledge to influence the systems whose effects we often bemoan.

Acknowledgments

The cooperation and assistance of the following agencies were instrumental in completing this study: La Clínica de los Campesinos, Wild Rose, Wisconsin; Laredo-Webb County Health Department, Migrant and Chronic Disease Divisions, Laredo, Texas; and Centro de Salud, Crystal City, Texas. Financial support during the writing of this article was provided in part under NIMH Grants 5T32 MH15741 and T32 MH14614. Beyond formal agency support, thanks are extended to many migrant laborers for their generous participation and to the families who provided shelter, insight, and social support. Further thanks are due to Arthur Rubel and Susan Abbott for helpful criticism of an earlier draft of this paper, and to Alan Harwood and two anonymous reviewers. The views expressed here are the responsibility of the author.

References

American Diabetes Association. 1974. Educational Pamphlet on Detection and Diagnosis of Diabetes: Plasma Glucose Procedures. Washington: American Diabetes Association.

Anderson, Barbara J., J. Philip Miller and Wendy F. Auslander. 1981. Family Characteristics of Diabetic Adolescents: Relationship to Metabolic Control. Diabetes Care 4: 586–94.

Axelrod, Julius and Terry D. Reisine. 1984. Stress Hormones: Their Interaction and Regulation. Science 224: 452–59.

Baer, Hans. 1982. On the Political Economy of Health. Medical Anthropology Newsletter 14: 1–17.

Baer, Hans, Merrill Singer and John H. Johnsen. 1986. Toward a Critical Medical Anthropology. Social Science and Medicine 23: 95–98.

Baker, L. and A. Barcai. 1970. Psychosomatic Aspects of Diabetes Mellitus. In Modern Trends in Psychosomatic Medicine, Vol. 2. O. W. Hill, ed. pp. 105–23. New York: Appleton-Century-Crofts.

Barglow, Peter, et al. 1986. Neuroendocrine and Psychological Factors in Childhood Diabetes Mellitus. Journal of the American Academy of Child Psychiatry 25: 785–93.

Bennett, Peter H., T. A. Burch and M. Miller. 1971. The High Prevalence of Diabetes in the Pima Indians of Arizona, U.S.A. *In* Diabetes Mellitus in Asia. Shozo Tsuji and Mashahisa Wada, eds. pp. 33–39. Amsterdam, Excerpta Medica.

Berkman, Lisa and S. Leonard Syme. 1979. Social Networks, Host Resistance and Mortality: A Nine-year Follow-up Study of Alameda County Residents. American Journal of Epidemiology 109: 186–204.

Berkowitz, Barry A., et al. 1980. Experimental Diabetes: Alternations in Circulating Dopamine-beta-hydroxylase and Norepinephrine. Journal of Pharmacology and Experimental Therapeutics 213: 18–23.

Bradley, Clare. 1979. Life Events and the Control of Diabetes Mellitus. Journal of Psychosomatic Research 23: 159–62.

Brown, Daniel E. 1981. General Stress in Anthropological Fieldwork. American Anthropologist 83: 74–92.

Bruhn, John G. 1974. Psychosocial Influences in Diabetes Mellitus. Postgraduate Medicine 56: 113–18.

Cassel, John. 1974. Psychosocial Processes and "Stress": A Theoretical Formulation. International Journal of Health Services 4: 471–82.

Cassens, Geraldine, et al. 1980. Alternations in Brain Norepinephrine Metabolism Induced by Environmental Stimuli Previously Paired with Inescapable Shock. Science 209: 1138–40.

Chakraborty, Ranajit, et al. 1986. Relationship of Prevalence of Non-insulin-dependent Diabetes Mellitus to American Indian Admixture in the Mexican-Americans of San Antonio, Texas. Genetic Epidemiology 3: 435–54.

Christensen, Niels Juel. 1974. Plasma Norepinephrine and Epinephrine in Untreated Diabetics, During Fasting and after Insulin Administration. Diabetes 23: 1–8.

Cobb, Sidney. 1976. Social Support as a Moderator of Life Stress. Psychosomatic Medicine 38: 300–14.

Cobb, Sidney, and Robert M. Rose. 1973. Hypertension, Peptic Ulcer, and Diabetes in Air Traffic Controllers. Journal of the American Medical Association 224: 489–92.

Cryer, Philip E. 1980. Physiology and Pathophysiology of the Human Sympathoadrenal Neuroendocrine System. New England Journal of Medicine 303: 344–46.

Curtis, George C., et al. 1978. Anxiety and Plasma Cortisol at the Crest of the Circadian Cycle: Reappraisal of a Classical Hypothesis. Psychosomatic Medicine 40: 368–78.

Danowski, T. S. 1963. Emotional Stress as a Cause of Diabetes Mellitus. Diabetes 12: 183–84.

Dohrenwend, Barbara Snell. 1970. Social Class and Stressful Events. *In* Psychiatric Epidemiology: Proceedings of the International Symposium. Edward H. Hare and John K. Wing, eds. pp. 313–19. New York: Oxford University Press.

_____1973. Social Status and Stressful Events. Journal of Personality and Social Psychology 28: 225–35.

Dunbar, Tony and Linda Kravitz. 1976. Hard Traveling: Migrant Farmworkers in America. Cambridge, MA: Ballinger Publishing Company.

Eaton, Cynthia. 1977. Diabetes, Culture Change, and Acculturation: A Biocultural Analysis. Medical Anthropology 1: 41–63.

Eaton, R. Philip and David S. Schade. 1978. Modulation and Implications of the Counter-regulatory Hormones: Glucagon, Catecholamines, Cortisol, and Growth Hormone. In Diabetes, Obesity and Vascular Disease, Part 1. Howard M. Katzen and Richard J. Mahler, eds. pp. 341–72. New York: Hemisphere Publishing.

Edward, Christopher and Aubrey J. Yates. 1985. The Effects of Cognitive Task Demand on Subjective Stress and Blood Glucose Levels in Diabetics and Non-diabetics. Journal of Psychosomatic Research 29: 59–69.

Elling, Ray H. 1981. Political Economy, Cultural Hegemony, and Mixes of Traditional and Modern Medicine. Social Science and Medicine 15A: 89–99.

Fatani, Hassan H., Siraj A. Mira and Ahmed G. El-Zubier. 1987. Prevalence of Diabetes Mellitus in Rural Saudi Arabia. Diabetes Care 10: 180–83.

Felig, Philip, et al. 1979. Hormonal Interactions in the Regulation of Blood Glucose. Recent Progress in Hormone Research 35: 501–32.

Fisher E. B., Jr., et al. 1982. Psychological Factors in Diabetes and its Treatment. Journal of Consulting and Clinical Psychology 50: 993–1003.

Fonner, Edwin, Jr. 1975. Mortality Differences in 1970 Texas Residents: A Descriptive Study. M.S. Thesis, School of Public Health, University of Texas Health Center at Houston.

Forsdahl, A. 1977. Are Poor Living Conditions in Childhood and Adolescence an Important Risk Factor for Arteriosclerotic Heart Disease? British Journal of Preventive Social Medicine 31: 91–95.

Frankenhaeuser, Marianne. 1971. Experimental Approaches to the Study of Human Behavior as Related to Neuroendocrine Functions. In Society, Stress and Disease. Lennart Levi, ed. pp. 22–35. London: Oxford University Press.

_____1975. Sympathetic-adrenomedullary Activity, Behavior and the Psychosocial Environment. In Research in Psychophysiology. P. H. Venables and Margaret J. Christie, eds. pp. 71–94. New York: Wiley.

_____1980. Psychoneuroendocrine Approaches to the Study of Stressful Person-environment Transactions. In Selye's Guide to Stress Research, Vol. 1. Hans Selye, ed. pp. 46–70. New York: Van Nostrans Reinhold.

Frankenhaeuser, Marianne and Anita Rissler. 1970. Effects of Punishment on Catecholamine Release and Efficiency of Performance. Psychopharmacologia 17: 378–90.

Friedland, William H. and Dorothy Nelkin. 1971. Migrant Agricultural Workers in America's Northeast. New York: Holt, Rinehart and Winston.

Gerich, J. E. and M. Lorenzi. 1978. The Role of the Autonomic Nervous System and Somatostatin in the Control of Insulin and Glucagon Secretion. In Frontiers in

Neurobiology, Vol. 5. William F. Ganong and Luciano Martini, eds. pp. 265–88. New York: Raven Press.

Giugliano, Dario. 1984. Morphine, Opioid Peptides and Pancreatic Islet Function. Diabetes Care 7: 92–98.

Glass, David C. and Jerome E. Singer. 1972. Urban Stress. New York: Academic Press.

Grant, I., et al. 1974. Recent Life Events and Diabetes in Adults. Psychosomatic Medicine 36: 121–28.

Haffner, Steven M., et al. 1986. Role of Obesity and Fat Distribution in Non-insulin-dependent Diabetes Mellitus in Mexican-Americans and Non-Hispanic Whites. Diabetes Care 9: 153–61.

Hamberg, Sol, Rosa Hendler and Robert S. Sherwin. 1980. Influence of Small Increments of Epinephrine on Glucose Tolerance in Normal Humans. Annals of Internal Medicine 93: 566–68.

Hauser, Stuart T. and Daniel Pollets. 1979. Psychological Aspects of Diabetes Mellitus: A Critical Review. Diabetes Care 2: 227–32.

Holmes, Thomas H. and Richard H. Rahe. 1967. The Social Readjustment Rating Scale. Journal of Psychosomatic Research 11: 213–18.

Jenkins, C. David, Michael W. Hurst and Robert M. Rose. 1979. Life Changes: Do People Really Remember: Archives of General Psychiatry 36: 379–84.

Kimball, Chase Patterson. 1971. Emotional and Psychosocial Aspects of Diabetes Mellitus. Medical Clinics of North America 55: 1007–18.

Knowler, William C., et al. 1981. Diabetes Incidence in Pima Indians: Contributions of Obesity and Parental Diabetes. American Journal of Epidemiology 113: 144–56.

Kuhn, Cynthia, et al. 1987. Exaggerated Peripheral Response to Catecholamines Contributes to Stress-induced Hyperglycemia in the ob/ob Mouse. Pharmacology, Biochemistry, and Behavior 26: 491–95.

La Clínica de los Campesinos. 1979. Wisconsin Migrant Health Project: FY 1978 Progress Report. Wild Rose, WI.

Lebovitz, Harold E. and Jerome M. Feldman. 1973. Pancreatic Biogenic Amines and Insulin Secretion in Health and Disease. Federation Proceedings 32: 1797–1802.

Lipowski, Z. J. 1977. Psychosomatic Medicine in the Seventies: An Overview. American Journal of Psychiatry 134: 233–43.

Locke Steven E. and Mady Hornig-Rohan. 1983. Mind and Immunity: Behavioral Immunology. New York: Institute for the Advancement of Health.

Lyndon Baines Johnson School of Public Affairs. 1977. Colonias in the Rio Grande Valley of South Texas: A Summary Report. Austin: University of Texas, Lyndon Baines Johnson School of Public Affairs.

Marmot, M. G., M. Kogevinas and M. A. Elston. 1987. Social/Economic Status and Disease. Annual Review of Public Health 8: 111–35.

Marmot, M. G., M. J. Shipley and Geoffrey Rose. 1984. Inequalities in Death: Specific Explanations of a General Pattern? The Lancet 5 May (i): 1003–6.

Mathew, Roy J., et al. 1981. Catecholamines and Dopamine-beta-hydroxylase in Anxiety. Journal of Psychosomatic Research 25: 499–504.

Mazze, Roger S., David Lucido and Harry Shamoon. 1984. Psychological and Social Correlates in Glycemic Control. Diabetes Care 7: 360–66.

McCarthy, R., C. Chiueh and Irwin Kopin. 1978. Spontaneously Hypertensive Rats: Adrenergic Hyperresponsivity to Anticipation of Electric Shock. Behavioral Biology 23: 180–88.

McWilliams, Carey. 1968. North from Mexico: The Spanish Speaking People of the United States. New York: Greenwood Press.

Mechanic, David. 1975. Some Problems in the Measurement of Stress and Social Readjustment. Journal of Human Stress 1: 43–48.

Mexican-American Policy Research Project. 1979. The Health of Mexican-Americans in South Texas. Austin: Lyndon Baines Johnson School of Public Affairs.

Morgan, Lynn M. 1987. Dependency Theory in the Political Economy of Health: An Anthropological Critique: Medical Anthropology Quarterly (n.s.) 1: 131–54.

Morsy, Soheir. 1979. The Missing Link in Medical Anthropology: The Political Economy of Health. Reviews in Anthropology 6: 349–63.

Nall, Frank C., II. and Joseph Spielberg. 1967. Social and Cultural Factors in the Response of Mexican-Americans to Medical Treatment. Journal of Health and Social Behavior 8: 299–308.

National Diabetes Data Group. 1979. Classification and Diagnosis of Diabetes Mellitus and Other Categories of Glucose Tolerance. Diabetes 28: 1038–57.

Neel, James V. 1962. Diabetes Mellitus: A "Thrifty" Genotype Rendered Detrimental by "Progress"? American Journal of Human Genetics 14: 353–62.

Nolasco, Margarita. 1978. Health and Disease in the Northern Border Area. In Modern Medicine and Medical Anthropology in the United States-Mexico Border Population. Boris Velimirovic, ed. pp. 49–59. Washington: Pan American Health Organization Publication Number 359.

Noth, R. H. and P. Mulrow. 1976. Serum Dopamine-beta-hydroxylase As an Index of Sympathetic Nervous System Activity in Man. Circulation Research 38: 2–5.

O'Dea, Kerin, R. M. Spargo and K. Akerman. 1980. Some Studies on the Relationship Between Urban Living and Diabetes in a Group of Australian Aborigines. Medical Anthropology 4: 1–20.

Paykel, Eugene S., B. Guiness and J. Gomez. 1976. An Anglo-American Comparison of the Scaling of Life Events. Journal of Medical Psychology 49: 237–47.

Peyrot, Mark and James F. McMurray, Jr. 1985. Psychosocial Factors in Diabetes Control: Adjustment of Insulin-treated Adults. Psychosomatic Medicine 47: 542–57.

Porte, Daniel, Jr. and R. Paul Robertson. 1973. Control of Insulin Secretion by Catecholamines, Stress, and the Sympathetic Nervous System. Federation Proceedings 32: 1792–96.

Rabkin, Judith G. and Elmer L. Struening. 1976. Life Events, Stress and Illness. Science 194: 1013–20.

Rivera, Tomás. 1975. When We Arrive. *In* Chicano Voices. Carlota Cárdenas de Dwyer, ed. pp. 150–54. Boston: Houghton Mifflin.

Rizza, Robert A., Lawrence J. Mandarino and John E. Gerich. 1982. Cortisol Induced Insulin Resistance in Man: Impaired Suppression of Glucose Production and Stimulation of Glucose Utilization Due to a Postreceptor Defect of Insulin Action. Journal of Clinical Endocrinology and Metabolism 54: 131–38.

Rotter, Jerome E. and David L. Rimoin. 1979. Genetic Heterogeneity in Diabetes: Difficulties in the Creation of Risk Tables. *In* Early Detection of Potential Diabetics: The Problems and the Promise. Gilman D. Grave, ed. pp. 3–39. New York: Raven Press.

Sarason, Irwin G., et al. 1985. Life Events, Social Support and Illness. Psychosomatic Medicine 47: 156–63.

Schade, David S. and R. Philip Eaton. 1980. The Temporal Relationship Between Endogenously Secreted Stress Hormones and Metabolic Decompensation in Diabetic Man. Journal of Clinical Endocrinology and Metabolism 50: 131–36.

Scheder, Jo C. 1981. Diabetes and Stress Among Mexican-American Migrants. Unpublished Ph.D. thesis, Department of Anthropology, University of Wisconsin, Madison.

Scheper-Hughes, Nancy and Margaret Lock. 1987. The Mindful Body: A Prolegomenon to Future Work in Medical Anthropology. Medical Anthropology Quarterly (n.s.) 1: 6–41.

Schmidt, Robert E., David M. Geller and Eugene M. Johnson, Jr. 1981. Characterization of Increased Plasma Dopamine-beta-hydroxylase Activity in Rats with Experimental Diabetes. Diabetes 30: 416–23.

Shamoon, Harry, Rosa Hendler and Robert S. Sherwin. 1980. Altered Responsiveness to Cortisol, Epinephrine and Glucagon in Insulin-infused Juvenile-onset Diabetes: A Mechanism for Diabetic Instability. Diabetes 29: 284–91.

Siegel, Sidney. 1956. Non-parametric Statistics for the Behavioral Sciences. New York: McGraw-Hill.

Singer, Merrill. 1986. Developing a Critical Perspective in Medical Anthropology. Medical Anthropology Quarterly 17: 128–29.

Singer, Philip. 1977. Introduction. *In* Traditional Healing: New Science or New Colonialism? Essays in Critique of Medical Anthropology. Philip Singer, ed. pp. 1–25. Buffalo, NY: The Conch Magazine, Ltd.

Skyler, Jay S. 1981. Psychological Issues in Diabetes. Diabetes Care 4: 656–57.

Slawson, Paul F., William R. Flynn and Edward J. Kollar. 1963. Psychological Factors Associated with the Onset of Diabetes Mellitus. Journal of the American Medical Association 185: 166–70.

Slesinger, Doris P. 1979. Health Needs of Migrant Workers in Wisconsin. Madison: University of Wisconsin, Department of Rural Sociology.

Society of Actuaries. 1978. Recommended Weight in Relation to Height. Bethesda, MD: Fogarty International Center, National Institutes of Health.

Stern, Michael P. 1985. Epidemiology of Diabetes and Coronary Heart Disease among Mexican-Americans. Transactions of the Association of Life Insurance Medical Directors of America 67: 79–90.

Stern, Michael P., et al. 1983. Does Obesity Explain Excess Prevalence of Diabetes Among Mexican-Americans? Diabetologia 24: 272–77.

Surwit, Richard S. 1983. Stress, Relaxation and the Behavioral Control of Blood Glucose. Unpublished manuscript, Department of Psychiatry, Duke University Medical Center.

Surwit, Richard S. and Mark N. Feinglos. 1983. The Effects of Relaxation on Glucose Tolerance in Non-insulin-dependent Diabetes. Diabetes Care 6: 176–79.

_____1987. Cognitive Functioning and Diabetes: A Reply. Diabetes Care 10: 136–37.

_____1988. Stress and Autonomic Nervous System in Type II Diabetes: A Hypothesis. Diabetes Care 11: 83–85.

Surwit, Richard S., Mark N. Feinglos and Albert W. Scovern. 1983. Diabetes and Behavior: A Paradigm for Health Psychology. American Psychologist 38: 255–62.

Szathmary, Emoke and Nasha Holt. 1983. Hyperglycemia in Dogrib Indians of the Northwest Territories, Canada: Association with Age and Centripetal Distribution of Body Fat. Human Biology 55: 493–515.

Thomas-Lycklama á Nijeholt, Geertje. 1980. On the Road for Work: Migratory Workers on the East Coast of the United States. Hingham, MA: Martinus Nijhoff Publishing.

Tokuhata, George K., et al. 1975. Diabetes Mellitus: An Underestimated Health Problem. Journal of Chronic Disease 28: 123–25.

U.S. Department of Health, Education and Welfare. 1978. Diabetes Data [compiled 1977]. Department of Health, Education and Welfare Publication No. (NIH)781468. Washington: U.S. Government Printing Office.

Usdin, Earl, Richard Kvetnansky and Irwin J. Kopin., Eds. 1976. Catecholamines and Stress. Bratislava: Proceedings of the International Symposium on Catecholamines and Stress (July 1975). Oxford: Pergamon.

Vague, Jean, et al. 1979. Clinical Features of Diabetogenic Obesity. In Diabetes and Obesity. Jean Vague and Philippe Vague, eds. pp. 127–47. Amsterdam: Excerpta Medica.

Waldhausl, Werner K., et al. 1987. Effect of Stress Hormones on Splanchnic Substrate and Insulin Disposal after Glucose Ingestion in Healthy Humans. Diabetes 36: 127–35.

Weiner, Herbert. 1981. Brain, Behavior and Bodily Disease: A Summary. In Brain, Behavior and Bodily Disease. Herbert Weiner, Michael A. Hofer, and Albert J. Stunkard, eds. pp. 335–69. New York: Raven Press.

Weinshilboum, Richard M. 1979. Serum Dopamine-beta-hydroxylase. Pharmacology Reviews 30: 133–66.

West, Kelly M. 1974. Diabetes in American Indians and Other Natives of the New World. Diabetes 23: 841–55.

Williams, Robert H. and Daniel Porte, Jr. 1974. The Pancreas. *In* Textbook of Endocrinology. 5th edition. Robert H. Williams, ed. pp. 502–626. Philadelphia: Saunders.

_____1981. The Endocrine Pancreas in Diabetes Mellitus. *In* Textbook of En-docrinology. 6th edition. Daniel Porte, Jr. and J. B. Halter, eds. pp. 716–843. Philadelphia: Saunders.

Willis, Thomas. 1679. Pharmaceutica Rationalis: Or Exercitation of the Operation of Medicines in Humane Bodies. The Works of Thomas Willis. London: Dring, Harper and Leigh.

Zimmet P., P. Taft, A.Guinea, W. Guthrie and K. Thoma. 1977. The High Prevalence of *Diabetes mellitus* on a Central Pacific Island. Diabetologia 13: 111–15.

CHAPTER 12

DIABETES AS A METAPHOR: SYMBOL, SYMPTOM, OR BOTH?

Terry Raymer

"That is the importance of language and stories: they give us a world view of who we are, they aren't just fables, we don't just 'learn a lesson' from them; it's about where our values come from and what shapes them."

> Paula Allen (Yurok, Karuk, and Hoopa) 2003, Personal interview.

"The people who occupy the top positions in science, religion, and politics have one thing in common: they are responsible for creating a technical language incomprehensible to the rest of us, so that we will cede to them our right and responsibility to think. They formulate a set of beautiful lies that lull us to sleep and distract us from our troubles, eventually depriving us of all our rights—including increasingly the right to a livable world…"

> Vine Deloria, c. 1997 Interview with Derrick Jensen, *The Sun*.

Summary of Chapter 12. The prevalence of diabetes is now increasing in *all* populations around the world. However, it disproportionately affects those populations not originally habituated to a more "western" lifestyle. While both touted and sought after, no substantial proof of a wholly "genetic" cause exists. In this discussion, I explore an empirical and intuitive view that the increasing incidence and prevalence of diabetes does not indicate a genetic or physiologic "aberration" of Indigenous Peoples. Rather, the burgeoning prevalence of diabetes is both representative and symptomatic of the disruption in the physiology *and* cultures of Indigenous Peoples around the world. Not only were traditional lifestyles physiologically adapted to a wide variety of environments around the world, but many aspects of these nations' cultures facilitated coping with the stresses and trauma of everyday life as well. Ironically, the erosion of the traditions and cultures devastated the ability for many Indigenous Peoples to weather the very stresses disrupting them.

Although somewhat unconventional, my perspective is based on knowledge gained from various colleagues as well as my experiences in a community of American Indians in Northwest California where I work. For contextual purposes, an overview of the epidemiological data precedes a brief discussion of current evidence for the "causes" of diabetes. I then describe how my experience with patients and the work of a medical anthropologist in the population where I practice have affected my views. These influences brought about a change in my approach to *all* patients. It has likewise al-

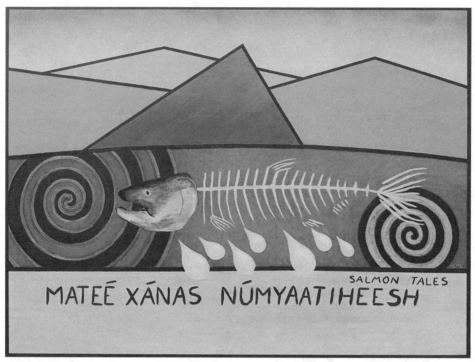

Artwork by Alme H. Allen, Karuk/Yurok artist from Northwstern California in response to the salmon kill that occured in the of Winter 2002 on the Klamath River resulting in the death of over 33,000 adult native salmon returning to their spawning grounds. The title is from a Karuk prayer and translates to "May It Be That We Live A Long Time Together." Acrylic on plywood c.2002. Private collection.

tered my attitudes toward diabetes and diseases in general. I go on to extrapolate how ideas born in my experiences can allow our society to view the epidemic of diabetes differently. Armed with this new perspective, I ask if there are different avenues we can explore to begin stemming the rising tide of diabetes by working with communities to apply traditional practices to the template of "modern" life. Finally I pose a deeper question: given the understanding of what needs to be accomplished, what will catalyze our actions toward those ends? Comprehending the relationships between the importance of reviving devastated traditions and cultures, the importance of a sense of "belonging," i.e. a spiritual knowledge (for lack of a better term) of one's place in their own world, and present day problems of physical and mental disease may help change our approach to diabetes and the health issues of our communities in general.

ఆ ఆ ఆ

Introduction

About five years ago someone asked me, "What's the most important problem in regard to the issues of diabetes today?" "Spirituality!" I spontaneously and quite unexpectedly answered. Trained in the Western scientific tradition and not a particularly religious creature, nothing had prepared me for the lessons and obstacles that would bring that particular sentiment bubbling to the surface. This chapter focuses on the empirical and intuitive process of my experience, infused with some acquired knowledge from the substantial body of literature on diabetes that led me to a new perspective on how to approach my patients and the escalating problem of diabetes.

In her fine book *Illness As Metaphor*, Susan Sontag (1979) disabuses us of the notion that illness is a metaphor in regards to the individual. Her thesis explores the concept that illness is neither a romantic representation of artistic temperament, nor is it the manifestation of self-punishment or years of repressed nature of the individual with the disease. In viewing diabetes as a metaphor, I do not wish to take issue with this premise. Rather, I have come to understand that diabetes represents just one dimension of how our lives have veered so far off course from the way our respective physiologies had harmoniously developed within specific environments over the millennia. For those populations not originally habituated to a more "western" lifestyle, it is just one more manifestation of how western society has insinuated itself between numerous Indigenous Peoples and the specific cultures they have honed for generations. And while the concept of "westernization" may be both vague and multifaceted, I think most would accept that the process has resulted in profound psychosocial and socio-economic changes in the cultures of Indigenous Peoples around the world. Any further discussion of "westernization" or "modernization" is beyond the scope of this chapter and has been explored by other authors (McGarvey 1999).

Throughout human history, thousands of culturally and ethnically diverse peoples have occupied the various continents and thrived in the particular environs unique to each location. This is not a romantic notion: for thousands of years numerous Indigenous Peoples around the world lived in balance with a wide variety of climates and geographies. For instance, peoples of what is now California used locally available resources to both make sense of and create the world in which they lived, resorting to their own cosmologies or world theories to help explain both the joys and the adversities of their lives. Surely, they encountered disease, misfortune, trauma, and war. Like many other Indigenous Peoples, they faced natural catastrophes, at times having to migrate, innovate, and adapt. At times, they most certainly were destructive either to their environs or to themselves. The burgeoning incidence of depression, substance abuse, and chronic diseases including diabetes, particularly in the adolescents, however, seems to be unprecedented in history. Therefore, diabetes can be viewed as a symbol for the disruption of many Indigenous Peoples' lives, as well as a symptom of that very same process.

Genetics and Lifestyle

Indeed, diabetes is increasing in both so-called developed and developing nations throughout the world. Among the numerous epidemiological studies and predictions, there is a projected 170% increase in diabetes in developing countries in the next 25 years (King et al. 1998). Although prevalence rates are increasing in all populations, Indigenous Peoples presently have the highest overall rates. Perhaps they represent the "canaries in the coal mine" rather than collectively somehow genetically predestined to get diabetes. The actual reasons for the increase in type 2 diabetes remain both elusive and complex; our work toward a complete understanding of this will no doubt continue for some time to come. However, several observations belie a simple "genetic" causation. Fifty to sixty years ago, type 2 diabetes was nearly nonexistent in American Indian populations. Lest we think this was merely a problem of poor diagnostic abilities or case finding, consider that type 2 diabetes prevalence increased 106% in the 15–19 year old American Indian/Alaskan Native populations alone from 1990-2001 (Rios Burrows et al. 2002). Geneticists understand that the basic structure of the human genome has not changed substantially for thousands of years. How can we reconcile this as a *genetic* problem?

The well-known case of two ancestrally similar peoples having two very divergent experiences with diabetes serves as an example to contradict a simple genetic explanation. The Pima of Arizona have very high rates of diabetes, while their ancestrally (i.e. genetically) common counterparts in the Sierra Madre Mountains in Mexico have less than one-sixth the prevalence of type 2 diabetes in their adult population. The population living in Mexico practices a more traditional lifestyle and has not been sequestered on a reservation or subjected to most of the changes characteristic of an intruding Western civilization. Several years ago at a conference I attended, a researcher I respect greatly said of the Mayacabo Pima living in the Sierra Madre with the same genetic ancestry as the Pima in Arizona, "They eat a starvation diet, no one can live like that." Yet they do. I do not know these people, but they survive, practice more traditional lifestyles and maintain a life coherent with their particular physiology. More importantly, they have been allowed to carry on their lives without most of the culturally traumatic intrusions the Pima in Arizona have endured.

This example presents an obvious dilemma: if the cause of diabetes is due to a genetic "defect," then how could it have become so prevalent in the past 50–60 years? While a "thrifty gene" has been postulated (Wendorf & Glodfine 1991; Neel 1982) but not found, this search may be quite off the point at this crucial time: we may expend terrific resources searching for a genetic holy grail that we could direct toward true prevention. If those with lightly pigmented skin live years out in the equatorial sun, many are apt to develop skin cancers, some more virulent than others (Elwood 2000, 2002); is there something inherently wrong with their genes for skin color? Or, has their environment become disadvantageous toward a characteristic which was previously benign or possibly beneficial? We may make efforts to stop depletion of the ozone layer, educate folks not to go out during peak ultra violet (UV) occurrence, wear appropriate attire, and offer any other preventive advice we know will make a difference. But we would not go looking for a genetic solution to the problem, and we certainly would not consider the person with the light skin as having something inherently wrong with their DNA. Lung cancer in people who smoke serves as a similar example: some may be "genetically" susceptible to lung cancer, but doesn't it make more sense to get folks to stop smoking?

Without further arguing the merits of "thrifty gene" and other such theories, I would at least posit that using such explanations with our patients to explain their illness is not helpful and likely harmful. It may even cause a kind of "genetic phobia" (Ferreira 1998 and chapters 3 & 18 in this book). Similarly, it serves no real benefit in how we view our patients while trying to care for them in a "holistic" sense. Arguably, there is a susceptibility that is a combination of both phenotype and genotype present in certain peoples around the world, yet even the use of a genetic explanation in our "internal language" hinders our own understanding of this disorder in relation to our patients. If we do not proffer genetic explanations to our patients, yet continue to harbor these notions, I fear we will only perpetuate some of the negative and counter-productive approaches to dealing with this ailment. We need a substantive change in our own perception of diabetes as health care providers and health educators if we are to shape future changes in health care delivery. We must ask ourselves how to accomplish this both on a professional and societal level.

So what about "lifestyle?" First, it is well documented that many lifestyle factors may be related to diabetes, especially among Indigenous Peoples. These include, but are not limited to:

- Excessive overall calorie load;
- Increase in saturated fats and trans-fatty acids;
- Excessive carbohydrate loads, particularly in so called "low-fat" diets;
- Elevated Body Mass Index (BMI, a measure of proportion of weight to height);
- Decrease in overall physical fitness and activity;
- Increasing amounts of "screen time" (TV, computer, etc.);
- Machine governed mobility (not only the automobile, but elevators, escalators, etc.);
- Marked changes in the school environment (e.g. money from soda sponsors, loss of physical activity programs);
- Unseen/unknown influences from "modern" and urban environments; the urban rates of diabetes are increasing faster than rural (King et al. 1998); and
- Smoking (unknown as yet if second hand smoke carries similar risks).

The Diabetes Prevention Program (DPP) showed that the same tenants used to treat diabetes, a relatively modest weight loss and an increase in regular aerobic activity, will prevent or forestall its onset (Knowler et al. 2002). The message seems much less complex than we try to make it. What if we employed these tenants early on in life? What if we had a national campaign akin to that used to curb smoking? Physical activity in mainstream American society has taken a backseat to mental activity. Most states do not require physical education in the schools and the data on television watching and increasing Body Mass Index in children is well known. Our "sedan and screen" lifestyle has become the major enemy of true "physical fitness." Physical activity to treat and prevent diabetes is not a punishment for having been "lazy." Computers, televisions, cars, and other conveniences like elevators are not inherently "bad." In the past, people generally did not "exercise" for health's sake; it was merely a daily living necessity.

So, it is simply the case that our bodies work better and more efficiently when we maintain *any* regular physical activity. Yet there are natural benefits to our emotional and spiritual health as well. To understand this is the easy part. We all know by now physical activity is beneficial; how and why we choose to incorporate it into our lives is the challenge. The juggernaut of mainstream American society propels us away from what is inherently a gift to our overall well being born out of the necessity to be physically active. At this point we must ask: why would we even choose to be more physically active? The section entitled *Complex and Obscure: Stress, Depression, and Cultural Trauma* explores some possible answers to this question.

Taking Food for "Granted?"

The weight and nutrition side of the equation is highly charged and I believe, unnecessarily controversial and artificially complex, as explored in many chapters of this book. We expend terrific amounts of resource and energy in over-dramatizing this discussion. We simply have ready access to excessive amounts of the wrong of foods. People like and eat fat for a reason. During times of need, it was the bulwark against caloric privation. It tastes good to us. The complex part is how, when we are stressed or otherwise dissociated from our own cultural context, we use food for some other purpose than sustaining and nourishing our body. To magnify this problem, western society in general has the abundance and separation from how food is actually obtained to allow us to take food for granted. In many societies, including most if not all American Indian peoples, eating was often (and still is in many cases) a ritualized and sacred event and closely linked to the origins of the food; the nature of obtaining food remained important from generation to generation. Gratefulness for having food was also expressed in a variety of ways. There was a spiritual context for eating: sustenance and nourishment outweighed satiety and gratification, as discussed in Part 2 of this volume. Resuming this context for food may be the only means to avoid the patterns of consumption so pervasive in our society today.

The histories of Indigenous Peoples around the world are replete with examples of how food is honored as a gift, and how dangerous it is to abuse that gift as well as the means by which it is obtained. In the Karuk, Tolowa, Weeot, Hoopa, and Yurok American Indian communities in northern California, songs, stories and dances incorporate the importance of gratitude and honoring gifts from the creator (Paula Allen, personal interview, Feb. 2003). Despite significant language differences, many of the mythical histories and ceremonies with their incumbent connotations are similar from community to community. Like many Northwest nations, salmon, local flora and fauna, the ocean, and rivers play key roles in their cosmologies. The following narrative certainly has many nuances and meanings, but it also embodies some aspects of gratitude, sharing, selflessness, community, and what those concepts mean to the survival and well being of a society.

The Greedy Father, as told by Paula Allen (Yurok, Karuk, and Hoopa)

This story is from a time long ago, the time of the First People.

There was famine in the village and families were not getting enough food to eat. The father and mother were worried about their children not getting enough to eat. The father told his family that he would fish tomorrow. The family went to bed that night with nothing to eat.

The next morning at dawn, the father left the village and walked to the family's fishing place to fish for salmon. He put his net made of iris fibers into the water and waited. After a while, he saw the trigger on the net quiver. He had caught a salmon!

He knew he should take the salmon home to his hungry family, but he was so hungry he decided to eat some. He cleaned the salmon, and carefully set the tail aside. He then built a fire and he cooked up that salmon. Then he sat there and at the entire fish!

He then realized what he had done, so he picked up the salmon tail and started home. As he approached the village he begin yelling to his family, "Here family, I have brought home a salmon tail, there were a lot of fish beggars on the trail home."

"Hurray, hurray" his children yelled, "we are going to have a salmon tail for dinner." The family was so happy to have food and that night they went to bed with their bellies satisfied.

The next morning the father again set out to fish for his family. And again, he caught a salmon. He knew he should take the whole fish home to his family, but he let his hunger get the best of him. Again, he carefully cleaned the fish and set aside the tail…and he again cooked and ate that whole salmon.

This time, he didn't feel as much guilt, after all his family was getting the salmon tail to eat and that part was really good. So as he approached the village he yelled, "Here family, I have brought home a salmon tail, there were a lot of fish beggars on the trail home."

His children were again happy, but as his wife prepared the fish for their evening meal she wondered if her husband was being truthful. The next morning as her husband set off to go fish for the family, she decided to follow him. She watched as he fished, and was shocked to see him clean, cook and then eat the entire salmon.

She quickly turned and walked back to the village. She gathered up her children and told them they had to leave because their father wasn't sharing the food with them.

Soon after, the father came into the village yelling, "Here family, I have brought home a salmon tail, there were a lot of fish beggars on the trail home."

There was silence. So he entered the family dwelling, again saying, "Here family, I have brought home a salmon tail, there were a lot of fish beggars on the trail home."

He looked around and saw they weren't there. He came out of the house, and noticed up on the hill his family was leaving the village. He yelled to them but they just kept going.

He followed after them. The wife yelled down to him, "You will eat alone because you would not share your food with your family." And they continued to travel up the hill, away from the village, and the husband followed. As he got closer to them he yelled for them to stop. But they kept going, the wife yelling to him, "You are going to do nothing but this: you will eat only mud from the creeks from now on because you were greedy, while your family will sit in front of rich people."

He was so upset he didn't know what to do. He thought, I will grab my youngest child and then they will stop. As he lunged for the little one, they turned into bear lily or bear grass plant. So then he lunged for his other child, and they turned into a hazel bush. He reached out for his wife and she turned into a pine tree.

And with that, he turned into a small gray bird, the moss eater, who eats from the mud next to creeks. And his family became the materials that are woven into the beautiful baskets used during ceremonial time. And during the deerskin dance, his family sits lined up in front of all the rich people.

In discussing this narrative, Paula Allen (personal interview, February, 2003) points out the importance of *sharing* the food, not simply the value of the food itself. She

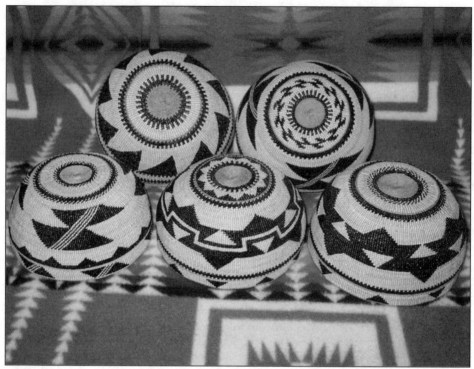

Yurok Women's Basket Hats made by Paula Allen's great-grandmother, Lena Reed McCovey.

notes the portrayal of the sacred relationships of the family and the inextricable links to the sharing of the food. There is a trust in breaking bread together and this was of particular importance with a perceived enemy. Sharing food involved a "process and a prayer" and this made violating trust much more difficult. Food meant more than simply assuaging hunger pains.

Paula Allen elaborated further in our discussion:

> In the past, before you went fishing, before you went hunting, you prayed and you fasted; taking that food was not simply to 'feed your hunger.' There was an intention, a consciousness of the process. Someone once explained it like this to me: when you stop to eat and actually think about it nourishing your body, it is not just eating to push away your hunger. The food is going to break down and nourish you and allow you to be alive. With Indian people traditionally, I do not necessarily think they even scrutinized it that explicitly, but they understood the spiritual aspect; and when they are doing our Jump Dance and our Deerskin Dance ceremonies, we pray for the food and we thank the creator for all the food that we have and we pray that we will have enough food for the coming year. So, there was a real intimate relationship with food.

She went on to explain that the Karuk word "ama" is fish or salmon,

> …but it really translates just to food…even when we say come to eat, we use that word for salmon and food interchangeably. So you can see the importance and the relationship we had with those things by how they were used in

the language. That is the importance of language and stories: they give us a world view of who we are, they aren't just fables, we don't just 'learn a lesson' from them; it's about where our values come from and what shapes them.

Or, I might add, what *deeper* truth might be learned from them?

Again, my purpose is not to romanticize any particular lifestyle. Yet we have lost so much of the connection between where our food comes from and its actual value, we have lost the awareness of what putting certain foods into our body means for the process of nourishing and maintaining our vibrancy. And when we succumb to corporate "supersizing" of our portions, allow ourselves to be fooled by "no-fat" calorie delivery devices, and ignore the simple correlation between elevated body mass index and high calorie diets, we do so with predictable results: western society in general is one of ever increasing unhealthy body weight. While I cannot predict all it will take to regain some of these "connections," we may begin by questioning the profit-driven calorie assault on society, especially on the youth. For example, schools allow Pepsi and Coke to vie as sponsors, and have gone so far as to expel students for questioning loyalty. What is nutritious about a Coke compared to a Pepsi? To quote a bit of Mark Morford (2001), a columnist for the on-line news magazine *SF Gate*:

> We allow…[the] unimaginably massive, world-dominated junk-food restaurant behemoth conglomerate[s] with enough marketing power to convince people that iceberg lettuce served in a plastic cup is a tasty idea, instead of being honestly and healthily pumped full of only the finest in mass produced, chemically injected, assembly line greaseball meat and sugar bombs and imitation flavorings and mutilated beef by-products the true sources of which the squads on Crime Scene Investigation probably couldn't trace.

Surely, this is a humorous caricature of the situation, but the fact is, we consume too much saturated fat and we eat more densely caloric carbohydrate than our systems require. Moreover, we do so at the expense of fruits, vegetables, and whole grain foods. Consider this from a caloric standpoint alone: McDonald's original burger, fries, and 12 ounce Coke contained 590 calories (a goodly sized portion of questionable health value). Today, a Super Size "Value" Meal delivers 1,550 calories. Such densely caloric diets with high saturated fat and trans fatty acid content may exceed the status of "unhealthy," they may actually poison certain physiologies. There is evidence that when some animals eat a diet high in saturated fat, amyloid deposits (a protein-like substance) develop in the insulin-producing beta cells of the pancreas. This supplants their insulin-producing capability and hence insulin reserve (Hull et al. 2003). One crucial and well known feature of type 2 diabetes is the loss of insulin reserve under conditions of increased demand. This can even occur in relatively "lean" folks with insulin resistance. Certainly it is possible that some ethnicities may be predisposed to this, but it does not make them genetically "defective."

While no one disputes the notion that an elevated body mass index is related to diabetes and insulin resistance, even this concept is subject to further scrutiny in light of at least one epidemiological study (Stern et al. 1983). In a subsequent related paper, "Elevated Incidence of Type 2 Diabetes in San Antonio, Texas, Compared With That of Mexico City," the risk of diabetes in the oldest cohort of Mexico City residents did *not* increase as the weight category increased from normal to "overweight," to "obese" as it did in the same age group in San Antonio (Burke et al. 2001). This was not adequately explained by higher case fatality rates or access to health care. The authors (Burke et al. 2001) speculate that this has to do with the practice of living a more traditional lifestyle; "Mexico appears to be in the midst of a transition from a traditional to a 'Westernized culture,' primarily affecting younger individuals, with the oldest individuals having lived most of their lives before this transition." Perhaps other factors are not taken into consideration in this kind of research related to the historical context of contact between Indians and Non-Indians in the United States and Mexico. Whatever it indicates, it continues to call into question standard notions about lifestyle and diabetes.

Finally, two final notes need highlighting in regards to nutrition. Certainly, we cannot ignore that economic factors inform food choices. In the United States, American Indians have had their usual means of obtaining food stripped from them in many ways both obvious and insidious and given instead commodities high in fat and starch content by the government. Even after no longer receiving or needing commodities, generations have had their perceptions and concepts of nutrition deeply altered by the distribution of this type of food. And lastly, I believe we must ask: what would compel more physiologically susceptible folks to eat such foods in the first place? Perhaps stated a bit simplistically, there is solace in eating for the depressed and oppressed, and additional solace in eating the very foods that may be harmful. For example, overeating among adolescents has been shown to be associated with negative psychological experiences (Ackard 2003). In some instances, it may be preferable to other, more destructive means of coping with intense, unremitting stress and there is physiologic evidence to support this (Dallman et al. 2003). Ann Bullock, a physician working with the Cherokee of North Carolina has mined the literature in depth and detail in this regard as it relates to the etiology of diabetes in American Indian populations. I discuss her exploration of this subject further in the section on stress and cultural trauma.

Gestational Factors

Somewhere around 4% of all pregnancies are complicated by gestational diabetes; these rates vary depending on the population studied and are as high as 15% in some American Indian/Alaska Native and Canadian First Nations populations (Benjamin et al. 1993, Engelgau et al. 1988, Rodrigues et al. 1999). Gestational diabetes mellitus (GDM) has many of the characteristics of type 2 diabetes and these women are at significant risk for developing type 2 diabetes later in life (Dornhorst and Rossi 1998). This is particularly true in American Indian populations (Benjamin et al. 1993). Moreover, the offspring of mothers with GDM are at increased risk of developing type 2 diabetes, glucose intolerance, and an elevated BMI as adolescents or young adults (Gillman et al. 2003; Pettit & Jovanovic 2001; Pettit et al. 1993). But an abnormal intrauterine environment may result in more insidious consequences for the future. Babies that are both large for gestational age (LGA or "macrosomic," which is not simply an overweight infant, rather an infant with a specific fat distribution and body-type) and small for gestational age (SGA) are at increased risk for diabetes, cardiovascular disease and features of the metabolic syndrome (Gillman et al. 2003; Lawlor et al. 2002; Mogren et al. 2001, Pettit and Jovanovic 2001; Valdez et al. 1994; Veening et al. 2002). Studies such as The San Antonio Heart Study have helped us recognize the particular risk for SGA babies, a somewhat unexpected finding (Valdez et al. 1994). To make a very complicated and not yet well-understood picture immediately accessible, it seems that the baby's intrauterine milieu helps determine the phenotype for life, i.e. how the genes are expressed, not the genetic make up per se. In other words, your intrauterine environment may permanently affect your physiology. I do not intend to demean these aspects of diabetes risk by distilling them to a few sentences; there is much in the literature discussing these topics and I think they are widely recognized as potential preventable risk factors.

So, while it seems that some physiologies are more or less susceptible to an altered intrauterine environment, the subsequent risk of diabetes in the infant who is LGA or SGA is not based solely on their respective "genotype." Many factors can affect the growth and development of an infant: nutritional status, smoking, disease processes like diabetes, maternal hypertension, and pre-eclampsia. While nutrition may contribute to SGA outcomes, this particular factor alone poses some ambivalence of effect as evidenced by the studies of the Siege at Leningrad compared to the Dutch Hunger Winter: those SGA babies from the Leningrad study were *no* more likely to develop glucose intolerance and features of the metabolic syndrome compared to a cohort before the war (Stanner et al. 1997). Yet those from the Dutch Hunger Winter *did* have increases in glucose intolerance, especially when nutritionally deprived in late gestation (Ravelli et al. 1998). However, all these factors may contribute in one way or another to the small for gestational babies who are later at risk for both diabetes and cardiovascular disease in ways we do not yet understand (Lawlor et al. 2002; Mogren et al. 2001; Power and Jeffris 2002; Valdez et al. 1994; Veening et al. 2002). Most importantly, given the possibility of certain genes being turned on or off based early physiologic experiences resulting in a predetermined phenotype, the environment one is subsequently exposed to may further determine how diabetes and the metabolic syndrome may manifest themselves in those individuals. So a small for gestational age child may grow up in relative poverty with socioeconomic forces steering them toward the path of diabetes, rather than away from it.

While no randomized control study has shown us that strict control of gestational diabetes will prevent diabetes later in life (nor would one likely be performed because of the ethical nature of doing such a study), it is presently accepted that rigorous control is the standard and may be beneficial in this regard. The factors that lead to intrauterine stresses on the fetus and fetal malnutrition certainly require addressing, yet this is a very complex issue and not simply one of making sure the mother gets adequate calories. Preventing such problems in the pregnancy and attending to the subsequent compounding socioeconomic factors will necessarily require a tremendous effort and significant resources. However, this topic is well beyond the scope of this discussion and is addressed by other authors (Benyshek et al. 2001). I do not think it is controversial *that* we must endeavor on this course, but the approach we take will be crucial. Our experiences and work in this field have lead some of us to believe we must consider the additional problems of chronic stress, depression, and cultural trauma as "risk factors" for diabetes as we set about this task. This is what we will explore next.

Complex and Obscure: Stress, Depression, and Cultural Trauma

While the factors previously discussed account for a substantial increase in diabetes in general, they may not completely account for the increasing rates of diabetes in American Indian populations or for the prevalence increases in many Indigenous Peoples throughout the world. The evidence that chronic stress, depression, and related "psychosocial factors" (again, for lack of a better term) have influenced the increasing rates of diabetes, the metabolic syndrome and cardiovascular disease continues to accumulate from epidemiological and neurobiological literature (Bjorntorp 1991a,b; Bjorntorp et al. 1999; Brunner et al. 2002; Chrousos 2000; Eaton 2002; Eaton et al. 1996; Keltikangas-Jarvinen et al. 1998; Obici et al. 2002; Rosmond et al. 1998; Taborsky et al. 1998). In her dissertation *Sweet Tears, Bitter Pills,* Mariana Ferreira (1996; see Ch. 3 in this book) explores how disruption of the normal fabric of culture has affected health and healing among the Yurok people in northern California. This study represents a story that has unfolded hundreds, perhaps thousands of times throughout the history of Indigenous Peoples as they encounter and cope with the intrusion of "western civilization." Indeed some of the ideas contained and expressed here were born out of that study. Prior to this, I viewed diabetes as largely a medical problem resulting from a mismatch of genetics and lifestyle. After reading *Sweat Tears, Bitter Pills* I began relating to my experience with patients and their families in a very different way. This allowed me to begin the work of changing my perceptions to address this ailment (and others) on an individual, community, and a societal level.

Several years later, after contemplating many interpersonal experiences with patients in relation to Mariana Ferreira's concepts, I heard Ann Bullock speak informally on this topic at a meeting of the Indian Health Service Area Diabetes Consultants. Ann Bullock is a physician who works with the Eastern Band of Cherokee in North Carolina and has arguably done more within the Indian Health Service to dispel the notion that diabetes is either the result of unfortunate genetics or simply a "bad" lifestyle. Dr. Bullock has marshaled a body of literature giving support to the views expressed in *Sweet Tears, Bitter Pills.* So what plausible evidence exists to support the notion that stress, depression, and cultural trauma might contribute to the astounding increase in type 2 diabetes, related diseases, and similar kinds of chronic conditions? It is impressive.

The concept that stress and social conditions may have profound effects on a population's health is no longer a novel nor abstract hypothesis, as shown in several chapters in this volume. In the study on Socioeconomic Factors, Health Behaviors, and Mortality, Lantz et al (1998) reveal that smoking, alcohol consumption, body mass index, and physical activity level explain only about 12–13% of the increased mortality risk in people with lower levels of education and income. While it is true these risk factors are more prevalent among those with more restricted socioeconomic status, they simply don't account for the premature morbidity and mortality found in these groups. In the companion commentary to this article, Dr. Redford Williams (1998) whose work in this arena is substantial, points out the logical inconsistency in our present approach to many of these diseases. To put it more bluntly, we simply cannot view "if we just get those poor, uneducated folks to eat better and exercise" as the treatment paradigm for the communities we serve. Heim et al. (2000) also showed quite convincingly in a recent study in the Journal of the American Medical Association (JAMA) that women with childhood abuse exhibit persisting alterations in their Hypothalamic-Pituitary-Adrenal (HPA) axis. There are other recent studies as well requiring us to question the notion that providing the socio-economically disadvantaged with a more healthy lifestyle will set them on a level playing field in regards to chronic disease outcomes (Chang et al. 2002; Poulton et al. 2002; Rozanski et al. 1999; Streeck-Fischer & van der Kolk 2002; Wong et al. 2002). Moreover, these pervasive, chronic, and abnormal life stresses consistently result in long term detrimental health effects, particularly in the absence of culture and community which may attenuate or negate those effects (Blaisdell 1993; Ferreira 1996, 1998, and in this book). The "Pima Pride" pilot study reveals ways in which we may start to reverse this trend and reinforces the relevance of doing so (Narayan et al. 1998).

Objective evidence also questions our current view and approach from a neurobiological perspective. In looking at Hemoglobin A1c (a measure of the body's ambient blood glucose for the past 2-3 months) in relation to social and environmental stress, Daniel et al. (1999) compared Caucasian as well as Greek migrants (presumably already to some degree "westernized") in Australia to several Indigenous Peoples from Australia (including Torres Strait Islanders) and Canada. This study certainly was more "hypothesis-generating rather than conclusive" as pointed out by the authors, but some connection seems to exist between the A1c levels and the effects of westernization on these populations whether they had diabetes, impaired glucose tolerance, or normal glucose tolerance. There are a number of studies and investigations relevant to insulin resistance and glucose metabolism and the role of stress induced activation of the sympathetic nervous system acutely and the neuroendocrine system of the HPA axis chronically (Bjorntorp et al. 1999; Brunner et al. 2002; Chrousos 2000; Keltikangas-Jarvinen et al. 1998; Obici et al. 2002; Taborsky et al. 1997). Many important relationships exist between stress and significant health factors such as smoking, depression, carbohydrate metabolism, and visceral fat deposition (Bjorntorp 1991a,b; Brunner et al. 2002; Rosmond et al. 1998). Visceral or "central adiposity" is widely accepted as a risk factor for diabetes and one of the key features of the metabolic syndrome, which is also associated with increased risk for cardiovascular disease and is usually present in type 2 diabetes (Bjorntorp 1991b). The metabolic syndrome itself is often evident long before the blood sugars actually begin to rise in those affected and cardiovascular disease may manifest before glucose intolerance or overt diabetes develops. Epidemiological evidence is also building for depression as an antecedent risk factor for diabetes, not a consequence of it (Eaton 2002; Eaton et al. 1996). In the past, many of us professionally supposed: "well, if I had diabetes, I'd probably be depressed as well." But once again, the picture seems to be much more complicated, although depression certainly has its own deleterious effect on the course of diabetes (Mazze et al. 1984; van der Does et al. 1996).

While it is important to point out support in the literature for the link between disorders like diabetes and depression, stress, and cultural trauma, my main purpose here is to explore some of our experiences as providers of medical care in these communities as it relates to our current knowledge. How might we gain a new perspective that allows us to better care for our patients? Indeed, in what ways can we work with our communities to repair the torn fabric of their respective cultures so that not only is there improved health, but also a significantly improved overall quality of life?

In my discussion with Paula Allen (personal interview, February 2003) after she related the story of The Greedy Father, reproduced above, I asked in what possible "detrimental" way has the relationship with food changed with the intrusion of western lifestyles and the disruption of her own culture. She conveyed the experiences of her two grandmothers and how their relationship to food changed with the some of the traumas they endured. Both grandmothers were sent to boarding schools. Her paternal grandmother signed the initial charter in the early 1970s for the clinic where Paula and I work: United Indian Health Services. This grandmother was widely active and influential in her community, and she had a deep sense of cultural pride. But Paula observed that despite all this, she did not have a way to express her sense of pride in her culture nor her self-esteem. Indeed, Paula states, "She was cut off from that…she was made to feel that she *was* less than other people." The alchemy of her diminished sense of self-esteem along with other factors such as the Great Depression and its attendant privation resulted in an altered relationship with food: it transformed food into something that was as much a comfort as it was nourishment and sustenance. Food as comfort may have had special significance in this regard, especially for women. It is much safer and more acceptable to eat than drink alcohol or act out in other, more destructive ways. In a sense, we may view this as a survival strategy in the face of daunting psychosocial circumstances.

Paula Allen then observed something reminiscent of Mariana Ferreira's work, a kind of corollary to the notion of food as self-comforting: "as a people, you can look at all of us like that, we could provide some comfort to our families by cooking for and feeding them, and we used what we had. That was an ingrained traditional concept: you used what you have." Ingredients that became readily available were white flour and lard, among other similar non-traditional foods. Paula goes on to describe how eating is so much a part of the culture, the importance of sharing food with others, and it appears critical to never "cut that piece of it off." The idea isn't so much of eating, but rather how relationships are nurtured around the social aspects of eating: "it can be a good thing, but because of what we have endured, the result isn't always physically healthy."

However, we know the story is so much more complex than that. Paula Allen then related another aspect of how cultural trauma might impinge on the advent of diabetes in her own community. Her maternal grandmother was sent to boarding school as well, but at the younger age of four, in part to accompany her sister who was made to go. I think it is difficult for us to understand or even imagine the effect that this kind of experience may have had on the generations of children subjected to it. Moreover, I had the privilege to see both of Paula's grandmothers in a capacity of physician here at UIHS. Without the intention of judgment or stereotype, I would observe that while one of her grandmothers might ostensibly fit the categorical "body type" of one with type 2 diabetes, the other was relatively lean. The point here is that the common thread is not "bad" eating habits or simply a sedentary lifestyle (I knew at least one of them to be quite physically active even in her later years), but rather a radical intrusion into their historical family and social structures. Both had type 2 diabetes.

These two elders' life histories do not "prove" anything, but they say much. Similar experiences have occurred over and over again in various permutations, each with its own set of circumstances, throughout Indigenous Peoples around the world. Many of us now believe it is possible to correlate these common experiences with the higher rates of diabetes, depression, alcoholism, traumatic death, and some other chronic diseases in the communities we serve. One could posit that the disruption of culture and social fabric leads to physiologic disturbances by way of neuroendocrine and sympathetic effects, as discussed earlier in this essay and in several chapters in this book. Moreover, intergenerational effects may be propagated in numerous ways including through the loss of what was normal parental mirroring and affect-reflections for any given society (Gergely and Watson 1996). Even if one rejects such theories, I believe it is still logical to see that if generations of children are taken from their parents, it is likely this will have a profound effect on subsequent generations in ways we may never imagine much less comprehend. Couple this with years of other historical traumas, racism, and poverty as well as the abuse and neglect that are so often a result of these societal poisons and it seems impossibly naïve to think that trying to convince those we serve to "exercise and eat right" will ever affect an appreciable change.

I have talked with many patients with similar stories to those of Paula Allen's grandmothers who understand their own illnesses through the lens of their past. Some of these folks have resigned themselves to the idea of a pre-destined, genetic cause. The sense of an inferior nature at the core, as well as an attendant feeling of guilt and shame often accompanies this resignation. But many individuals and communities are standing against the ideas of purely genetic and "bad" lifestyle causes to change the course of their destinies, not only in regards to diabetes, but the survival of their cultures and traditions. While avoiding the pitfalls of "romanticizing" a traditional lifestyle (few of us would choose a pre-electric, pre-automobile return to the wilderness under any circumstances!), many communities are beginning to regain their cultural practices and knowledges. This is evident in the Yurok, Tolowa, Wiyot, Karuk, Hoopa, and many other California Indian communities with participation in traditional ceremonies, such as dances and games, gathering of food as well as materials for medicines and their arts, basketry and weaving, in conjunction with many other community oriented activities. While we as health care providers may not have the knowledge to effect some of these changes, we can honor this effort and attempt to facilitate this process for individuals and the communities we serve. We can work in the spirit of cooperation toward these goals and incorporate fresh perspectives into our practices. This will allow us to eschew sterile concepts of "non-compliance" and "denial" in dealing with our patients; hopefully, it will allow us to gain new insights into the difficulties faced by those we serve.

So what does the notion of "spirituality" have to do with these current issues surrounding diabetes? Time and again those of us working in this field have observed that there is not a lack of knowledge of what must be done to treat and prevent diabetes. But the legacy of historical trauma superimposed on the present day problems of poverty, racism, and a myriad other psychological and socioeconomic problems preclude simple answers and approaches. Indeed, our futile endeavors to inform people to simply "exercise and eat right" exemplify our ineffectiveness to affect change in our communities. What would make people want to change their behaviors? I believe people need a sense of belonging in their communities and in their "world." A community member who is both Yurok and Hoopa recently spoke of the dilemma faced by many in her own culture: they could either abandon many of their traditional practices to become successful in the dominate society, or they could retain their heritage and run the risk of societal and economic failure. She pointed out that the corollary to this dilemma is that many of those who were successful at traditional practices were neither honored nor attained

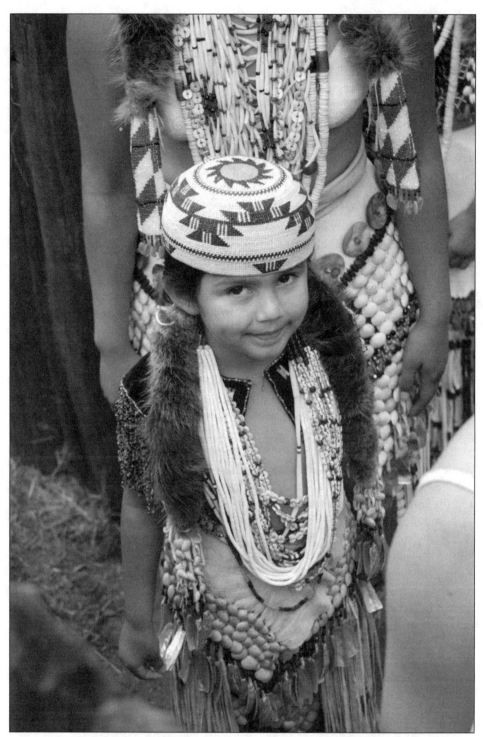

Paula Allen's daughter Ty'ithreeha at age 5, participating in a Brushdance Ceremony.

the status (i.e. the sense of place in their world) that they most certainly would have in their traditional societies. Without oversimplifying, I would point out that similar dilemma's have faced millions of Indigenous Peoples around the world with intrusions into their respective cultures. Such circumstances set up conflicts within individuals as well as families and communities that can only serve to fuel the fires of chronic disease, poor mental health, and substance abuse now so prevalent in many of these populations.

In order to begin changing this destructive course, we all must work to restore the connection between the spiritual as viewed by individuals and communities in relation to their physical and emotional well being. We should work with communities to establish these connections in the ways *they* know are best, based on *their* histories, knowledges, practices, and ultimately lifestyles. The time of imposing patronizing solutions on a variety of Indigenous Peoples' cultures and their communities is past. There remains a challenge: to overcome the "catch 22" of needing a sense of place in the world and a vehicle to attain that, while at the same time having a sufficient sense of one's place in the world to want to take that path in the first place. The magic of a beginning is conjuring this change, but it requires much nurturing. As more tradition and culture is brought back into the context of present day lifestyles, I believe a sense of spirituality reflected by the knowledge of one's place in the world and a feeling of belonging will occur to restore both mental and physical well being.

Conclusion?

The shortcoming of my discussion is that I have posed more questions than offered direct solutions; they are not mine to offer. Individuals and their communities must be active participants of the solutions we propose. I am acutely aware that it is one thing to ponder these issues in an academic manner even while trying to gain a new perspective; it is quite another to live within communities and cultures so profoundly affected by the problems delineated. We cannot begin to comprehend the weight of the effect on the spirit of the individuals and communities in which they live.

The dominant biomedical culture tends to view disease largely as a physiological disturbance of the body. We have evolved a rudimentary concept of how our mind both responds to and influences bodily disturbances. What we sometimes ignore, and at other times debate, is the inseparable nature of the spirit in regards to these problems of the mind and body. We persist in splitting up and analyzing our mind, body and spirit as three separate entities. I believe many would dispute the wisdom of this atomization. The spirit, or soul if you will, is simply dressed up in the garb of the mind and body, but they are all one, inextricable, and that is how they act and respond. As we approach the conundrum of diabetes in the world, it is my contention that we must not only incorporate the understanding of this inseparable nature of the mind-body-spirit, but we should simply view them as perceptual manifestations of the same entity, as medical anthropologists have proposed in this anthology of critical writings.

My intention here is not to career off into a metaphysical treatise on the condition of man. Whatever religious or philosophical convictions we might engender is less important than viewing that the approach to some solutions on diabetes must have an inclusive perspective or else we may find ourselves winning a few minor skirmishes with medicines and admonitions (the "allopathic model") only to lose the entirety of the "war." Discovering very effective medications to target insulin resistance may find us using them by the age of 21 in 30% of the world's population. Even if we did find a genetic "cause," we may pluck out several "defects" from the human genome only to discover under different conditions or unforeseen circumstances that we miss them dearly.

Type 2 diabetes has been with us for millennia, primarily described in agrarian, less perpetually mobile societies and in relatively "older" individuals. It is doubtful we will completely eradicate this illness from the world. Yet many cultures and peoples throughout the world existed for generations without the devastating harvest we now reap. Rather than focus on a purely medicinal or genetic solution for this disease and many others like it, I propose we return to the communities and families for whom we care, *our* communities and families, and attempt to rediscover the wisdom of their cultural traditions. Our present-day society must re-establish our interconnectedness with food as a nurturing substance, not for our bodies alone, but for the body-mind-soul. Our efforts should include healing of the oppressed and colonized peoples in a modern day context. This is not to naïvely suggest a return to lifestyles unattainable in today's society. But we can apply the sustaining concepts of those traditions to the template of modern life. This is a challenging notion, but I believe not impossible. The hope of this possibility depends on including our communities and their knowledges and practices in our solutions; to disregard them, I fear, will have the devastating consequences we are only now beginning to experience. To continue the present course of viewing diabetes as purely a genetic and lifestyle problem places in peril those we serve and the health of humankind as a whole.

Acknowledgments

I would like to thank Twila Sanchez for her contribution, patience, and bearing in assisting me with these ideas (i.e. putting up with me). Thanks to Paula Allen for sharing her insights, thoughts, and family stories and thanks also to Ann Bullock, Mariana Ferreira, Karen Moulton, Dwight Pargee, and Rachel Robinson for their inspiration and ideas as well as their dedicated work in regards to diabetes in American Indian peoples. Finally, a dedicated thanks to all my patients past, present, and future; you have been my greatest teachers.

References

Ackard, D. M., D. Neumark-Sztainer, M. Story and C. Perry. 2003. Overeating among Adolescents: Prevalence and Associations with Weight-Related Characteristics and Psychological Health. Pediatrics 111(1): 67–74.

Benjamin, Evan, D. Winters, J. Mayfield and D. Gohdes. 1993. Diabetes in Pregnancy in Zuni Indian Women. Prevalence and Subsequent Development of Clinical Diabetes after Gestational Diabetes. Diabetes Care 16(9): 1231–35.

Benyshek, Daniel C., J.F. Martin and C.S. Johnston. 2001. A Reconsideration of the Origins of the type 2 Diabetes Epidemic among Native Americans and the Implications for Intervention Policy. Medical Anthropology 20(1): 25–64.

Björntorp, Per. 1991a. Visceral Fat Accumulation: The Missing Link between Psychosocial Factors and Cardiovascular Disease? J Intern Med. 230(3): 195–201

_____1991b. Metabolic Implications of Body Fat Distribution. Diabetes Care 14(12): 1132–43.

Björntorp, Per, G. Holm and R. Rosmond. 1999. Hypothalamic Arousal, Insulin Resistance and Type 2 Diabetes mellitus. Diabet. Med. 16: 373–83.

Blaisdell, R. K. 1993. Health Status of Kanaka Maoli (Indigenous Hawaiians). Asian Am Pac Island J Health. 1(2): 116–60.

Brunner, E. J., H. Hemingway, B.R. Walker, M. Page, P. Clarke, M. Juneja, M.J. Shipley, M. Kumari, R. Andrew, J.R. Seckl, A. Papadopoulos, S. Checkley, A. Rumley, G.D. Lowe, S.A. Stansfeld and M.G. Marmot. 2002. Adrenocortical, Autonomic, and Inflammatory Causes of the Metabolic Syndrome: Nested Case-control Study. Circulation 106(21): 2659–65.

Burke, J.P., K. Williams, S.M. Haffner, V. Gonzalez and M.P. Stern. 2001. Elevated Incidence of Type 2 Diabetes in San Antonio, Texas, Compared with that of Mexico City, Mexico. Diabetes Care 24(9): 1573–78.

Chang, P.P., D.E. Ford, L.A. Meoni, N.Y. Wang and M.J. Klag. 2002. Anger in Young Men and Subsequent Premature Cardiovascular Disease: The Precursors Study. Arch Intern Med. 162(8): 901–6.

Chrousos, G. P. 2000. The Role of Stress and the Hypothalamic-Pituitary-Adrenal Axis in the Pathogenesis of the Metabolic Syndrome: Neuro-endocrine and Target Tissue-related Causes. Journal of Obesity (Suppl. 2)24: S50–55.

Dallman, Mary, N. Pecoraro, S.F. Akana, S.E. La Fleur, F. Gomez, H. Houshyar, M.E. Bell, S. Bhatnagar, K.D. Laugero and S. Manalo. 2003. Chronic Stress and Obesity: A New View of "Comfort Food." Proc Natl Acad Sci.(USA) 100(20): 11696–701.

Dornhorst, Anne and Michela Rossi. 1998. Risk and Prevention of Type 2 Diabetes in Women with Gestational Diabetes. Diabetes Care (Suppl. 2)21: B43–49.

Daniel, M., K. O'Dea, K.G. Rowley, R. McDermott and S. Kelly. 1999. Glycated Hemoglobin as an Indicator of Social Environmental Stress among Indigenous versus Westernized Populations. Prev Med. 29(5): 405–13.

Eaton, W. W. 2002. Epidemiologic Evidence on the Comorbidity of Depression and Diabetes. Journal of Psychosomatic Research 53(4): 903–6.

Eaton, W. W., H. Armenian, J. Gallo, L. Pratt and D.E. Ford. 1996. Depression and Risk for Onset of type II Diabetes. A Prospective Population-based Study. Diabetes Care 19(10): 1097–1102.

Elwood, J. M. 2002. Developing Areas in Cancer in New Zealand. Jpn J Clin Oncol 32 (Suppl): S43–51.

Engelgau, Michael M., W.H. Herman, P.J. Smith, R.R. German and R.E. Aubert. 1988. The Epidemiology of Diabetes and Pregnancy in the U.S. Diabetes Care 18(7): 1029–33.

Ferreira, Mariana. 1996. Sweet Tears and Bitter Pills. The Politics of Health among the Yuroks in Northern California. Unpublished Doctoral Dissertation, University of California—Berkeley and University of California—San Francisco.

_____1998. Slipping Through Sky Holes. Yurok Perceptions of the Body in Northern California. Culture, Medicine and Psychiatry 22(2): 171–202.

Garbe, C., G.R. McLeod and P.G. Buettner. 2000. Time Trends of Cutaneous Melanoma in Queensland, Australia and Central Europe. Cancer 89(6): 1269–78.

Gergely, G. and J.S. Watson. 1996. The Social Biofeedback Theory of Parental Affect-mirroring: The Development of Emotional Self-awareness and Self-control in Infancy. Int J Psychoanal. 77(6): 1181–212.

Gillman M.W., S. Rifas-Shiman, C.S. Berkey, A.E. Field and G.A. Colditz. 2003. Maternal Gestational Diabetes, Birth Weight, and Adolescent Obesity. Pediatrics 111(3): 221–26.

Heim, Christine, D.J. Newport, S. Heit, Y.P.Graham, M. Wilcox R. Bonsall, A.H. Miller and C.B. Nemeroff. 2000. Pituitary-Adrenal and Autonomic Responses to Stress in Women after Sexual and Physical Abuse in Childhood. JAMA 284(5): 592–97.

Hull, R. L., S. Andrikopoulos, C.B. Verchere, J. Vidal, F. Wang, M. Cnop, R.L. Prigeon and S.E. Kahn. 2003. Increased Dietary Fat Promotes Islet Amyloid Formation and Beta-cell Secretory Dysfunction in a Transgenic Mouse Model of Islet Amyloid. Diabetes 52(2): 372–79.

Keltikangas-Jarvinen, L., N. Ravaja, K. Raikkonen, A. Hautanen and H. Adlercreutz 1998. Relationships between the Pituitary-Adrenal Hormones, I=Insulin, and Glucose in Middle-aged Men: Moderating Influence of Psychosocial Stress. Metabolism 47(12): 1440–49.

King, H., R.E. Aubert and W.H. Herman. 1998. Global Burden of Diabetes, 1995–2025: Prevalence, Numerical Estimates, and Projections. Diabetes Care 21(9): 1414–31.

Knowler, William C., E. Barrett-Connor, S.E. Fowler, R.F. Hamman, J.M. Lachin, E.A. Walker, and D.M. Nathan. 2002. Diabetes Prevention Program Research Group Reduction in the Incidence of type 2 Diabetes with Lifestyle Intervention or Metformin. N Engl J Med. 346(6): 393–403.

Lantz, Paula M., J.S. House J.M. Lepkowski , D.R. Williams, R.P.Mero and J. Chen. 1998. Socioeconomic Factors, Health Behaviors, and Mortality: Results from a Nationally Representative Prospective Study of US Adults. JAMA 279(21): 1703–8.

Lawlor, Debbie A., G.D. Smith and E. Shah. 2002. Birth Weight of Offspring and In-sulin Resistance in Late Adulthood: Cross Sectional Survey. BMJ 325 (7360): 359.

Mazze, Roger S., D. Lucido and H. Shamoon. 1984. Psychological and Social Correlates of Glycemic Control. Diabetes Care 7(4): 360–66.

McGarvey, Stephen T. 1999. Modernization, Psychosocial Factors, Insulin and Cardiovascular Health. *In* Hormones, Health and Behavior: A Socio-ecological and Lifespan Perspective. C. Panter-Brick and C.M. Worthman, eds. pp. 244–80. Cambridge: Cambridge University Press.

Mogren, Ingrid, U. Högberg, B. Stegmayr, B. Lindahl and H. Stenlund. 2001. Fetal Exposure, Heredity and Risk Indicators for Cardiovascular Disease in a Swedish Welfare Cohort. International Journal of Epidemiology 30: 853–62.

Morford, Michael. 2001. Notes and Errata, August 29, SF Gate. [columnist, sfgate.com/San Francisco Chronicle]

Narayan, K. M., M. Hoskin, D. Kozak, A.M. Kriska, R.L. Hanson, D.J. Pettitt, D.K. Nagi, P.H. Bennett and W.C. Knowler. 1998. Randomized Clinical Trial of Lifestyle Interventions in Pima Indians: A Pilot Study. Diabet Med. 15(1): 66–72.

Neel, James V. 1982. The Thrifty Genotype Revisited. *In* The Genetics of Diabetes Mellitus. J. Kobberling and R. Tattersall, eds. pp. 283–93. London: Academic. (Serono Symposium No. 47).

Obici, S., B.B. Zhang, G. Karkanias and L. Rossetti. 2002. Hypothalamic Insulin Signaling is Required for Inhibition of Glucose Production. Nat Med. 8(12): 1376–82.

Pettitt, David J. and L. Jovanovic. 2001. Birth Weight as a Predictor of type 2 Diabetes mellitus: The U-shaped Curve. Curr. Diab. Rep. 1(1): 78–81.

Pettitt, David J., R.G. Nelson, M.F. Saad, P.H. Bennett and W.C. Knowler. 1993. Diabetes and Obesity in the Offspring of Pima Indian Women with Diabetes during Pregnancy. Diabetes Care 16(1): 310–14.

Poulton, Richie, A. Caspi, B.J. Milne, W.M. Thomson, A. Taylor, M.R. Sears and T..E. Moffitt. 2002. Association between Children's Experience of Socioeconomic Disadvantage and Adult Health: A Life-Course Study. Lancet 360: 1640–45.

Power, C. and B. Jeffris. 2002. Fetal Environment and Subsequent Obesity: A Study of Maternal Smoking. Int'l. Journal of Epidemiology 31: 413–19.

Ravelli, A. C. J., J.H.P. van der Meulen, R.P.J. Michels, C. Osmond, D.J.P. Barker, C.N. Hales and O.Bleker. 1998. Glucose Tolerance in Adults after Prenatal Exposure to Famine. Lancet 351: 173–77.

Rios Burrows, Nilka, K. Acton, K. Moore, L. Querec, L.Geiss and M. Engelgau. 2002. Trends in Diabetes Prevalence Among American Indian and Alaska Native Children, Adolescents, and Young Adults. American Journal of Public Health 92(9): 1485–90.

Rodrigues, S., E. Robinson and K. Gray-Donald. 1999. Prevalence of Gestational Diabetes mellitus among James Bay Cree Women in Northern Quebec. Canadian Med Assn J 160(9): 1293–97.

Rosmond, Roland, M. Dallman and P. Bjorntorp. 1998. Stress-Related Cortisol Secretion in Men: Relationships with Abdominal Obesity and Endocrine, Metabolic and Hemodynamic Abnormalities. J Clin Endocrinol Metab. 83(6): 1853–59.

Rozanski, Alan, J.A. Blumenthal and J. Kaplan. 1999. Impact of Psychological Factors on the Pathogenesis of Cardiovascular Disease and Implications for Therapy. Circulation 99: 2192–217.

Sontag, Susan. Illness as Metaphor. NY: Vintage Books.

Stanner, S. A., K. Bulmer, C. Andrès, O.E. Lantseva, V. Borodina, V.V. Poteen and J.S. Yudkin. 1997. Does Malnutrition *in utero* Determine Diabetes and Coronary Heart Disease in Adulthood? Results from the Leningrad Siege Study, a Cross-Sectional Study. BMJ 315(7119): 1342–48.

Stern, M. P., S.P. Gaskill, H.P. Hazuda, L.I. Gardner and S.M. Haffner. 1983. Does Obesity Explain Excess Prevalence of Diabetes among Mexican Americans? Results of the San Antonio Heart Study. Diabetologia 24(4): 272–77.

Streeck-Fischer, A. and B.A. Van der Kolk. 2000. Down Will Come Baby, Cradle and All: Diagnostic and Therapeutic Implications of Chronic Trauma on Child Development. Aust N Z J Psychiatry 34(6): 903–18.

Taborsky, Gerald Jr., Peter J. Havel and Daniel Porte, Jr. 1998. Stress-Induced Activation of the Neuroendocrine System and its Effects on Carbohydrate Metabolism. *In* Diabetes Mellitus, Theory and Practice. 5th Edition. D. Porte, Jr. and R. S. Sherwin, eds. pp. 141–68. Appleton and Lange, Publ.

Valdez, R., M.A. Athens, G.H. Thompson, B. S. Bradshaw and M.P. Stern. 1994. Birthweight and Adult Health Outcomes in a Biethnic Population in the USA. Diabetologia 37(6): 624–31.

Veening, M. A., M.M. Van Weissenbruch and H.A. Delemarre-Van De Waal. 2002. Glucose Tolerance, Insulin Sensitivity, and Insulin Secretion in Children Born Small for Gestational Age. J Clin Endocrinol Metab 87(10): 4657–61.

Van der Does, F. E., J.N. De Neeling, F.J. Snoek, P.J. Kostense, P.A. Grootenhuis, L.M. Bouter and R.J. Heine. 1996. Symptoms and Well-being in relation to Glycemic Control in type II Diabetes. Diabetes Care 9(3): 204–10.

Wendorf, Michael and Ira D. Goldfine. 1991. Archeology of NIDDM, Excavation of the "Thrifty" Genotype. Diabetes 40: 161–65.

Williams, Redford B. 1998. Lower Socioeconomic Status and Increased Mortality: Early Childhood Roots and the Potential for Successful Interventions. JAMA 279(21): 174.

Wong, M. D., M.F. Shapiro, W.J. Boscardin and S.L. Ettner. 2002. Contribution of Major Diseases to Disparities in Mortality. N Engl J Med 347(20): 1585–92.

CHAPTER 13

THE SPIRIT'S CELL: REFLECTIONS ON DIABETES AND POLITICAL MEANING

Jo C. Scheder

"I looked at the candy for a while and gave it to my father. He looked at it for a while, too, and handed it back to the detective.

"I'm sorry, Detective Clayton," my father said. "But my son and I are diabetics."

"Oh, sorry," the detective said and looked at us with sad eyes. Especially me. Juvenile diabetes. A tough life. I learned how to use a hypodermic needle before I could ride a bike. I lost more of my own blood to glucose tests than I ever did to childhood accidents.

"Nothing to be sorry for," my father said. "It's under control."

The detective looked at us both like he didn't believe it. All he knew was criminals and how they worked. He must have figured diabetes worked like a criminal, breaking and entering. But he had it wrong. Diabetes is just like a lover, hurting you from the inside. I was closer to my diabetes than to any of my family or friends. Even when I was all alone, quiet, thinking, wanting no company at all, my diabetes was there. That's the truth."

> from Sherman Alexie, 1993, *The Lone Ranger and Tonto Fistfight in Heaven*. NY: Harper-Collins, pp. 221–22.

Summary of Chapter 13. The theory of illness causation proposed here is related to a "physiology of oppression." It insists on an examination of the ideology of health care delivery, which itself is built upon presumptions of etiology. Discordant ideologies, or discordances between ideology and experience, operate as fundamental interlopers in health practices and deliveries. A re-envisioning of illness causation, and subsequently a revision of health care delivery and preventive efforts, focused on political issues, is necessary.

☙ ☙ ☙

Prologue and Perspective

Everyone familiar with diabetes knows that it is a complicated metabolic condition. But diabetes is more than that. It is a complicated *social issue* that has become flattened and over-simplified. That it remains a recalcitrant and entrenched illness suggests that

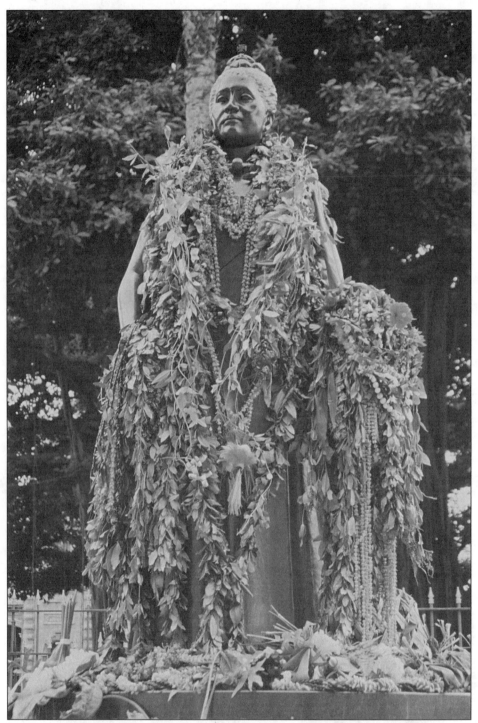

Queen Lili'uokalani statue draped in leis on 100th Anniversary of her overthrow.

it needs to be re-complicated and re-contemplated. One version of that re-thinking involves life stress, neuroendocrinology and political meaning—a daunting tangle of race/ethnicity, inequality, gender, colonialism, history, memory, identity, culture, daily micro-aggressions, mind-body medicine, and public health presumptions and explanatory models. It doesn't have to be daunting, however, as the re-thinking also offers a clarity of insight and a path that appreciates the tangles.

That clarity and path come from an integrative mind-body perspective, as several chapters in this book indicate. New developments in health and medical research continue to open the way to this fuller understanding of diabetes as a product of life experience. These newer studies, wittingly or not, are built on the longtime efforts by a very few diabetes researchers, such as Richard Surwit and Mark Feinglos (1983 and 1988), who have persistently shown physiological links between diabetes and stress, and who have repeatedly demonstrated improved glucose control through stress management (2002). Recently a Dutch study found stressful life events to be related to diabetes risk (Mooy 2002). Researchers at Sweden's Karolinska hospital announced findings that stress, in the form of loneliness, bullying and financial worries, brought a four-fold greater risk for diabetes (Agardh et al. 2003; *Nordic Business Report*, 22 January 2002). New research at the University of Chicago implicates sleep deficit in insulin resistance and potentially in diabetes onset (Cobb 2002; Spiegel et al. 1999; Van Cauter 1999). Sleep disturbance can be induced by corticosteroids—a class of stress hormones (Glaser and Kiecolt-Glaser 1998; Brunner 1997).[1]

Concurrently, there is a new international health focus on social/political forces in mental health. This comes in part from sequelae of conflict in Rwanda, South Africa, Sri Lanka, the former Yugoslavia, and is eloquently presented in the series on social suffering edited by Veena Das and collaborators (2001). They write of subtle violence, soft violence, and the burden of living in a hostile world. Scheper-Hughes (1992) writes of Brazilian shantytowns, everyday violence, and the dangers of living in a place where hope has vanished. Luhrman (2000: 158) writes of the Parsis of Bombay, exemplars of "quiet trauma" and its persistence several generations later, of the impact of colonialism on the collective self, the unchanged cultural ideal of moral selfhood, but the changed expectations—or possibility—of their fulfillment.

But we need not look far away. In Luhrman's work, we see parallels for particular generations of American Indians, Native Hawaiians, Mexican-Americans. Becoming a "good Parsi" under British rule involved a transformation of Parsi attributes to reflect the "English gentleman" and therefore be deemed worthy of status in colonial society, and eventual Parsi ambivalence about the Quit India anti-colonial movement and their subsequent decay in social status and birthrate, increase in mental health problems and poverty, a "shift to despair in community self-perception" (2000: 166), and the next generation's mixture of pride and shame in their identity.

---

1. The stress hormone cortisol suppresses immunity, and raises blood glucose by accelerating the conversion of fats and proteins to glucose. Excess cortisol promotes central body obesity and hyperglycemia (Thibodeau and Patton 1997). A team at Umea University in Sweden, in collaboration with Scottish researchers, demonstrated how fatty tissue enzymatically increases the production of cortisol, which in turn leads to increased glucose availability (Rask et al. 2001; *Obesity, Fitness and Wellness Week* 2002). Researchers in the Netherlands reported a cortisol-resistant gene variant in humans, which was related to lower blood levels of glucose and insulin (Van Rossum 2002).

Yet, what are the private feelings of individual community members, and how do variations across communities also contribute to variations in health and diabetes prevalence?

"Native American populations at greatest risk for developing type 2 diabetes today are the ones which endured the most extreme and extended periods of political and economic oppression in the late nineteenth an early twentieth centuries" (Benyshek 2002). Samoans have been differentially affected by diabetes in a pattern that Kunitz (1994) has traced to different parameters of nineteenth century colonial administration and land tenure in Western and American Samoa, respectively.

Contemporary chronic diseases are sometimes mislabeled "diseases of civilization." Rather, they are diseases of colonialism—and that's a very big difference. We consider our world to be "post-colonial"—a convenient but misleading label, marking a change in the official location of governance. Colonialism does not end with changes in government, however, and the residual effects on psyche and spirit do not evaporate/dissipate with time. Witness recent work on "post-colonial" and "post-apartheid" Africa in playwright Wole Soyinka's *The Burden of Memory, the Muse of Forgiveness*, or Jennifer Cole's *Forget Colonialism?*, or the afore-mentioned trilogy on suffering and violence from Das, Kleinman, Lock, Ramphele and Reynolds (2001). What happens to the energies of trauma? By the laws of physics, energies transform, but how?

What we in America ask of the oppressed, however, is to "forget it, get over it, move on." But like Sri Lanka and South Africa, flagrant hostilities end but one must live forever with the perpetrators, the tormentors. As if nothing had happened. If dominant America remembers Pearl Harbor, why deny the Cheyenne the memory of Sand Creek? Why deny Mexican Americans the memory of round-ups and deportations? Why deny African Americans the memory of slavery, segregation, lynching ? Why deny Hawaiians the memory of usurpation and colonial domination?

New "indigenist stress-coping models" look at health in contexts of colonialism, considering "historical trauma" and the "soul wound" of discrimination, where identity, culture, spiritual coping and traditional practices serve as buffers between stress and health outcomes, and where stress is understood to encompass "unresolved grief and mourning related to loss of land and place and the negotiation of invisibility in urban settings (Walters 2002: 523).

This is not just about cultural memory—it is about the continuing fact of everyday racism, of privilege and barriers, of glances and expectations, of slights and reflexive anticipations. These are assaultive, what Bourdieu (1977) referred to as symbolic violence, maintained inherently in systems of inequality and domination.

The "Spirit's Cell" refers to the neuroendocrine cell biology of emotional life, to the spirit of a people as played out in cellular processes underlying joy, anger, triumph, grief, trust, fear, stress, health, to political awareness and the imprisonments of colonialism, and to the intangible substance of traumatic memory. The cell walls include conventional models of health promotion and disease prevention. We have only begun to examine what Mariana Ferreira (1998, and this volume) calls "the political dimension of emotion"—an examination that promises rich understanding if approached through a clustering of anthropology, psychology, history, and mind-body medicine.

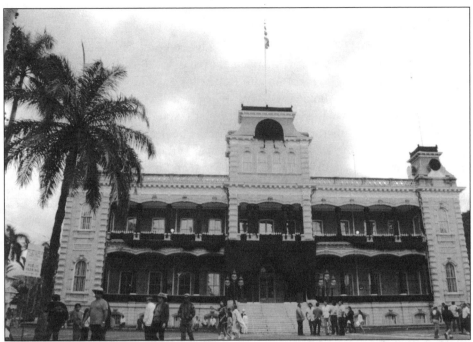

Iolani Palace draped in mourning for *Onipa'a*, the 100th anniversary of the illegal overthrow of the Hawaiian Nation. Honolulu, 1993.

Paths to "Untangling"

Current work on the psychophysiology of emotion reveals patterns of neuroendocrine reactivity to emotional repression that are suggestive of a mechanism for chronic health effects of emotional stress (Miller et al. 1996).

A provocative study by Surwit and collaborators (2002) showed that hostility was related to fasting glucose levels independent of body mass index (BMI) in African-Americans, but not in Caucasians. This suggests that BMI is a necessary factor mediating stress and diabetes in Caucasians (who are by far the population from which diet/obesity models of diabetes derive), but that stress alone—in the form of hostility—can elevate glucose levels regardless of BMI for African-Americans. In other words, stress is a more potent diabetes risk for members of a "minority" population than for the dominant group in U.S. society. The authors modestly suggest: "It is also possible that certain groups, such as African-Americans, might be both more metabolically vulnerable to stress as well as more exposed to stressful environmental stimuli. This might help explain the racial disparity in diabetes observed in this ethnic group...further study of these differences may contribute to understanding the mechanisms of the significant racial disparity in the prevalence of diabetes in African-Americans" (Surwit et al. 2002).

Metabolic vulnerability to stress can come from exposure. Individuals exposed to chronic psychological stress develop heightened reactivity, entering the physiological response more readily, quickly and intensely, and take longer to recover from it (Pike et al. 1997; Pruessner et al. 1997). Gabarino and Kostelny (1997) write of developmental damage to children from the accumulation of risk, from the impact of chronic community violence. Are these processes coming together in the findings of Richard Surwit and his collaborators?

A growing number of studies focus on the adverse health effects of the subjective experience of racism (cf. Clark et al. 1999; Harrell et al. 1998; Krieger 1999; Noh et al. 1999). Following findings that African Americans scored higher than Euro-Americans on measures of psychological distress (Neighbors 1984), Thompson (2002) examined impact of racism as a specific source of stress, focusing on the experience of daily racism and the "microaggressions" that must be dealt with or overlooked. She found that African Americans reported significantly more experiences of racial discrimination and higher impact of discrimination than Euro-Americans.

Ewart and Suchady (2002) look at health effects of the emotional stress of coping with poverty, how stress and emotion relate to neighborhood conditions, and connect these chronic difficulties to immune or cardiovascular vulnerability. The researchers combine a measure of perceived neighborhood disorder and exposure to violence with an experimental evocation of stress. They found that stress-related attitudes and emotions were more closely related to adolescents' perceptions of "proximal environmental conditions and events"—their experiential daily reality—than to broader structural indices of deprivation.

Residents of disadvantaged neighborhoods live with daily fear—of burglary, assault, injury. Ross and Mirowsky (2001) examined whether living in a disadvantaged neighborhood damages health, over and above the impact of personal socioeconomic characteristics. Among their findings: residents of disadvantaged neighborhoods had feelings of "chronic foreboding," worse self-reported health, worse physical functioning, and more chronic conditions. The association was mediated entirely by perceived neighborhood disorder and resulting fear (e.g., neighborhood effect did not lead to limitation of outdoor physical activity). They summarized their findings succinctly: "The daily stress associated with living in a neighborhood where danger, trouble, crime and incivility are common apparently damages health." They talk about "the centrality of imminent danger" and call for "a *bio-demography of stress* that links chronic exposure to threatening conditions—with physiological responses that may impair health" (2001: 272).

We know physiologically that chronic foreboding and frequent terror repeatedly flood the body with adrenal hormones that directly undermine health. A threatening environment—and fear itself—can invoke physiological responses that increase susceptibility to pathogens and accelerate the degradation of physiological systems (Fremont and Bird 2000; McEwan 2000; Taylor et al. 1997).

The experience of discrimination as a stressful life event has received scant but increasing attention (Kessler and Neighbors 1986; Miller 1992; Williams et al. 1997). Cultural and intra-cultural differences in the perception and understanding of discrimination and stressful life events—the appraisal of the stressor—are pertinent to understanding variation in health outcomes. Komaroff, Masuda and Holmes (1968) reported that Mexican-Americans, African-Americans and Euro-Americans differed in the amount of adjustment required by events. Mexican-Americans and American Samoans share stress perceptions of certain events, but differ on others (Scheder 1983c). Cervantes and Castro (1985) posit that disruption of social support networks is associated with greater expression of illness for Mexican-Americans, consistent with ratings by Mexican American respondents that migratory and social mobility life events require more change as they disrupt extended family networks. R. Hough and collaborators (1981; Hough 1985) found a stress effect for Mexican-Americans even if the stressful event happened to their significant others rather than themselves. Poss and Jezewski (2002) found that *susto* (fright) was a significant theme in Mexican Americans' explanatory model of type 2 diabetes.

In addition, Ross and Mirowsky (2001) call for a transfer of psychoendocrinology from lab and clinical studies to large scale social and demographic surveys, field-testing the hypothesis that the chronic release of stress hormones links experience to poor health, and doing this in the worlds in which people live. The migrant farmworker study did this on a smaller scale in 1979–81 (Scheder 1988, 1981). The Hawaii-Samoa Stress Study did this in the 1980s (Baker et al. 1986; Howard 1986; Scheder 1983a, 1983b). Much of this is old news. The amount of current interest is what's new (House 2002; Williams 2002).

So, why now? Perhaps we finally understand "diabetes" as a monolithic label for a multi-causal condition, and for which one-size-fits-all etiological explanations are inappropriate. Perhaps because of the increased knowledge of stress and health, development of neighborhood effects theory, incipient attention to sociopolitical awareness as an antidote to stress, increased attention to racial/ethnic health disparities, new understandings of stress hormones and fat metabolism, stress and immune compromise, infection and diabetes risk, or growing acceptance of complementary and alternative healing and their underlying spirit/emotion and energy-based philosophies?

Maybe the timing is right. Maybe we have the methodological tools and conceptual understanding. Maybe we just finally have the right words. For whatever reasons, research on stress and diabetes has found new life.

The key challenge is not in plumbing diabetes as an endocrine or public health problem, however, but as a political problem, and on at least two fronts. One is the politics of life, of social inequality, daily struggle, historical memory. The other is the politics of explanatory modeling and the ideologies of causation, prevention and treatment that determine everything else about how diabetes is researched and clinically treated. The politics of daily life transforms select peoples into "high risk diabetes populations." The politics of health science prevents that understanding. The challenge for diabetes work is to embrace stress physiology and its embeddedness in the experience of discrimination—racism, post/neo-colonialism, and other forms and effects of subjugation, and its generated emotional concomitants, whether those be traumatic memory, neighborhood disorder, race stress, daily microaggressions, cultural alienation, or compromised identity. That is the portal to finding effective glycemic control, and it requires community action.

But where then to situate prevention and control? We can still look to individual, community, and institutional efforts. Understanding racism's effects on a cellular level. Mind-body medicine and political action. Expanding on evidence that political awareness promotes better health. Grappling conceptually, methodologically and morally with the intellectual arrogance whereby medicine and health education seek to define and dominate others' experience.

There is violence in non-recognition (Ewing 2000). The absence of empathy for others' experience, encouraged by acculturation into the health professions, contributes to the lack of imagination in health research. That has produced a quarter century of health promotion that has shown, more than anything else, that the key to diabetes for Indigenous Peoples and communities of color surely does not lie in diet and exercise.

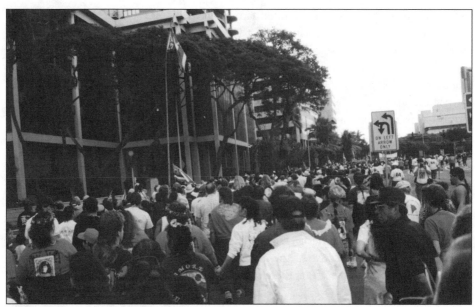

As part of *Onipa'a* Centennial commemorations, an estimated 15,000 marchers gather to trace the route to Iolani Palace taken by US Marines in 1893.

Contemporary American society expects people to make lemonade out of lemons. How much sugar do you have to add to make it drinkable? What are the costs of all that sugar?

The Spirit's Cell: A Physiology of Oppression[2]

Discordances between ideology and experience are fundamental interlopers in health practices, from prevention and treatment delivery to patient adherence. State-validated versions of health care delivery, seen in health promotion, screening programs, access to health care and the like, presume a conception of illness etiology based largely on personal agency, and clouded by patient-blaming accusations of "non-compliance" or "denial" (see Humphery, this volume). These are the very assumptions of causation and course which critical medical anthropologists critique. If the ideological foundations of health remain mired in the model of individual actions, and do not consider social location and the physiological effects of oppression, then the majority of the population will remain outside the benefits of that model. What is necessary is a re-envisioning of illness causation, and subsequently a new vision of health care delivery and prevention efforts, built on political understanding.

At issue is a "physiology of oppression," spun off from research in stress, neuroimmunology, endocrinology, and psychophysiology. It is a perspective that recognizes the power of the everyday, the lingering and cumulative decay of existential reality. It is the constant, lived experience of oppression that erodes the body as well as the spirit.

2. An earlier version of the second half of this chapter was presented at the 1995 annual meeting of the American Anthropological Association, Washington, DC, under the title "Critical Analysis in Biocultural Theory."

A "physiology of oppression" provides an investigative tool and a conceptual framework. It evades reductionism and individuation by focusing on structural, macro processes including the individual's conditions of existence, while remaining equally concerned with experience, phenomenology and hormones.

The biological data are voluminous, longstanding, and exponentially increasing (Freund and McGuire 1999). For example: Research since the late 1960s and early 1970s has suggested that the requirement for frequent readjustment to instability in the lives of lower-income people is a key stressor leading to adverse psychological or health outcomes (Holmes and Rahe 1967; Dohrenwend 1973). Physiological studies suggest that habituation to unpredictability and intermittent stress does not develop (Edwards and Yates 1985). Bodies do not "get used to" repeated stress—including stressors that are erratic, sporadic and ongoing.

What happens to diabetes work when we consider that these daily experiences and microaggressions may represent recurrent neuroendocrine mini-spikes? As more is learned about the human biopsychological mechanisms which translate this lived oppression into glucocorticoid dysregulation, catecholamine disturbances, or T-cell suppression, the inescapable conclusion emerges: the pathogen is internalized oppression, and the mechanism involves neuroendocrine responses to living inside of inequality.

This conception of etiology then challenges the prevailing ideology of health care delivery. A "physiology of oppression" emphasizes that current experiences of illness are not new typologies or changed patterns, or isolated events disconnected in time from our collective past. They are part of a long process. And they are determined by differential power relations. Controlling the definition of diabetes, or the definition of disease risk, are also displays of power.

The core construct of "The Spirit's Cell" is simple: social and political conditions have practical and physiological effects on morbidity and mortality that can be measured and connected. The process is exemplified in the experience of Indigenous Peoples.

I will try to illustrate the position by describing a specific example of a people whose health status is bound to social and political causation, to an etiology which not only resists standard models of health care delivery, but for whom these models are etiologically and therapeutically irrelevant and ultimately damaging—if not lethal. The people: Native Hawaiians.

Native Hawaiian Health

Among Hawaii's people, Native Hawaiians have the lowest life expectancy, and the highest mortality rates for all of the major causes of death (heart disease, cancer, stroke, accidents, diabetes, infections, bronchitis, emphysema), as well as for infant mortality and suicide. Breast cancer incidence for Native Hawaiian women is higher than that of African American women and more than twice that of Korean and Vietnamese women (Miller et al. 1996).

One-third of Native Hawaiian women are diabetic (Women of Color Health Data Book 1998). Diabetes mortality is 200 percent higher among Hawaiians than the combined US rate for all race/ethnicities. Native Hawaiians have the highest percentage of

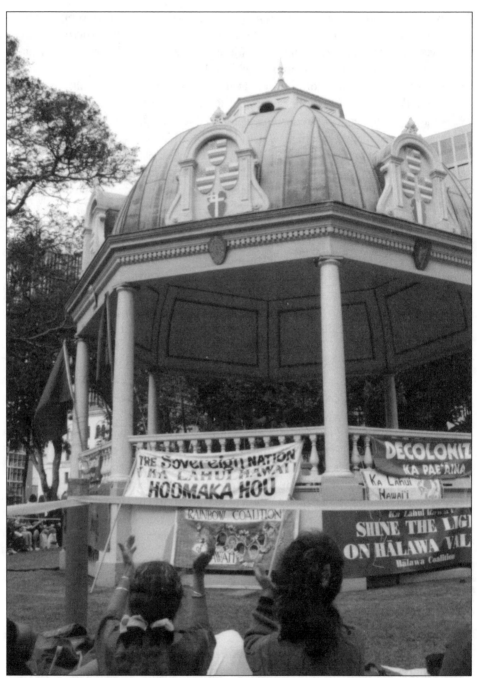

Iolani Palace Bandstand was the setting for Hawaiian chant, hula, and speeches at the Onipa'a Commemoration.

population below the poverty level in Hawai'i (14 percent), highest unemployment, highest representation in service jobs, and highest rate of incarceration. Waianae, a predominantly Hawaiian community on O'ahu, has the lowest socioeconomic status in the state (Blaisdell 1993).

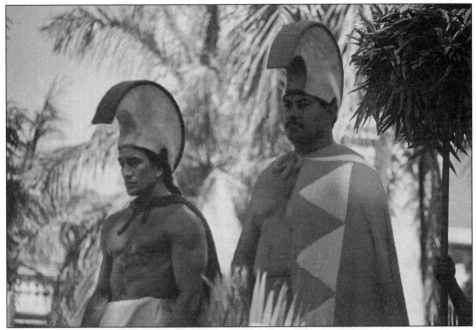

Men on float at 1995 Kamehameha Day parade.

Let's trace the process of illness and colonialism, beginning with western contact. Captain James Cook's descriptions from 1778 attest to the vigor and vitality of the Hawaiian people at the time of the first European contact, whom Cook described as "possessing much liveliness" and having "strong and well-proportioned bodies" (Cook 1778). Hawaiians were physically robust.

The Hawaiian population collapse during the 19th century was a result of cultural violence, aided by introduced pathogens. The *new* susceptibility to disease among formerly robust people coincided with cultural devastation, and the assault of explorer, missionary and trader sensibilities that undermined the cosmological cohesion that supports physical vitality (Scheder 1998, and this volume). In other words, the epidemics—the rate of genocide—in those early years occurred in a psychological milieu which we now understand as having specific physiological effects, hastening immune impairment, elevating blood sugar through familiar biochemical pathways, and activating physiological stress responses to the experiential state of oppression: fear, anger, unpredictability, lack of control over events. The cumulative experience of stressful life events, loss, grief, despair and bereavement constitutes a process that continues today and is reflected in the current health statistics.

How is the past relevant to today? Colonialism remains. Post-statehood Hawai'i is characterized by a tourism- and military-based economy; commercialization of Hawaiian culture; destruction of sacred sites (e.g., from military practice bombing and freeway construction); land occupation by military installations (30% of the state land is under military control); and evictions of Native Hawaiian communities to make way for housing developments for upper classes and outsiders, for resorts and golf courses. Meanwhile, the cost of living in Hawai'i is 40% higher than in continental America, and the median house price is 340,000 U.S. dollars

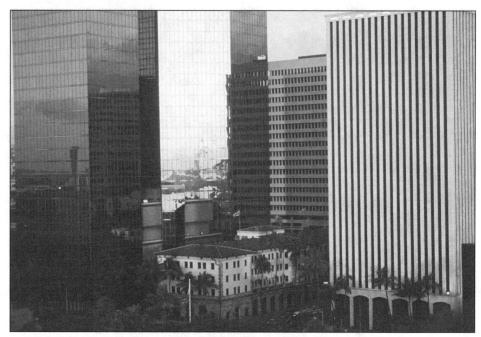

Honolulu Cityscape, 1996.

What does this say to health care? Kuumeaaloha Gomes, a Native Hawaiian public health activist, makes clear the political economic connection between land and health, and brings that perspective to the public health model of causation: "In talking about health, you must talk about food, so you must talk *lo'i* (taro gardens)—and so you've got to talk golf courses, and so you've got to talk foreign investment."

Taro lands have been converted to golf courses and other commercial developments. Corporate acquisition has turned healthful taro and its natural product, *poi*, into pancake mix and deep fried chips for upscale markets. The loss of taro lands goes beyond the displaced families and the diminished supply of the crop—it cuts to the core of the continued colonial hegemony. This too must be recognized as fundamental to illness etiology. "We cannot isolate health from socioeconomic status and government issues. The policy arena is where change will happen. We must address land issues, access to land" (Gomes 1992).

Will a solution to Native Hawaiian health problems be found in "cultural sensitivity" by the biomedical system? Will a solution simply be the training of more Native Hawaiian health professionals? Not in the context of enculturation into a "professional" culture, as demonstrated in Hawai'i: even Native Hawaiian health professionals are replicating the western bureaucracy and public health approaches, but using Hawaiian labels. Local health education programs adopt some of the language of Hawaiian knowledges and practices, but wrap them around the default approach of regulating behavior.

What they add is a cultural sensitivity clause, effectively perpetuating the idea that it is culture and not political economy that creates and continually re-creates both health risk exposures and barriers to improved health. Nowhere do they deal with cultural and spiritual loss, or the struggle against political and economic subordination.

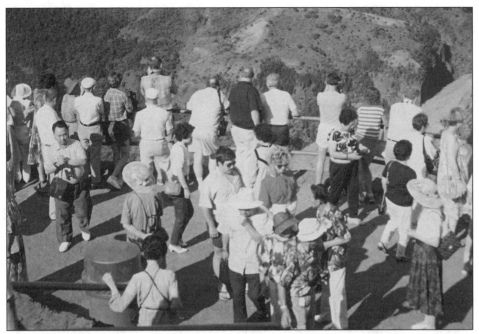

Tourists at Waimea Canyon, Kauai, near the restricted access Barking Sands Military Reserve.

For example, the concept of *lokahi*, a unity or connection and balance between all things, is invoked only outside of the political ramifications of neo-colonialism's effects on *lokahi* and health.

Compulsory *Aloha*

In Hawai'i, an aspect of the health costs of colonialism is the repression of anger, fostered by community pressure to maintain an image of "*aloha* spirit" consonant with the tourist industry's fantasy of what it means to be "Hawaiian" (Trask 1994; Scheder 1996). The idea is that Hawaiians must show "*aloha*" to visitors and maintain that public posture at all times. *Aloha* is complicated and rich, deep in its meaning and cultural ancestry. Love, generosity, empathy, grace, kindness and affection are integral cultural elements. Sincerity of intent is fundamental, emanating from the *na'au*, a constellation of "heart," mind, and affection (literally intestines; Ito 1999: 8). *Aloha* is given freely, but it is based in a cultural history of reciprocity in which *aloha* is extended by all members. "*Aloha* spirit" is an invention of modern commerce, a perversion of the Hawaiian concept of *aloha* into a guise of subservience. Indeed, the Aloha Marketplace in Waikiki, the bazaar in which the Visitor Industry sells trinkets and "goodwill," provides an unwitting self-description of the selling of Hawaiian culture, the marketing of *aloha*, the commodification of spirit and soul. Tourists and other outsiders are frequently perceived as *maha'oi*: invasive, persistent, disrespecting of boundaries. "Compulsory *aloha*" denies the reality of lived experience, and imposes yet another layer of

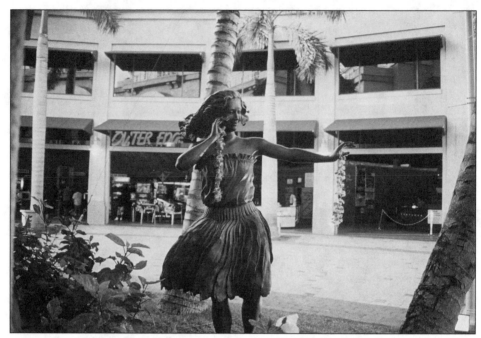

Hula dancer statue at entrance to Aloha Marketplace.

social control, cognitive dissonance, control over the expression of emotion, and psychophysiological challenge. The "*aloha* spirit" campaign has invaded public life throughout Hawai'i, no longer constrained to the tourist industry but now a generalized tool of social control, down to the ubiquitous "Live *Aloha*" bumper stickers.

Which leads back to the physiology of oppression. In a study of personality and glycemic control, Lane et al. (2000) found higher levels of blood glucose in association with higher altruism scores, and with lower scores for expressed anxiety and angry hostility. They speculate that the tendency to focus on the needs of others instead of oneself could prove to be a risk factor for poor glycemic control through neglect of self-care. This leads, alternatively, to a question of interactive effects of the contexts and meanings of altruism and the non-expression of emotion, and glycemic control.

Hawaiian culture and ethnopsychology emphasize social relationships. *Hihia*, which literally means "entanglements," refers to interpersonal conflicts and escalating hurtful emotional exchanges, potentially leading to illness and death (Ito 1999: 7). As Ito presents in her research with Hawaiian women in Honolulu, these relationships and their moral implications of correct behavior and intent are indelibly present in what she terms "culture-as-lived," and which the women vividly describe in their daily lives.

The continuing colonialism reveals the processual nature of domination. As social and cultural oppressions are embedded in historical process and continuity, so is health. As stated at the outset, a "physiology of oppression" emphasizes that current experiences of illness are not new typologies or changed patterns, or isolated events disconnected in time from our collective past.

Accordingly, the profile of morbidity in Hawai'i has "progressed" from the stark death scenes beginning in the late 18th Century missionary era, through the disguised decay of the late 19th Century colonial consolidation, to the contemporary perseverance of chronic morbidity under late 20th/early 21st Century statehood. These problems are not amenable to the public health models of cause, prevention, or health care delivery.

So—where then is the possibility of *rapproachment,* of reconciliation? Surprisingly, a hint or two of progressive insight have surfaced in the government health literature describing federal guidelines on "intentional injury." The National Committee for Injury Prevention and Control points out (1989: 1): "...the burden is borne disproportionately by the poor and minorities. Underlying social, environmental and economic conditions exacerbate these disparities. Programs to prevent injuries must recognize this and work to improve the conditions that lead to this burden." This applies to neuroendocrine illness as well, as these chronic disorders must be recognized as disproportionate burden, and critically re-conceptualized as cultural and spiritual injuries.

Daily microaggressions are like bullets. They are like a torturer's electrodes, constantly attached, expected but unpredictable in timing, voltage and source. They are not sought out but they requite constant vigilance. During my 2003 summer course on race and ethnicity, two African American men tried to explain this vigilance to their predominantly Euro-American classmates, and how (white) accusations of "pulling the race card" deny the everyday reality of life as a person of color in America. In the previous fall semester an African-American student told how her Euro-American partners in a class project did not even look at her during planning meetings, and during a car ride talked in her presence about how the declining atmosphere at their high school alma mater—her alma mater, too—was due to the African-American students there; in her part-time job as a department store clerk, she was instructed to watch the ethnic minority customers, specifically, for shoplifting. In a 2002 session with first year medical students, an African-American patient was asked to name the most important thing that doctors should know about her, culturally. Her response: "That I could not get waited on today at the jewelry counter."

The long-term effects of coping with discrimination, of living with historical memory, of the perceived environment and opportunities, are critical to poor health. The people at greatest risk have been telling this story for years. Deborah McDowell , in her analysis of "loss, grief, and the politics of memory" at the 2003 University of Wisconsin centennial symposium honoring W.E.B. DuBois' *Souls of Black Folk*, spoke of the problem of leaving emotions outside of history, and proposed a "provisional history of emotion under the dead weight of social degradation."

As Ito learned from 1990s Hawaiian women, "The ties that bind are in one's heart, one's *na'au*; ties of memories, of history, of hostilities, of love. One cannot patch or cover over the emotions intensely shared. One cannot depart" (Ito 1999: 38).

What is needed is a transformative view of health and the solutions to ill health. This can come from a redefining and restructuring of etiologic understanding. I would argue that for real meaning and legitimacy, there could be no other reconciliation.

Acknowledgments

I wish to thank Mariana Leal Ferreira and Gretchen Chesley Lang for fueling the expansion and updating of this paper through their invitation to contribute, their gracious patience and encouragement, and their commitment in presenting critical perspectives to an audience of affected communities and health practitioners. To my colleagues in activism and scholarship in Hawai'i, especially Haunani-Kay Trask, David Stannard, John Witeck, and Joyce Chinen, *mahalo nui loa* for your many and ongoing years of impassioned dedication to the struggle, and for your friendship, kindness, generosity, and intellectual sparks.

References

Agardh, Emilie E. , Anders Ahlbom, Tomas Andersson, Suad Efendic, Valdemar Grill, Johan Hallqvist, Anders Norman and Claes-Goran Ostenson. 2003. Work Stress and Low Sense of Coherence is Associated with type 2 Diabetes in Middle-aged Swedish Women. Diabetes Care 26(3): 719–25.

Baker, Paul T., Joel M. Hanna and Thelma S. Baker, eds. 1986. The Changing Samoans: Behavior and Health in Transition. New York, NY: Oxford University Press.

Benyshek, Daniel. 2002. Type 2 Diabetes and Fetal Origins: The Promise of Prevention Programs Focusing on Prenatal Health in High Prevalence Native American Communities. Paper presented at the Annual Meeting of the American Anthropological Association, 2002.

Blaisdell, Kekuni. 1993. The Health Status of Kanaka Maoli (Indigenous Hawaiians). Asian American and Pacific Islander Journal of Health (manuscript version).

Bourdieu, Pierre. 1977. Outline of a Theory of Practice. Richard Nice, Trans. Cambridge: Cambridge University Press.

Brunner, Eric. 1997. Stress and the Biology of Inequality. British Medical Journal 314: 1472–75.

Cervantes, R.C. and F.G. Castro. 1985. Stress, Coping, and Mexican-American Mental Health: A Systematic Review. Hispanic Journal of Behavioral Sciences 7(1): 1–73.

Clark, R., N.B. Anderson, V.R. Clark and D.R. Williams. 1999. Racism as a Stressor for African Americans: A Biopsychosocial Model. Am. Psychol. 54: 805–16.

Cobb, Kristin. 2002 Missed ZZZ's, More Disease? Skimping on Sleep May be Bad for Your Health. Science News 162: 152–54.

Cole, Jennifer. 2001. Forget Colonialism? Sacrifice and the Art of Memory in Madagascar. Berkeley, CA: University of California Press.

Cook, James. 1778 (1967). The Journals of Captain James Cook on His Voyages of Discovery. Vol. 3. The Voyage of the Resolution and Discovery 1776–1780. J.C. Beaglehole, ed. The Hakluyt Society. Cambridge: Cambridge University Press.

Das, Veena, Arthur Kleinman, Margaret Lock, Mamphela Ramphele and Pamela Reynolds. 2001. Remaking a World: Violence, Social Suffering, and Recovery. Berkeley, CA: University of California Press.

Dohrenwend, Barbara Snell. 1973 Social Status and Stressful Events. *In* Psychiatric Epidemiology: Proceedings of the International Symposium. Edward H. Hare and John K. Wing, eds. pp. 313–19. New York, NY: Oxford University Press.

Edwards, Christopher and Aubrey J. Yates. 1985 The Effects of Cognitive Task Demand on Subjective Stress and Blood Glucose Levels in Diabetics and Non-diabetics. Journal of Psychosomatic Research 29: 59–69.

Ewart, C. K. and S. Suchday. 2002. Discovering How Urban Poverty and Violence Affect Health: Development and Validation of a Neighborhood Stress Index. Health Psychology: 21(3): 254–62.

Ewing, Katherine Pratt. 2000. The Violence of Non-recognition: Becoming a 'Conscious' Muslim Woman in Turkey. *In* Cultures Under Siege: Collective Violence and Trauma. Antonius C.G.M. Robben and Marcelo M. Suarez-Orozco, eds. pp. 248–71. Cambridge: Cambridge University Press.

Ferreira, Mariana Leal. 1998 Slipping Through Sky Holes: Yurok Body Imagery in Northern California. Culture, Medicine & Psychiatry 22: 171–202.

Fremont, Allen M. and Chloe E. Bird. 2000. Social and Psychological Factors, Physiological Processes, and Physical Health. *In* The Handbook of Medical Sociology. Fifth Ed. Chloe E. Bird, Peter Conrad and Allen M. Fremont, eds. pp. 334–52. Upper Saddle River, NJ: Prentice Hall.

Freund, Peter E.S. and Meredith B. McGuire. 1999. Health, Illness, and the Social Body: A Critical Sociology. Third edition. pp. 29, 88–89. Upper Saddle River, NJ: Prentice-Hall.

Garbarino, J. and K. Kostelny. 1997. What Children Can Tell Us about Living in a War Zone. *In* Children in a Violent Society. Joy D. Osofsky, ed. pp. 32–41. New York, NY: Guilford Press.

Glaser, Ronald and Janice K. Kiecolt-Glaser. 1998. Stress-associated Immune Modulation: Relevance to Viral Infections and Chronic Fatigue Syndrome. American Journal of Medicine 105: 35s–42s.

Gomes, Kuumeaaloha. 1992. Personal communication.

Harrell, F.E., M.M. Merritt and J. Kalu. 1998. Racism, Stress and Disease. *In* African American Mental Health. R.L. Jones, ed. pp. 247–80. Hampton, VA: Cobb and Henry Publishers.

Holmes, Thomas H. and Richard H. Rahe. 1967. The Social Readjustment Rating Scale. Journal of Psychosomatic Research 11: 213–18.

Hough, R.L. 1985. Life Events and Stress in Mexican-American Culture. *In* Stress and Hispanic Mental Health: Relating Research to Service Delivery. W.A. Vega and M.R. Miranda, eds. pp. 110–46. Rockville, MD: U.S. Department of Health and Human Services.

Hough, R.L., W. McGarvey, J. Graham and D. Timbers. 1981. Cultural Variation in the Modeling of Life Change-Illness Relationships. Working paper, Life Change and Illness Research Project, Neuropsychiatric Institute, University of California, Los Angeles, CA.

House, James S. 2002. Understanding Social Factors and Inequalities in Health: 20th Century Progress and 21st Century Prospects. Journal of Health and Social Behavior 43(2): 125–43.

Howard, Alan. 1986. Questions and Answers: Samoans Talk about Happiness, Distress, and Other Life Experiences. In The Changing Samoans: Behavior and Health in Transition. Paul T. Baker, Joel M. Hanna,and Thelma S. Baker, eds. pp. 174–202. New York, NY: Oxford University Press.

Ito, Karen L. 1999. Lady Friends: Hawaiian Ways and the Ties that Define. Ithaca, NY: Cornell University Press.

Kessler, R.C. and H.W. Neighbors. 1986. A New Perspective on the Relationships among Race, Social Class, and Psychological Distress. Journal of Health and Social Behavior 27: 107–15.

Komaroff, A.L., M. Masuda and T.H. Holmes. 1968. The Social Readjustment Rating Scale: A Comparative Study of Negro, Mexican and White Americans. Journal of Psychosomatic Research 12: 121–28.

Krieger, Nancy. 1999. Embodying Inequality: A Review of Concepts, Measures and Methods for Studying Health Consequences of Discrimination. Int. J. Health Services 29: 295–352.

Kunitz, Stephen J. 1994. Disease and Social Diversity: The European Impact on the Health of Non-Europeans. New York, NY: Oxford University Press.

Lane, James D., Cynthia C. McCaskill, Paula G. Williams, Priti I. Parekh, Mark N. Feinglos and Richard S. Surwit. 2000. Personality Correlates of Glycemic Control in Type 2 Diabetes. Diabetes Care 23 (9): 1321.

Luhrmann, T.M. 2000. The Traumatized Social Self: The Parsi Predicament in Modern Bombay. In Cultures Under Siege: Collective Violence and Trauma. Antonius C.G.M. Robben and Marcelo M. Suarez-Orozco, eds. pp. 158–93. Cambridge: Cambridge University Press.

McDowell, Deborah. 2003. Now That He is Gone I Sweep the Veil Away and Cry: W.E.B. DuBois, "The Souls of Black Folk", and the Poetics of Mourning. Centennial Symposium, University of Wisconsin-Madison, April 10–12, 2003.

McEwan, Bruce S. 2000. Allostasis and Allostatic Load: Implications for Neuropsychopharmacology. Neuropsychopharmacology 22(2): 108–24.

Miller, F.S. 1992. Network Structure Support: Its Relationship to the Psycho-Social Development of Black Females. In The Psycho-Social Development of Minority Group Children. G. Powell, ed. pp. 275–306. New York, NY: Brunner/Mazel.

Miller BA, L.N. Kolonel, L. Bernstein, et al. 1996. Racial/ Ethnic Patterns of Cancer in the United States, 1988–1992. Bethesda, Md: National Cancer Institute. NIH publication 96-4101.

Miller, T.Q., T.W. Smith, C.W. Turner, M.L. Guijarro and A.J. Hallet. 1996. A Meta-Analytic Review of Research on Hostility and Physical Health. Psychological Bulletin 119: 322–48.

Mooy, Johanna M., Hendrik de Vries, Peter A. Grootenhuis, Lex M. Bouter and Robert J. Heine. 2000. Major Stressful Life Events in Relation to Prevalence of Undetected type 2 Diabetes: The Hoorn Study. *Diabetes Care* 23: 197–201.

National Committee for Injury Prevention and Control. 1989. Injury Prevention: Meeting the Challenge. New York, NY: Oxford University Press.

Neighbors, H.W. 1984. The Distribution of Psychiatric Morbidity in Black Americans. Community Mental Health Journal 20: 169–81.

Noh, S., M. Beiser, V. Kaspar, F. Hou and J. Rummens. 1999. Perceived Racial Discrimination, Depression, and Coping: A Study of Southeast Asian Refugees in Canada. Journal of Health and Social Behavior 40: 193–207.

Nordic Business Report. 2002. Swedish Study Shows Connection between Diabetes and Stress. January 22, 2002.

Obesity, Fitness and Wellness Week. 2002. Umea Scientist Honored for Article on Stress Hormone and Diabetes. May 11, 2002, p.8.

Pike, Jennifer L., Tom L. Smith, Richard L. Hauger, Perry M. Nicassio, Thomas L. Patterson, John McLintick, Carolyn Costlow and Michael R. Irwin. 1997. Chronic Life Stress Alters Sympathetic, Neuroendocrine, and Immune Responsivity to an Acute Psychological Stressor in Humans. Psychosomatic Medicine 59: 447–57.

Poss, Jane and Mary Ann Jezewski. 2002. The Role and Meaning of *susto* in Mexican Americans' Explanatory Model of Type 2 Diabetes. Medical Anthropology Quarterly 16(3): 360–77.

Pruessner, Jens C., Jens Gaab, Dirk H. Hellhammer, Doris Lintz, Nicole Schommer and Clements Kirschbaum. 1997. Increasing Correlations between Personality Traits and Cortisol Stress Responses Obtained by Data Aggregation. Psychoneuroendocrinology 22: 615–25.

Rask, E., T. Olsson, S. Sodergerg, R. Andrew, D.E.W. Livingsone, O. Johnson and B.R. Walker. 2001. Tissue-Specific Dysregulation of Cortisol Metabolism in Human Obesity. Journal of Clinical Endocrinology and Metabolism 86(3): 1418–21.

Ross, Catherine E. and John Mirowsky. 2001. Neighborhood Disadvantage, Disorder, and Health. Journal of Health and Social Behavior 42: 258–76.

Scheder, Jo C. 1981. Diabetes and Stress Among Mexican-American Migrants. Unpublished PhD Dissertation. University of Wisconsin, Madison.

_____1983a. Migration, Stress, and Changing Health Patterns Among Mexican-Americans and Samoans. Presented at 43rd Annual Meeting, Society for Applied Anthropology, San Diego, CA.

_____1983b. Chronic Disease and 'Disorders of Adaptation' in Migrant and Modernizing Populations Session. Presented at 52nd American Association of Physical Anthropologists Annual Mtgs., Indianapolis, IN.

_____1983c Stress, Life Events and Health Among Samoans and Mexican-Americans. Presented at 82nd Annual Meeting, American Anthropological Association Annual Mtgs., Chicago, IL.

_____1988. A Sickly-Sweet Harvest: Farmworker Diabetes and Social Equality. *Medical Anthropology Quarterly* (n.s.) 2(3): 251–77.

_____1996. Co-Opted Aloha and the Body in Struggle. Presented at the 95th American Anthropological Association Annual Mtgs., San Francisco, CA.

_____1998. The Death of Health: Cosmology and Emotion in Colonial Depopulation. Presented at the 97th American Anthropological Association Annual Mtgs., Philadelphia, PA.

Scheper-Hughes, Nancy. 1992. Death Without Weeping: the Violence of Everyday Life in Brazil. Berkeley, CA: University of California Press.

Soyinka, Wole. 1999. The Burden of Memory, the Muse of Forgiveness. New York, NY: Oxford University Press.

Spiegel, K., R. Leproult and E. Van Cauter. 1999. Impact of Sleep Debt on Metabolic and Endocrine Function. Lancet 354(9188): 1435–39.

Stannard, David E. 1989. Before the Horror: The Population of Hawai'i on the Eve of Contact. Honolulu, HI: University of Hawai'i Press.

Surwit, Richard S. and Mark N. Feinglos. 1983 The Effects of Relaxation on Glucose Tolerance in Non-Insulin-Dependent Diabetes. Diabetes Care 6(2): 176–79.

_____1988. Stress and Autonomic Nervous System in Type II Diabetes: A Hypothesis. Diabetes Care 11(1): 83–85.

Surwit, Richard S., Mark N. Feinglos, et al. 2002 Stress Management Improves Long-Term Glycemic Control in type 2 Diabetes. Diabetes Care 25(1): 30–34.

Surwit , Richard S., Redford B. Williams, Ilene C. Siegler, James D. Lane, Michael Helms, Katherine L. Applegate, Nancy Zucker, Mark N. Feinglos, Cynthia M. McCaskill and John C. Barefoot. 2002. Hostility, Race, and Glucose Metabolism in Nondiabetic Individuals. Diabetes Care 25(5): 835–39.

Taylor, Shelly, Rena L. Repetti and Teresa Seeman. 1997. Health Psychology: What is an Unhealthy Environment and How Does It Get under the Skin? Annual Review of Psychology 48: 411–47.

Thibodeau, Gary A. and Kevin T. Patton. 1997 The Human Body in Health and Disease, 2nd edition. New York, NY: Mosby.

Thompson, Vetta L. Sanders. 2002. Racism: Perceptions of Distress among African Americans. Community Mental Health Journal 38(2): 111–19.

Trask, Haunani-Kay. 1993 Lovely Hula Hands. *In* From a Native Daughter. pp. 179–97. Monroe, ME: Common Courage Press.

Van Cauter, Eve and K. Spiegel. 1999. Sleep as a Mediator of the Relationship between Socioeconomic Status and Health: A Hypothesis. Ann N Y Acad Sci 896: 254–61.

Van Rossum, E.F. 2002. A Polymorphism in the Glucocorticoid Receptor Gene, Which Decreases Sensitivity to Glucocorticoids *in vivo*, is Associated with Low Insulin and Cholesterol Levels. Diabetes 51(10): 3128–34.

Walters, Karina. 2002. Reconceptualizing Native Women's Health: An "Indigenist" Stress-coping Model. American Journal of Public Health 92(4): 520–24.

White, Carolynne J. 1995. Native Americans at Promise: Travel in Borderlands. *In* Children and Families "at Promise." Swadener, Beth Blue and Sally Lubeck, eds. pp. 163–84. State University of New York Press.

Williams, David R. 2002. Racial/Ethnic Variations in Women's Health: The Social Embeddedness of Health. American Journal of Public Health 92(4): 588–97.

Williams, D.R., Y. Yu, J. Jackson and N. Anderson. 1997. Racial Differences in Physical and Mental Health: Socioeconomic Status, Stress, and Discrimination. J Health Psychol. 2: 335–51.

Women of Color Health Data Book: Adolescents to Seniors. 1998. Bethesda, MD: Office of Research on Women's Health. NIH Publication 98-4247.

Chapter 14

Love in Colonial Light: History of Yurok Emotions in Northern California[1]

Mariana Leal Ferreira

Summary of Chapter 14. Mollie Ruud was a Yurok fisherwoman born on the Yurok Indian Reservation in northern California in the late 1920s. Mollie was always a very active defender of the rights of her People, especially the water and fishing rights of the Yurok Tribe on the Klamath River. After suffering multiple physical and emotional abuses at the Chemawa Boarding School for Indian children in Oregon, Mollie Ruud spent her young adult life working as a fisherwoman, fish filleter, and chambermaid on and around the Yurok "rez." I start with Mollie's lifetime perspective on fishing rights at the turn of the 21st century and then go back in time, presenting the elder's opening statement about her early childhood on the rez until her compulsory eight-year incarceration at Chemawa in the 1940s. As Mollie's life narrative unfolds, diabetes mellitus is brought into discourse in such a way as to call our attention to the historical and political context or background in which the disorder and its complications originate. As the main protagonist of this chapter, Mollie Ruud unveils the intrinsic links between diabetes and oppression, pointing directly to the perverse ways in which colonialism and genocide have placed Indigenous Peoples at heightened risk for the disorder. During our multiple encounters since 1994 at her home on the reservation and at tribal meetings, ceremonial dances, salmon festivals, and unfortunately in hospitals given her ill health, Mollie Ruud's life history clearly revealed powerful connections between traumatic events and her twenty-plus year experience with type 2 diabetes. The elder's narrative leads us in the direction of the broader Yurok community's perceptions of the strong relationship between emotional suffering and the emergence of diabetes in northern California. Here in this essay, this association is shown to be statistically positive in a genealogical analysis of 20 Yurok extended families, traced back to the 1850s and including 1702 individuals—extending the discussion on trauma presented earlier in this book in Chapters 3 and 18. The quantitative analysis supports the qualitative ethnographic data, confirming the validity of Mollie Ruud and many other Yurok

---

1. All cartoons and line drawings in this chapter are by Yurok artist Sammy Gensaw. Reproduced with permission.

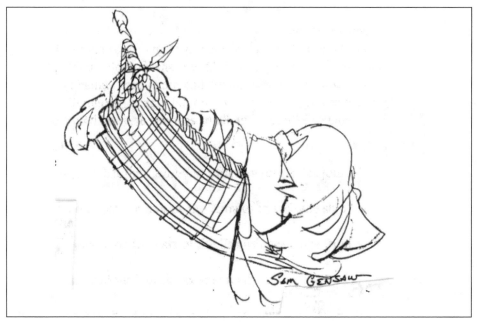

Yurok child in a baby basket.

women's theory about the emotional causes of diabetes. Our conclusion: Yurok individuals who experienced a major traumatic event—confinement in boarding schools, prisons, juvenile halls and foster homes, military experiences, premature death of family members, and/or sexual abuse—have a much higher probability of developing type 2 diabetes because of emotional suffering. On the other hand, those families and individuals who are engaged in networks of social support can manage their sentiments more effectively and are thus able to assure emotional liberty, seen here as a protective factor against diabetes. Physiologically speaking, we contend that type 2 diabetes is an outcome of emotionally stimulating claims in terms of the arousal of the autonomic nervous system and the endocrine system. Emotional suffering and emotional liberty are proposed as conceptual ideas that can help redefine the diabetes question in terms of what we call a politically meaningful history of emotions.

Introduction

Mollie Ruud: "Indian people have always been closely watched and controlled"

Fish sure is a hot issue around here. People get all worked up when it comes to fishing rights and regulations on the reservation. My blood sugar always goes up just to think of it, especially after a fish meeting. And everyone is involved in this war, in one way or another. 'Cause it is a war, you know...the

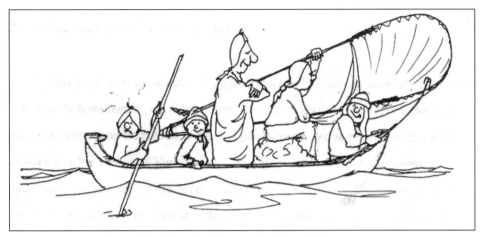

Yurok family fishing on the Klamath River.

feds were here with their machine guns…They arrested a whole bunch of people, knocked people on the head, twisted women's arms around. They came down on people with their big guns and if it weren't for these lawyers that went up to them and said, "We're lawyers, we're lawyers. Don't do anything to these people," they would've killed us.

You'd think that if we are a Tribe, we'd be able to make our own fishing regulations on the Klamath River. But it's not the case. Even though we won our fishing rights back in 1973, the federal government still gets to make all the regulations. They say we'd have to own 50 percent of our reservation to regulate anything, and we own less than 10 percent! Can you believe that?…Now, how come we get only 3 salmon per dip net? Having to get a California State license to fish? No drift-netting? No salmon snagging with an eel hook, either? The papers say sport fishermen are getting a bigger fishing season, and so are shore fishermen. So we are here, and we're being asked to cut back on our season, while non-Indians are getting more time. The federal government has no right to say what we should do if they allow non-Indians to sport fish and commercial fish on our river.

My hair dances on the back of my neck just to think of all these regulations. It's like you spend your whole life being closely regulated, controlled, every single thing you do, every step you take you are watched…All my life I've felt like I was under supervision of some kind, and this has an effect on people, I'm sure. Indian people, it seems to me, have always been closely watched and controlled, all our lives, all our lives.

On January 17, 1995, Mollie Ruud and I drove back to her house in Requa after attending a fish meeting at the Yurok Tribal Office in Klamath, Northern California. In her usual loud and bold voice, Mollie reiterated some of the thoughts she had voiced at the meeting. The Yurok elder seemed to be worked up; she was agitated and angry. "I need to get home and take my insulin first thing. I don't feel good." As we crossed

Highway 101 on the way to her house in Requa where the Klamath River runs into the Pacific Ocean, she continued: "I bet you fishing has made a lot of people diabetic around here. It's just too much."[2]

I had just watched Mollie and a few other Yurok women engage in a forceful discussion among themselves and with the fish biologist of the Yurok Tribe, on the management and regulation of the gill-net fishery on the Klamath River. Most of the people present at the meeting were women, including the Chairperson of the Yurok Council and a council member. Like Mollie, they protested vehemently against the set of governmental regulations on fishing, while trying to devise new strategies to increase Yurok control of fishing on the reservation.

As they passionately debated how to manage their own chinook, coho, and steelhead salmon harvests,[3] I learned of their struggle to win back aboriginal fishing rights lost in 1892. By Executive Order, the Klamath River Reservation established in 1855 was opened "to settlement, entry, and purchase under the laws of the United States granting homestead rights." Yuroks could apply, "at any time within one year...to the Secretary of the Interior for an allotment of land." But the Secretary of the Interior could also "reserve...any tract...upon which any village or settlement of Indians is now located" for settlement, entry or purchase (*Mattz v. Arnett* U.S. Supreme Court decision No. 71-1182 of 6/11/73). Today, logging companies alone own 85 percent of the Yurok Reservation, while another 5 percent is in the hands of other private owners.

The U.S. Allotment Act (aka Dawes Act) and consequent termination of Indian reservation status in 1892 banned Indigenous subsistence and ceremonial fishing on the Klamath River and its tributaries in northern California until 1973. Raymond Mattz, a Yurok fisherman from Requa, a Yurok village located on the mouth of the Klamath River and the Pacific Ocean, fought in court for 12 years (*Mattz v. Arnett* U.S. Supreme court case No. 71-1182) to see Yurok territory regain its "Indian country" status according to federal law. However, the new set of federal regulations on "Indian Fishing," published in 1978, favored non-Indian ocean sport fishery, commercial troll fishery and river sport fishery, over Yurok gill-net and drift-net fishing rights.[4] It pro-

---

2. The Klamath River Reserve was created by Executive Order in 1855. In 1864 another section of Yurok aboriginal land became a part of the Hoopa Valley Indian Reservation (known as the 12-mile "Square"), which was set apart for Yuroks and other Northern California populations. In 1891, a further part of Yurok territory was added to the Klamath River Reserve, when "The Extension" to the Hoopa Reservation was set aside by executive order. This statutory reservation extension, which became the Yurok Reservation after the Yurok-Hoopa split in 1963 (described in the *Jessie Short* case), extends from the mouth of the Klamath River, including the old Klamath River Reserve, about 50 miles inland, encompassing the river and its bed, along with one mile on both sides of the river. Today, only 5% of the Yurok Reservation is owned by Yuroks, while approximately 85% is in the hands of timber companies. The remaining 10% is in the hands of other private owners. (Sources: The Yurok Constitution pp. 2, and the Yurok Tribe.)

3. The Klamath River system used to have a fairly large run of chinook (king) salmon (*Oncorhynchus tshawytscha*), coho (silver) salmon (*Oncorhynchus kisutch*), and steelhead rainbow trout (*Salmo gairdneri gairdneri*). However, this run has declined significantly because of habitat changes brought about by mining, logging, damming, and pesticide spraying (source: Yurok Tribal Fisheries Program).

4. A gill net is "a flat net suspended vertically in the water with meshes that allow the head of a fish to pass but entangle the fish when it seeks to withdraw." A drift net or a pole net is "a gill net

hibited commercial fishing on the reservation, restricted the use of fishing gear, demanded strict compliance with fish-catch reporting to the U.S. Fish and Wildlife Service and imposed penalties (fees, jail terms and suspension of tribal fishing rights) for violations of the regulations.

According to Mollie Ruud,

> It was like, "OK, you've got the right to fish now, but we're going to tell you how." We didn't like that, them telling us when and how we could fish, how much fish we needed for subsistence, what ceremonial fishing meant. Right after [the Department of Interior] published the regulations, the feds came down on us real hard, acting like a bunch of wild hogs, beating the shit out of everybody. We'd fool them pretending we were gill netting, but it was just a line stretched out with corks on it, no web hanging on the net. They'd go furious and come down on us even harder, taking our nets, arresting everybody, getting real tough. They wanted us to fish at night not to bother the tourists during the day. Unbelievable. But we didn't give in. They declared war on us. It was a pretty amazing spectacle of their military power.

War indeed it was to the federal government. Yurok resistance to enforcement efforts of the 1978 Indian Fishing Regulations on the Klamath River was met with a "strike force" of special agents, U.S. Park Police and Bureau of Indian Affairs officers. On the part of the Yuroks there were, according to the Chief of the Division of Law Enforcement, "constant attempts to harass, provoke and intimidate officers," such as "cursing....Spitting....Occult threats of death, disease, impotence....Biting. Sand in the face. Passive resistance and refusal to identify. Wrestling, punches thrown...Roadblocks." Some of the 134 Indians arrested by the special agents were considered "criminal types with long arrest records. Heavy alcohol and drug use was common...Outside radical left wing influence was apparent." The U.S. "Command Organization" thus felt the need for "SWAT and riot control training," including defensive tactics, riot control tactics, use of tear gas and mace, firebomb defense, air support, anti-sniper tactics and equipment—tuned-up and sighted-in AR-15 and M-16 rifles, and riot guns.[5] (A sniperscope is an optical device used during World War II, for use especially with a rifle that allows a person to see targets better in the dark.)

According to the Yuroks, however, the U.S. strike force did not produce "a notable improvement in compliance" as the director of the Division of Law Enforcement believes it did. Determining the catch taken by the Indian gill-net fishery, for example, is also in the best interest of the Yuroks, whose fishing practices include an awareness of spawning seasons and the danger of overfishing wild stocks. Reporting the harvest of salmon and steelhead to the BIA is also aimed at showing the public that the Yuroks are not responsible for depleting wild stocks of fish and that they do have a fishery

---

which is not staked, anchored or weighted, but drifts free" (Rules and Regulations of Indian Fishing, Federal Register, vol. 44, no. 55, March 20, 1979, pp. 17148–49).

5. "Analysis of Klamath River Fishery Enforcement Project—1978." Memorandum in reply to FWS/LE ENF 1-04, June 22, 1979, from the Chief of Division of Law Enforcement to the Director of the U.S. Fish and Wildlife Service (pp. 1–7).

management program. This, in turn, prevents the federal government from imposing further restrictions on Yurok fishermen (Tripp 1976). These management strategies are far from being totally compliant with federal rules and regulations. That power is not only repressive but also productive, is well known. What else has this power produced? Frank McCovey, a Yurok fisherman who confronted the U.S. strike force on several occasions in 1978, puts it this way: "Situations like this make me mean." [6] Mollie Ruud agrees: "They've made people so mad, so angry, so much hatred brought into our hearts…It's like they make you hate the world, be angry all the time. You just can't stand being under all this control."

The Social and Political Context Where Diabetes Originates

Throughout our frequent encounters in the 1990s until the moment of her death on June 4, 2004, Mollie Ruud also spoke about her early childhood on the Yurok Reservation, boarding school experiences in Salem, Oregon, and work in fish canneries in Northern California. Her reminiscences included moments of her brothers', mother's, grandmother's and close friends' lives on or near the reservation. Whether she spoke about her "wild little Indian" childhood, life on the rez, feelings at the off-reservation Chemawa Boarding School for Indian kids, the fish filleter routine, alcohol and drug abuse, or her perceptions on diabetes, I saw the issue of "control" weaving these seemingly diversified experiences together. Control on the part of individuals who, like Mollie, "tried to keep my dignity as a person when they tried to make me into an animal"; control on the part of the Yuroks as a community to regain what they call their "aboriginal rights"; control on the part of the United States government to discipline and rehabilitate individuals and populations. As Yurok tribal member Robert McCoy explained at a 1979 fish meeting:

> Control means that they are going to control, and I'm talking about the Bureau of Indian Affairs here. They are going to control every aspect of whatever you Indians do. They have had control for a hundred years or more and they are still going to maintain that control, so control means that there is an overall plan and the plan is the fishing regulations, as a part of that plan…They want to take control away from the Court of Claims. They do not want you, as individuals, to be qualified by the Court of Claims because then we would probably have justice. Now, if they can take that control away from the courts and they come up with their own regulations…they will have complete control over everything that happens to you people…What they are doing is control you until you can't even breathe like they've been doing for years and years.[7]

---

6. Deposition to a community meeting promoted by the Bureau of Indian Affairs on the "Regulations Governing Indian Fishing on the Hoopa Indian Reservation in Northern California, including the Square and the Extension [the Yurok Indian Reservation]," Jan. 21, 1979, in Arcata, CA (p. 28).

7. Deposition to a community meeting promoted by the Bureau of Indian Affairs on the "Regulations Governing Indian Fishing on the Hoopa Indian Reservation in Northern California, includ-

Mollie Ruud's life experience brings together elements of the overall plan of control Robert McCoy explains above. Her narratives speak of a generalized carceral or penal system, developed in many European countries and in the United States to discipline and punish individuals. Much like hers, a considerable proportion of Yurok biographies of the 1800s and 1900s involve boarding schools, reservations, prisons, mental homes, hospitals, TB wards, forced labor camps, rehabilitation centers and so forth. Work in canneries, logging camps, mills, factories and rich homes in San Francisco are also part of the more subtle mechanisms of the nineteenth and twentieth-century penal reform to "rehabilitate" individuals. The transformation of the madman, the vagabond, the criminal and the sick—categories which the "savage Indian," in one way or another, fit easily into—called for a very specific political tactic: deprive individuals of liberty through imprisonment and forced labor.

The constraints and privations, obligations and prohibitions Mollie Ruud speaks about are characteristic of this penal system, which has transformed physical punishment into an "economy of suspended rights" (Foucault 1995: 11). Rather than rehabilitation, the disciplinary "training" Mollie and many other Yuroks have gone through in the last 200 years has *produced* sickness, delinquency, despair and other forms of emotional suffering. While the purpose of such disciplinary mechanisms, it is widely believed, is to lead *away* from prisons, hospitals and reformatories, the histories of 20 Yurok extended families, show an opposite trend. Most of the Yuroks held in local jails, state prisons and mental homes, as well as those who suffer from diabetes and related illnesses, alcoholism, drug abuse and domestic violence, spent their childhood in boarding schools, juvenile detention centers, forced labor camps, and the like (see chapters 3 and 18 in this volume).

A close look at the life experiences of eight generations of Yurok individuals, dating back to the gold rush in the 1850s, contextualizes the emergence of premature deaths, drug abuse, alcoholism, domestic violence, suicides and degenerative diseases in Northern California. This genealogical approach treats Yurok narratives about their past and present experiences as historical events and correlates the perceptions of such events with neuroendocrine patterns of emotional response. The correlations Mollie has drawn allow us to spatialize diabetes on the social and political body, rather than exclusively on the physical one. Forced labor, confinement, and murder are also treated here as diseases.

As Mollie Ruud and many other individuals narrated in detail Yurok life experiences, I myself often thought of a question formulated by the physician Wilhelm Reich in his study on fascism: after centuries of exploitation, why do people still tolerate being humiliated and enslaved? As Reich remarks, "The astonishing thing is not that some people steal or that others occasionally go out on strike, but rather that all those who are starving do not steal as a regular practice, and all those who are exploited are not continually out on strike" (Reich 1970, cited in Deleuze and Guattari 1977: 29). While Reich himself did not provide a satisfactory explanation of this phenomenon, Michel Foucault (1995: 301–2) offers an answer in *Discipline and Punish*: The most important effect of the new penal system is that "it succeeds in making the power to punish natural and legitimate, in lowering at least the threshold of tolerance to penalty. It tends to efface what may be exorbitant in the exercise of punishment." In other words, it

---

ing the Square and the Extension [the Yurok Indian Reservation]," Jan. 21, 1979, in Arcata, CA (pp. 16–18).

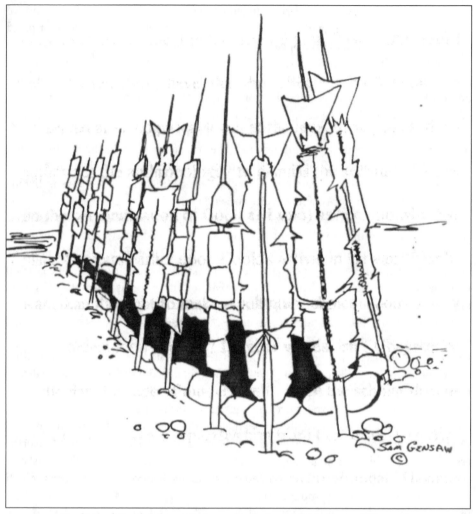

Traditional Yurok Salmon Barbecue on Redwood Sticks around Charcoal.

makes violence more readily accepted and tolerated. Yurok women's articulation of their own bodies and local histories, however, attests to their role as powerful and active sentient beings, capable of engaging in struggles, constructing resistances and mobilizing resources. The tactics and strategies the Yuroks themselves have devised to organize themselves as a federally recognized tribe, to manage the reservation's natural resources and to operate United Indian Health Services and now the Potawot Health Village illustrate this ability (see chapter 18 in this book).

Let us now go back to Mollie Ruud's childhood in the 1930s on the Yurok Indian Reservation.

Mollie Ruud: "I just can't handle freedom"

I remember when I was young, there was no electricity and we had to pack our water. We didn't have an outhouse, either. But we were happy. I couldn't wait for the evening when grandma would make acorns and we'd fight over the rocks, to scrape the acorn off them.[8] That was sooooo good, and we had so much fun! I can remember when electricity first came. We just went nuts over these light switches, on and off, on and off…

Also, we used to get rocks and sticks and throw them at the cars that went down the road. We'd hide in the bushes, that was pretty fun. We were like wild little Indians. That's all we did, play in the brush. We never had wagons or ropes. We used to swing in the branches, and if we were lucky enough to find an old piece of cardboard box, we'd sit on it and slide down the hills. We were such bratty kids! There were these warty toads, they'd hide in the bark. We'd dig them out to play. We'd poke their behinds to see how far they jumped! All we did was play in the brush, and it was a lot of fun.

Below our house, there was this island, a little creek and a bridge. We'd play around in the creek and we learned how to swim, all by ourselves. Once we begged our mother to go across the river in grandpa's dugout, and she finally let us. Right in the middle of the river, we fell overboard. Then we ducked underneath the boat and hid there for a while. We sure did get a whipping for that!

The other thing we liked to do was play tourist. Just a few days ago, I saw tourists playing around with salmon. They use non-barbed wire so the fish is not really hooked, but they can play around with it and still pretend they're really fishing. I guess it's a feeling. By the time they let the fish go, the animal is so tired that it usually dies. You can see the fish floating on their bellies. I think this is the worst law they've ever made. Can you imagine, they can't fish out of season, but pretending is allowed. Giving tourists the pleasure! So in those days, 50 or 60 years ago, we watched them do that. And we, too, I mean, all the kids that lived on this side of the river, we wanted to do the same. We just loooooved to play tourist on the Klamath. Grandpa had this dugout. We'd paddle to the cove, hook a fish and yard it right in, then we'd let it go. But then grandpa would get mad at us and say we couldn't play with food. He said we were spoiling food, that food is sacred and if the whites go around sport fishing, we don't do that. He said in Indian, "if you get a fish you have to pull it in the boat immediately. No playing around." Naturally, we cried. See, I was just six or seven. So sometimes we'd bring the fish home, to make winter food. Grandma would dry it so we'd have food in the winter. Oh, but these are good memories!

Now, there was some work we had to do, too. Mom worked at the Requa cannery filleting fish all day. She had us sit under the cannery, my brother and I, to get the brains of the fish the white men discarded. It was awful under there, muddy and stinky, with all the fish guts floating about. We'd crawl in that water under the cannery, it was really gross. We'd carry this sack and we'd have to do it everyday. We had to fill up that sack so we'd fight to see who could fill up that sack first. But we wanted those fish heads. We didn't get to eat the fish Mom filleted. We couldn't afford it. And it came from our very own river! So

8. Hot rocks are placed inside a basket or pan to cook the acorn soup. See recipe ahead.

we took the sack home, and we'd lay those salmon heads on berry leaves, smoke them a little bit and dry them. Then in the winter we'd boil them and eat them. Oh, they smelled so bad! They really stunk! But they were clean and we liked them. I guess when you don't have much food, you appreciate things differently.

The old cannery was built in this cove at the mouth [of the Klamath River], near Windy Point. That's where the resort is now, where the whites deal all the dope. They blew Windy Point up with dynamite and made it into a resort for tourists, but now it's just a cover up for all the dope trafficking, one of the biggest in the area. And everyone knows about it, too.

But then it happened. Mom told us that sooner or later the day would come, when they would take us away to school, to boarding school, and that we had to go. It was so scary, but we thought we'd be able to hide in the bushes when the truck came for us. We even had a secret hideout!...Some folks would hide their kids 'cause they didn't want them to go through all that pain, or else 'cause they needed them at home to help them out. Uncle Scott, they hid him. True, they found him later and he had to go. Now he's in a mental home, after years and years of redwood logging. But Mom, I guess she did-n't really want us 'cause she was always too doped up. She herself had been dragged to Chemawa Boarding School and to Hoopa Boarding School. She was so troubled, into drinking and drugging all the time after she got out, I guess she just didn't care about us or even about herself. So when the day came, she made my brother and I get into the cattle truck and off we went. Eight years away from home, can you imagine? Eight looooong years, a life-time, it seemed to me. No visits, no letters, no nothing. Just like being in prison, Chemawa to me was a prison, a jail house. Like Pelican Bay [State Prison]. Gray, dark, cold. I shiver just to think of it. When I got out, I was 16. I just went wild, wild. I couldn't handle all that freedom, just couldn't handle freedom.

Mollie Ruud, like several other Yurok women and men I met, often refer to board-ing schools as prisons, reservations as concentration camps, medical practices as mil-itary interventions, and negotiations with the federal government as battles or wars. Their analogies are not unfounded. Although the U.S. Office of Indian Affairs was transferred from the War Department to the new Department of Interior in 1849, mil-itary strategies and tactics have always guided the education, supervision and protec-tion of Indigenous Peoples by the United States government. The violent disruption of American Indians' social life since the Gold-Rush in northern California is well doc-umented (Adams 1995; Heizer & Mills 1991 [1952]); ITEPP 1999; Ferreira 1996, 1998, 1999; Nelson Jr. 1978; Rawls n/d; Thompson 1991[1916]). The perverse effects of the continuing genocide of Indigenous Peoples in the state since the 1850s include severe depopulation (90-95%), a dramatic decrease in life expectancy due to alcoholism and violence, and a tremendous rise, especially since the 1950s, in the incidence of degen-erative diseases, such as type 2 diabetes. As discussed in Chapter 18, between 1950 and 1969, Yurok life expectancy was at its lowest—36.4 years. Diabetes, in turn, is known

A word on genocide: *Geno*, Latin for a people or tribe; *Cide*, for killing. Genocide, or the killing or murder of an entire people. In 1948 the United Nations General Assembly adopted the term as "denial of the right of existence of an entire human group," adding in 1994, beyond the act of outright murder, also the "destruction and extermination of culture." In the *Convention on the Prevention and Punishment of the Crime of Genocide,* adopted by Resolution 260 (III) A of the United Nations General Assembly on December 9, 1948, five attributes are said to pertain to genocide: (a) Killing members of the group; (b) Causing serious bodily or mental harm to members of the group; (c) Deliberately inflicting on the group conditions of life calculated to bring about its physical destruction in whole or in part; (d) Imposing measures intended to prevent births within the group; (e) Forcibly transferring children of the group to another group. The widely documented history of Indigenous Peoples in California prove that *all* of these attributes pertain to Californian Indigenous nations. The United States has signed, but still not ratified, the UN Convention on Genocide.

to be a major risk factor for cardiovascular disease—the leading cause of death for American Indians and Alaska Natives (Ellis and Campos-Outcalt 1994).

The similarity Mollie Ruud evokes between fishing and forced labor, boarding schools and confinement is the starting point from which a novel network of analogies can be traced linking diabetes, emotional suffering, and emotional liberty. This network of analogies or equivalences springs from a close consideration of the genealogies of 20 Yurok extended families, traced back to the 1850s and including 1702 individuals (see Ferreira, Chapter 3). Traumatic experience generated by the process of colonization and genocide—boarding school confinement, premature death of a loved one, racial discrimination, among other shocking or distressing events, places the Yurok and other Indigenous Peoples in northern California at high risk for diabetes and correlated illnesses. The fur trade, the gold rush, and federal Indian policies broadly speaking (relocation onto reservations and termination of tribal status, among others) tragically disrupted social networks of support and, therefore, the emotional liberty of California peoples, while exterminating entire populations all together. As defined by anthropologist W. Reddy (1999), emotional liberty is the ability to manipulate or manage one's emotions. It involves freedom to change goals in response to bewildering, ambivalent situations, and to undergo conversion experiences and life-course changes involving numerous contrasting incommensurable factors. What emotional liberty means for the Yurok People, and the role played by love in light of the current diabetes epidemic is what Mollie Ruud and I have attempted to explain in this chapter.

Studies in medical anthropology, as discussed in most chapters of this book, show that colonization and genocide are, in themselves, responsible for the rise of many disorders, including depression, alcoholism, drug abuse, domestic violence, and diabetes all over the world. Survivors of the Jewish Holocaust have suffered from these ailments as well, and so have victims of war crimes and other horrendous tragedies (Baider et al. 2000; Farmer 2003; Malkki 1995; Pérez-Sales et al. 2000; Scheper-Hughes and Bourgois 2004). It is not surprising that California Indigenous nations refer to their contact history since the gold rush as the California Holocaust (ITEPP 1999). In a similar vein, The American Holocaust Project, as envisioned by the Dakota actor and activist Floyd Red Crow Westerman, addresses the continuing genocide of American Indians and the deliberate ahistorical consciousness that denies how legacies of the past linger into the present lives of Indigenous Peoples in the United States (Pino and Ferreira, forthcoming).

As we shall see next, Yurok individuals who experienced a major traumatic event—confinement in boarding schools, prisons, juvenile halls and foster homes, military experiences, premature death of family members, and/or sexual abuse—have a much higher probability of developing type 2 diabetes.

Illness Narratives, Traumatic Experience, and Type 2 Diabetes

Mollie Ruud's life experience is in no way unique but very similar and in some ways identical to the trajectories of other Yurok women who were born in northern California during the first half of the twentieth century. These women associate the onset of type 2 diabetes with traumatic experiences they have been through or of which they hold memories. Lydia Thompson, as I shall call her, was a Yurok elder who died in 1998 in her mid fifties of multiple organ failure—heart, kidney, and liver, as a result of type 2 diabetes. Mollie Ruud and Lydia Thompson grew up together on the rez and their life histories have many points in common. Much like Mollie's, Lydia's life narrative places diabetes into discourse in such a way as to call our attention to the context or background in which the disorder and its complications originate:

> I just can't get over all the beatings and rapings we went through in boarding school. I have nightmares. The children screamed at night, little children missing their parents. We were beaten up for any little thing we did, even for being hungry. We were kept locked up in a dark room if we spilled anything, slapped in the face for speaking Indian, beaten up if we dared to look the matrons in the eye. It was just horrible. My blood sugars go up just because I am thinking about it. In fact, I got diabetes when I learned that my son was going to be sent to Chemawa. It is just like being sent to prison.

Chemawa is the boarding school in southern Oregon most Yuroks, Tolowas and Wiyots were confined to, and, in some cases, are still sent to. It is now a therapeutic school for "troubled Indian kids." In addition, Lydia's association between school and prison is not unwarranted: Off-reservation boarding schools for Indians in the United States were fashioned after 18th century prison models. The order was to "kill the Indian in him and save the man," according to Lieutenant Pratt, the founder of Carlisle, in Pennsylvania—the first boarding school for American Indians built in the U.S. (Ferreira 1996).

The importance of life histories in advancing new findings about Indigenous Peoples' health cannot be overstated. This is what several authors in this book show quite clearly because we take what Indigenous Peoples think, say, feel, and do very seriously (see Lang, Chapter 9, in particular). The collection of life experiences or personal trajectories are of key importance to Indigenous Peoples' emotional liberty because:

1. personal trajectories can elucidate the ways in which Indigenous Peoples think about the world in which they live and help create;

2. life-histories illuminate the emotional structure of a way of life;

3. life-histories can generate oral-history workshops and/or be used to document and produce important educational materials to be used by the different tribes (in local schools and cultural centers, if the community and research partners feel this is desirable);

4. the process of narrating personal trajectories may constitute a therapeutic act in itself (when conducted appropriately, following specific guidelines), because it may provide a coping mechanism for grieving and dealing in a systematic way with one's emotions.

Paying close attention to personal illness narratives like Mollie's and Lydia's, and life-histories of members of 20 Yurok extended families enabled us to detect novel associations between the emergence of symptoms of diabetes and/or its diagnosis. Here, trauma is seen not only as a clinical concept but as a social dimension of ill health. Traumatic experience produces feelings of powerlessness, which materialize in the women's self-images of worthlessness, a sense of being under tight control and imprisoned in their life situation, and emotional suffering (Strandmark 2004). No longer able to resort to family or community support, as the California gold rush disrupted the basic tissues of social life that bond people together, destructive feelings of alienation, anguish, shame for being an "Indian" and guilt take over, and the individual's autonomy and existence are threatened.

Ethnographic Research Methods: Correlating Qualitative and Quantitative Information

The way in which Mollie Ruud's life experience correlates traumatic events and the onset of diabetes type 2 is in no way exceptional but extraordinarily similar to the trajectories of Yurok men and women in northern California in the 19th and 20th centuries. In order to analyze the way in which diabetes was contextualized and given meaning by Yurok individuals, extensive qualitative data were obtained during 128 home visits conducted on, and on the outskirts of, the Yurok Reservation in Humboldt and Del Norte Counties in northern California in the late 1990s. Personal data of central collaborators and extended family members were organized into genealogical charts using Cyrillic software. The resulting family trees represent 8 generations of 20 Yurok families, with a total population of 1702 people. Generation 1 is situated during the California Gold Rush (1850–60) and Generation 8 from 1990 to date. The first documented cases of diabetes among "Indian women" appeared in 1901 (Ferreira 1998, 1999, and chapter 3 in this volume).[9]

---

9. Entries in the Hoopa Valley Health and Sanitary Records (HVHSR) of 1901 and 1902 show three unidentified Indian women being diagnosed as "diabetic". A recipe for a "Drink for Diabetics" ("Acidi citrici, Glycerini, Spts. vini gallici and Aqu_ destil. Use as a drink") can already be found in the 1896 HVHSR. Insulin became one of the medications dispensed on a regular basis at the Hoopa Valley Agency in the 1930s. This is precisely the decade when Yurok individuals born as of 1890 (Generation 3 in Fig. 2) showed the first signs and symptoms of the disorder. The Hoopa Valley Agency provided medical assistance to the Hupas, Yuroks and other Indians confined in the Hoopa Valley

For this particular study, 544 individuals between the ages of 45–81 were randomly selected from (1) the Diabetes Registry of United Indian Health Services (UIHS)[10] in Trinidad, California, and (2) the broader Yurok community in order to trace the correlation between trauma and diabetes. Life-histories and interview responses reflecting traumatic factors related to the onset and/or diagnosis of type 2 diabetes were marked and organized into topic areas. Typical comments regarding emotional response to adverse life conditions included "shocking," "dreadful," "awful," "disgusting," "wicked," "terrible," "sinful," "offensive," "sentenced me to death," "hardened my heart," "made me angry," "destroyed my sole," killed my hope," "killed my spirit." Events associated with these emotional responses, as in Mollie Ruud's memories of her childhood, were classified into eight trauma types to further clarify the meanings of traumatic memory and experience. Trauma types positively associated with the onset and/or diagnosis of diabetes in this study, as shown ahead in Figure 14.1, are:

1. Boarding School (BS) confinement—between 1890–1940, BS attendance was compulsory for Yurok children aged 8–16;

2. Death of a loved one—Yurok life expectancy decreased from 60.6 years in generation 3, to 36.4 years in generation 6;

3. Local jail, juvenile hall or high security state prison confinement (including Folsom, San Quentin and Pelican Bay prisons);

4. Sexual and/or physical abuse (forced sexual contact and beatings by custodians, foster parents and other caretakers);

5. Army, Navy and/or War experience (WW I, II, Korean and Vietnam wars);

6. Foster home—a disproportionate number of children in foster care placement in northern CA were, and still are American Indians;

7. Forced/induced labor—individuals were trapped in a debt-system in fish, logging and steel industries;

8. Overt racial discrimination—"Indian blood" and its fractions define Indian identity in the U.S., and are used to justify or excuse Indian failures; and

9. Multiple—2 or more of the trauma types listed above.

The apparent connection between traumatic experiences and the onset and/or diagnoses of type 2 diabetes prompted us to test for the statistical correlation between diabetes and trauma categories. A logistic regression was employed to determine any effect of trauma on the odds of an individual being diagnosed with diabetes in a sample of 544 individuals born between 1870 and 1969 (generations 3 to 6). The data were coded in a

---

Indian Reservation Reserve, in northern CA. Yurok ancestral territory was part of this reservation until 1963, when the Yurok Reservation (YR) acquired independent status. The YR extends from the mouth of the Klamath River on the Pacific about 50 miles inland, encompassing the river and its bed, along with one mile on both sides of the river.

10. UIHS is the primary health care provider for American Indian families in Humboldt and Del Norte Counties. The service area covers approximately 5,000 square miles (Hoopa Reservation not included as it has its own health program). The service population is estimated to be 12,000 American Indians and Alaska Natives. The current client population for all health services is over 14,000 and over 35,000 encounters are made annually.

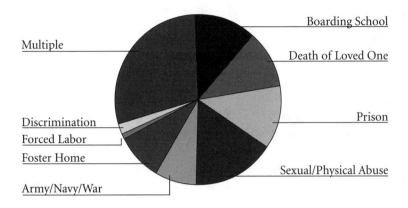

Figure 14.1   Trauma types for Yurok individuals born after 1890.

binary fashion, first for diabetes, with a one (1) expressing the presence of diabetes type 2 in the individual, and a zero (0) representing absence of diabetes. A similar coding is used for the presence (1) and absence (0) of trauma in each individual. The results of this test were highly significant. The test produced an odds ratio of 165.6, which means that practically all individuals experiencing trauma suffered or are suffering from diabetes. The remaining question becomes: what protects the very few that experienced trauma and did or do not suffer from diabetes? How did these individuals make it through?

The correlation between trauma and type 2 diabetes in Yurok communities for generations 3 to 6 (1870 to 1969) is shown in Figure 14.2. In Figure 14.2, Generation 6 shows a low prevalence of diabetes since individuals in that generation (1950–69) have only recently been diagnosed, or are in the process of developing the first symptoms of the disorder. A full 80% of patients with diabetes at UIHS are 45 or older, and, of

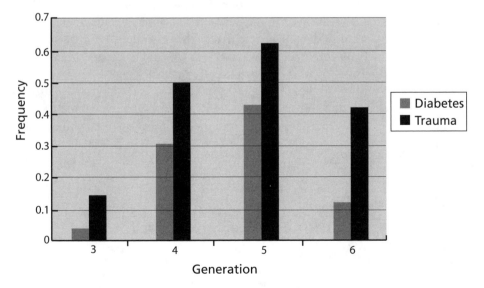

Figure 14.2   Correlation between trauma and diabetes for Yurok generations 3 (1890–1909), 4 (1910–1929), 5 (1930–1949), and 6 (1950–1969).

these, 42.5% are aged 65 or above (IHS 2000: 1). Because individuals in generation 6 have suffered traumatic experiences, we suggest that prevalence rates will rise steadily for this generation.

Our findings show that traumatic experience is an important risk factor for diabetes mellitus among the Yuroks in northern California. Statistically speaking, there is a strong, positive correlation between trauma and type 2 diabetes in Yurok communities for individuals born between 1870 and 1969. For younger generations, it is true that the sources of trauma have changed, to a certain extent: American Indian youth in Humboldt and Del Norte County are now faced with a) school failure, b) the risk of removal from home, c) out-of -home placement in non-Indian foster care, d) the risk of violence, dysfunctional families who are dealing with depression, alcoholism, substance and tobacco abuse, spousal and/or sexual abuse, and, e) the risk of suicide. According to the Department of Social Services of Humboldt County, 22.3% of children in foster care placement are American Indian. Countywide statistics reveal disproportionate numbers of American Indian youth (20–30%) detained in the Juvenile Hall (UIHS 2000).

Tragic but true: traumatic memory itself (thinking about the tragedies one's parents, uncles, grandparents or loved ones went through) is, in itself, traumatizing. Recent studies show that second-generation Holocaust survivors' react to current adverse life situations with extreme distress (Pérez-Sales et al. 2000). Ethnographic research conducted in Humboldt and Del Norte counties also indicated that individuals with a history of childhood sexual or physical abuse, and early parental loss, also exhibited more symptoms of depression and anxiety (Ferreira 1996, 1998; see also Chapter 18 in this volume). It has been proven that early adverse experiences play a preeminent role in the development of neurological disorders in adult life, thereby contributing to vulnerability to mental illness (Heim et al. 2000; Mullen et al. 1996; Nemeroff 1999; Stein et al. 1996). Women with a history of childhood sexual or physical abuse, for instance, exhibit more symptoms of depression and anxiety, and more frequently attempt suicide than women without a history of childhood abuse (Heim et al. 2000). Childhood abuse also predisposes to the development of anxiety disorders in adulthood, including panic disorder and generalized anxiety disorder (Portegijs et al. 1996; Stein et al. 1996). Early parental loss, whether due to parental separation or premature death has also been found to increase the risk for major depression in case control and epidemiological studies (Agid et al. 1999; Brown & Dollery 1984; Furukawa et al. 1999; Mullen et al. 1996; Okley-Browne 1995; Roy 1985). In all these studies, nervous system hyperreactivity appears as a persistent consequence of childhood abuse that may contribute to the predisposition for type 2 diabetes, as indicated elsewhere in this book (see Scheder Chapters 1 & 11; McGrady & Grower-Dowling Chapter 15).

Emotional Experience and the Autonomic Nervous System

In the summer of 1998, Mollie Ruud and I met again at her home on the Yurok Indian Reservation. After a delicious bowl of acorn soup Yurok neighbors had sent our way, Mollie showed me her blood sugar log in her One Touch machine:

Recipe for Acorn Soup

Pick your acorns in the fall, when they're nice and fresh. The butts should be white, separated from the hats. Check for holes, because you don't want any worms. Be respectful as you do your picking, since you are walking on sacred ground, gathering food the Creator has placed here for us. I myself always ask for His permission when I do any gathering. That's what the old folks, my mother and aunties, taught me.

Find a warm place to store the acorns because they have to be dry for you to crack them. Like near the stove. You can feel they're getting drier. In a few days crack them open and grind them. We used a stone pestle, but nowadays a meat grinder is fine. Grind them real fine and put the flour into a leaching basket, the kind that will let the water run through but that will hold the flour. If you don't have a basket use a white flour sack or something like that to hold the flour and let the water run through. Cover the basket with the same kind of flour sack material and pour water through it. Leaching can take up to a few days, depending on how bitter the acorns are. You've gotta taste the flour until it's got all that bitter out of it.

When it's finally sweet, sweet as water, the acorn meal is ready to be cooked. We used hot rocks inside the basket to cook the soup, and we'd stir them quick with a paddle so the soup would cook evenly, and so the rocks wouldn't burn the basket. But today you can add the water and acorn meal to a pan and cook it over a stove. Or add the hot rocks to a regular pan. Whatever. Oh! It's so good! And don't you add any sugar or salt, as that will spoil it. It's already very sweet, and we appreciate it that way. (Recipe by Yurok elder Aileen Figueroa, 1995)

The fishing situation still makes my sugars go up. Take a look. This whole month I was up in the 200s all the time because now it is the pesticide spraying from the timber companies and all the debris from cutting the trees that run into the river and kill the fish. My diabetes will never get better, no matter how much insulin I take. I get home and see the salmon floating on their bellies because of all the pollution in the water? It's totally upsetting.

—*Oh my. Tell me how your body feels.*

My body? My body's worn out, tired, sore, full of holes all these needles I stick myself with have made. What I do is: I never think about myself. I hurt and I just try to get it out of my mind. Like I can have sharp pains on my breast and then I just forget about it. When you live your whole life with people beating the shit out of you that's what happens to you, you want to give up. Thing is, you can put the hurt out of your mind and just feel numb, but you can't stop the sugar from eating you from the inside. It eats you up. I know I am a wreck for everything I've been through and see what I've got: diabetes.

Since I became a diabetic, things have gotten much worse, my health has gone down hill. I've had so many infections, both vaginal and urinary. So I take antibiotics to prevent infections. It's like another pill killing everything inside me. I take 12 different pills a day! This is how I take care of my life: taking pills, lots of pills everyday! Would you say I am in control of my health? I don't think so, we Indian people have never been in control of anything. I run out of medicine, what happens? I get a pretty bad spell, my urine turns gray and the infections pop right back. I've run out of life and now I can't run out of medicine. It's the end.

—What do you think would help your diabetes?

> I'm hopeless, are you talking about me? What am I going to do, go back in time
> and fix my life? Fix my family, you know I was part of a broken family, the
> boarding school and all that. There's no hope for me. I never really had a fa-
> ther or a mother—she was always too drunk. I was raised by matrons that beat
> me in the face, yelled at by my bosses, even in jail, always punished for being
> an Indian. Now you see how much trouble the kids are in today? Doing all
> kinds of drugs, getting into car wrecks. Everyone knows why these kids are in
> trouble but does anyone care? Who really cares if Indian kids are in trouble?
>
> Now, ask yourself: have you seen families around here doing real good? Out of
> trouble, folks that do not have cancer or diabetes? They are rare in your stud-
> ies, aren't they? That's always made me think: how do some folks get through?

Social and behavioral scientists have noted that statements like Mollie's about emotions in social life occur most frequently as part of, or else appear to designate, specific
scenarios or relationships (Averill 1994; De Sousa 1987; Reddy 1999; Rosaldo 1984;
Wierzbicka 1994). The fish and boarding school scenarios Mollie uses to situate her narrative illuminate how the elder's emotions give meaning to her diabetes experience. Mollie's life experience demonstrates how emotions involve widespread activations of
thought materials variously called "appraisals," "cognitions," "judgements," or "knowledges" about, broadly speaking, the continuing history of oppression of the Yurok People. Whether conscious or semi-conscious, the knowledges or appraisals created by individuals like Mollie—"I can't stand being controlled" or "I just can't handle freedom"—
have been shown to arouse the autonomic nervous system (ANS) or the endocrine system, raise and sustain blood sugars in the context of war, confinement in boarding
schools, mental homes and state prisons, and sorcery accusations that provoke grief,
fear, anger, anxiety, and depression (Averill 1994; Dashiff and Bartolucci 2002; Ferreira
1998, 1999; Lévi-Strauss 1963; Papageorgiou et al. 2000; Stephen 1999. See also Scheder,
and McGrady and Gower-Dowling in this volume). Most importantly, the woman argues that forced labor and confinement have wounded her ability to manage her emotions, allowing for emotional suffering to set in.

In addition, statements like Mollie's involving the diagnosis or treatment of diabetes
are themselves emotionally charged, because they touch deeply upon issues of self-
knowledge, body-imagery, and social identity. To say "I am diabetic" may be a way of
refusing to cooperate with someone or a request for a change in a relationship. To say
"I am pure-blood" or "I am quarter-blood" confirms social membership to a community that is at high risk for diabetes. To say "I've been good" suggests compliance with
collective actions of diabetes prevention, while "I've been bad" implies lack of self-control which potentially generates communal goal conflicts. In the medical field, recent
studies on genes and self-knowledge have shown that information about one's genetic
construction makes a large difference in the way people think about themselves and
relate to people around them. Diagnoses of psychiatric disorders, such as PTSD (post-
traumatic stress disorder), and of chronic diseases, such as cancer and diabetes, can
also penetrate people's lifeworlds and become real, shaping the self-knowledge of patients, clinicians and researchers (Weir et al. 1995).

In spite of more than a century of rigorous scientific research showing that diabetes mellitus originates in the nervous system (Bernard 1877; Canguilhem 1991; Daniel et al. 1999; Lustman 1981; Surwit and Feinglos 1988; Szathmary and Feinglos 1988), critical studies addressing the emotional causes of the ailment have been largely ignored and received very little support from the medical community. Why do studies that look at health disparities among ethnic minorities privilege instead the physiological aspects of the disorder, aiming interventions exclusively at the physical, biological body? Why has the so-called genetic makeup of Indigenous Peoples always been blamed for the diabetes epidemic—as if there could be such a thing as a global "Indigenous genotype"—when the definition of "Indigenous" is in itself controversial and when considerable efforts in trying to find a genetic cause for type 2 diabetes have remained unsuccessful (US DHHS 2000: 12–13), as discussed in this book? As critical scholars and health professionals, we see very clearly in our research and daily work how perverse links between political ideology and medical technology seriously affect Indigenous Peoples. By political ideology we are referring to, among other things, the racist politics of Indigenous identity in the United States: 1) when it comes to Indigenous *rights*, only those individuals who meet minimum blood quantum requirements (1/4, 1/8, 1/16, etc.) are *allowed* to be enrolled members of a federally recognized tribes and receive federal benefits; but 2) whatever one's blood fraction is, "Indian heritage" figures prominently in the medical literature as a risk factor for a gamut of both degenerative and infecto-contagious disorders, diabetes included. Medical technology, in turn, uses clinical, biological knowledge about diabetes to efficiently develop products and supplies that meet the bureaucratic and capitalistic demands of the current health care model it both feeds from and helps support. "Indian people" are now big clients of the gigantic diabetes industry. The political and economic gains of the medical corporation are enormous. With corporatism of the medical-care delivery system, the pharmaceutical industry, as well as medical equipment suppliers, have made diabetes a lucrative opportunity. The medical costs of diabetes reached 91.8 billion dollars in 2003, with approximately half of this figure attributable to the direct medical cost of diabetes care and the other half credited to indirect costs, such as disabilities, work loss, and premature mortality (IDF 2003).

Mollie's thoughts on pharmaceuticals in 2000:

> I feel like a slot machine, popping pills like quarters, dimes and nickels into my mouth. We all wish we'd strike it rich gambling around here in these casinos. But who does? The machines are tight, real tight, they aren't letting you win easy, just swallow up your money. You think you have a chance, you hear stories about folks who get a few grand. But most people? Nothing! Spend all their money in the casinos, they can't help it. That's what the government gave us Indian people for development, casinos![11]

> I'm hooked on gambling too, just like these damned pills. Now you tell me, how many people actually get cured? I don't see anyone around here, all my

---

11. Gaming on U.S. Indian Reservations was officially regulated after Congress passed the Indian Gaming Regulatory Act (IGRA) in 1988. This legislation requires gaming tribes to have compacts with their respective state governments specifying the types of gaming permitted on reservation lands.

Figure 3　Copy of Mollie Ruud's medicine tab for September–October, 2000.

DISPENSING HISTORY				
Fill Date	Drug	Qty	Prescriber*	Price
10/11/00	VIOXX 25MG TABLET	30.00		80.75
10/03/00	HYDROCODONE/APAP 5/500 TA	40.00		15.55
10/03/00	SULFAMETHOXAZOLE/TMP DS T	20.00		22.10
10/03/00	NEURONTIN 400MG CAPSULE	90.00		130.35
10/03/00	CLOTRIMAZOLE 1% CREAM	30.00		18.40
09/15/00	NITROFURANTOIN MCR 100MG	30.00		39.10
09/15/00	QUININE SULFATE 325MG CAP	30.00		8.75
09/15/00	AVANDIA 4MG TABLET	30.00		80.00
09/15/00	ACCUPRIL 40MG TABLET	60.00		66.00
09/15/00	HYDROCHLOROTHIAZIDE 25MG	30.00		5.60
09/15/00	FOLIC ACID 1MG TABLET	30.00		6.15
09/15/00	PREVACID 30MG CAPSULE DR	30.00		121.45

*The prescriber's name has been omitted.　　　　　　　　[total cost: 594.20]

relations are dying off and they sure take a lot of pills! If it weren't for Medicare, I couldn't afford it. But if you look at these prices [showing her monthly medicine list] they add up to a lot of money, more than 500 bucks a month. Who pays the bill? The government pays the pharmaceutical companies, who are making big bucks on us Indian people. Just like mining or logging or fishing and now casinos. So every time I pop a pill I feel like a gambler: I close my eyes and hope to hit the jackpot, that my diabetes will go away forever.

Hitting the Jackpot: Love, Solidarity and Generosity

What are the protective factors that safeguard a small number of individuals against the perverse social and neurological effects of traumatic memory and experience? I often thought of this question when I met other women who, like Mollie, also spoke of their traumas: boarding schools and prisons, rapings and beatings, violent deaths, despair and fright, but who nevertheless made it through their old age relatively healthy as compared to many of their friends and relations. What enabled these women to withstand such hardships? "I guess their faith is one reason, and also the world renewal ceremonies helped them. Indian doctors also came and doctored them," reasoned Joy Sundberg, the Chairwoman of the Trinidad Rancheria and member of United Indian Health Services Board of Directors. I also asked Yurok singer Aileen Figueroa in 1996 why, like a few other women, she indulged in recollections of sweet times, despite all the suffering she, too, had gone through since the early 1920s. How come you are so sweet and speak so fondly of a past which you experienced so little of, while most of your life you've gone through incredible horrors, I asked? Aileen's response: "Believe me, it's because of love. If it weren't for love, I couldn't stand the way it feels inside my heart."

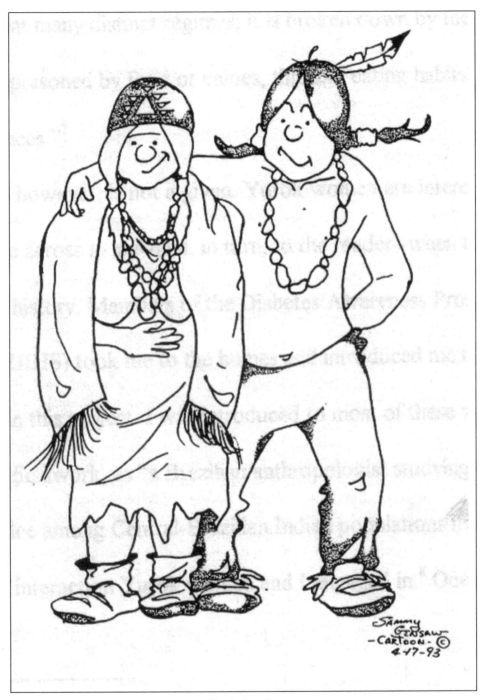

Yurok Couple.

In October 2003, I asked Mollie Ruud again if she had any further insights on why a select number of individuals she knows or knew survived in relatively good health despite all the hardships they went through, while the vast majority developed diabetes and correlated illnesses.

The last time you asked me that question I started thinking about it a lot....
my life as a wild little Indian, remember? There was so much happiness, I
guess because we felt good inside. That didn't last too long for me, it doesn't
last too long for Indian people around here. You know all about my life,
wouldn't you say I should have died a long time ago after Chemawa, a broken
family, and Cassie's death... Why have I lasted so long? I'm sturdy like a redwood, like I said, I was conceived behind a redwood tree! But there's something else, and that is the love that man [her husband Reidar Ruud] has given
me. Whenever I felt angry, really pissed off, wanting to give up, what happens? There he is, right by my side, ready to help me. Not many women I
know were lucky enough to find love in their lives.

—*What happens to people who aren't as fortunate, how do they deal with problems in
their lives?*

They go find happiness in casinos, drinking, smoking, even fighting with
their relations, things we didn't use to do before. Not like this. Or they take
pills, medicine that make them feel good, like tranquilizers. Look at all the
people doped up around here! I myself have to admit that when I was un-
happy, that's what I felt like doing, too. But when I got back home, well, I
even had a home! And food, a beautiful garden and a clean bed! Because I
have a generous man that cares for me so much! That's what I am thinking,
that some folks that get through life feel good about themselves and have a
bunch of people caring about them. They don't seem to be dying from diabetes to me.

Mollie directed me to the lives of some of her relatives in northern California who
have been spared from the signs and symptoms of type 2 diabetes. In these families,
as shown in a few of the Yurok genealogies here examined, "life's problems never
seem to get out of hand," as Mollie put it. A close look at the social relationships and
professional lives of these individuals seems to indicate that social well-being stems
from strong family ties and positive personal achievements (schooling, jobs, marriage, intense ceremonial life). Mollie explained, citing a family in Requa she felt very
close to:

You know these kids right here [pointing to a family tree] have always felt like
they were loved, that's how I see it. I know all of their elders very well, we are
all related. It made a difference in their school grades, too, and most of them
have good jobs and feel proud of being Yurok. Not that they've only lead the
good life, no! Suicide, drugs, you name it! But most have always come through
one way or another because of love and tradition. Love is part of Indian culture.

Mollie is right. Love is an intrinsic part of Indigenous Peoples' cultures, as it is of
any society's culture. As we well know, one of the major components of culture is
knowledge (Barth 1995). According to local Yurok community members, knowledge
encompasses how people see and feel about themselves and others around them, and
what people do in their daily lives (Ferreira 2002, UIHS 2002). But what kind of love
are we talking about and where does it stem from? For the present purpose, love is de-

fined as having the stimulation that one desires, which includes having an emotional bond with a person for whom one yearns, as well as having sensory stimulation that one desires (Komisaruk and Whipple 1998).

Anthropologists have shown that generosity and solidarity are cultural characteristics that Indigenous Peoples have in common across the globe. More importantly, generosity and solidarity have been shown to tighten social bonds in Indigenous societies worldwide (Ferreira 1997; Lévi-Strauss 1969; Mauss 1990 [1950]; O'Nell 1996; Trompf 1994). Yurok life histories suggest that when generosity and solidarity prevail within families and communities, individuals tend to be more supportive of one another. Their achievements—passing grades in a course, a new job, the creation of ceremonial regalia, etc.—are praised by their relatives, friends and acquaintances leading to the development and/or maintenance of high self-esteem and empowerment. In turn, when one does not find her/himself supported in the face of adversity—poverty, death of a family member, sickness, etc., it becomes increasingly difficult to cope with these situations. The absence of coping mechanisms, including the ability to grieve over personal losses in a culturally accepted way, leads to feelings of worthlessness, self-blame, and anger (Dressler and Bindon 2000; O'Nell 1996; Reddy 1999). Like many other Yurok men and women, Mollie could never get over the fact that her 21-year-old only daughter Cassie died of cancer in 1987 allegedly due to timber companies' pesticide spraying on the Yurok reservation (Ferreira 1996, 1998, chapter 3 in this book). Until the day of her own death in June 2004, Mollie would not let go of any of her daughter's belongings, and numerous photos which decorated her trailer house in Requa. Not only did the elder blame timber companies and the U.S. government for the death; she also blamed herself for it and was never able to fully grieve over and thus recover from her daughter's premature passing. The affection, love, and support of family and community members provide the safeguard against loneliness, and offer culturally sanctioned mechanisms of grieving, which Mollie seemed to lack in part.

Neglected for centuries by experimental sciences, love and social attachment have recently become the topic of extensive neuroscientific research to elucidate their biological mechanisms (Bartels and Zeki 2004, 2000; Comings and Blum 2000; Marazziti and Cassano 2003; Porges 1998). Love and its main component, social attachment, are seen as highly significant experiences for the brain's "reward system," responsible for the release of dopamine—a neurotransmitter that carries signals between neurons (nerve cells) in the nervous system. Dopamine is commonly associated in the literature with the 'pleasure system' of the brain, providing feelings of enjoyment and reinforcement that motivate us to do, continue doing, or stop doing certain activities. In this respect, love is directly involved in decision making-processes. Other neuroendocrine theories attribute health benefits to loving relationships. Love and social attachments are shown to provide a sense of safety, and reduce anxiety or stress (Bechara and Naqvi 2004; Carter 1998; Komisaruk & Whipple 1998; Wash et al. 1987). For social scientists, too, emotions are conceived as to offer cultural and individual specific interpretations of social action, and to provide culture and specific motivations for social action—all in a language that is strongly bound in relations of power (Averill 1994; De Sousa 1987; Lutz 1985, 1990; Lutz and Abu-Lughod 1990; Shkilnyk 1984). Generosity and solidarity, the fundamental axes of love in Indigenous societies, have the ability to create pleasurable and desirable sensations that help overcome grief in situations of great distress or emotional shock—experiences and sentiments that Yurok

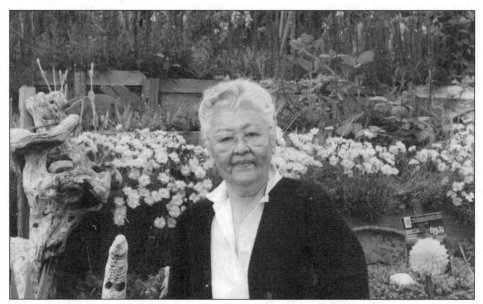

Mollie Ruud. Photo: Mariana L. Ferreira, 1996.

women, Mollie in particular, have shown to trigger the sign and symptoms of diabetes (see also chapters 3 and 18 in this volume).

It is important to demonstrate the significance of the neuroendocrine perspective for a political history of emotions that links oppression, domination, and diabetes. We have shown that diabetes is an endocrinological disorder, which originates in the nervous system. Advances in the neurosciences of emotions should help elevate emotional suffering and emotional liberty to the status of scientific concepts that allow for a critical understanding of diabetes as an indicator of emotional distress.

A Politically Meaningful History of Emotions

In this chapter, Mollie Ruud has taught us to see that a politically meaningful history of emotions has the power to illuminate historical and political factors that place Indigenous Peoples at particularly high risk for type 2 diabetes. The identification of traumatic risk factors and their intrinsic meanings for the different Indigenous communities can be instrumental in delaying the onset of diabetes mellitus and its related complications. Such a history of emotions calls for a radical shift in the definition of diabetes, elevating the centrality of affection and the political dimension of sentimental expression as core analytic concepts and methodological tools. Poverty, unemployment, premature death, depression, malnutrition, substance abuse and domestic violence are some of the pervasive psychological, social, political and economic issues identified by the authors in this book that trigger emotional suffering among Indigenous Peoples globally. Traumatic memory—involving forced removal, boarding school and reservation confinement, and racism, among other experiences—should also be considered variably important in structuring risk for diabetes mellitus among the Yurok and other Indigenous Peoples in the United States if we consider the emotionally charged context of Indigenous life and identity on and around reservations and rancherias in northern California, and in the rest of the country, broadly speaking.

Showing how emotions change over time, and how they relate to projects of sovereignty and liberation, in the context of oppression and domination can be instrumental in building a conceptual and theoretical framework to understand the centrality of love, desire, and social relationships in the promotion of social justice and emotional well-being. Mollie Ruud's life narrative is precisely about the love of her people, her desire for sovereignty, and her struggle for justice and freedom in light of a history of colonization. Adopting the image of emotion as discursively produced, as we followed Mollie Ruud's life history in this essay, encourages us to attend to the pragmatic, political and historical dimensions of emotional experience, focusing on the ways in which power relations and discourses of emotion are tied together (Lutz and Abu-Lughod 1990).

The narratives and genealogies of Yurok families here considered play the role of recording a history of love in colonial light: a political history of emotions, ideas, and spiritual concepts; a history of love, anger, sorrow and ecstasy; a history of emotional suffering as it is played out in the desire for liberty and peace; a history of how Yurok love, as a force, has also reacted against itself, giving rise to distress and mortifications as manifested in the high incidence of alcoholism, drug abuse, domestic violence, and diabetes.

As Yurok poet Pudoh Jene says in "In My Heart":

Walking in faith, we believe in love.
Like a blossom, we bloom, we grow, bringing out the best of us.
In our lives we all need the fun of new beauty and new love
In our hearts there is always room.

This is my secret:
Sometimes love doesn't love love;
it is not a personal fault;
we make mistakes in who we choose to love.
Sometimes the one we choose to love doesn't love the love you have to offer.
Sometimes love doesn't love love.

      Pudoh Jene, a Yurok from the Klamath, 1995

Acknowledgments

My dearest Mollie, thank you very much for opening my student eyes to the real causes of diabetes in Yurok country. You have made a great contribution to the history of Yurok people and to the lives of Indigenous Peoples around the world! Thank you, Reidar Ruud, for always being there for your amazing woman. Your love for her shines through you and contaminates us all. Lavina Bowers, many thanks for introducing me to Mollie and for taking me on home visits on and around the Yurok rez. I am also deeply indebted to all my Yurok acquaintances and friends for showing me the real power of Yurok love. To my advisor at the University of California at Berkeley, Nancy Scheper-Hughes, I owe much of the critical insights on diabetes research conveyed in this book. Fieldwork was supported by the Brazilian agencies CNPq—Conselho Nacional para o Desenvolvimento Científico e Tecnológico, FAPESP—Fundação para o Amparo à Pesquisa do Estado de São Paulo and UIHS—United Indian Health Services. Finally, I greatly appreciate all the friendship and trust of my larger family at United Indian Health Services in northern California. Muito obrigada!

References

Adams, David W. 1995. Education for Extinction. American Indians and the Boarding School Experience. Lawrence, Kansas: University Press of Kansas.

Agid, O., B. Shapira and J. Zislin. 1999. Environment and Vulnerability to Major Psychiatric Illness: A case Control of Early Parental Loss in Major Depression, Bipolar Disorder and Schizophrenia. Molecular Psychiatry 4: 163–72.

Averill, J. 1994. Emotions Unbecoming and Becoming. In P. Ekman and R. Davidson, eds. The Nature of Emotions: Fundamental Questions. Oxford: Oxford University Press.

Baider, L. T. Peretz, P.E. Hadani, S. Perry, R. Avramov and A.K. De-Nour. 2000. Transmission of Response to Trauma? Second-Generation Holocaust Survivors' Reaction to Cancer. American Journal of Psychiatry (6): 904–10.

Bartels, A. and S. Zeki. 2004. The Neural Correlates of Maternal and Romantic Love. Neuroimage 21(3): 1155–66.

_____2000. The Neural Basis of Romantic Love. Neuroreport 11(17): 3829–34.

Barth, Fredrik. 1995. Other Knowledge and Other Ways of Knowing. Journal of Anthropological Research. 51: 65–67.

Bechara, A. and N. Naqvi. 2004. Listening to Your Heart: Interoceptive Awareness as a Gateway to Feeling. Nature Neuroscience. 7(2): 102–3.

Bernard, Claude. 1877. Leçons sur le Diabète et la Glycogenèse Animale Londre, Madrid: Librairie J.-B. Baillière et Fils.

Brown, M.J. and C.T. Dollery. 1984. Adrenaline and Hypertension. Clinical Experiments in Hypertension. 6(1-2): 539–49.

Canguilhem, Georges. 1991. The Normal and the Pathological. New York: Zone Books.

Carter, C.S. 1998. Neuroendocrine Perspectives on Social Attachment and Love. Psychoneuroendocrinology 23(8): 779–818.

Comings, D.E. and K. Blum. 2000. Reward Deficiency Syndrome: Genetic Aspects of Behavioral Disorders. Progressive Brain Research. 126: 325–41.

Daniel, M., K. O'Dea, K. Rowley, R. McDermott and S. Kelly. 1999. Glycated Hemoglobin as an Indicator of Social and Environmental Stress among Indigenous Versus Westernized Populations. Preventive Medicine 29: 405–13.

Dashiff C. and A. Bartolucci. 2002. Autonomy Development in Adolescent with Insulin Dependent Diabetes mellitus. Journal of Pediatric Nursing. 17(2): 96–106.

Deleuze, Gilles and Felix Guattari. 1977. Anti-Oedipus. Capitalism and Schizophrenia. New York: The Viking Press.

De Sousa, R. 1987. The Rationality of Emotion. Cambridge, MA: MIT Press.

Dressler, William and James Bindon. 2000. The Health Consequences of Cultural Consonance: Cultural Dimensions of Lifestyle, Social Support, and Arterial Blood Pressure in an African Community. American Anthropologist 102(2): 244–60.

Ellis, J.L. and D. Campos-Outcalt. 1994. Cardiovascular Disease Risk Factors in Native Americans: A Literature Review. American Journal of Preventive Medicine 10(5): 295–307.

Farmer, Paul. 2003. Pathologies of Power. Health, Human Rights, and the New War on the Poor. Berkeley, CA: University of California Press.

Ferreira, Mariana K. L. 2002. A Place of Our Own. Cultural Integrity, Social Inequality, and Community Health. Report, Potawot Health Village, United Indian Health Services, Arcata, CA. Documentation, Evaluation, and Dissemination. California Endowment, Grant # 1998/233.01.

_____1999. Corpo e História do Povo Yurok. [Body and History of the Yurok People] Revista de Antropologia Universidade de São Paulo vol 41 (2): 17–39.

_____1998. Slipping Through Sky Holes. Yurok Perceptions of the Body in Northern California. Culture, Medicine and Psychiatry 22(2): 171–202.

_____1997. When 1 + 1 ≠ 2: Making Mathematics in Central Brazil. American Ethnologist. 24(1): 132–47.

_____1996. Sweet Tears and Bitter Pills. The Politics of Health among the Yuroks in Northern California. Unpublished Doctoral Dissertation, University of California at Berkeley and University of California at San Francisco.

Foucault, Michel. 1995. Discipline and Punish. The Birth of the Prison. New York: Vintage Books.

Furukawa, T.A., A. Ogura, T. Hirai, S. Fujihara, T. Kitamura and R. Takahashi. 1999. Early Parental Separation Experiences among Patients with Bipolar Disorder and Major Depression: A Case Control Study. Journal of Affective Disorders 52: 85–91.

Heim, C., J. Newport, S. Heit, Y. Graham, M. Wilcox, R. Bonsall, A. Miller and C. Nemeroff. 2000. Pituitary-Adrenal and Autonomic Responses to Stress in Women after Sexual and Physical Abuse in Childhood. JAMA 284(5) 592–97.

Heizer, R. and J. Mills. 1991 [1952]. The Four Ages of Tsurai. A Documentary History of the Indian Village on Trinidad Bay. Berkeley, Los Angeles and London: University of California Press.

IDF—International Diabetes Federation. 2003. 18th International Diabetes Federation Press Conference, Aug. 24, 2003. Le Palais des Congres de Paris, France.

Indian Health Service (IHS). 2000. California Area: Assessment of HIS Diabetes Care. Fiscal Year 1999.

Indian Teacher and Educational Personnel Program (ITEPP). 1999 . Northwest Indigenous Gold Rush History—The Indian Survivors of California's Holocaust. Arcata: Humboldt State University.

Komisaruk, B.R. and B. Whipple. 1998. Love as Sensory Stimulation: Physiological Consequences of its Deprivation and Expression. Psychoneuroendocrinology 23(8): 927–44.

Lévi-Strauss, Claude. 1963. The Sorcerer and His Magic; The Effectiveness of Symbols. In Structural Anthropology. New York: Basic Books.

_____1969. The Principle of Reciprocity. In The Elementary Structures of Kinship. Needham R, ed. pp. 52–68. Boston: Beacon Press.

Lustman, P., R. Carney and H. Amado. 1981. Acute Stress and Metabolism in Diabetes. Diabetes Care. 4(6): 658–59.

Lutz, Catherine. 1990. Engendered Emotion: Gender, Power, and the Rhetoric of Emotional Control in American Discourse. In Language and the Politics of Emotion. C. Lutz and L. Abu-Lughod, eds. Cambridge: Cambridge University Press.

_____1985. Depression and the Translation of Emotional Worlds. In Culture and Depression. Arthur Kleinman and Byron Good, eds. Berkeley, Los Angeles and London: University of California Press.

Lutz, Catherine and L. Abu-Lughod, eds. 1990. Language and the Politics of Emotion. Cambridge: Cambridge University Press.

Malkki, Liisa. 1995. Purity and Exile: Violence, Memory, and National Cosmology among Hutu Refugees in Tanzania. Chicago: University of Chicago Press.

Marazziti, D. and G.B. Cassano. 2003. The Neurobiology of Attraction. Journal of Endocrinological Investigation 26(3): 58–60.

Mauss, Marcel. 1990 [1950]. The Gift. The Form and Reason for Exchange in Archaic Societies. New York, NY: W. W. Norton.

Mullen, P.E., J. Martin and J. Anderson. 1996. The Long-term Impact of the Physical, Emotional, and Sexual Abuse of Children: A Community Study. Child Abuse and Neglect 20: 7–21.

Nelson Jr., Byron. 1978. Our Home Forever. A Hupa Tribal History. Hoopa, CA: The Hupa Tribe.

Nemeroff, C.B. 1999. The Preeminent Role of Early Untoward Experience on Vulnerability to Major Psychiatric Disorders: The Nature-Nurture Controversy Revisited and Soon to be Resolved. Molecular Psychiatry. 4: 106–8.

O'Nell, Theresa. 1996. Disciplined Hearts. History, Identity and Depression in an American Indian Community. Berkeley: University of California Press.

Okley-Browne, M.A., P.R. Joyce, J.E. Wells, J.A. Bushnell and A.R. Hornblow. 1995. Disruptions in Childhood Parental Care as Risk Factors for Major Depression in Adult Women. Australian NZ Journal of Psychiatry 29: 437–48.

Papageorgiou V., A. Frangou-Garunovic, R. Iordanidou, W. Yule, P. Smith and P. Vostanis. 2000. War Trauma and Psychopathology in Bosnian Refugee Children. European Child Adolescent Psychiatry. 9(2): 84–90.

Pérez-Sales P., T. Durán-Pérez and R.B. Herzfeld. 2000. Long-term Psychosocial Consequences in First-degree Relatives of People Detained, Disappeared or Executed for Political Reasons in Chile. A Study of Mapuce and Non-Mapuce Persons. Psicothema 12: 109–16.

Pino, Manuel & Mariana Ferreira, eds. (forthcoming) Take Our Word For It. Indigenous Peoples of Turtle Island. Wadsworth Publishing Co.

Porges, S.W. 1998. Love: An Emergent Property of the Mammalian Autonomic Nervous System. Psychoneuroendocrinology 23(8): 837–61.

Portegijs, P.J.M., F.M.H. Jeuken , F.G. van der Horst, H.F. Kraan and J.A. Knottnerus. 1996. A Troubled Youth: Relations with Somatization, Depression and Anxiety in Adulthood. Family Practitioner 13: 1–11.

Rawls, James. n/d. Indians of California. The Changing Image. Norman and London: University of Oklahoma Press.

Reddy, W. 1999. Emotional Liberty: Politics and History in the Anthropology of Emotions. Cultural Anthropology. 14(2): 256–88.

Rosaldo, Michelle. 1984. Toward an Anthropology of Self and Feeling. In Culture Theory: Essays on Self, Mind and Emotion. R. Shweder & R. LeVine, eds. Cambridge: Cambridge University Press.

Roy, A. 1985. Early Parental Separation and Adult Depression Arch Gen Psychiatry 42: 987–91.

Scheper-Hughes, Nancy and Philippe Bourgois, eds. 2004. Violence in War and Peace. An Anthology. Malden, MA: Blackwell Publishing.

Shkilnyk, Anastasia. 1984. A Poison Stronger than Love : The Destruction of an Ojibwa Community. New Haven: Yale University Press.

Stein, M.B., J.R. Walker and G. Anderson. 1996. Childhood Physical and Sexual Abuse in Patients with Anxiety Disorders in a Community Sample. American Journal Psychiatry 153: 235–39.

Stephen, M. 1999. Witchcraft, Grief, and the Ambivalence of Emotions. American Ethnologist 26(3): 711–37.

Strandmark, M. 2004. Ill Health is Powerlessness: A Phenomenological Study about Worthlessness, Limitations and Suffering. Scandinavian Journal of Caring Sciences 18(2): 135–44.

Surwit, R. and M. Feinglos. 1983. The Effects of Relaxation on Glucose Tolerance in Non-Insulin-dependent Diabetes. Diabetes Care 6(2): 176–79.

———1988. Stress and Autonomic Nervous System in Type II Diabetes. A Hypothesis. Diabetes Care 11(1): 83–85.

Szathmary, E.J.E. and R.E. Ferrell. 1990. Glucose Level, Acculturation, and Glycated Hemoglobin: An Example of Biocultural Interaction. Medical Anthropology Quarterly 4: 315–41.

Thompson, Lucy. 1991 [1916]. To the American Indian. Reminiscences of a Yurok Woman. Eureka, CA: Cummins Printing Co. Reprinted by Heyday Books, Berkeley, CA.

Trompf, G.W. 1994. Payback: The Logic of Retribution in Melanesian Religions. New York, NY: Cambridge University Press.

United Indian Health Services (UIHS). 2000. Department of Child and Family Services, Arcata.

_____2002. Potawot Health Village. A Place Of Our Own. Arcata, CA: United Indian Health Services.

U.S. Department of Health and Human Services (DHHS). 2000. Healthy People 2010. (Conference Edition, in 2 Volumes). Washington DC.

Walsh, A., J.A. Beyer and T.A. Petee. 1987. Love Deprivation, Wechsler Performance Greater than Verbal Discrepancy and Violent Delinquency. Journal of Psychology 121(2): 177–84.

Weir, R., S. Lawrence and E. Fales, eds., 1994. Genes and Human Self-Knowledge. Historical and Philosophical Reflections on Modern Genetics Iowa City: University of Iowa Press.

Wierzbicka, A. 1994. Cognitive Domains and the Structure of the Lexicon: The case of Emotions. *In* Mapping the Mind: Domain Specificity in Cognition and Culture. L. Hirschfeld and S. Gelman, eds. Cambridge: Cambridge University Press.

CHAPTER 15

RELAXATION AND STRESS REDUCTION FOR PEOPLE WITH DIABETES MELLITUS

Angele McGrady and Kim Grower-Dowling

More than two thousand years ago, the Greeks understood intuitively that emotions and health are one. The Greek god of healing, Asclepius,...symbolized all that was essential in this balance—healthy diet, pure water, exercise and support of friends and family. Essential, too, were the emotions and soothing activities that calmed them —sleep, music, and prayer.

from Esther Sternberg, *The Balance Within* (2001: 3).

Summary of Chapter 15. Chronic psychological and socioeconomic stress has profound effects on normal physiological function and increases the risk for illness. In people with diabetes, stress increases blood glucose, accelerates the risk for development of complications, as well as interfering with self-care and adherence to treatment recommendations. Relaxation helps to counteract the effects of stress, thus helping people with diabetes to maintain more normal blood glucose levels. Several types of relaxation are discussed, and one relaxation exercise is presented in detail. All types of relaxation have the capacity to assist the person with diabetes to decrease sympathetic over-arousal, the physiological activation of the heart, blood vessels and muscles that comprises the stress response. As a result of regular use of relaxation techniques, the body relaxes and the mind and spirit become quiet. A brief literature review on the effects of relaxation facilitated by imagery, biofeedback or powerful words is presented, with specific reference to glycemic control and the metabolic syndrome.

ò. ò. ò.

Introduction

People with Diabetes Mellitus (DM) are affected by both acute and chronic psychological stress. Stress mobilizes the autonomic nervous system (sympathetic division) to prepare the body for a physical response, comprising, in part, increased blood pressure, heart rate, skeletal muscle tension and respiratory rate. Glucose is released from hepatic stores of glycogen into the blood stream, but insulin production may be compromised, or the tissues may be resistant to insulin. In the absence of an appropriate, acute, musculoskeletal response to the specific stress (commonly known as flight or fight), blood glucose levels rise, while cellular glucose availability remains constant or decreases. Another pathway through which stress elevates blood glucose is via the endocrine system. Hormones from the adrenal cortex and medulla participate in the stress response, prolonging the mobilization of the excess blood glucose. Since the hormones cortisol and aldosterone and the catecholamines circulate in the blood stream, the response to a single severe stressor can continue for hours (Ganong 1997). When persons with DM are challenged by chronic stress, both the sympathetic and endocrine systems remain in their active mode, resulting in sustained hyperglycemia and behavioral impediments to good self care. Details of the psychophysiology of the stress response are beyond the scope of this chapter, but excellent reviews are available for the interested reader (Surwit and Schneider 1993; Cacioppo 1994; Dantzer 1991).

Certain types of stress affect people with DM differently than people with other stress related disorders, such as headaches and irritable bowel syndrome. Low socioeconomic status (SES), defined as low educational and employment level and low income is associated with more severe DM (Wolk and Orth-Gome 1997). Persons of low SES are more likely to have an unhealthy life style. Daily diet, especially consumption of foods that have high sugar and fat content, has severe implications in DM where total caloric intake and sugar content of foods must be closely monitored. Difficulties in coping with adverse living conditions or stressful situations sometimes leads to the use of alcohol, nicotine, or other mind-altering drugs as a substitute for regular meals. Alcohol, because of its high sugar content, raises blood glucose quickly. Smoking serves as a portal for nicotine, a potent vasoconstrictor, to enter the circulatory and respiratory systems. The long term effects of nicotine and tar are well known; however, in less than a few minutes, nicotine produces constriction of the arterioles, already sensitized by hyperglycemia, which in turn increases the risk for cardiovascular disease (ADA 2000). Even in non-diabetic individuals, lower level of employment, lack of social support and unhealthy coping are correlated with higher values of glycohemoglobin (Feldman and Steptoe 2003). These characteristics are common in Indigenous communities worldwide, as discussed in other chapters of this book.

Life events and daily hassles in people with DM increase the risk for worsening of the disorder. Individuals must devote time and energy to coping with stressful events thus decreasing the available time for daily self care of DM. Multiple life events in the preceding year, such as marriage, divorce, illness of a loved one, significant increase or decrease in income, whether positive or negative, increases the likelihood of illness, and increases utilization of services. (McGrady et al. 2003). Chronic, unremitting stress, from which no escape is obvious, produces anxiety and/or depressed mood. Negative affect and chronically elevated anxiety are related to poorer metabolic control (Wiebe et al. 1994). Mood disorders have a higher prevalence in people with DM than in the general population (Anderson et al 2001). Depressive symptomatology (for example, consistent sadness, tearfulness, and sleep disturbances) was associated with higher glycohemoglobin levels in native Hawaiians (Grandinetti et al. 2000). A large study of Japanese men showed an association between moderate or severe depression and higher risk for onset of type 2 diabetes (Kawakami et al. 1999). Indigenous Peoples attempting to adapt to so-called western culture are at significantly higher risk for elevated glycohemoglobin concentrations (Daniel et. al. 1999).

In summary, stressors are contributing factors to the development and progression of type 2 diabetes as well as increasing risk for frequently co-morbid conditions such as hypertension and hyperlipidemia (McGrady et al. 2003). The task of controlling blood glucose is in itself a major, chronic, stressor that is compounded by lack of time for exercise, incomplete understanding of healthy food choices and infrequent access to health care providers, problems that abound in Indigenous communities. Depression, if present, with its symptoms of loss of motivation and interest is likely to present further barriers to self-care. In contrast, positive coping can counteract the effects of stress. Relevant aspects of positive coping are the acknowledgement that personal resources are sufficient to manage the challenge or that social support is available. In studies of patients with chronic pain, coping skills training helps to de-emphasize the despair often associated with daily pain, while teaching effective, positive coping (Keefe 1996). Therefore, strategies to decrease the impact of stress, such as daily relaxation and increasing social support are recommended components of the diabetes self care package. Support groups, talking circles, oral history workshops and other related activities as portrayed in this book are important components in prevention and treatment of diabetes.

Relaxation assists persons with DM to manage both the acute and chronic psychophysiological effects of stress. Some relaxation strategies can be learned from books and audiotapes without the assistance of a health care provider. Persons with DM must be motivated to practice the techniques until mastery is achieved and then develop the ability to incorporate daily relaxation to calm the mind and decrease physiological responses to stress.

However, for individuals suffering from diabetes who are challenged with chronic stress, who suffer from depressive symptoms or anxiety, relaxation therapy should be offered in the context of a therapeutic relationship. The provider becomes aware of recent traumatic situations, such as premature death in the family—a common occurrence for Indigenous Peoples whose life expectancy is still very low due to the negative effects of colonization—and helps the person with DM deal with the strong resultant emotions. For severe mood or anxiety disorders, cognitive-behavioral psychotherapy is recommended to assist the person with DM to resolve conflict, develop adaptive coping and then integrate relaxation into the overall diabetes management plan. In addition, the use of relaxation is recommended for use during stress to decrease its impact on blood glucose. The sources of acute, daily stress and life factors producing chronic stress should be identified in a dialogue between the individual and the provider. Then, reasonable recommendations for integrating the relaxation response into the person's daily life can be made.

Part 1. Types of Relaxation

The mind-body interventions include a broad spectrum of therapies based on the premise that thoughts, emotions and beliefs can influence physiological function. Modalities that have been utilized to assist persons with DM comprise relaxation therapy, breathing training, yoga, tai chi, biofeedback and hypnosis (Rice 2001). The "Relaxation Response" was introduced to the public by Herbert Benson in the mid-seventies and quickly became a best seller (Benson 1975). Stress was named as the culprit in increasing risk and incidence of hypertension. A list of types of relaxation techniques and their associated effects on heart rate, blood pressure, muscle tension, respiration and oxygen consumption was provided. Then, instructions for generating the relaxation response were explained in detail. Regular, daily practice of the response was recommended to maintain the physiological and psychological benefits. Given the effectiveness of relaxation therapy, more educational initiatives should be directed to make this favorable technique better known and more accessible to Indigenous Peoples across the globe.

In this section, six methods of relaxation are described. Some research studies have attempted to identify the primary effective component, or active ingredient, in a treatment package that comprises various types of relaxation, supportive therapy and education. It is important to remember, however, that in the clinical setting, the provider will be trained in multiple techniques and will use them in combination, choosing the type(s) of relaxation based on client skill, preference and literature-based efficacy reports for the person's particular concern.

Breathing Therapy

Rhythmic, slow inhalation and exhalation of air within the respiratory system is characteristic of relaxed breathing. When breathing is even, deep and diaphramatic, muscle tension is reduced and the relaxation response is induced (Davis 1995). Recommended breathing rates are usually significantly lower than usual breath speed and average 6-8 breaths per minute. Deep breathing training is incorporated into all forms of relaxation discussed in this chapter and is applicable to many psychophysiological disorders (Gevirtz and Schwartz 2003). Deep breathing is the easiest method of relaxation and can be learned independently by those without significant physical or psychological problems.

Autogenic Relaxation

> …what is unique about autogenic training, as a form of autonomic self-regulation…is…the emphasis…on 'self control' and 'patient administered' (Linden 1990: 6).

The word autogenic means "self generated" indicating relaxation must come from within and cannot be imposed on one person by another. This type of passive relaxation, originated by German psychiatrist and neurologist Johann Heinrich Schultz, consists of concentrating on specific words and phrases designed to decrease tension in skeletal muscle and to reduce the activation of the sympathetic nervous system. The mind and body learn to answer to instructions to relax muscles in the lower and upper body and to warm the hands. The goal is to achieve balanced activity of the sympathetic and parasympathetic parts of the autonomic nervous system and to calm the mind. When balance is attained, the individual feels well physically and emotionally,

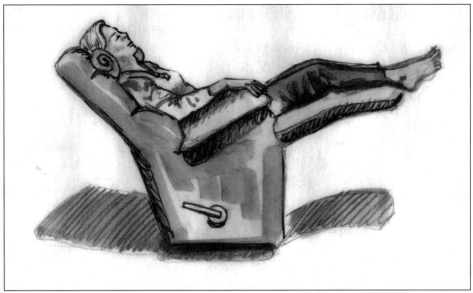

Person in relaxed position suitable for practice of autogenic training. The body is well supported and the eyes are closed. Drawn by Kim Grower-Dowling.

diverted from the mental, emotional and physical toll of stress. Using autogenic relaxation, persons with DM can learn to exert control over the neural and hormonal responses to stress (Linden 1990).

The process of autogenic relaxation involves systematically responding to directives, originating either from the individual's memory, an audiotape or the therapist's voice, to relax, feel heavy and warm, or similar sensations, working from feet up to the head. When overall relaxation is achieved, the individual stretches, prepares to become more alert, and arises refreshed. Autogenic relaxation can be practiced at home or in the clinic; ideally, it should be learned and practiced in a place with minimal distractions, lying in a darkened room in a comfortable position conducive to muscular relaxation (Figure 1). Once the sensation of relaxation is familiar to the person with DM, relaxation can be induced after brief sessions of about 5 minutes. Even single autogenic suggestions such as, "I feel calm" or "I feel quiet" are useful (Davis 1995). The quiet, dark, ideal environment becomes less important once the techniques are learned.

Progressive or Neuromuscular Relaxation

In the early twenties, physician Edmund Jacobson first promoted the benefits of progressive relaxation (Jacobson 1929); the technique was subsequently modified to shorten the training period and adapt the process to specific musculoskeletal disorders (Bernstein and Carlson 1993). By methodically tensing and relaxing the muscles from feet to head, the person learns to be aware of and to differentiate between physical feelings of muscle tension and muscle relaxation. The relaxation response is reinforced by longer periods of relaxation than of tension so that the person achieves sensations of rest and rejuvenation (Everly and Lating 2002). That feeling of relaxation is to be stored away in the body's memory to be recalled when stress occurs. Similarly to autogenic relaxation, acquiring a command of progressive relaxation demands multiple practice sessions and a quiet environment with supportive furniture. Once learned, even sessions under less than ideal circumstances may effectively diminish the psychophysiological stress responses (Davis 1995).

Yoga

Yoga combines controlled physical postures with breathing training and meditation to produce harmony between an individual's *material* (physical) and *nonmaterial* (mind and soul) entities (Patel 1993). There are four basic paths in yoga: karma yoga, the unfolding of mind and soul; hatha yoga, the physical path; gnyana yoga, the intellectual path; and bhakti yoga, the devotional path. The ultimate goal, 'raja yoga,' combines all of the above segments.

Meditation practice in yoga promotes focusing on an individual task and devoting full energy to it. A task may be as simple as focusing on a single object, or perhaps the person's own breathing. The purpose of the task is to become fully aware of it through all senses and thus, be able to concentrate on it alone. Learning to singly focus, to the exclusion of all other thoughts, is essential to progressing in the four basic paths of yoga.

In order to exercise each muscle of the body, over 200 balanced postures need to be learned. Practice of these postures increases suppleness, tones the body and organs, and slows degeneration associated with aging or illness. The most common is illustrated in Figure 2. *Sukhasana,* or "easy pose", is a starting position which strengthens the lower back area and helps the individual focus on breathing and awareness of the body; sitting cross-legged with a straight spine, rest arms on legs with hands on knees, palms upward. *Trikosana,* or "triangle pose", improves an individual's balance and concentration, as well as stretches the spine; standing with feet parallel, spread about three feet apart, turn the left foot out about 90 degrees and the right foot out about 45 degrees. With an inhalation, position the arms parallel with the floor, left downward and right upward. With an exhalation, turn head to left and look downward toward fingers, stretch until fingertips touch inside of calf. Turn head to look upward at right hand, take several deep breaths, straighten up and repeat procedure on opposite side. *Ushtra asana,* or "camel pose", is a passive, head-down backbend that is especially effective for relaxation and quieting the mind. On the ground, with knees apart and ankles at the side of the buttocks, stand up on knees with arms at sides. Feet lay with soles up behind the body. Bend gently backward and grasp left heel with left hand and right heel with right hand. (If you cannot reach your heels, wood blocks positioned next to your feet are helpful.) One book to consider is Judith Lasater's book, *Relax and Renew.* The web is also a good source; two sites to seek out are: <www.yogajournal. com> and <www.yahooyoga.com>.

In a controlled study of 149 persons with type 2 diabetes, yoga practice produced a fair to good reduction in blood sugar levels (Jain et al. 1993). This may be due to any of the following components of yoga practice: reducing stress; instilling discipline, i.e. maintaining a healthy diet; changing hormone balance; or changing biochemical balance (Sahay 1986). It is important to remember that according to eastern medicine, yoga is done in the context of a complete lifestyle that promotes health and well-being,

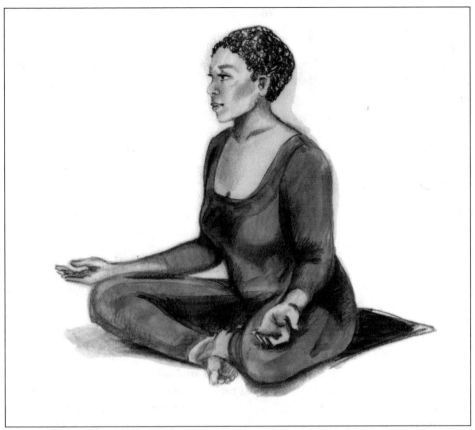

Person in position to practice yoga. Eyes can be open or closed. Drawn by Kim Grower-Dowling.

including balanced diet, exercise and proper usage of medicines and other appropriate self-care, such as blood glucose monitoring.

Transcendental Meditation

In 1969, Maharishi Mahesh Yogi (1969), widely regarded as the foremost scientist in the field of consciousness and founder of the Maharishi University of Management, developed the Transcendental Meditation (TM) method from the ancient Vedic tradition that originated in India. Throughout chronicled history, meditation has been used as a way to alter consciousness in a healthful way, to promote spiritual awareness, and enhance a sense of well-being. TM is meant to develop the vastly untapped potential for creative intelligence. Three phases continually cycle during a TM session (Travis 1999): first, awareness transitions from an alert, top-level of consciousness to quieter, more complex thinking; deepening to more profound thought; finally, after 'stress release,' returning to top-level consciousness. The technique emphasizes repetition of a word or sound and is usually practiced twice daily, approximately 20 minutes each time. Most individuals can adequately learn proper technique with instruction from a qualified teacher in about six hours (Riedesel 1979).

In several studies (Eppley et al. 1989; Alexander et al. 1989, 1991), TM was shown to be superior to other forms of relaxation in reducing the psychological effects of stress such as anxiety (Delmonte 1987) as well as to modulate chronic hypertension that has developed during a stressful life style. During meditation, an individual enters a deeply restful state. Typically, blood pressure, oxygen use, respiration and heart rates are decreased (Wallace et al. 1971; Allison 1970; Wallace 1970), the experience of stress is relieved, and blood glucose levels are lowered in diabetic patients (Heribeto 1988). It has also been suggested that TM may be a means of unburdening individuals from deeply imprinted traumatic events and stressors in addition to relief from daily hassles (Bloomfield 1976). Once the effects of the trauma are ameliorated, the individual is then able to progress to a healthier state.

Mindfulness Meditation

While there are different forms of meditation, all include passive concentration or focus on a target, a stimulus, something that serves as a focal point. Mental inhibitions are loosened and the individual may release thoughts that are no longer useful. Freeing a person of these roadblocks is the initial step that empowers them to move toward healing and better health. Distracting thoughts are gently moved out of consciousness so that the mind can return to the initial focus. "Mindfulness meditation" (Kabat-Zinn 1990) is the form commonly used in clinical settings. First taught by Buddha over 2,500 years ago, mindfulness means complete awareness and acceptance of each individual moment (Waring 2000). This pure awareness allows for the most powerful concentration. The person with DM practicing mindfulness meditation will notice decreased skeletal muscle tension, slowing of the heart beat and breathing rate, although the focus is not any of these specific responses. Mastery is not emphasized, but rather, the individual continues through the process of meditation, accepting rather than directly controlling physiological and psychological states (Everly and Lating 2002).

Studies on Psoriasis patients (Kabat-Zinn 1990) who use mindfulness meditation have shown a healing rate approximately four times faster than those who don't meditate, yet both groups received the same standard care including phototherapy. Mindfulness may alter cellular activity, increasing regeneration or may act to enhance the benefits of prescribed medical therapy.

Part 2. Enhancement of the Relaxation Response

...the power of the imagination far exceeds that of the will. It is hard to will yourself into a relaxed state, but you can imagine relaxation spreading through your body, and you can visualize yourself in a safe and beautiful retreat.

Davis et al. 1995: 55

Relaxation can be facilitated by the use of feedback, powerful words or imagery.

Healing Words

Powerful words can enhance the relaxation experience during actual practice of relaxation and can also be used as cues to recall the sensation of relaxation during other times when formal practice is not taking place. The person actively engaged in relaxation with or without biofeedback is already using key words, like "relax, heavy, calm and quiet". As described by Goldman (2001) words can contribute to healing. Words that have specific meanings to an individual with DM can be incorporated into relaxation and used as a stimulus for imagery. "Mending" refers to an "improvement in health or condition" that does not necessarily imply cure or unreasonable expectations, but suggests the possibility for progress in controlling blood glucose and decreasing the risk of complications. "Smile" indicates pleasure, and the act of smiling relaxes the muscles of the face and produces physiological changes in heart rate indicative of lowered tension. Links have been demonstrated between facial expression, the activity of the autonomic nervous system and mood. Artificially placing the muscles of the face in configurations associated with anger, joy, fear or contentment brings about the actual feelings and physiological manifestations of the positive or negative emotions (Ekman 2003). Smiling during the day may assist in generalization of the relaxation response.

Imagery

Guided imagery, a form of visualization, is a cognitive intercession used to heal the mind and body. Guided imagery uses both positive images created in one's own mind and powerful words that may assist in the production of that imagery. It may be used for general relaxation or focused on healing. All the senses are used to create images in the mind of restoring comfort and balance in an area that has been producing a negative response to harmful stimuli (Lyon and Taylor 2003). Imagery may be guided by oneself or a leader; can be interactive; be additive, such as looking forward to a goal; or be subtractive, such as taking away physical or emotional pain (Rossman and Bresler 1993).

An advantage to guided imagery is that it may be practiced almost anywhere and it is available to anyone, regardless of education or socio-economic status. In the first phase of imagery, the person uses a combination of controlled breathing and muscle tension release. Once relaxation is achieved, visualization is implemented to control pain, rehearse an event, or provide healing (Ford-Martin 2001). Some types of imagery as simple as visualizing a pleasant scene; at the other end of the spectrum are complex, intensive protocols directed at speeding the healing after surgery or directing healing energy towards a painful limb.

Recent research has indicated that guided imagery is useful in motor movement rehabilitation after stroke (Stevens and Stoykov 2003), anxiety reduction and stress management. Successful results may depend on individual's ability to create images in their minds and then effectively utilize them.

Biofeedback

Recently, it has been found that people can have extraordinary control over their body, including those functions previously thought to be under involuntary control.

Samuels and Samuels (1975: 66, 70)

Biofeedback is a way of providing data or information to the person about the level of physical tension in the muscles or any other physiological function. Visual or auditory information helps the person to gain awareness of the increases or decreases in the activity of groups of muscles (Figure 3). With biofeedback, sensors are attached to the surface of the skin; these sensors are designed to pick up the small electrical signals emanating from the body systems. As nerves transmit information to muscles, to the heart or to the digestive system, the electrical potential can be monitored from the surface of the body. The most familiar example of this is the electrocardiogram (EKG), a recording of the electrical events occurring during contraction and relaxation of the heart muscles as well as the frequency of the heart beat. When a person is shown his/her EKG, he or she can increase or decrease heart rate by changing breathing pattern, by moving, or by thinking of pleasant or stressful things (Schwartz and Schwartz 2003). The capacity to modulate physiological functions, however, is influenced by the range of the system itself, and the homeostatic properties of the system being controlled. In other words, there is a center in the brain that controls heart rate; this center depends on information from the heart itself, from blood vessels and substances in the blood, in addition to the person's emotional state. The ability of the person to control their heart rate is limited by the speed at which the nerve cells are able to respond, the capacity of the heart to pump blood and the physiological limits at which the cardiovascular system can function.

With positive reinforcement and practice, individuals suffering from diabetes can learn to control their heart rate or other physiological process. Biofeedback is often used in concert with relaxation therapy to help the person learn how to relax more quickly. Biofeedback always requires an instrument that measures the function of interest and gives out a fluctuating sound or series of lights that indicate increases or decreases. Numbers of training sessions needed to achieve mastery range from 5-12 depending on how quickly the person grasps the concept, the level of motivation to practice and the extent of emotional distress or the presence of psychiatric illness.

People with diabetes, as several chapters in this book have indicated, often have chronic psychological stress due to the diagnosis of DM, difficulty in achieving good glycemic control or the fear of complications. Biofeedback and relaxation can be useful tools in lessening the effects of stress, and increasing the sense of personal efficacy over blood glucose. The person with DM who feels helpless about the long-term consequences of the disease is likely to have less of a commitment to diet, exercise and medication. Success at biofeedback as evidenced by steadily decreasing muscle tension levels, or increasing hand temperatures serves as a powerful reminder that the person can control at least some of their physiological functions. The provider then utilizes this evidence to promote regular monitoring of blood glucose, adherence to diet and exercise and daily dosing of medication. Empowerment refers to a person's belief that blood glucose control is possible and

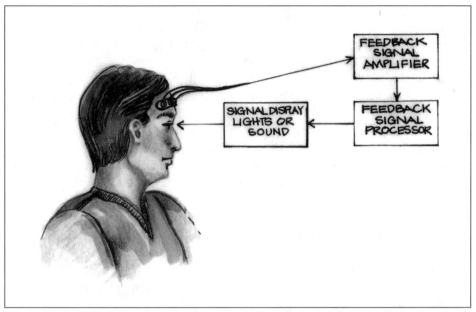

Scheme for biofeedback. Muscle tension is monitored from the forehead. The biofeedback equipment amplifies and processes the electrical activity from the forehead muscles. The signal is displayed in visual or auditory format (fluctuating lights or sounds). Drawn by Kim Grower-Dowling.

the tools to achieve normalcy are within reach (Anderson 1995). A positive, empowering, healing relationship between provider and the patient with DM helps create a healing environment, in which the person with DM believes that the disease can be managed.

Research shows that many life stressors and negative affect predict utilization of services, as does the patient's perception of their physician as warm and caring (Nagel et al. 2003). Negative affect refers to a tendency to experience and report unpleasant emotions, a prevailing attitude that contradicts the expectation of positive outcome. For the provider, teaching the skills of physical relaxation and quieting of the mind and spirit should be part of the management plan. For the person with DM, learning to meditate, or relax by other means can be as important as maintaining a healthy diet and regular exercise in overall glycemic control. Although the latter can be taught in a nonjudgmental manner, by refraining from blaming the individual for being overweight or not exercising, the patient often interprets diet, exercise and more general life style recommendations as punishment or disciplinary action from the provider. In contrast, the experience of relaxation is most often positive, decreasing anxiety and improving mood, allowing individuals to be in control of their own well-being.

Part 3. Autogenic Relaxation Process and Benefits

Autogenic relaxation is a form of psychophysiological self-regulation. The body and mind may be trained to be aware of tension, then to respond to directives to relax through suggestion. The aim of this form of passive relaxation, in contrast to relaxation involving movement (progressive or yoga) is to assist an individual in achieving or maintaining a relaxed state, even when stressed, by merely recalling the sensation of relaxation learned in previous sessions. The following script contains phrases that are intended to prompt a sense of deep relaxation through physical feelings of heaviness, warmth or floating (Davis et al. 1995; Linden 1990, 1993).

Once an appropriate and comfortable practice space is found, one without disturbances such as pets, electronics, or other people, 15–20 minutes of relaxation may begin. Head, neck, and back should be supported while either sitting up or lying down. Preferably, glasses, shoes and any tight clothing should be removed before starting relaxation. As the individual begins the relaxation process, it is helpful to make a mental note of any part of the body that is experiencing particularly high levels of tension or pain. That area may receive extra attention during the session.

As the exercise begins, gently close the eyes. If the eyes are forced shut, tension will remain in the forehead area and it will be more difficult to focus on the process of relaxation. Attention now turns to breathing; notice the pace and depth. The most benefit comes from deep, slowly and evenly paced breathing that comes from the lowest part of the lungs in the area of the diaphragm. This should be used throughout the session. After several of these breaths, let the last one out through a partially opened mouth as the autogenic practice starts.

Working up from the feet to the head and then back down the body to the feet usually ensures a complete, relaxing and refreshing exercise. There is no hurry. As an individual becomes more familiar with the phrases and the process, it is usually easier to prevent becoming distracted. Whatever physical, emotional or mental responses occur should be allowed but attention should always be directed toward the phrases.

It is not unusual to actually fall asleep at some time during the sessions when first learning the exercise. This is good if it is part of a practice at bedtime or when the exercise is being used to decrease insomnia. Falling asleep at other practice times, however, is not beneficial. It becomes important to try to stay awake in order to recognize the physical and mental sensations of the relaxed state; they need to be remembered so they become easier to recall in times of stress.

Some sensations have come to be associated as normal or common during the relaxation response: lightness, floating and tingling, or great heaviness and comfortable warmth. In first learning the techniques, some individuals experience pain or brief feelings of anxiety. Generally, these disappear as an individual continues to practice. If they persist, pain or anxiety should be discussed with a practitioner trained in relaxation therapy.

Once the exercise area with low light is found, the individual is in a comfortable position with support and legs uncrossed, the eyes gently closed and the deep breathing begun, start with the phrases, allowing for a pause between them:

I feel quite quiet…Quiet and relaxed…Quiet, relaxed and comfortable…

My feet feel heavy…Heavy and relaxed….Heavy, relaxed and comfortable…

My feet and ankles feel heavy…Heavy and relaxed…Heavy, relaxed and comfortable…

My ankles and legs feel heavy and relaxed…Heavy, relaxed and comfortable…

My legs, knees and hips feel heavy, warm, relaxed and comfortable…Warm, relaxed and comfortable…

My hips and lower back feel heavy, warm, relaxed and comfortable…Relaxed and comfortable…

My lower back, stomach and whole central portion of my body feel heavy and relaxed… Heavy, warm, relaxed and comfortable…

My stomach and central portion of my body feel heavy…Heavy and relaxed…Heavy, relaxed and comfortable…

My hands, arms and shoulders feel heavy…Heavy and relaxed…Relaxed, warm and comfortable…

My arms and shoulders feel heavy, warm, relaxed and comfortable…Relaxed and comfortable…

My shoulders, neck and jaws feel heavy…Heavy and relaxed…Heavy, warm and relaxed…

My neck, jaws and mouth feel heavy and relaxed…Heavy, relaxed and comfortable…

My jaws, mouth and forehead feel heavy and relaxed…Heavy, relaxed and comfortable…

My mouth, forehead and eyelids feel heavy and relaxed…Heavy, warm and relaxed…

My mouth, forehead, eyelids and scalp feel smooth…Smooth and relaxed, Smooth, relaxed and comfortable…

My whole face and neck lose their tension…tightness melts away…I am heavy, warm, relaxed and comfortable…

Imagine a white light…a white, healing light shining down on my body…

The white light is shining down on my head and shoulders…Healing white light is shining down…Penetrating beneath the skin…

The white light is beneath my skin, seeking out all areas that need healing…

The white light is at my _____ (name part of body)…The white light is covering my _____ (part) with protection and healing…

The white light is pushing out the pain and protecting my _____ (part)…

I feel quite relaxed…Relaxed, warm and comfortable…

My whole head and neck feel relaxed, warm and comfortable…

My shoulders, arms and hands feel heavy and relaxed…Heavy, relaxed and comfortable…

My whole back feels relaxed…Relaxed, heavy and warm…Warm and comfortable…

My stomach, hips and lower back feel relaxed…Relaxed, heavy and warm…Warm and comfortable…

My hips, legs and knees feel relaxed…Relaxed, heavy and warm…Warm and comfortable…

My legs, knees and feet feel relaxed…Relaxed, heavy and warm…Warm and comfortable…

My feet and ankles feel relaxed…Relaxed, heavy and warm…Warm and comfortable…

My whole body feels relaxed…Relaxed, heavy and warm…My whole body feels relaxed and warm…(Adapted from Davis et al. 1995; Linden 1990)

I will store this feeling in my memory, so I may use it at another time…

Now prepare to become more alert. Note how the sensation of relaxation feels. As practice continues at other times, the sensation may be recalled more easily; relaxation will begin sooner. Take several deep, slow breaths, using the diaphragm and exhale through the mouth. Gently stretch the body and open the eyes, feeling relaxed and refreshed.

When beginning practice of relaxation, several sessions per week will introduce the learner to the script and the sensations that develop during that time. Eventually, the individual will memorize the phrases and customize them to their own particular needs. As the individual becomes more experienced, brief practices a couple of times a day will provide benefit and almost become automatic. Practice times should fit where the individual feels most comfortable. Some prefer immediately before predicted stressful events, immediately after unknown stressful events, or as a healthy way of beginning and ending the day. With practice, the relaxation sensation is generalized to everyday life and can be recalled at any time during the day. A few deep breaths, use of powerful words, remembering a pleasant image, briefly smiling can help quiet the body, mind and spirit.

Since type 2 diabetes is a progressive illness, different than healing a physical injury, relaxation must be practiced on an ongoing basis to maintain the greatest benefit. Autogenic relaxation heightens an individual's sense of internal locus of control (Sharp et al. 1997). When an individual believes the power of control over a situation is coming from within, that sense of empowerment allows them to direct their self-care compliance to factors that directly contribute to blood glucose levels such as exercise, diet and stress management.

Part 4. Effects of Relaxation on Diabetes Mellitus

When a threat is discerned, whether emotional or physical, individuals affected by diabetes are likely to tense muscles and activate the sympatho-adrenal-medulary stress response system. Ongoing stress has been linked to several illnesses such as essential hypertension (Robinson 1979), pain and stiffness, headaches (Levinthal 1987), and heart disease (Porte 2003; Stansfeld 2002).

Since Benson's seminal work on the relaxation response (Benson 1975), applications of relaxation based therapy to decreasing symptoms of illness as well as promoting wellness have been published in the scientific literature and made accessible to the public. Literature reviews and statistical meta-analysis have supported the use of relaxation with biofeedback, deep breathing, imagery or integrated into psychotherapeutic paradigms. Several examples are in the therapy of migraine and muscle tension headache (Baskin 2003), and essential hypertension (Linden 1994, 2001; McGrady 1994).

Case studies have supported the benefits of relaxation therapies for persons with diabetes in improving well-being, and gaining a greater sense of control over their diabetes. However, prior to the publication by Surwit and collaborators (2002), neither biofeedback nor relaxation had been consistently shown to lower average blood glucose or glycohemoglobin in type 2 DM. Suggestions were that certain types of patients, those with excessive sympathetic nervous system activity were the best candidates for biofeedback therapy (Lane et al. 1993), or that relaxation training could improve glucose tolerance (Jablon et al. 1996). The randomized controlled study of stress management compared to an education control (Surwit et al. 2002) showed significantly lower glycohemoglobin values in the trained patients. However, positive effects required longer than six months to be achieved. Preliminary results from our laboratory (McGinnis 2003) suggest that 10 sessions over three months of biofeedback and relaxation therapy are associated with decreased average blood glucose and glycohemo-globin in comparison to an education control group.

It is important to note, however, that participants with clinical depression dropped out of our research protocol in large numbers. Furthermore, those who completed the pro-tocol did not demonstrate a reduction in blood glucose from either behavioral treatment or education if the depressive symptoms were moderate to severe. Nonetheless, there is encouraging evidence that depressive symptoms in persons with DM do respond to anti-depressant medication or to cognitive behavioral therapy (Goodnick et al. 1995; Lustman et al. 1998). In summary, it is less likely that relaxation therapy with or without biofeed-back will relieve clinical depression and in fact, mood disorders may inhibit beneficial ef-fects of relaxation on blood glucose. Depression must be treated with antidepressants or cognitive behavioral therapy before a relaxation therapy program can be successful.

Biofeedback and relaxation have other noteworthy benefits to the person with DM, for example improvement in poor circulation and decreased blood pressure. Thermal biofeedback offers information to the person with DM about the temperature of the hands and feet. With practice, the person is able to warm the hands and the feet by as much as 10 degrees Fahrenheit. Rice and Schindler (1992) provided evidence of in-creased blood flow to the feet and associated decreased pain in a group of patients with DM trained with thermal biofeedback.

Research in relaxation-based therapies in disorders often co-existing with DM, such as essential hypertension is also relevant. McGrady and Linden (2003) reviewed the lit-erature on biofeedback and relaxation effects in high blood pressure and found that improvements did occur in trained patients in comparison to untrained controls. De-creases in blood pressure were maintained over the long term in more than half of the trained patients. Muscle tension and thermal biofeedback, relaxation therapy and home practice of relaxation were associated with significant decreases in systolic and diastolic blood pressure. Transcendental meditation was also shown to be beneficial in decreasing blood pressure in African Americans with essential hypertension who were trained in groups instead of individually (Alexander et al. 1996; Schneider 1995).

Behavioral modification, including relaxation training was associated with signifi-cant reduction in fear of complications of diabetes. Trained participants were more ac-cepting of their diabetes, more willing to perform proper self-care and decreased their negative self talk and criticism over slight omissions in routine (Zettler 1995).

Summary

A vast literature supports the use of relaxation in stress related disorders either as a personal self help tool or as adjunctive therapy in an overall provider-designed management plan. Various types of relaxation, enhanced by biofeedback, imagery or healing words have been applied to type 2 diabetes. Although randomized con-trolled clinical trials targeting average blood glucose are few, results are encouraging. Persons with DM are well advised to implement a relaxation program on their own or to seek a trained practitioner if co-morbid medical or psychiatric problems are present. Health care providers for individuals affected by diabetes are recommended to offer relaxation training as one of the four pillars of control, in addition to diet, exercise and medication. The person with DM may benefit from relaxation in many ways, such as reduction in anxiety, fear, and physiological stress responses. Reductions in blood glucose, improved peripheral circulation and decreased risk for complications of the disease because of lower blood glucose are reasonable goals. In addition, the mental calm that comes with regular relaxation practice may help the person with DM to see a clearer path to self management with diet, exercise and medication.

References

Alexander, C. N., E.J. Langer, R.I. Newman, H.M. Chandler and J.L. Davies. 1989. Transcendental Meditation, Mindfulness, and Longevity: An Experimental Study with the Elderly. Journal of Personality and Social Psychology 57: 950–64.

Alexander, C. N., M.V. Rainforth and P. Gelderloos. 1991. Transcendental Meditation, Self Actualization and Psychological Health: A Conceptual Overview and Statistical Meta-Analysis. Journal of Social Behavior and Personality 6(5): 189–247.

Alexander, C. N., R.H. Schneider, F. Staggers, W. Sheppard, B.M. Clayborne, M. Rainforth, J. Salerno, K. Kondwani, S. Smith, K.G. Walton and B. Egan. 1996. Trial of Stress Reduction for Hypertension in Older African Americans. Hypertension 28: 228–37.

Allison, J. 1970. Respiratory Changes during Transcendental Meditation. Lancet 1(7651): 883.

American Diabetes Association. 2001. American Diabetes Association Clinical Practice Recommendations. Diabetes Care 24 (Suppl. 1): S1–S33.

Anderson, R.M., M.M. Funnell, P.M. Butler, M.S. Arnold, J.T. Fitzgerald and C.C.Feste. 1995. Patient Empowerment. Diabetes Care 18: 943–49.

Anderson, R.J., K.E. Freedland, R.E. Clouse and P.J. Lustman. 2001. The Prevalence of Comorbid Depression in Adults with Diabetes. Diabetes Care 24: 1069–78.

Baskin, S.M. and R.E. Weeks. 2003. The Biobehavioral Treatment of Headache. In Handbook of Mind-Body Medicine for Primary Care. Donald Moss, Angele McGrady, Terence C. Davies and Ian Wickramasekera, eds. pp. 449–55. Thousand Oaks, CA: Sage Publishers.

Benson, Herbert, with Mariam Z. Klipper. 1975. The Relaxation Response. New York: William Morrow and Co., Inc.

Bernstein, D.A. and C.R. Carlson. 1993. Progressive Relaxation: Abbreviated Methods. In Principles and Practice of Stress Management, 2nd Ed. Paul M. Lehrer and Robert L. Woolfolk, eds. pp. 53–88. New York: Guilford Press.

Bloomfield, H.H. and R.B. Kory. 1976. Happiness: The TM Program, Psychiatry and Enlightenment. New York: Simon and Schuster.

Cacioppo, J.T. 1994. Social Neuroscience: Autonomic, Neuroendocrine, and Immune Responses to Stress. Psychophysiology 31: 113–28.

Daniel, M., K. O'Dea, R.G. Rowley, R. McDermott and S. Kelly. 1999. Glycated Hemoglobin as an Indicator of Social Environmental Stress among Indigenous versus Westernized Populations. Preventive Medicine 29: 405–13.

Dantzer, R. 1991. Stress and Disease: A Psychobiological Perspective. Annals of Behavioral Medicine 13(4): 205–10.

Davis, Martha, with Elizabeth R. Eshelman and Matthew McKay. 1995. The Relaxation and Stress Reduction Workbook. Oakland: New Harbinger Publ.

Delmonte, M.M. 1987. Constructivist View of Meditation. American Journal of Psychotherapy 41(2): 286–98.

Ekman P. 2003. Emotions Revealed. Times Books. New York: Henry Holt and Company.

Eppley, K., A. Abrams and J. Shear. 1989. The Differential Effects of Relaxation Techniques on Trait Anxiety: A Meta-Analysis. Journal of Clinical Psychology 45: 957–74.

Everly, G.S. and J.M. Lating, eds. 2002. Neuromuscular Relaxation. In A Clinical Guide to the Treatment of the Human Stress Response, 2nd Ed. New York: Kluwer Academic.

Feldman, P.J. and A. Steptoe. 2003. Psychosocial and Socioeconomic Factors Associated with Glycated Hemoglobin in Nondiabetic Middle-Aged Men and Women. Health Psychology 22(4): 398–405.

Ford-Martin, Paula A. 2001. Guided Imagery. In The Gale Encyclopedia of Medicine, 2nd Ed. Jacqueline L. Longe, ed. pp. 1325–26. Farmington Hills, MI: Gale Group.

Ganong, W.F. 1997. Review of Medical Physiology, 18th Ed. Greenwich, CT: Lange Medical.

Gevirtz, R.N. and M.S. Schwartz. 2003. The Respiratory System in Applied Psychophysiology. In Biofeedback, A Practitioner's Guide, 3rd Ed. Mark S. Schwartz and Frank Andrasik, eds. pp. 212–24. New York: Guilford Press.

Goldman, Caren. 2001. Healing Words. New York: Marlowe and Co.

Goodnick, P.J., J.H. Henry and V.M. Buki. 1995. Treatment of Depression in Patients with Diabetes Mellitus. Journal of Clinical Psychiatry 56: 128–36.

Grandinetti, A., J.K. Kaholokula, K.M. Crabbe, C.K. Kenui, R. Chen and H.K. Chang. 2000. Relationship Between Depressive Symptoms and Diabetes Among NativeHawaiians. Psychoneuroendocrinology 25: 239–46.

Heriberto, C. 1988. The Effects of Clinically Standardized Meditation on type II Diabetics. Ph.D. Dissertation. Adelphi University. The Institute of Advanced Psychological Study.

Jablon, S.L., B.D. Naliboff, S.L. Gilmore and M.J. Rosenthal. 1996. Effects of Relaxation Training on Glucose Tolerance and Diabetic Control in Type II Diabetes. Applied Psychophysiology and Biofeedback 22: 155–69.

Jacobson, Edmund. 1938. Progressive Relaxation. Chicago: University of Chicago Press.

Jain, S.C., A. Uppal, S.O.D. Bhatnagar and B. Talukdar. 1993. A Study of Response Pattern of Non-Insulin Dependent Diabetics to Yoga Therapy. Diabetes Research and Clinical Practice 19: 69–74.

Kabat-Zinn, Jon. 1990. Full Catastrophe Living: Using the Wisdom of Your Body and Mind to Face Stress, Pain and Illness. New York: Delacorte Press.

Kawakami, N., N. Takatsuka, H. Shimizu and H. Ishibashi. 1999. Depressive Symptoms and Occurrence of Type 2 Diabetes Among Japanese Men. Diabetes Care 22: 1071–76.

Keefe F.J., P.M. Beaupre and K.M. Gil. 1996. Group Therapy for Patients with Chronic Pain In Psychological Approaches to Pain Management. Robert J. Gatchel and Dennis C. Turk, eds. pp. 259–82. New York: Guilford Press.

Lane, J.D., C.C. McCaskill, S.L. Ross, M.N. Feinglos and R.S. Surwit. 1993. Relaxation Training for NIDDM. Diabetes Care 16: 1087–94.

Lasater, Judith. 1995. Relax and Renew: Restful Yoga for Stressful Times. Berkeley, CA: Rodnell Press.

Levinthal, Carol. 1987. The Effects of Indirect Hypnosis, Direct Hypnosis, and Progressive Relaxation on the Primary and Secondary Physiological Symptoms of Chronic Headache. Ph.D. Dissertation, Department of Education, University of Cincinnati.

Linden, W. 1990. Autogenic Training, A Clinical Guide. New York:Guilford Press.

_____ 1993. The Autogenic Training Method of J.H. Schultz. In Principles and Practices of Stress Management, 2nd Ed. Paul M. Lehrer and Robert L. Woolfolk, eds. pp. 89–137. New York: Guilford Press.

Linden, W. and L.A. Chambers. 1994. Clinical Effectiveness of Non-Drug Therapies for Hypertension. A Meta Analysis. Annals of Behavioral Medicine 16: 35–45.

Linden, W., J.W. Lenz and A.H. Con. 2001. Individualized Stress Management for Primary Hypertension: A Randomized Trial. Archives of Internal Medicine 161: 1071–80.

Lustman, P. J., K.E. Freedland, L.S. Griffith and R.E. Clouse. 1998. Predicting Response to Cognitive Behavior Therapy of Depression in Type 2 Diabetes. General Hospital Psychiatry 20: 302–6.

Lyon, Debra E. and Ann G. Taylor. 2003. Nursing Education for Mind-Body Nursing. In Handbook of Mind-Body Medicine for Primary Care. Donald Moss, Angele McGrady, Terence C. Davies, and Ian Wickramasekera, eds. pp. 449–55. Thousand Oaks, CA: Sage Publications, Inc.

MacLean, Christopher R.K., Kenneth G. Walton, Stig R. Wenneberg, Debra K. Levitsky, Joseph P. Mandarino, Rafiq Waziri, Steven L. Hillis and Robert H. Schneider. Effects of the Transcendental Meditation Program on Adaptive Mechanisms: Changes in Hormone Levels and Responses to Stress After 4 Months of Practice. Psychoneuroendocrinology 2(4): 277–95.

Maharishi Mahesh Yogi. 1969. Maharishi Mahesh Yogi on the Bhagavad-Gita: A New Translation and Commentary. Baltimore: Penguin Books.

McGinnis, R., A.V. McGrady, K. Grower-Dowling and J. Malhotra. 2003. Impact of Mood on Outcome of Biofeedback-assisted Relaxation Therapy in Type 2 Diabetes Mellitus. Symposium presented at Association for Applied Psychophysiology and Biofeedback Annual Meeting. Jacksonville, Florida (March).

McGrady, A.V. 1994. Effects of Group Relaxation Training and Thermal Biofeedback on Blood Pressure and Related Psychophysiological Variables in Essential Hypertension. Biofeedback and Self-Regulation 19(1): 51–66.

McGrady, A., R. Bourey and B. Bailey. 2002. Metabolic Syndrome. *In* Handbook of Mind Body Therapies in Primary Care. Donald Moss, Angele McGrady, Terence C. Davies and Ian Wickramasekera, eds. pp. 275–97. Thousand Oaks, CA: Sage Publishers.

McGrady, A.V. and W. Linden. 2002. Biobehavioral Treatment of Essential Hypertension. *In* Biofeedback, A Practitioner's Guide, 3rd Ed. Mark S. Schwartz and Frank Andrasik, pp. 382-408. New York: Guilford Press.

McGrady, A. V., D. Lynch, R. Nagel, R. and E. Wahl. 2003. Application of the High Risk Model of Threat Perception to Medical Illness and Service Utilization in a Family Practice. Journal of Nervous and Mental Disease 191: 255–59.

McGrady, A. V. and J. Horner. 1999. Role of Mood in Outcome of Biofeedback Assisted Relaxation Therapy in Insulin Dependent Diabetes Mellitus. Applied Psychophysiology and Biofeedback 24: 79–88.

Nagel, Rollin W., Angele V. McGrady, Denis J. Lynch, Denis J. and Elmer F. Wahl. 2003. Patient-Physician Relationship and Service Utilization: Preliminary Findings. Primary Care Companion Journal of Clinical Psychiatry 5: 15–18.

Patel, Chandra. 1995. Yoga-Based Therapy: *In* Principles and Practices of Stress Management, 2nd ed. Paul M. Lehrer and Robert L. Woolfolk, eds. pp. 89–137. New York: Guilford Press.

Porte, Daniel, Jr., Robert S. Sherwin and Alain Baron, Alain, eds. 2003. Ellenberg and Rifkin's Diabetes Mellitus. New York: Pantheon Books.

Rice, B.I. 2001. Mind-Body Interventions. From Research to Practice/Complementary and Integrative Medicine. Diabetes Spectrum 14(4): 213–15.

Rice, B. I. and J.V. Schindler. 1992. Effect of Thermal Biofeedback-Assisted Relaxation Training on Blood Circulation in the Lower Extremities of a Population with Diabetes. Diabetes Care 15: 853–58.

Riedesel, Brian C. 1979. Toward Full Development of the Person. Personnel and Guidance Journal 57 (7): 332–37.

Robinson, Richard J. 1979. The Effects of Progressive Relaxation on Diastolic Blood Pressure, EMG, and Self-Report Indices of Anxiety among Male Hypertensives. M.A. Thesis, Department of Psychology, University of Dayton.

Rossman, M. L. and D.E. Bresler. 1993. Interactive Guided Imagery, 6th Ed. Mill Valley, CA: Academy for Guided Imagery.

Sahay, B. K. 1986. Yoga and Diabetes. The Journal of the Association of the Physicians of India 34(9): 645–48.

Samuels, Mike and Nancy Samuels. 1975. Seeing with the Mind's Eye. New York: Random House Inc.

Schneider, R. H., F. Staggers, C.N. Alexander, W. Sheppard, M. Rainforth, K. Kondwani, S. Smith and C.G. King. 1995. A Randomized Controlled Trial of Stress Reduction for Hypertension in Older African Americans. Hypertension 26: 820–27.

Schwartz, N. M. and M.S. Schwartz. 2002. Definitions of Biofeedback and Applied Psychophysiology. In Biofeedback: A Practitioner's Guide, 3rd Ed. Mark S. Schwartz and Frank Andrasik, eds. pp. 27–42. New York: Guilford Press.

Sharp, Conni, David P. Hurford, Julie Allison, Rozanne Sparks and Bradley P. Cameron. 1997. Facilitation of Internal Locus of Control in Adolescent Alcoholics Through a Brief Biofeedback-Assisted Autogenic Relaxation Training Procedure. Journal of Substance Abuse 14(1): 55–56.

Stansfeld, Stephen and Michael Marmot, eds. 2002. Stress and the Heart: Psychosocial Pathways to Coronary Heart Disease. London: BMJ Books.

Stevens, J.A. and M.E. Stoykov. 2003. Using Motor Imagery in the Rehabilitation of Hemispheres. Archives of Physical Medicine and Rehabilitation 84(7): 1090–92.

Sternberg, Esther M. 2001. The Balance Within. New York: W.H. Freeman and Company.

Surwit, R.S. and M.S. Schneider. 1993. Role of Stress in the Etiology and Treatment of Diabetes Mellitus. Psychosomatic Medicine 4: 380–93.

Surwit, R.S., M.A. van Tilburg, N. Zucker, C.C. McCaskill, P. Parekh, M.N. Feinglos, C.L. Edwards, P. Williams and J.D. Lane. 2002. Stress Management Improves Long-term Glycemic Control in Type 2 Diabetes. Diabetes Care 25: 30–34.

Travis, Frederick. 1995. Autonomic and EEG Patterns During Eyes-Closed Rest and Transcendental Meditation TM Practice: The Basis for a Neural Model of TM Practice. Consciousness and Cognition 8: 302–18.

Wallace, R. K. 1970. Physiological Effects of Transcendental Meditation. Reviste Brasileire de Medicine 8: 397–401.

Wallace, R.K., H. Benson and A F. Wilson. 1971. A Wakeful Hypometabolic Physiologic State. American Journal of Physiology 221: 795–99.

Wamala, S.P., A. Wolk and K. Orth-Gomer. 1997. Determinants of Obesity in Relation to Socioeconomic Status Among Middle-aged Swedish Women. Preventive Medicine 26(5): 734–44.

Waring, Nancy. 2000. Mindfulness Meditation: Studies Show That Awareness Practices Promote Healing. Hippocrates 14(7): XX.

Wiebe, D.J., M.A. Alderfer, S.C. Palmer, R. Lindsay and L. Jarrett. 1994. Behavioral Self-regulation in Adolescents with Type l Diabetes: Negative Affectivity and Blood Glucose Symptom Perception. Journal of Consulting and Clinical Psychology 62(6): 1204–12.

Zettler, A., G. Duran, S. Waadt, P. Herschbach and F. Strian. 1995. Coping with Fear of Long-term Complications in Diabetes Mellitus. Psychotherapy and Psychosomatics 64(3-4): 178–84.

CHAPTER 16

COMMUNITY EMPOWERMENT FOR THE PRIMARY PREVENTION OF TYPE 2 DIABETES: KANIEN'KEHÁ:KA (MOHAWK) WAYS FOR THE KAHNAWAKE SCHOOLS DIABETES PREVENTION PROJECT

*Ann C. Macaulay, Margaret Cargo, Sherri Bisset, Treena Delormier,
Lucie Lévesque, Louise Potvin and Alex M. McComber*

Vision Statement of the Kahnawake School Diabetes Prevention Project

All Kahnawakero:non (the people of Kahnawake) are in excellent health. Diabetes no longer exists. All the children and adults eat healthily at all meals and are physically active daily. The children are actively supported by their parents and family who provide nutritious foods obtainable from family gardens, local food distributors and the natural environment. The school program, as well as local organizations, maintain programs and policy that reflect and reinforce wellness activities. There are a variety of activities for all people offered at a wide range of recreational facilities in the community. All people accept the responsibility to co-operatively maintain a well community for the future Seven Generations.

KSDPP Community Advisory Board 1995

Summary of Chapter 16. This chapter outlines the experiences of an innovative and continuing program for the primary prevention of type 2 diabetes developed in the Kanien'kehá:ka (Mohawk) community of Kahnawake, near Montreal, Canada. In the early 1990s community members and community researchers entered into a partnership with academic researchers, to develop the Kahnawake Schools Diabetes Prevention Project (KSDPP). This project aims to mobilize the community for the promotion of healthy lifestyles, with the long-term goal of preventing diabetes and so ensuring good health for present and future generations of Kanien'kehá:ka (The Seven Generations). Throughout this process, the community of Kahnawake has taken the lead for the direction of the project, incorporating Kanien'kehá:ka traditions into decision-making at all levels and ensuring sensitivity to cultural ways.

Successful components of developing the project were documenting the local prevalence of diabetes and complications associated with diabetes and returning these results to the community, using community-based participatory research to develop the community-researcher partnership, developing a Code of Research Ethics to guide this partnership from intervention to dissemination of results, ensuring community members are equal partners with the researchers, integration of intervention and evaluation teams to create synergy, being responsive to changes with organisational and programmatic flexibility, and building local capacity by making the project a learning opportunity for all. The numerous, multi-faceted interventions in the elementary schools are reinforced by multi level community interventions that are developed to promote living in balance. Strategies of teaching, enabling, reinforcing, networking and role modeling aim to develop individual capabilities. Interventions are often effected in partnership with other community organisations, with ideas either originating from the project or initiated by other organisations. Evaluation of community governance shows that decision-making is considered to be shared among multiple community partners. Throughout this initiative sharing an interest for keeping children healthy has continually reinforced the collective responsibility of the Kanien'kehá:ka for the Seven Generations. The Seven Generations is an Aboriginal concept referring to the seven generations following the present. It is used in a way so as to require the present generation to give serious consideration to present words and actions—to consider the effect that current decisions will have looking seven generations to the future.

    ❧ ❧ ❧

Introduction

Demographically, Aboriginal peoples in Canada represent a small segment of the overall population. Approximately 3 percent of the Canadian population self-identify as Aboriginal in origin. Of the 1,192,600 Aboriginal persons living in Canada, 507,200 are Registered Indians, 57,000 Inuit, 205,800 Metis, and 422,600 are classified as non-status/other. Aboriginal peoples live in 596 bands and 2284 reserves across Canada. There is considerable linguistic diversity among Aboriginal peoples living in Canada with 11 major language groups and more than 58 dialects. The Aboriginal population in Canada is 10 years younger than the general population with an average age of 25.5 years. Forty-four percent of the Aboriginal population is under age 20 compared to 28 percent of the national population (Statistics Canada 2003).

While Aboriginal peoples in Canada represent a small percentage of the overall population, they are over-represented in the prevalence of type 2 diabetes. For Aboriginal peoples, the national age-adjusted rate of type 2 diabetes is three to five times greater than in the general population (Young et al. 2000; Bobet 1998; Anonymous 1999) and in some communities the age-adjusted rate for the entire community is as high as 26 percent, with half of individuals aged 50 having developed diabetes (Harris et al. 1997).

These elevated rates of type 2 diabetes are in turn causing high rates of complications of cardiovascular risk factors such as elevated blood lipids (Harris et al. 1997), cardiovascular disease, such as heart attacks and strokes (Anand et al. 2001; Harris et al. 2002; Howard 1999), high blood pressure (Young et al. 2000; Anonymous 1999), amputations and poor peripheral circulation (Fabitz 1999), and kidney failure leading to kidney dialysis (Young et al. 2000). These complications contribute to prolonged suffering and premature death (Mao et al. 1992). Additional concerns are a younger average age of onset of type 2 diabetes (Bobet 1998) and increased rates of gestational diabetes (Harris et al. 1998). No longer just a disease of adulthood, the diagnosis of type 2 diabetes in young children and adolescents leads to diabetes complications in young adults (Dean 1998). As in the general population, screening of community members repeatedly uncovers previously undiagnosed cases of diabetes (Harris et al. 1997; Delisle and J.M. Ekoë 1995), so the current known figures may represent a conservative estimate.

In Aboriginal communities, chronic diseases such as diabetes are considered indicative of the negative socio-cultural changes, the long term results of colonisation, disempowerment (Friedman and Starfield 2003; Israel, et al. 1997; Joe 2001; Durie 2003), decreased land base, loss of traditional ways, social stressors, and a lifestyle that is increasingly mechanized and no longer includes the former high level of physical activity for daily living. Nutrition is also changing from traditional foods that are closely connected to the land to highly refined foods available in abundance in numerous stores. The results of changes in physical activity and traditional eating patterns are high rates of obesity in adults (Young 1996) and children (Hanley et al. 2000), which in turn predisposes to diabetes.

Given that diabetes is a population-wide problem in Aboriginal communities, there is an urgent need for implementing a population approach to diabetes prevention. Such an approach aims to lower exposure to risk factors across the whole population (Rose 1985), as opposed to only focussing on those at high risk. This approach parallels the traditional Aboriginal philosophy of ensuring well-being for all, in contrast to providing benefits for a few (Bird 2002). A population approach can emphasize the full range of influences on a community, including society's political context and the role of public policies and laws directed toward multiple sectors, enfranchisement, and community empowerment (Friedman and Starfield 2003). Research driven by a population approach recognises the multiple levels of influence on diabetes prevention (i.e. personal, family, school, workplace, organizations, neighborhood, community, inter-community, health care system, regulatory policies, local and external governments) rather than limiting its focus on the individual (Smedley and Syme 2001). One population-level approach to community health utilizes community participation to ensure that locally identified program needs are founded on and incorporate local traditions, values and culture (Israel et al. 1998). For Aboriginal communities the importance of restoring control for health has been clearly stated in Canada by the report of Royal Commission of Aboriginal Peoples (1996) and on an international level in the context of cultural revitalization (Smith 1999). It is within this context of cultural revitalization that we present the Kahnawake Schools Diabetes Prevention Project (KSDPP).

Primary Prevention of Type 2 Diabetes

This chapter outlines the experiences of an innovative program developed for the primary prevention of type 2 diabetes with the Kanien'kehá:ka community of Kahnawake, near Montreal in Canada. The key to the success of this project has been the ongoing community commitment to the central vision that type 2 diabetes is a preventable disease (Harris and Zinman 2000). The people of Kahnawake have taken a collective responsibility to prevent the development of diabetes in its future generations.

The Kahnawake Schools Diabetes Prevention Project (KSDPP) is demonstrating that this can be accomplished when a community comes together at all levels to incorporate community traditions and values into such a project and works towards living in balance. Drawing upon its participatory democratic roots (Alfred 1995), KSDPP reflects the active participation of community members as professionals and part of the extended family in decision-making related to community-based diabetes prevention, as expressed by one community health professional:

> [Traditionally] we operated under what is called a direct democracy, we actively sat in and problem solved and built consensus around the direction our communities, our clans wanted to go. We used our collective wisdom, our communities were learning systems and from there we used that wisdom to make our decisions and to plan the future of our communities and how we were [going to] function. So if you take it now to service delivery, what I see happening is that it's a practice that's been inherent in us.

With the people of Kahnawake directing the course of the project, KSDPP is more accurately a reflection of the values of Kahnawakero:non (the people of Kahnawake);values, a strength of the people working together to take control, to protect and promote the health of the present and future generations of Kanien'kehá:ka (Seven Generations). This is the story of KSDPP—a story of community empowerment and cultural revitalisation—told in the hope that it will inspire other communities to begin their journey.

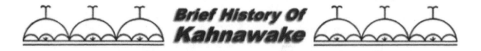

The Mohawks of Kahnawake are members of the Six Nations Iroquois Confederacy or as is common in their Kanien'kehá:ka language, members of the Haudenosaunee "People of the Longhouse". They have existed as a sovereign nation long before the arrival of Columbus and the European settlers (approximately 1300 years). The Mohawks taught the European settlers how to survive the northern climate, how to live off the land and new ways of governing themselves democratically.

As the Mohawks influenced the European way of life, European practices and beliefs also affected them. By signing a peace treaty with the Haudenosaunee, first in 1667 and again in

1700, the French were secured in fulfilling their two main objectives: securing a military and political alliance and establishing Christian missions in Mohawk territory. Reduced tensions led many French settlers to move onto Mohawk territory, with the Mohawks acting as a buffer between the French and the other five members of the Iroquois Confederacy: the Oneida, Onondaga, Cayuga, Seneca, and Tuscarora nations. Jesuit missionaries, determined to "civilize" the Mohawks, established Christian missions with the sole intent to convert the natives. The Francis Xavier mission is an example and testimony to this process. Many forms of spirituality now exist on the reserve, Traditional Beliefs, Catholics, Protestants, and some Jehovah's Witness as well.

The Iroquois People are unique because of their social and political structure. They are governed by the Great Law, an accord among the Six Nations of the Confederacy that bans bloodshed and ensures peace as a way of life. The Iroquois social system is both matrilineal and a matriarchy, the bulk of the political power lies with the women of the society. Family names and clans are passed down through the mother to the daughter and so any children then belong to the mother's clan. It should be noted that in this social structure, both men and women were considered equal, neither being superior to the next. The traditional political system also relies heavily on the clan structure. The decisions are made through consensus of the people, making the Iroquois Confederacy one of the world's first true democracies. Thomas Jefferson studied and later presented the political structure of the Iroquois Confederacy to the thirteen colonies. The American democratic system as we know it today is based upon the values and beliefs of the Iroquois people.

The Mohawks of Kahnawake have appeared prominently throughout history, not only in North America but in the world as well. Military allegiances with Mohawk warriors were coveted by many Dutch, French, British, and later American generals throughout the colonial wars. Later in World War I and World War II, the Mohawks contributed many soldiers and support personnel. Once again, many volunteered for Korean, Vietnam, and Gulf wars. Although Kahnawake Mohawks have a strong warrior tradition not all our exploits have been through conflict. In 1884, 56 Mohawks from Kahnawake helped the British map and navigate the cataracts of the Nile river in Egypt; our reputation as expert boats-men of the St. Lawrence river earned us this contract. In the 1860s, the men of Kahnawake took up the trade of Ironwork, building bridges first, then moving on to ships and skyscrapers. The skill of our men in this trade has become world renowned, structures made with Mohawk blood, sweat and tears range from Mexico to Greenland and Alaska to Turkey. The Mohawks also excel in sports. Alwyn Morris was our first Olympian, participating in the Los Angeles 1984 games in the sport of kayaking. Our second Olympian, Waneek Horn-Miller, was co-captain of the Women's Water Polo team at Sydney 2000 Olympic games.

Although this document mentions the exploits of mainly our men, much credit is due to our Mohawk women for these successes. Without the women tending their families' needs with their men absent, and raising the men mentioned in the first place, our mark in history would not be as significant or noticeable. With this said, all the Mohawks of Kahnawake share a proud past and look forward to an even prouder future.

Located on the website of the Mohawk Council of Kahnawake
<www.kahnawake.com>
where it is reprinted from a document courtesy of
The Kahnawake Tourism Information Office

Traditionally, tionhnhehkwen (the foods needed to be healthy) were obtained through agriculture, fishing, hunting and gathering. Agricultural staples included corn, beans, and squash, named the Three Sisters. The Three Sisters are rooted in the story of creation that tells of their nurturing properties. In addition to providing good nutrition, these foods store through the winter and so ensure the survival of the women and the next generation. In the late 19th century agricultural and trading practices were gradually replaced as men became involved in the structural steel industry across diverse locations in North America. These are the famous high steel workers who built many of the early bridges and buildings in the major cities in the USA. By the 1950s, farming, local fishing and food gathering virtually disappeared due to expropriation of community lands and most of the riverfront to build the St. Lawrence Seaway, increase participation of men in the iron-working industry, and people acquiring employment in nearby Montreal.

Kahnawake, situated across the St. Lawrence River approximately nine miles southwest of Montreal, has a population of 7200 (2002). An additional 1868 people live outside the community. Men continue to work in construction with an increase of men and women in local white-collar careers stimulated by community development, and high numbers of students gaining further education at trade schools, colleges and universities. While the Mohawk Council of Kahnawake is the federally recognized government of the community, traditional government through the Longhouse system is still strong. Community strengths include decentralisation of power with control through locally elected boards of directors, endorsed by the Mohawk Council of Kahnawake, governing community education services (1967), health services (1970), youth recreation (1972), social and community services (1972) and the Kahnawake local court (1979). Community control of local services came as community leaders successfully negotiated for greater autonomy from the federal government of Canada. Through this high level of community governance came programs developed by the community specifically for the community. As in the past, the women of Kahnawake have taken a leadership role in many community initiatives related to protecting and promoting the health of the present and future generations of children. Their active involvement in the governance and program implementation of KSDPP illustrates cultural continuity in their traditional maternal role in caring for the children, voiced by a Kahnawake community member:

> One thing I have to say here, in Kahnawake, in this community, education has always led the way. Who was the first group to say to the government: No, we're not following that policy? It was the school committee. The school committee, those women of the school committee were the first ones to say to the government: No, we're not doing that…

In the 1990s local economic development services, together with a new community co-operative banking system, rapidly facilitated a variety of new community owned small stores and businesses (Macaulay 2003). Today Kahnawake is recognised as one of the leading Aboriginal communities in Canada.

Origins of the Kahnawake Schools
Diabetes Prevention Project

In the early 1980s a young Kanien'kehá:ka doctor, together with one of the established family physicians working in Kahnawake, undertook a chart review that documented a prevalence of type 2 diabetes among 45–64 year-old persons living in

Kahnawake that was twice that of the Canadian population (Montour and Macaulay 1985). Their second study showed that for this same age group, almost half of those with diabetes also had severe heart disease as a complication of diabetes. In addition, persons with diabetes had six times the complications of heart disease, stroke, kidney complications and amputations than those without diabetes. This study also documented very high rates of obesity in both those with diabetes and those without diabetes (Macaulay, Montour, and Adelson 1988; Montour, Macaulay, and Adelson 1989).

From these baseline studies, the physicians had planned a third research initiative to document the predisposing factors leading to the complications of diabetes in Kahnawake. At the same time, due to a promise they made to return research results to the community, they began, in the spring of 1987, a series of presentations which would change both their own, and the community's perceptions of diabetes. Contacts with community members including elders and community leaders in health, education, culture and politics were made through several formal one-hour presentations, and a radio presentation followed by radio phone-ins (Montour and Macaulay 1988). In response to these presentations, key community members and elders requested that action be taken to prevent diabetes:

> People came to us and asked us to do something. Do something about diabetes. That was their reaction (Family physician working in Kahnawake).

Moreover, based upon these research results and other observations concerning the increasing rates of obesity of the school children, the type of preventive action requested was specific:

> They're finding that more and more children are coming to school already obese, because of their change of lifestyle…they're looking at trying to prevent children from having diabetes…everybody understands that we all come together for the welfare of the children (Kahnawake community member).

In response to this request, the family physicians changed track from a clinical orientation focussing on diabetes complications, to a diabetes primary prevention agenda centred upon the children. As a family physician working in Kahnawake stated: "We realized this was a much more important topic with which to get involved." The community reaction was part of a process in which key community members shifted their perceptions about diabetes as being not only a threat to individuals, but also a threat to the community. This process, described as "legitimizing diabetes as a community health issue" embodies structural, social and cultural community conditions, along with a set of strategies alerting the community to the research findings (Bisset et al. 2003).

Prior to the presentations in 1987, diabetes was described as being a pervasive health problem that was encountered daily, and perceived as something to live with, when a community member said: "If you didn't get it you were lucky" and if you did you would eventually require the care of a physician and the diabetes education team. This familiarity with diabetes, together with an increased awareness that diabetes risk factors such as obesity were increasingly manifested among the school children, set the stage to raise levels of consciousness about a familiar problem. The baseline studies uncovering a relative health disparity within Kahnawake were presented in an open, interactive forum, allowing key community members to 'self-diagnose' diabetes as a relevant health issue. Where:

> Just hearing it spoken and seeing the figures had a big impact, as peoples' own results were given back to them (Family physician working in Kahnawake).

The impact of this message was an unexpected consequence of two physicians with credibility, sending a message through various channels, strategically directed to different levels of the community in a culturally appropriate way. Three factors set the stage for KSDPP. First, community-level solutions to this health problem were not imposed nor suggested. Traditionally, Kanien'kehá:ka

> ...actively sat in, and problem-solved and built consensus around the direction our communities, as our clans wanted to go. We used our collective wisdom" (Kahnawake community member).

Secondly, the credibility of the messengers influenced the reception of the message in Kahnawake. Credibility was facilitated by one messenger being Kanien'kehá:ka, both having occupational status *"Letters behind your name"* (Kahnawake community member), espousing Aboriginal values, and caring for community wellness. Lastly, the message raised consciousness around an emotional issue. The elders spoke openly about being fixed in their ways of eating, being frequently overweight, having already undergone heart by-pass surgery or suffering from a stroke or amputation of a limb, and that for them it was *"too late"* (Kahnawake community elder). They, however, wished for a different future, one free of diabetes, for future generations, and so specifically asked that any new program focus on the young to protect their children and grandchildren from carrying the same burden of disease (Montour and Macaulay 1988). This request was facilitated by the well established and comprehensive diabetes education program, developed and coordinated by a Kanien'kehá:ka nurse educator at the community hospital, for those already diagnosed with diabetes (Macaulay, Hanusaik and Delisle-Diabo 1988).

From the elders' request the seeds were sown for what was to become the Kahnawake Schools Diabetes Prevention Project (KSDPP). The new goal was to establish a research project with both intervention and evaluation components. To accomplish this goal the community-based professionals from health and education, who had also developed early research skills, first came together and then invited academic researchers from two neighboring universities to join the team for their expertise in health promotion design and program evaluation.

> I think Kahnawake was very lucky that there was another family physician and myself to start the research. You know, most research is academic, it's bench research and it's Ivy League people in their towers coming down to the poor masses (Kahien'kehá:ka family physician).

After seven years of discussions and unsuccessful grant applications, in a time when there was little monies available for health promotion, KSDPP was finally launched in 1994 funded through a national research grant (Macaulay et al. 1997). A doctoral thesis has since documented that it was a national lobby effort for diabetes in the early 1990s, including the physicians from Kahnawake backed by the original Kahnawake data, which had convinced a national research granting agency to release grant monies specifically for diabetes in Aboriginal peoples (Rock 2003).

> My involvement was with the Canadian Diabetes Advisory Board, which was struck in the mid '80s. We were an advisory committee to the Minister of Health, to report to him on the state of diabetes in the nation. So, this was not just Aboriginal, it was national and from that group spun off the national competition for Aboriginal diabetes research, which is what funded KSDPP (Kahien'kehá:ka family physician).

For KSDPP the academic researchers were absolutely essential as they contributed their academic expertise to developing the initial grant proposals to secure national research funding. These grant proposals were a first collaborative success whereby academic content and Kanien'kehá:ka ways were integrated after community reviews. The strength of the final and successful proposal was reflected in the partnership forged by all the researchers with community members and community organizations.

A Participatory Approach
to Community-based Research

From the beginning, KSDPP was planned as a community-based participatory research project, where researchers and community members would partner to share expertise in support of a vision to prevent diabetes (Green et al. 1995; Macaulay et al. 1999; Reading 2002; Gibson, Gibson and Macaulay 2001). While framed as participatory research by academic researchers, the underlying philosophy of KSDPP converged with a longstanding tradition of consensus decision-making by the Kanien'kehá:ka. This participatory approach is the opposite to 'helicopter' research where researchers make decisions on behalf of the community, and the voice of community members is not equally heard (Model Tribal Research Code. With Checklist for Tribal Regulation for Research for Indian Health Boards 1999). This 'helicopter' way of research had also been experienced in Kahnawake.

> In the past outside research teams had swooped down from the skies, swarmed all over town, asked nosey questions that were none of their business and then disappeared never to be heard of again (Kanien'kehá:ka family physician).

KSDPP Community Advisory Board

Building on a rich history of community control, the KSDPP Community Advisory Board (CAB) was formed to direct the intervention and research components. In keeping with traditional practices of the Kanien'kehá:ka, CAB is based on voluntary participation with representation of community members from all walks of life. The volunteer members have varied in age from 26 to 80 years. Membership includes representatives from various community organizations, such as health, social services, education, the environment office, the cultural center, spiritual groups, the Kahnawake Youth Center, as well as interested community members. These members are very dedicated, the strength of their commitment guided by the need to protect and promote the health of the Seventh Generation and from experiencing, first hand, the toll that diabetes has taken on themselves and close family members.

> MY STORY? How do I put into words someone's life? What name do you give the space in a family that is missing a daughter? What comfort can you give to a mother who outlives her child? What do you say to nieces and nephews who depend on Kairwah Ienné (Aunty Sarah) to make the best homemade bread in the whole wide world? What happened to the cousin who was always dependable to help in any way she could? Where did the friend go who would always save seats for everyone at the bingo hall? Where is the Grandmother who dropped by every day just for hugs and kisses because she considered them a bonus? What answer do you give to grandchildren who say that she's not even 60 years old, therefore she's not even old enough to die? Where did she go? How do you explain to a four-year-old that she's not just playing at sleeping? How do you say to her that Ma was in the hospital for six months because of a broken arm resulting from a car accident? How can you explain Ma missed you so much that she would ask about you every day? Explain to a child that hospital rules don't allow a four year old visitation, especially when Ma's arm was turning gangrene so badly that the whole room smelled like you wanted to get sick. Can anyone explain how a nurse who was at her bedside since the day she came to the hospital broke down and ushered the four-year-old right through the security guard, daring him to say something or make a move to try to stop them because she was determined that Ma would see her grandchild for the first time in six months because she was a model patient and deserved it! Can you imagine the look on Ma's face when she saw that four-year-old with her handful of picked flowers? Where do you put those kind of memories? What do you think about the day she came home from the hospital? There was so much to do, so many people to visit, so many places to go. She was like a bird set free from a cage. How many hours did she count to midnight? There she was at the window in the moonlight, very visible. I asked her : "Ma, why are you still awake?" Ma said: "I can't sleep I'm so happy to be home." What do you do when that happiness is broken. Ask yourself the question, why didn't she wake up the next morning? We will be asking that question every day for the rest of our lives. Dare we ask if diabetes is a killer? (Amelia Tekwatonti McGregor, 2003)

CAB members meet monthly to direct the project. Their tasks are all encompassing and include:

- ensuring cultural relevance of the project;
- promoting KSDPP objectives in their homes and organizations;
- role-modeling healthy lifestyles;
- advising on the design and implementation of research protocols;

- shaping the interpretation of research results;
- reviewing abstracts, scientific articles and this book chapter;
- participating in the dissemination of project activities and research results to both Aboriginal and scientific audiences;
- co-teaching with researchers on participatory research and ethics at academic institutions, national and international workshops; and
- participating in administrative activities i.e. reviewing applications and interviewing candidates for KSDPP positions.

CAB members actively participate in the life and direction of the project, as shared by a CAB member:

> If there's a general community event we're [CAB members] also asked to volunteer some time or some food. I mean there are always phone calls coming in once a month, can you make soup or sandwiches. For example, the trade show at the arena this summer, there was a booth there so they asked CAB members to go in and volunteer some time. So there's also direct involvement from the CAB members representing KSDPP.

CAB has incrementally taken a more active role in the life and direction of the project. Nine years since its inception, KSDPP, which was originally linked with the Kahnawake Education Centre, has now become an independent organization. As of 2003, CAB has formed an executive committee to provide the leadership required to govern the project.

The KSDPP Code of Research Ethics

One of the first major achievements of the community-researcher team was in developing a code of research ethics, a code that continues to provide researchers and community members with a set of guidelines for negotiating issues. In 1994, CAB and researchers came together to formalise the partnership and develop guidelines to promote the sharing of leadership, power, and decision-making among all team partners. At this time, the primary partners included community members, community-based researchers and academic researchers. The development of this code began with a review of the literature and other research codes. The KSDPP Code of Research Ethics (www.ksdpp.org) is founded on two policy statements: 1) the Kanien'kehá:ka of Kahnawake are sovereign to make decisions about research in Kahnawake, and 2) research should benefit and contribute to community empowerment

> …because we've got a guide for research, we don't have to keep repeating that all the time, make sure that you do this, make sure you do that. We know that it's written right into the agreements. Plus we have the new research council, so we know that the research is going to be done right and that it's going to be owned by the community of Kahnawake. It's for us, not just to help a student out there do a paper and we never see them again (Kahnawake community member).

The KSDPP Code of Research Ethics continues with an understanding of the principles of participatory research: all the partners should be involved at all stages of the research process: design, implementation, data analysis and interpretation, and dissemination of the results. All partners contribute ideas and resources that strengthen the project and its outcomes.

The document begins by outlining the obligations of the academic researchers, community researchers and the community throughout the research process. It ensures that the data are owned by the community and must be returned to them after analysis is complete. It also ensures that the research benefits the community, as voiced by one CAB member:

> I think it's been to look at the work that's being done, to try to set some guidelines to make sure that the work is work that the community benefits from and that we're comfortable with it and that is acceptable to the community.

One innovative section states that any new researchers wishing to join the team, be they students or established researchers, must be accepted by both the community and the researchers. This means that new senior researchers cannot automatically join the team, and researchers do not alone have the authority to bring a student into the team or give the KSDPP data to a student to analyse. All students are first invited to meet with CAB, to discuss their proposals which can then be accepted, modified or rejected by CAB. For any study, once data has been analysed, the results are first interpreted by the entire team, and then returned to the community of Kahnawake, before dissemination outside of the community. If the community and researchers do not agree on the interpretation of the findings, then the dissemination process allows for dissension and the inclusion of two different interpretations of the findings in the same oral dissemination or publication. As far as we know, this last clause is unique and, to date, has not been applied. Developing the KSDPP Code of Research Ethics took a period of eight months. At the time, this seemed very long. In retrospect, the discussions and negotiations were important steps to understanding academic and community cultural practices and to building trust among team members. Both steps were necessary to develop the concept of equal partnership blending together different types of expertise, with no partner having authoritative status (Macaulay, Delormier et al. 1998).

The KSDPP Code of Research Ethics showed foresight in developing clauses that protected not only individuals, but the entire community from potential stigmatization, which reflects current developments in ethics to develop guidelines to protect the collectivity or community (Weijer et al. 1999; Guideslines for Ethical Research in Indigenous Studies 2000). In the words of another CAB member:

> Help the researchers, O Wise Ancestors, when they sit in their universities and do not look into the eyes or see the faces of those they research. We must educate the researchers to see that we are a people who must be involved from the beginning of any research. We want an equal partnership with involvement in the decision making process. In our project, the moral and ethical guidelines (Code of Research Ethics) are an important component to empower all the community participants and researchers to work together in a successful relationship. Through this empowerment comes the owner-

ship and the commitment to work together for a healthier community. As Onkwehonwe (The Real People), we ask our Ancestors to help us to 'look inwards' to ourselves, our culture and our spirituality for a healthy lifelong journey.

The KSDPP Code of Research Ethics has been used as a model by the Kahnawake Onkwatakari'tahshera Health and Social Services Research Council (the Kahnawake research council which reviews all research requests), other Aboriginal projects and organizations in North America. (Alaska Native Science Commission: Code of Research Ethics 1997; First Nation and Inuit Regional Longitudinal Health Survey 1999. Code of Research Ethics; Appendix 4 (A-54) http://www.naho.ca/fnc/rhs) and has served the project well for the last nine years. KSDPP is currently revising the Code to include guidelines for knowledge translation, new aspects concerning the storage of tapes and qualitative data, the enhanced review process of abstracts and scientific articles before public dissemination, and to ensure that KSDPP is up to date with concepts from other guidelines developed in the last nine years by Indigenous organizations and national granting agencies (Weijeret al.1999; Guideslines for Ethical Research in Indigenous Studies 2000).

Kahnawake Schools Diabetes Prevention Project

The KSDPP Model of Community-based Intervention

KSDPP embodies an integrated community wide (ecological) and (w)holistic approach to diabetes prevention. Like many other Aboriginal cultures, the worldview of the Kanien'kehá:ka is based on the complex web of relationships that exist between people, animals, spirits, natural forces, plants and landforms that comprise the ecosystem (Battiste 2000; Battiste and Youngblood 2000; Dei et al. 2000; Smith 1999). The interdependence of life forces that forms the basis of the Kanien'kehá:ka worldview is combined with a (w)holistic view of health emphasising living in balance, the ideas of which are reflected in the continuity of the circle which has no beginning and has no end. (Bopp and Project. 1985; Montour 2000; Morgan and Slade 1997) The circle represented by the Medicine Wheel symbolizes the ideals of interconnectivity, (w)holism and living in balance, that mirror the way Aboriginal peoples strive to live their lives. (Bopp and Project 1985)

How does KSDPP respect and incorporate Kanien'kehá:ka culture? A qualitative analysis of the KSDPP intervention shows that the implementation of diabetes prevention activities is directed toward living in balance (Delormier et al. 2003). Living in balance signifies being well in mind, body, emotion and spirit, embodied in the KSDPP Vision Statement that introduces this chapter and the traditional Aboriginal philosophy of health (Bird 2002).

The vision statement clearly outlines living in balance through a positive attitude, healthy living and the overall community goals needed to support a future free of diabetes. Each year at the annual KSDPP community day this vision is re-visited, to maintain the energy needed to continue to 'walk the talk'.

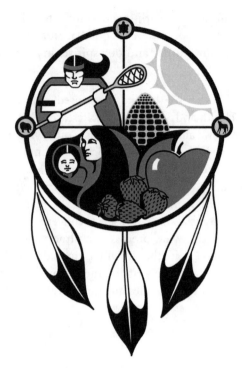

The logo for KSDPP, designed by Kim Delormier—a community artist—embodies the vision for KSDPP.

The circle is the main symbol found in Onkwehon:we cultures. It represents life: the past, present and future, no beginning or end. There is strength and unity in the circle. **The three clans** of the Mohawks of Kahnawake sit on the circle. The bear, wolf and turtle represent the unity of the people in preventing diabetes in the future generations. **The lacrosse player** symbolizes in importance of daily physical activity through the traditional Iroquois game of lacrosse. **The sun**, our elder brother with his life giving energy and strength reminds us that we all possess this energy and strength in the wellness journey for ourselves, families and community.The food represents the importance of healthy eating. The corn is one of the Iroquoian lifegivers or 'Three Sisters' , the strawberries are the first fruit of the season in the Northeast, while the apples last the longest on the trees into the fall. *The elder and child* reminds us that the wellness of our future generations is everyone's responsibility as Onkwehon:we. **The eagle feathers** represent the gifts of the eagle, the brother who flies highest and closest to the Creator. His vision, wisdom and courage are gifts that we each possess. **The colour purple** is known to us as a healing colour (<www.ksdpp.org>).

It is with an ecological and holistic approach to health that KSDPP aims to decrease the future occurrence of type 2 diabetes, through the short-term goals of increasing healthy eating and daily physical activity, and the adoption of a positive attitude. How does this unfold in the context of community practice? An ecological approach to diabetes prevention, such as employed by KSDPP (Delormier 2003), recognizes that the adoption of healthy behaviours can be enhanced if consistent messages are provided in multiple settings, such as school, home, community, and through multiple sources, including teachers, parents, and media (Killip 1987).

There is a general consensus that an ecological approach provides a more comprehensive framework than just individual-level approaches. Some of the limitations of the earlier individual approaches were associated with a tendency to attribute behavior change failures to shortcomings on the part of the individual, i.e., "blaming the victim" (Pearce 1996). By contrast the ecological approach espoused by KSDPP harmonizes with Kanien'kehá:ka values of involving the entire community (i.e., organisations, families and individuals), and of creating opportunities for participation and capacity-building. Moving towards a diabetes-free future requires that the intervention contain a host of multi-target, multi-setting intervention strategies designed and implemented by the community for the benefit of community. As requested by the elders, the project focuses on the current and future generations of children. Implementing interventions in the school are not seen as sufficient to modify the health trajectories of children. Children require ongoing support from those who nurture and shape their development. The following describes the interventions in the elementary schools and the community and how the two elements of the KSDPP intervention are intertwined in the overall goal of reaching the whole community.

> We always keep our focus on the children and that it's important to give them some kind of role model (Kahnawake community member).

Elementary Schools' Interventions to Educate Young Children

At the heart of the KSDPP model is a health education curriculum (described below) that is supported by extra-curricular activities in schools. The majority of elementary school children attend an English language school or a Kanien'kehá:ka immersion school in the community, where since 1994 the total number of children in Grades 1 to 6 has varied from 401 to 458. The schools are under the direction of the Kahnawake Education Centre, which is governed by the Kahnawake Combined Schools Committee and whose members are parents of children from kindergarten to high school.

In partnership with the schools and the community hospital, KSDPP supported the introduction of a new health curriculum into the elementary schools, with the goal of having this curriculum delivered by the teachers (as opposed to health care professionals). The Kateri Memorial Hospital Centre Health Education Program for Diabetes Prevention(c) was created by a dietitian and two community health nurses from the community owned hospital, with input from the teachers and KSDPP staff. The curriculum was written in English and then translated into Kanien'kehá:ka for the Kanien'kehá:ka immersion school, with sections on nutrition, fitness and physical activity, diabetes and healthy lifestyles. The 10, 45-minute lessons per year for Grades 1 through 6 use practical experiences in addition to inter-active and cooperative learning techniques. Lessons incorporate traditional learning styles with hands on interactions and high visual content, and include story telling, games, food tasting, experiments, puppet shows, crafts and audiovisual presentations. The nutrition section discusses healthy eating, balanced meals, healthy snacks, avoidance of high fat foods, nutrients and their roles, label reading, factors influencing eating habits, body image and healthy weight. This section incorporates traditional foods, as well as foods commonly eaten in the community. The fitness section includes the benefits of different types of activity: aerobic, strength building and flexibility and emphasizes the pleasure of daily physical activity. The last section links lifestyle to disease, describes diabetes with its consequences and how it can be prevented.

During the first year, in order to increase knowledge and build capacity, the community health nurses and the dietitian delivered the curriculum in the presence of classroom teachers, who are mainly from the community and themselves parents and grandparents. Then the teachers received training and by year three began to deliver the program themselves with the support of the KSDPP intervention team (Macaulay et al. 1997).

> I think because the teachers are the ones that are the closest to the children, the teachers have to be the ones that…need to be taught. They need to know, we need to know about this disease (Kahnawake community member).

KSDPP successfully lobbied the Kahnawake Combined School Committee to reinforce the schools' nutrition policy that had been introduced prior to KSDPP.

> Well, we were always concerned about the quality of foods that children were bringing into the school with the high sugar content and a high fat content, and so it was a decision made by administration that we would just not allow children to bring things that were not healthy for them. And it took a lot of work. First we tried persuasion, education and information, and when that didn't work fully, then we started to take things away from kids or if they brought things into the schoolyard, any junk food, we took it away from them (Kanien'kehá:ka educational leader).

Therefore the nutrition policy ensures that children bring only healthy foods to schools for lunches and snacks. Junk food is not allowed, and there are no machines selling sodas and other convenience foods in the schools (Macaulay et al. 1998).

> And now for the Nutrition Policy in the schools: we have made a better list for teachers to understand. Teachers want to know what can be brought in and what's not allowed. When there is a parent-teacher night we try to reinforce the nutrition policy with the parents. We've rated different snacks that kids bring to school, to show parents what was healthy (KSDPP intervention team member).

Other KSDPP school initiatives have included healthy breakfasts and lunches prepared by parents for staff and students, snow sculpture contests to increase wintertime physical activities, and a one mile run 'Racers for Health' in the early summer which now attracts 100 to 200 students from other Kanien'kehá:ka communities.

KSDPP is different from many other programs in showing that the teacher's role is not limited to just classroom teaching. Many of the teachers have assumed a major role: in addition to delivering the health education program, many teachers reinforce the messages by walking with the children in the school grounds before school or at recess, making sure that all classroom treats are healthy snacks and role-modeling healthy lifestyles. Some teachers incorporate health education program lesson plans into other studies, such as using food label reading in their math class. Currently, KSDPP is developing a health curriculum for pre-school children, and will begin to work more closely with families of this age group.

Community Interventions to Promote Living in Balance

Another KSDPP goal is to ensure that the immediate and extended families acquire the same knowledge as the children, so that they are well-positioned to be good role-models and to support their children. To complement the school based program, community wide interventions are designed to increase community awareness, to develop positive attitudes towards healthy lifestyles and to provide all ages, families and extended families fun opportunities to eat healthily and be physically active. It also underlines that learning is not limited to the classroom, and that schools do not operate in isolation from the community, but rather offer support to and in turn are supported by the community (Killip et al. 1987). Healthy living is supported by healthy community environments, and another early success of KSDPP was to develop a partnership with other organisations to plan and build a new one mile recreation path along the water front where people can walk, jog, bike and roller blade in a safe and positive environment.

Community interventions are actively promoted through a variety of channels. KSDPP uses the local radio for numerous public service announcements, and conducts talk shows where listeners can phone in with their questions. We have used regular half-page advertisements in the local newspaper to provide short and behavior-oriented information about healthy lifestyles, and to advertise upcoming activities. Now there is a new TV channel in the community that KSDPP will start to use.

KSDPP undertakes intervention activities to offer good opportunities for families to be physically active and eat healthily throughout the year. For example, community walks with incentives for the families with the most participation and the earliest registrations, bowling parties, food tasting events, cooking classes, food demonstrations, walks for young mothers with baby carriages, walking for all ages including elders at the arena in cold weather, roller blading for the youth, and family sledding parties in the wintertime. Many of these events include a healthy meal, such as soups, chili and sandwiches. Meals are frequently prepared by the participants as food is central to tradition and the opportunity is there to role model healthy food preparation and healthy eating.

> We keep the messages the same, but change the colour of the table cloth and the paper it is printed on…it keeps it interesting to put a new look or twist on a repeated activity, but we are always looking to try something totally new (KSDPP intervention team member).

Interventions are planned to reach as many people as possible not only at invitational community events but also by meeting people in their own environments. This may involve chatting with the men when they pick up their coffee at 5 or 6 am at a local coffee shop, and visiting community organizations during the workday to bring information to both men and women about making healthy food choices and being physically active. From the beginning KSDPP chose to build on pre-existing strengths and thus to partner and support existing community groups and events that could help attain the KSDPP goals. Partnering with organizations such as the Kahnawake Youth Centre, co-sponsoring walking clubs (e.g., Mohawk Miles), and attending health and harvest fairs, and several sporting competitions has been critical to promote capacity building and sustainability. By coming together under the umbrella of a same community event, partners created opportunities to optimize community resources to promote healthy behaviours (Levesque et al. 2003):

> We had started to work together on different initiatives, because we are all promoting health. It was better for us to join forces rather than doing individual work. It reinforces everything we are doing…itt makes [carrying out activities] so much more fun if everyone does a little bit and it makes the booth all that more exciting (KSDPP intervention team member.).

From qualitative evaluation of the interventions, we have found that most KSDPP interventions are planned and implemented in collaboration with other community groups. For example, in 1996-97 two-thirds of the collaborations around physical activity interventions occurred in response to invitations received by KSDPP from other community groups (Levesque 2003, In Press). This suggests that KSDPP is well accepted and is perceived as a good health promotion community resource. We hypothesize that this proportion may increase as KSDPP continues to expand (Potvin et al. 2003). KSDPP is a good example of community mobilization, where a community actively chooses to solve a community problem (Green and Kreuter 1991; Ottawa Charter of Health Promotion 1986).

Examples of the strategies applied by the KSDPP intervention team to promote participation in intervention activities are shown below.

1. **Continuity of the message from activities, settings and population groups.** A teacher appreciation breakfast was offered at school, and a few weeks later a pot-luck breakfast buffet was coordinated for the children. Later in the spring a mother's day illustration contest reflecting on healthy breakfast for mom was held among the children at school to reinforce the message; all participants' names were entered into a draw with a winner from each of 53 classes taking home a basket of healthy breakfast groceries for their mom.

2. **Taking the message to the people.** During parent teacher interviews at the schools, booths were set up and intervention staff invited parents to participate in the booth activities.

3. **Incentives to engage participation and reinforce the message.** The walking club offers incentives as participants reach intermediate levels on the way to their ultimate completion goal. Incentives included water bottles, rain coats, t-shirts and work-out gear.

4. **Capitalizing of pre-existing events, occasions and opportunities.** The annual community harvest fair, organized by the Environment Office, was co-hosted with KSDPP to take advantage of this food centered, local event to promote KSDPP messages

5. **Using multiple strategies in a single intervention.** A nationally coordinated community walk of 7km commemorates the work of a dedicated diabetes prevention worker who died tragically in British Columbia. After the walk, a healthy lunch donated by CAB is offered. Age appropriate incentives are given to all participants, with chances to win prizes for a draw i.e. a bike for children and wagon of healthy groceries for adults.

6. **Responding to concerns raised by the community.** Participation in the monthly meetings of the Kahnawake diabetes working group informs KSDPP of areas of needed intervention activities.

7. **Embedding culture into the intervention.** Having meals offered at events that are provided by community volunteers reflects the importance of eating together and sharing food among family.

8. **Creating a social environment for participation.** Walks are organized so that families as well as co-workers can walk together.

9. **Blending old with new activities.** Setting up informative and interactive booths at strategic community locations is a KSDPP time tested activity and many new ways of doing this are always in the works.

10. **Collaborating with community organizations and groups.** Where an event was being planned by a new youth group, KSDPP became involved with sponsoring the snacks for the evening and providing support to the youth to prepare the food.

Using these practices KSDPP has become embedded in the dynamic social, recreational and educational structures of the community. In all these activities community knowledge and ideas are incorporated throughout (Delormier et al. 2003). This is a very 'bottom up' project and the participatory research team supports the community vision. Because KSDPP intervention staff and CAB members are all Kanien'kehá:ka, the intervention activities, together with the accompanying decision making, all naturally incorporate local values and Kanien'kehá:ka traditions.

Reflections on the KSDPP Model

In KSDPP the intervention and research components have been integrated to strengthen the overall project (Potvin et al. 2003). Both the intervention team and research assistants for the evaluation team are based in Kahnawake, in contrast to many research projects where evaluation teams are university based. However, there are also researchers who work outside of the community and only attend research team meetings in the community. Research needs to answer academic questions, but should not be answering hypothetical questions developed outside the community. Research is richer when community context is informing the research questions (Koelen et al. 2001), and the intervention team has been strengthened by assimilating research concepts and developing community researcher skills. The KSDPP research component is seen as integral to the project. For example, in 1997 the overall impact and visibility of KSDPP were decreased in that year, as lack of funds prevented school data collections. Compared to three previous years, parents were not asked to sign consent forms, the evaluation team was not in the schools to measure the children and incidentally answer many questions, children did not complete questionnaires or run in the fitness tests. This confirmed to us that the annual KSDPP evaluation activities were a constant reminder to students, teachers and parents.

Another priority for KSDPP has been to build local capacity and promote sustainability. KSDPP provided training in specific skills, such as collecting anthropometric data, telephone surveys and data entry, and summer students to assist in research projects. After working as a research assistant one community member has enrolled as a PhD candidate, another used KSDPP data to complete her Masters' degree before entering medical school, and others collaborate or play leading roles with national agencies. Team members co-present and run workshops to scientific and non-scientific audiences, which both builds capacity and sends a strong message through role-modeling the research partnership to others (Potvin et al. 2003). Today KSDPP employs 11 full time people including 9 community members, and hires additional community members at times for specific tasks such as data collection.

Challenges

KSDPP was implemented in an era of scarce research funding and needed to find new funding sources after the first three-year research grant ended. Due to early success of the project and a high level of community support (Macaulay et al. 1998), three community organizations (the Mohawk Council of Kahnawake, Kahnawake Shakotiia'takehnhas Community Services, and the Kahnawake Education Center) chose to continue funding for one year, but could only afford to support continuation of the intervention component and the two community staff positions. The evaluation component, together with the position of the evaluation coordinator, were necessarily discontinued. In the following two years both intervention and evaluation components were funded by private foundations combined with community contributions. This critical period of bridge funding allowed KSDPP to continue, and two years later the team was well positioned to apply for innovative national research grant monies designated for university-community partnerships, which led to five years of infrastructure funding. This history certainly documents the precariousness of long-term community based research projects needed to accomplish lifestyle changes, and underlies the importance of promoting early capacity building and sustainability.

Participatory research promotes learning, respect and trust of both researchers and community. Internally, priorities and activities evolve requiring discussions between the various partners. It requires commitment, time and more time, and continued and ongoing negotiation processes. Over the years challenges have included deciding on priorities, reconciling community and academic timelines, adapting to changing different funding environments, community questions, opportunities and agendas, changing personnel, academic sabbatical leaves, academic students with different interests, and individual strengths and varying time commitments. Other Aboriginal communities recognize that Kahnawake is creating innovative approaches to diabetes prevention; this is a source of pride in the community.

Reflecting on Community Governance

KSDPP is one of the few community-based prevention programs showing evidence of sustainability. Indeed, the driving and sustaining forces of KSDPP are borne from active community participation in designing the intervention program to developing the Code of Research Ethics to committing to local capacity-building and overseeing the financial administration of the project. The strength of the community in shaping and directing the project builds on the strong history of the Kanien'kehá:ka in reclaiming their right to governance.

Speaking from the voice of a researcher, those who participate in KSDPP on a day-to-day basis quickly come to know that ideas require discussion which often result in something that reflects what neither the community nor the academic researchers initially put on the table. The end result often reflects something in between, an accommodation of academic and community interests for mutual benefit. This is where KSDPP departs from many other projects. History tells us that Aboriginal communities are dissatisfied with the "helicopter research" alluded to earlier in this chapter. While the impetus for many community intervention research projects has come from external academic influences with transference of ownership to community with time, our experience suggests that communities like Kahnawake can direct the process from the inception. KSDPP quantitative research shows quite clearly that community partners have been perceived as the primary owners of KSDPP since the beginning and that they carry the greatest influence across all domains of project functioning (Cargo et al. 2003).

To date the discourse in health promotion literature has revolved around the "transference of ownership" from academic researchers to community partners, particularly for researcher-initiated projects (Bracht 1994). This discussion is not relevant for KSDPP because the project was initiated by community members and leaders, who then invited academic researchers to join the partnership for their expertise in community research. Indeed it is almost the opposite, where community partners have had a major impact on the academic researchers.

Conclusion

Social justice is about having the same opportunities and choices, without discrimination as others in a society. This has not been the case and has been difficult to achieve for Indigenous Peoples because of the history of governmental and colonial racism. KSDPP shows an example of a community taking responsibility to ensure a healthy future, by confronting the many challenges it faces to restoring a well community.

The high level of ongoing community commitment and the shared community decision-making of KSDPP have been critical to the success and longevity of this project. Other key factors are the integration of the intervention and evaluation components. KSDPP may be considered innovative from both an intervention and research perspective for implementing an "ecological model" and for espousing an "empowerment" philosophy. KSDPP is now offering training in community mobilization for diabetes prevention to other Aboriginal communities. We believe that other communities will need to adapt the Kahnawake experiences, to build on their own pre-existing strengths and to incorporate their own traditions and values.

We have reflected on some of the reasons for success earlier in this chapter. Other reasons likely include the pre-existing strengths such as community control of health, education and other services, sharing the early research results with the community, a pre-existing comprehensive diabetes education program developed within the local hospital, health professionals from Kahnawake, other health professionals with long service in the community, always keeping the community informed and external academic researchers who espoused community control of this project.

However, we postulate that the predominant reason for longevity and success is that Kahnawake applied traditional approaches to problem-solving and did not just adopt an outsider model or philosophy to diabetes prevention. Community ownership of KSDPP is in keeping with the strong autonomous roots that characterizes the Kanien'kehá:ka (Alfred 1995, 1984) and with current approaches to implementation of community interventions (Barnes 2000). With respect to program characteristics, the Kanien'kehá:ka community of Kahnawake gathered around the issue of diabetes prevention, agreeing that it should not be viewed as socially disparaging and, that, as a disease, diabetes posed a threat to the well being of those faces yet to come. Sharing an interest for keeping children healthy reinforces the collective responsibility of the Kanien'kehá:ka for the Seven Generations (Alfred 1995). This may reflect a timely fusion of Kanien'kehá:ka culture with its emphasis on participatory democracy (Morgan and Slade 1997; Wallace 1946) and the value of social justice underlying health promotion (Ottawa Charter of Health Promotion 1986).

Acknowledgments

We wish to thank KSDPP CAB members Amelia Tekwatonti McGregor and Vera L. Goodleaf for their detailed discussion and review of this chapter, and Kathryn Phillips for reviewing an earlier draft. We also thank Gisele Guilbault, MSc for her contribution to KSDPP through detailed analysis of the physical activity interventions in 1996-1997. Special thanks to Ashley Ross, Geraldine Sky and Joyce Rice for varying and significant supporting roles.

Funding: Since 1994 KSDPP is or has been funded through the Canadian Institutes of Health Research-CIHR (#838-2000-1015), National Health Research and Development Program- NHRDP (#6605-4188-ND and 6605-4187-ND), Social Sciences and Humanity Research Council of Canada-SSHRC (#828-1999-1021), Canadian Diabetes Association-CDA (two grants), Community of Kahnawake, Private Foundations and Aboriginal Diabetes Initiative-ADI (Health Canada).

M. Cargo and L. Lévesque were funded by the Medical Research Council of Canada through Postdoctoral Fellowship awards (MRC H5-55050-AP009992 and MRC H5N-1018-57385) and Louise Potvin was funded by the Medical Research of Canada through a Scientist award (MRC H3-17299-AP007270).

Lucie Lévesque: (#9804H5N-1018-57385), Margaret Cargo: (#H5-55050-AP009992) and Louise Potvin: (CHSRF-CIHR Research Chair)

Please visit <www.ksdpp.org> for further information on KSDPP. This includes a 25 minute video of the experiences of KSDPP, the KSDPP Code of Research Ethics, Three Sisters Cookbook, information on intervention activities and research findings. For information and purchase of the KMHC Health Education Program for Grades 1 through 6, please contact Sheila Arnold, Community Health Unit, Kateri Memorial Hospital Centre, Box 10, Kahnawake, PQ J0L 1B0, Canada.

We thank the editors of *Pimatziwin: Journal of Health in Aboriginal and Indigenous Communities* for permission to build on Table 1, which was originally published as Delormier, Treena, Margaret Cargo, Rhonda Kirby, and Alex McComber in 2003. Activity Implementation as a Reflection of Living in Balance: The Kahnawake Schools Diabetes Prevention Project. *Pimatziwim: Journal of Health in Aboriginal and Indigenous Communities* 1(1): 45–163.

References

Alaska Native Science Commission: Code of Research Ethics. 1997. Alaska Native Science Commission. <www.nativescience.org>.

Alfred, Gerald R. 1995. Heeding the Voices of Our Ancestors: Kahnawake Mohawk Politics and the Rise of Native Nationalism. Toronto: Oxford University Press.

Anand, Sonia S, Salim Yusuf, Ruby Jacobs, Darlene A. Davis, Qilong Yi, Hertzel Gerstein, Patricia A. Montague and Eva Lonn. 2001. Risk Factors, Atherosclerosis, and Cardiovascular Disease Among Aboriginal People in Canada: The Study of Health Assessment and Risk Evaluation in Aboriginal Peoples (SHARE-AP). The Lancet 358: 1147–53.

Barnes, H.M. 2000. Collaboration in Community Action: A Successful Partnership between Indigenous Communities and Researchers. Health Promotion International 15: 17–25.

Battiste, Marie, ed. 2000. Reclaiming Indigenous Voice and Vision. Vancouver: UBC Press.

Battiste, Marie and J. Henderson Youngblood. 2000. Protecting Indigenous Knowledge and Heritage: A Global Challenge. Saskatoon: Purich Publishing Ltd.

Bear, L.L., M. Boldt and J.A. Long, eds. 1984. Pathways to Self Determination. Toronto: University of Toronto Press.

Bird, Michael E. 2002. Health and Indigenous People: Recommendations for the Next Generation. American Journal of Public Health 92(9): 1391–92.

Bisset, Sherri, Margaret Cargo, Treena Delormier, Ann C. Macaulay and Louise Potvin. 2003. Legitimizing Diabetes as a Community Health Issue: A Case Analysis of an Aboriginal Community in Canada. Health Promotion International 19(3): 317–26.

Bobet, Ellen. 1998. Diabetes Among First Nations People. Aboriginal Peoples Survey 1991. Ottawa: Minister of Public Works and Government Services.

Bopp, Judie and Four Worlds Development Project. 1985. The Sacred Tree. 2nd Ed. Lethbridge, Alta.: Four Worlds Development Press.

Bracht, Neil, J.R. Finnegan, C. Rissel, R. Weisbrod, J. Gleason, J. Corbett and S. Veblen-Mortenson. 1994. Community Ownership and Program Continuation Following a Health Demonstration Project. Health Education Research 9: 243–55.

Cargo, Margaret, Lucie Lévesque, Ann C. Macaulay, Alex McComber, Serges Desrosiers, Treena Delormier, Louise Potvin, with KSDPP Community Advisory

Board. 2003. Community Governance of Diabetes Prevention: A Reflection of Cultural Values; Kahnawake Schools Diabetes Prevention Project (KSDPP). Health Promotion International 18(3): 177–87.

Dean, Heather J. 1998. NIDDM-Y in First Nation Children of Canada. Clinical Pediatrics (Feb): 89–96.

Dei, G.J.S., Budd L. Hall and D.G. Rosenberg. 2000. Indigenous Knowledge in Global Contexts. University of Toronto Press, pp. 3–20.

Delisle, Hélène F. and Ekoé J.M. 1995. Prevalence of Non-Insulin Dependent Diabetes Mellitus and Impaired Glucose Tolerance in Two Algonquin Communities in Quebec. Diabetes Care 18: 1255–59.

Delormier, Treena, Margaret Cargo, Rhonda Kirby and Alex McComber. 2003. Activity Implementation as a Reflection of Living in Balance: The Kahnawake Schools Diabetes Prevention Project. Pimatziwim: Journal of Health in Aboriginal and Indigenous Communities 1(1): 45–163.

Durie, Mason H. 2003. The Health of Indigenous Peoples. British Medical Journal 326: 510–11.

Fabitz, R.R., A.N. Sidway, O. Go O, E.T. Lee, T. Welty, R.B. Devereux and B.V. Howard. 1999. Prevalence of Peripheral Arterial Disease and Associated Risk Factors in American Indians: The Strong Heart Study. American Journal of Epidemiology 149(4): 330–38.

First Nation and Inuit Regional Longitudinal Health Survey. 1999. Code of Research Ethics; Appendix 4 (A-54) <www.naho.ca/fnc/rhs>.

Friedman, D.J. and Barbara Starfield. 2003. Models of Population Health: Their Value for US Public Health Practice, Policy, and Research. American Journal of Public Health 93(3): 366–69.

Gibson, Nancy, Ginger Gibson and Ann C. Macaulay. 2001. Community-based Research: Negotiating Agendas and Evaluating Outcomes. In The Nature of Qualitative Evidence. J. Morse, J. Swanson and A. J. Kuzel, eds. Thousand Oaks: Sage Publications.

Green, Lawrence W., M.A. George, Mark Daniel, C. J. Frankish, Carol P. Herbert, W. R. Bowie and M. O'Neill. 1995. Participatory Research in Health Promotion: Institute of Health Promotion Research. Royal Society of Canada.

Green, Lawrence W. and Marshall W. Kreuter. 1991. Health Promotion Planning: An Educational and Environmental Approach. Mountain View, CA: Mayfield Publishing Company.

Guidelines for Ethical Research in Indigenous Studies. 2000. The Australian Institute of Aboriginal and Torres Islander Studies. <www.aiatsis.gov.au>.

Hanley, Anthony J., Stewart B. Harris, Joel Gittelsohn, Thomas M. Wolever, Brit Saksvig and Bernard Zinman. 2000. Overweight among Children and Adolescents in a Native Canadian Community: Prevalence and Associated Factors. American Journal of Clinical Nutrition 71(3): 693–700.

Harris, Stewart B., L. E. Caulfield, M. E. Sugamori, E. A. Whalen and Beth Henning. 1997. The Epidemic of Diabetes in Pregnant Native Canadians. Diabetes Care 20(9): 1422–25.

Harris, Stewart B., Joel Gittelsohn, Anthony J. Hanley, A. Barnie, Thomas M. Wolever, J. Gao, A. Logan and Bernard Zinman. 1997. The Prevalence of NIDDM and Associated Risk Factors in Native Canadians. Diabetes Care 20(2): 185–87.

Harris, Stewart B. and Bernard Zinman. 2000. Primary Prevention of Type 2 Diabetes in High-risk Populations.[comment]. Diabetes Care 23(7): 879–81.

Harris, Stewart B., Bernard Zinman, Anthony J. Hanley, Joel Gittelsohn, Robert A. Hegele, P. W. Connelly, B. Shah and J. E. Hux. 2002. The Impact of Diabetes on Cardiovascular Risk Factors and Outcomes in a Native Canadian Population. Diabetes Research and Clinical Practice 55(2): 165–73.

Howard, B.V., E.T. Lee, L.D. Cowan, R.B. Devereux, J.M. Galloway, O.T. Go, W.J. Howard, E.R. Rhoades , D.C. Robbins, M. Sievers and T. Welty. 1999. Rising Tide of Cardiovascular Disease in American Indians: The Strong Heart Study. Circulation 99: 2389–95.

Israel, Barbara A., Amy J. Schulz, Elizabeth A. Parker and A. B. Becker. 1998. Review of Community-based Research: Assessing Partnership Approaches to Improve Public Health. Annual Review of Public Health 19: 173–202.

_____1997. It Takes a Community: Framework for the First Nations and Inuit Fetal Alcohol Syndrome and Fetal Alcohol Effects Initiative. Ottawa: Health Canada. Minister of Public Works and Government Services.

Joe, Jennie R. 2001. Out of Harmony: Health Problems and Young Native American Men. Journal of American College of Health 49: 237–42.

Killip, Diana C., S.R. Lovick, L. Goldman and Diane D. Allensworth. 1987. Integrated School and Community Programs. Journal of School Health 57: 437–43.

Koelen, M.A., L. Vaandrager and C. Colomer. 2001. Health Promotion Research: Dilemmas and Challenges. Journal of Epidemiology and Community Health 55: 257–62.

Lévesque Lucie, Gisele Guilbault, Treena Delormier and Louise Potvin. 2004. Unpacking the Black Box: A Deconstruction of the Programming Approach and Physical Activity Interventions Implemented in the Kahnawake Schools Diabetes Prevention Project. Health Promotion Practice (in press).

Macaulay, A.C., S.B. Harris, L. Lévesque, M. Cargo, E.Ford, J. Salsberg, A.M. McComber, R. Fiddler, R. Kirby , A.J.G. Hanley, L.Potvin, B. Zinman, J. Gittelsohn, K. Phillips and O. Receveur. 2003. Primary Prevention of Type 2 Diabetes: Experiences of Two Aboriginal Communities in Canada. Can J Diabetes 26(3): 464–75.

Macaulay, Ann C., Gilles Paradis, Louise Potvin, Edward J. Cross, Chantal Saad-Haddad, Alex M. McComber, Serges Desrosiers and Rhonda Kirby. 1998. Primary Prevention of Type II Diabetes in First Nations: Experiences of the Kahnawake Schools Diabetes Prevention Project. Canadian Journal of Diabetes Care 22(3): 44–49.

Macaulay, Ann C., Laura E. Commanda, William L. Freeman, Nancy Gibson, Melvina L. McCabe, Carolyn M. Robbins and Peter L. Twohig. 1999. Participatory Research Maximises Community and Lay Involvement. BMJ 319 (7212): 774–78.

Macaulay, Ann C., Nancy Hanusaik and Deborah Delisle-Diabo. 1988. Diabetic Education Program in the Mohawk Community of Kahnawake, Quebec. Canadian Family Physician 34: 1591–93.

Macaulay, Ann C., Louis T. Montour and Naomi Adelson. 1988. Prevalence of Diabetic and Atherosclerotic Complications among Mohawk Indians of Kahnawake, PQ. CMAJ Canadian Medical Association Journal 139(3): 221–24.

Macaulay, Ann C., Gilles Paradis, Louise P. Potvin, Edward J. Cross, Chantal Haddad-Saad, Alex M. McComber, Serge Desrosiers, Rhonda L. Kirby, Louis T. Montour, Donna L. Lamping, Nicole Leduc, and Michele Rivard. 1997. The Kahnawake Schools Diabetes Prevention Project: Intervention, Evaluation, and Baseline Results of a Diabetes Primary Prevention Program with a Native Community in Canada. Preventive Medicine 26: 779–90.

Mao, Y., B. W. Moloughney, R. M. Semenciw and H. I. Morrison. 1992. Indian Reserve and Registered Indian Mortality in Canada. Canadian Journal of Public Health. Revue Canadienne de Sante Publique 83(5): 350–53.

Model Tribal Research Code, with Checklist for Tribal Regulation for Research for Indian Health Boards. 1999. Albuquerque: American Indian Law Center. American Indian Law Center, Inc. P.O. Box 4456—Station A, Albuquerque, NM, 87196, USA.

Montour, Louis T. 2000. The Medicine Wheel: Understanding "Problem" Patients in Primary Care. The Permanente Journal 4(1): 34–39.

Montour, Louis T., Ann C. Macaulay and Naomi Adelson. 1989. Diabetes mellitus in Mohawks of Kahnawake, PQ: a Clinical and Epidemiologic Description. CMAJ Canadian Medical Association Journal 141(6): 549–52.

Montour, Louis T. and Ann C. Macaulay. 1985. High Prevalence Rates of Diabetes mellitus and Hypertension on a North American Indian Reservation. Canadian Medical Association Journal 139(10): 1110–11.

_____1988. Diabetes mellitus and Atherosclerosis: Returning Research Results to the Mohawk Community. Canadian Medical Association Journal 139(3): 201–2.

Morgan, D.L. and M.D. Slade. 1997. Aboriginal Philosophy and its Impact on Health Care Outcomes. Australia and New Zealand Journal of Public Health 21: 597–601.

National Steering Committee for the First Nations and Inuit Regional Health Survey. 1999. Final Report. Canada.

Ottawa Charter of Health Promotion. 1986. Canadian Journal of Public Health. Revue Canadienne de Sante Publique 139: 425–30.

Pearce, N. 1996. Traditional Epidemiology, Modern Epidemiology, and Public Health. American Journal of Public Health 86: 678–83.

Potvin, Louise, Margaret Cargo, Alex M. McComber, Treena Delormier and Ann C. Macaulay. 2003. Implementing Participatory Intervention and Research in Communities: Lessons from the Kahnawake Schools Diabetes Prevention Project in Canada. Social Science & Medicine 56(6): 1295–305.

Reading, Jeff. 2002. Improving the Health of Future Generations: the Canadian Institutes of Health Research, Institute of Aboriginal Peoples' Health. American Journal of Public Health 92(9): 1396–1400.

Rock, Melanie. 2003. Sweet Blood and Social Suffering: Rethinking Cause-Effect Relationships in Diabetes, Distress and Duress. Medical Anthropology: Cross-Cultural Studies in Health and Illness 22(2): 131–74.

Rose, Geoffrey. 1985. Sick Individuals and Sick Populations. International Journal of Epidemiology 14(1): 32–38.

Royal Commission on Aboriginal Peoples. 1996. Report of the Royal Commission on Aboriginal Peoples Ottawa, Canada <www.ainc-inac.gc.ca/ch/rcap/index_e. html>.

Smedley, B. D. and S. L. Syme, Eds. 2001. Promoting Health. Intervention Strategies from Social and Behavioral Research. National Academy Press.

Smith, Linda Tuhiwai. 1997. Decolonizing Methodologies: Research and Indigenous People. Zed Books Ltd.

Statistics Canada. 2003. Aboriginal Peoples of Canada: A Demographic Profile. 2002 Census. Ottawa.

_____1999. Final Report:, Final Report.

Wallace, P.A. 1946. The White Roots of Peace. Philadelphia: University of Pennsylvania Press.

Weijer, Charles. 1999. Protecting Communities in Research: Philosophical and Pragmatic Challenges. Cambridge Quarterly of Healthcare Ethics 8(4): 501–13.

Weijer, Charles, Gary Goldsand and Ezekliel J. Emanuel. 1999. Protecting Communities in Research: Current Guidelines and Limits of Extrapolation. Nature Genetics 23: 275–80.

Young, T. Kue. 1996. Obesity Among Aboriginal Peoples in North America: Epidemiological Patterns, Determinants, and Consequences. In Progress in Obesity Research. A. Angel, H. Anderson, C. Bouchard, D. Lau, L. Leiter and R. Mendelsohn, eds. London: John Libby.

Young, T. Kue, Jeff Reading, Brenda Elias and John D. O'Neil. 2000. Type 2 Diabetes mellitus in Canada's First Nations: Status of an Epidemic in Progress. [erratum appears in CMAJ 2000 Oct 31; 163(9):1132]. CMAJ Canadian Medical Association Journal 163(5): 561–66.

CHAPTER 17

"I'M TOO YOUNG FOR THIS!": DIABETES AND AMERICAN INDIAN CHILDREN

Jennie R. Joe and Sophie Frishkopf

Summary of Chapter 17. Type 2 Diabetes Mellitus is now endemic in a growing number of American Indian communities in the United States. Mortality and associated morbidities from the disease, such as cardiovascular complications, retinopathy, and neuropathy are taking a toll on individuals with the disease, their families, and their communities in terms of quality of life, cultural survival, and cost of care.

As the number of American Indian adults diagnosed with Type 2 diabetes increases, the incidence rates of the disease are also growing among American Indian children and youth, some as young as eight years of age. Most of the children who are at risk of developing diabetes not only have a strong family history of the disease but also are often overweight, have signs of insulin resistance, and were born to mothers with gestational diabetes. Treatment for children with Type 2 diabetes typically mirrors that for adults, including an emphasis on weight reduction through diet and exercise.

This chapter summarizes the growing epidemic of Type 2 diabetes in American Indian children and the need to address the problem. The authors discuss the Wellness Camp for Indian Children with Diabetes as one intervention/ prevention strategy that is geared to children between the ages of 10 and 15. The camp, established in 1991, began with a modest goal of teaching children about diabetes within a familiar cultural context. Ten years later, campers continue to learn about what the common complications associated with the disease are, how diabetes can be prevented, and how persons with diabetes can manage to live with the disease.

The authors advocate that intervention/prevention strategies for minority children with Type 2 Diabetes need a culturally appropriate curriculum, a curriculum that not only builds on the cultural strengths of the children but also helps them experience healthy food and fun ways to increase physical activity.

❧ ❧ ❧

"I'm too young for this," remarked 11 year-old Joseph[1] as he and his peers from one southern Arizona tribal community lined up to fill out a registration form at a recent Native American Research and Training Center (NARTC) Summer Wellness Camp for Indian Children with Diabetes. As he submitted his registration form, he again repeated that he was too young to have diabetes and that he shouldn't have been asked to attend the camp. One of the camp volunteers gently took Joseph aside and told him that the medical team at the camp will help determine if there is a diabetes problem. Seeming reassured by this brief conversation, Joseph joined the other boys as they gathered their belongings to take to their assigned cabins.

The reaction of Joseph on the first day at camp is not unusual. Many children have difficulty accepting their diagnoses, especially children with type 2 diabetes whose symptoms are not as dramatic or immediately life threatening as are those experienced by children with type 1 diabetes.

Joseph's parents noted on the camp application that Joseph would be entering the fifth grade and is the second of four children. Joseph, however, is the first child in his family to be diagnosed with type 2 diabetes. When he arrived at camp, Joseph had been on medication for a few months but apparently was still not convinced that he had diabetes, and he believed that the diagnosis was a temporary one. Joseph's denial is perhaps influenced by his parents' reluctance to accept the diagnosis. He mentioned that he did not think he had diabetes because he did not feel sick and that his family thought he was too young to get diabetes.

The additional medical background supplied by Joseph's pediatrician indicates that Joseph's parents have been instructed to help Joseph lose weight by encouraging him to exercise and to eat a healthy diet, a recommendation that would be familiar to Joseph's mother, who had gestational diabetes with her last pregnancy. She was subsequently diagnosed with type 2 diabetes after the birth of her fourth child.

Joseph's camp referral also carries the following handwritten footnote from his pediatrician: "Joseph needs to learn more about diabetes!" The footnote message is a common reason given by providers for referring children to camp, especially those who are newly diagnosed. The referral also serves, at least indirectly, as a way to remind the parents that their child has a very serious health problem that needs special attention.

As type 2 diabetes increases among American Indian youth such as Joseph, there is a growing concern not only about how to stop this epidemic but also how to effectively help these children, especially those who face the early onset of a number of diabetic complications that will greatly impact their quality of life. This chronic disease, once found only among adults, is taking a toll not only on the children with the disease but also on their families. For many families, it has become a devastating intergenerational disease.

While diabetes treatment and education programs for adults are well established, similar programs do not exist or are not readily available for children with type 2 diabetes. This chapter discusses the Summer Wellness Camp for Indian Children with Diabetes as one approach to addressing this problem. The camp was initiated to help provide a comfortable and fun environment for American Indian children, where they

---

1. Not his real name.

can learn more about the disease, about self-care, and about how to prevent or delay onset of complications that often accompany this disease. This chapter also highlights some of the other interventions that have been utilized to address the increasing incidence of pediatric type 2 diabetes. At the center of this story about childhood diabetes, however, are children like Joseph, who despite all the clinical encounters and the efforts at diabetes education, refuse to accept their diagnosis and therefore increase their already high risk for early onset of secondary complications.

Type 2 Diabetes

Type 2 diabetes is a complex metabolic disorder with a heterogeneous etiology that includes an array of possible social, behavioral, environmental, and genetic causes. According to the American Diabetes Association (ADA) (2000), diabetes affects over 15 million adults in the United States. Despite the considerable scientific advances in understanding and treating type 2 diabetes, some major questions about this disorder remain unanswered, including the reason why type 2 diabetes is devastating increasing numbers of American Indian communities and other indigenous populations worldwide. Because onset of type 2 diabetes is now occurring at younger ages among ethnic minority populations such as the American Indians, the human and economic consequences are greater and more devastating for these groups.

A number of theories have been suggested to explain this unusual disease burden for American Indians, ranging from genetic predisposition to environmental or forced cultural change (Neel 1962; Dabelea et al. 1998; Dean et al. 1992; Jones 1998; Narayan 1997; Joe and Young 1994). Understandably, research into the biological explanation for Type 2 diabetes continues to receive the most attention, especially by the National Institutes of Health (NIH) researchers who have been studying type 2 diabetes for several decades among the Pima Indian tribe in Arizona. Despite progress made in the Pima studies, tribal leaders impatiently ask why NIH has yet to find a cure for diabetes (Sevilla 1999). Questions such as these underscore the desperation and frustration felt by the Pima and other tribal communities plagued by diabetes.

Pediatric Type 2 Diabetes

Childhood type 2 diabetes is rapidly being recognized as a worldwide problem, and in the United States, the type 2 diabetes epidemic has become particularly visible in ethnic minority children. Prior to the 1990s less than four percent of pediatric diabetes cases nationally were diagnosed as type 2 diabetes, but recent epidemiological data indicate that this percentage has soared to 45% (ADA 2000; Pinhas-Hamiel et al 1996). ADA reports that the rate of type 2 diabetes among junior high school students in Tokyo increased from 7.3/100,000 in 1976-80 to 13.9/100,000 in 1991-95 (ADA 2000). In addition, Kitagawa and colleagues (1994) report that this increase in type 2 diabetes among Japanese school children has been marked by a parallel increase in childhood obesity.[2] Similar epidemiological trends for type 2 diabetes have been observed among aboriginal children in Australia and among children and adolescents in Libya and Bangladesh (ADA 2000). An increase in obesity and a decrease in physical activity among these children have been identified as key contributors to this epidemiological shift in type 2 diabetes among youth (ADA 2000).

The increase in type 2 diabetes among American Indian children has been noted by a number of health care providers from different regions of the United States. Although type 2 diabetes was first reported in American Indian teenagers in 1979, similar morbidity trends have also been observed since 1979 among African American and Hispanic youth in the United States (Mazur et al. 1998). Similar observations have also been made for First Nations' youth in Canada (Dean et al. 1992; Harris et al., 1996). These and other epidemiological data confirm that type 2 diabetes is becoming a major public health problem for many minority youth.

The prevalence of type 2 diabetes in children and adolescents in these communities, however, is not uniform. The incidence and prevalence vary within and across different ethnic populations. For example, the prevalence rate of type 2 diabetes for Pima Indian youth (ages 15–19) is reported at 50.9/1,000 compared to 4.5/1,000 for the general American Indian population and 2.3/1,000 for Canadian Ojibway Indians in Manitoba (Fagot-Campagna et al. 2000). These investigators report that the prevalence of Type 2 diabetes increased among Pima Indian adolescents 6-fold between the following two intervals: 1967–76 and 1987–96 (Fagot-Campagna et al., 2000). Researchers have observed that the problem was especially significant for pre-adolescent Pima children, ages 10 to 14. The federal Indian Health Service (I.H.S.) also reports a 54% increase in the prevalence rate of type 2 diabetes among Indian youth, ages 15–19 between 1996 and 1998 (ADA 2000). As noted above, this growing type 2 diabetes epidemic among youth is not unique to tribes but is occurring among the youth of other indigenous populations internationally (Fagot-Campagna et al., 2000).

Risk Factors and Complications

Risk factors for type 2 diabetes in youth include high levels of insulin in the bloodstream (hyperinsulinemia), obesity, impaired glucose, strong family history of type 2 diabetes, gender (prevalence is higher in females), maternal diabetes, high or low birth weight, and bottle feeding (ADA 2000; IHS National Diabetes Program 2000; Mazur et al. 1998). Acanthosis nigricans, velvety hyperpigmented patches in intertriginous areas, is a marker indicating both hyperinsulinemia and a high risk for diabetes.

Foremost among the early risk factors for diabetes, however, is obesity. A 1994 national survey showed that American Indian children had the highest prevalence of obesity among all other ethnic groups. Studies indicate that the obesity that begins early in childhood is centrally distributed, and this central deposition of adipose tissue is an indicator of susceptibility to diabetes (Story et al. 1998).

---

2. Eighty per cent of these children with diabetes were obese, a predominantly female phenomenon. Type 2 diabetes with no accompanying obesity is also common in females (Kitagawa et al., 1994).

Several biological factors are thought to help explain this population-based difference. Resting energy expenditure (REE), for example, may explain some of the differential rates of type 2 diabetes in black and white children (Kaplan et al 1996). Fasting insulin concentrations have also been found to vary across ethnic groups. For example, Pima Indians have higher fasting insulin concentrations at an earlier age than Euro-American children, indicating susceptibility to type 2 diabetes for Pima children (Pettitt et al. 1993). Blackett and colleagues (1996) also found obesity was associated with early onset of elevated lipid levels among their sample of a Plains Indian population. As noted earlier, these researchers also felt that adiposity combined with genetic predisposition is an important predictor of type 2 diabetes in children, especially since researchers have found that insulin sensitivity improves with weight loss in obese children (Walker 1995).

Once diabetes develops, the difficulties experienced by children diagnosed with the disease are similar to those experienced by adults who are diabetic. For instance, obesity often keeps many children sedentary and, like adults, they also experience the frustrations that often accompany the vicious weight loss—weight gain cycle. Obesity, poor self image, and the frustration of trying to manage their diabetes often trigger severe bouts of low self-esteem for many of these children and youth. Moreover, as with many adults with diabetes, the absence of life threatening symptoms also fuels denial among these children (Mazur et al. 1998).

Diabetes, however, poses unique difficulties for children. For example, the chance of a misdiagnosis (type 1 diabetes instead of type 2 diabetes) is higher in children than in adults, especially as some medical providers have been slow to acknowledge that type 2 diabetes can occur in children (Mazur et al. 1998). The danger of delaying diagnosis and treatment may result in a poorer prognosis because onset of diabetes at an earlier age increases the likelihood of early onset of diabetes-related complications (Fagot-Campagna et al. 2000). Type 2 diabetes can be more destructive when onset begins in youth because these youth begin to experience complications before age 30 (Mazur et al., 1998; Lindner 2000), thus diminishing their quality of life at earlier ages. The array of possible complications includes cardiovascular disease, blindness, end-stage kidney disease, and amputation of extremities.

Based on a presentation at an ADA conference about secondary complications associated with type 2 diabetes in youth, D. Brown (2002) of the *Washington Post* reported that seven of 89 First Nations' (Indian) youth in Canada diagnosed with type 2 diabetes before age 17 had died prematurely. Those surviving reported earlier onset of complications such as blindness and amputation. Many of the young women in this group reported problems with pregnancies, including miscarriages and stillbirths.

Social and Political Factors

The tendency toward obesity in American Indians is greatly influenced not only by biological and genetic factors, but also by social, economic, and political factors that are frequently ignored by some researchers and health care providers. The American Indian poverty rate is alarmingly high: 31.6% of American Indians live below the poverty level, a rate that is 2.5 times greater than that of the general U.S. population

(IHS 2000; Story et al. 1998), placing the American Indian population at greater risk for poor health. Unemployment for American Indians is twice that for the general population, and the median income is two-thirds that of the U.S. general population. High school dropout rates are 35% for American Indian youth compared to 25% for the U.S., all races (IHS National Diabetes Program 2000). Moreover, the American Indian and Alaska Native life expectancy is below the national average, despite a median age of 27.7 (compared to 35.5 for the US, all races) and a population in which 33% are under age 15 (IHS 2000).

Not surprisingly, the risk of nutrition-related health problems is greatest among economically disadvantaged populations such as American Indians and Alaska Natives, where the elderly and the young are especially vulnerable. Story and colleagues (1998) have speculated that hunger and obesity are causally related: consumption of cheap, high-fat foods along with physiologic adaptation to a chronic food shortage may well increase the percentage of body fat. In this study, 87.6% of American Indian households reported having access to a sufficient quantity of food, but 49% noted that the foods they had access to were not always the kinds they wanted. Twelve percent reported they sometimes did not have enough to eat, and among this group, 81% said they were without food or did not have enough money to purchase food an average of 5.5 days per month. Two-thirds of the households that reported not having enough to eat also said they skipped meals an average of 4.2 days per month due to food shortage (Story et al. 1998).

Under conditions of poverty, diabetes care and/or diabetes prevention is frequently not a priority when families or individuals are faced with other pressing problems or economic hardships (Steve Ponder, M.D., email communication, November 29, 2000). Physician recommendations (including proper and timely food intake, low fat diet, and reduction in calories) are not realistic because they are expensive for low-income populations: families may not be able to afford a low-fat diet, assuming that family members are willing to live on such a diet. Moreover, the individual with diabetes may not feel sick, may believe that the therapy does not have any effect, or may perceive adverse effects when the therapy is accompanied by weight gain (Jones 1998).

One also would not expect poor, two-parent working households, with limited time and money, to provide opportunities for their children to engage in exercise requiring equipment or payment of fees (Ilene Fennoy, email communication, December 1, 2000). In a study of parents with children aged 4–6, Claus and colleagues (1999) identified factors, mostly related to lifestyle (i.e., food choices and exercise), which could influence the success of a diabetes prevention program for Indian children. The sample of parents for this study was recruited from an I.H.S. clinic waiting room, and when the parents were queried, most indicated that lack of time would prevent them from having their children participate in an exercise program. It is also interesting to note that half of these parents did not believe that their child was at risk for diabetes.

Lack of fiscal resources and facilities contribute to the growing epidemic of diabetes in many low-income tribal communities. Physical education may not be available to schoolchildren, especially in rural isolated communities where schools have limited budgets (Ilene Fennoy, email communication, December 1, 2000). In addition, dietary counseling is not generally available in these rural communities, and access to quality foods is also limited. Instead of a healthy diet, many low-income families in some of these communities have to rely on dry or canned government surplus commodity foods (high in fat and calories) for most meals. Moreover, with the seizure of Indian lands, the level of physical activity among American Indian communities declined as traditional reliance on hunting and farming has given way to more sedentary occupations (I.H.S., 2000).

Corporate influences are also pernicious when it comes to enhancing diabetes susceptibility. Advertising campaigns for unhealthy foods often directly target those most predisposed to develop type 2 diabetes and those who are least knowledgeable about healthy nutrition. Children, in particular, are targets for this kind of marketing: companies offer them toys in exchange for the purchase and consumption of unhealthy foods (Steve Ponder, M.D., email communication, November 29, 2000; Ileana Vargas, personal communication, December 1, 2000). The soda companies are another notorious example of marketing gone astray. According to a report on National Public Radio, the soft drink industry has been candid about its marketing strategy, namely that it specifically gears its advertising campaigns toward children (Hall 1999). When the USDA attempted to lower its guidelines on the maximum amount of soda to be consumed by children, the soda companies successfully lobbied against these recommendations (Ileana Vargas, personal communication, December 1, 2000).

There are also other factors to consider. One study of low-income mothers in Cincinnati, Ohio, found that mothers do not define overweight/obesity in their preschool aged children according to established height/weight measurements (Jain et al. 2001). Instead, factors such as whether their children are teased about their weight or whether they have any physical limitations are used to determine whether the children are overweight. If children are active and have a healthy diet and a good appetite, they are not considered overweight. Rather than describing children as overweight, mothers describe them as "thick" or "solid." They also feel that weight gain is an inherited tendency rather than a result of environmental factors. Mothers state that they are limited in their ability to influence their children's diets because their influence is challenged by other family members, and they have trouble denying a child food if the child is hungry despite having just eaten (Jain et al. 2001). The authors conclude that since mothers may differ in their opinions of what constitutes overweight, focusing on a goal of healthy diet and exercise (seen as indicators of good health by both doctors and mothers) may be more effective than labeling children as overweight (Jain et al. 2001).

Today, the focus of diabetes prevention programs for children in many tribal communities is placed on increasing physical activity and nutrition education for all of the children without singling out those who are overweight. Most programs also do not advertise their services as intended for weight loss but rather as helping to improve fitness. The other goal is to get children to learn to like a variety of physical activities and to understand why exercise is necessary for maintaining good health. Programs that reinforce positive messages are seen as more culturally appropriate than those emphasizing the dangers of obesity or diabetes, i.e., less is said about obesity and the negative consequences of obesity. This is not to say that adolescents, especially adolescent girls, are not concerned about their weight. They are. In fact, in this culture as well as in others, adolescent girls more so than adolescent boys, tend to view exercise and physical activity as a helpful way to lose or to control weight. Adolescent girls are therefore more willing to try numerous ways to lose weight, including dangerous behaviors that may lead to anorexia or bulimia.

ndian children and youth respond to the adult-centered diabetes education and prevention strategies in different ways. Those who have experienced some success with
weight loss are more likely to be motivated to continue while others who fail to see
positive results in a short time are less likely to remain motivated. Invariably, those
children who are severely overweight and therefore would have the most gain from
these interventions usually have more difficulty, not only with the intervention, but
also because they are less likely to experience rapid weight loss and therefore less likely
to remain motivated without considerable support and encouragement. This is especially true when a child's weight loss goals are unrealistic. Children who are severely
overweight need specialized intervention programs that are long term as well as flexible. These programs must be flexible because often the severely overweight children
also have other health problems, such as asthma, which may limit the type or the intensity of physical exercise they are able to perform.

Childhood/Youth Culture and Diabetes

As a child grows older, an increasing percentage of his or her daily activity is spent
with other children in a social environment that has its own boundaries. For example,
it is not uncommon to find some children with diabetes avoiding socializing with other
children because they are teased for being different (Liddane 2001). To fit in, these
children will find a way not to appear different. They want to eat what their friends eat
no matter how unhealthy it is or whether it is counter indicated, i.e., food or snacks
with high fat and caloric content (Jones 1998; Mazur et al. 1998). The desire not to
appear different is especially important to some adolescents, resulting in indifference
to their own health situation. Sometimes, this indifference also serves as a rebellion
against an authoritative voice (Jones 1998; Casper and Offer 1990).

In one study, Wake and colleagues (2000) examined the psychosocial well being of children and youth (ages 5–17) with and without diabetes. The researchers found interesting
differences between the self-reported information provided by the children below age 12
and the information provided by their parents. Data from parents indicated that children
with routinely high glucose as indicated by hemoglobin A1c (HbA1c) are more likely to
have poor psychosocial scores than those in the normative sample. Children with diabetes,
however, reported health statuses that did not differ greatly from that of their peers who
did not have diabetes. Although the results of this study suggest that youth with diabetes
perceive their health to be similar to that of their peers, the investigators caution against
making this assumption, noting that some of these youth with diabetes may not have
wanted to present themselves as being "different" from their peers. The investigators also
suggest that even among young children in the primary grades, diabetes has a greater effect on a child and the child's family's well-being than may be realized (Wake et al. 2000).[3]

Results of studies such as that by Wake and her co-investigators (2000) indicate
that health educators developing culturally relevant diabetes intervention or preven-

---

3. The study measured factors such as self-perceived physical functioning, bodily pain, mental
health, self-esteem, general health, parent time with the child, family activities, and family cohesion
(Wake et al 2000).

tion programs targeting children and their families need to pay equal attention to the culture of childhood as well as to the child's family's traditional or ethnic culture. As with all cultures, the culture of childhood, according to Goodman (1970), is learned, shared, and transmitted. A child learns this culture from his or her childhood peers and siblings, or from adults, through a process that is learned but not necessarily taught. For example, the child learns for his or her daily interaction with others the "patterned (customary) ideas and expectations about the nature, capacities, and proper behavior of children" (Goodman 1970: 9). Where and in what context this learning takes place, however, changes as the child matures. The child is often shaped and re-shaped as his or her network of friends, mentors, and role models also change.

The degree to which some of these lessons are learned or rejected are also influenced by the child's age, gender, and culture (Davis et al. 1993). The cultural lens, for example, may place a child and his/her family's perspective of obesity at odds with that held by health care providers. In some cultures, childhood obesity may not be seen as a risk factor but is viewed as a marker of a child who is well provided for. Conversely, thinness in children (where thinness is not a family trait) might be perceived as the result of neglect or undernourishment due to severe poverty.

In addition to differing views about body image and the role of obesity in health, there may also be differing views about diabetes (Gittlesohn et al. 1996). Despite long-term utilization of allopathic medicine by tribal communities in the United States, chronic diseases such as diabetes remain poorly understood, especially because it is one of the diseases that cannot be cured by allopathic medicine or by traditional tribal healing practices. Moreover, the concept of a chronic disease or a lifelong health ailment is not usually a part of most traditional tribal health beliefs and practices. Furthermore, the orientation of most traditional tribal healing practices emphasizes *why* a health problem developed and gives less attention to how a health condition might have occurred. Within this cultural framework, the development of childhood diabetes might be attributed to breech of a taboo or a violation of a cultural rule by one or both of the child's parents. In addition, the traditional categories of disease causalities for most tribes do not include obesity as an etiology. Although there are taboos against eating certain foods, these foods generally do not include sugar, fat, or processed foods.

It is difficult, therefore, for many tribal members to accept the idea of obesity as a health risk. In fact, almost every tribe has one or more food sources considered sacred, and these are symbolized in various ceremonial or religious activities. Salmon, bowhead whale, maize, buffalo, and the acorn are examples of foods considered sacred by various tribes across the U.S. One only has to observe a buffalo or deer dance and/or see the observance of sacred rituals by a whaling crew as they prepare for a bowhead whale hunt to understand the significance and sacredness of these foods.

Health educators developing effective interventions or prevention programs for American Indian and Alaska Native children must therefore pay attention to the culture of childhood, to socio-cultural phenomena, and to the child's familial or tribal heritage. Some would also say there is also a culture of diabetes, but it does not have the same significance to children as it does to adults whose lifestyles have been slowly altered or disabled by diabetes and its complications. This is not to say the culture of diabetes will not have a similar significance to children in the future. It is beginning to have significance, but for the most part, this significance is still invisible.

Cultural Competency from Within and Without

Today, the significant push nationally for cultural competency is aimed at health care providers, especially those serving the culturally different. Attaining cultural and linguistic competency is seen as an important investment for health care providers because it is a way to improve health outcomes for diverse populations and to enhance efforts to address racial and ethnic health disparities. According to guidelines from the Office of Minority Health (OMH), cultural and linguistic competency means that providers and their health organizations not only have to learn these skills but also have to practice what they have learned so that they understand and respond to a patient's needs within the context of that patient's unique culture (2001). For the patient, the benefits of receiving culturally competent health care include greater comfort and satisfaction with the health care services and the sense that they are being treated with respect and understanding.

How one goes about developing cultural competency, however, is not always clearly articulated, albeit there seems to be some general agreement that cultural competency is best learned through building and working in partnerships with various cultural groups (Gilliland et al. 1998). The interaction with the group or community targeted for the intervention therefore serves as a living classroom where knowledgeable cultural experts informally teach as they help plan and establish strategies that are most likely to be accepted by their communities, i.e., strategies that take into account local cultural practices, values, and beliefs.

Although the national cultural competency agenda is predominantly aimed at health care providers or organizations serving racial or ethnic minority communities, similar needs are also being expressed from within the racial and ethnic minority communities. In some cases this interest is motivated by the desire of the group or the community to address widening internal cultural gaps within their communities that are challenging existing strategies or interventions. Some strategies may be seen as unworkable because the idea of "one size fits all" is no longer appropriate. Another motivation driving community interest might be the community's own commitment to self-determination, which includes improving the health of their communities. Both of these examples apply to many American Indian and Alaska Native Tribal communities, especially those investing in various culturally relevant prevention and intervention programs.

Intervention/Prevention Programs for Children/Youth

An important outcome of tribal communities' involvement in managing their own health care services has been the emphasis they have placed on prevention. One of the most visible of these prevention/intervention efforts targets diabetes. Because cultural relevancy is central to each of these tribal efforts, each community has tailored its prevention/intervention programs so that they are culturally sensitive, culturally relevant, or linguistically appropriate for its diverse tribal populations. If one were to observe these programs, however, it would be apparent that the way these programs are organized and/or the approaches that are implemented are not likely to differ significantly from similar programs in non-tribal communities. The reasons are that tribal programs in disseminating or promoting prevention information have borrowed extensively from majority culture, although the borrowed approaches have been modified to meet local needs. Examples include radio programs, videos, brochures given out at supermarkets, personalized letters, and phone calls.

No matter how generic, the message is usually delivered in the tribal language, using storytelling or familiar icons from tribal legends. Typically, the artwork utilized with the messages is also familiar, i.e., tribal designs or motifs. Wherever possible, personnel make sincere efforts to deliver the message personally. The one-on-one interaction is preferred because the messenger is able to adjust or adapt the message to meet the needs of the individual. This one-on-one approach not only conveys a personal concern about the receiver's health, but also follows cultural practices that ask that important news or concerns be delivered face-to-face.

Most tribal diabetes prevention programs have elected to create public awareness about the need to prevent diabetes. Community events are offered to encourage members of the community to increase their physical activities and to attend specially scheduled nutrition education presentations that promote ways to shop and prepare healthy meals. Increasing numbers of fitness and "wellness" centers now dot the reservations, providing a place for various exercise programs. Some prevention endeavors have also targeted specific age groups or may focus primarily on individuals who have been diagnosed with diabetes, with the goal of preventing or delaying onset of secondary complications.

A number of these prevention and intervention programs have targeted children and youth (Rosenbloom et al. 1999). Unfortunately, despite the success of some of these pilot programs, many are no longer offered because of lack of funding. *STOP Diabetes*, a pilot project that was implemented in 1995 on the Winnebago reservation for Winnebago adolescents (Marlow et al. 1998), is an example of one such program. Adolescents took classes on diabetes and diabetes prevention, which were based on a curriculum that emphasized exercise and good nutrition. The young people, once trained, worked with other youth in the community and, in accordance with Winnebago principles of education, the adolescent instructors were asked to lead by example rather than through direct instruction. While the investigators did not discuss the outcome evaluations of this approach, they did report that the post-test scores of the youth who served as role models demonstrated a significant gain in their knowledge about diabetes.

McKenzie et al. (1988) have described a pilot intervention study that was designed to develop a culturally appropriate primary intervention program for Mexican American children at risk for type 2 diabetes (McKenzie et al. 1998). Thirty-seven Mexican American children (ages 7–12) with at least one parent or grandparent with type 2 diabetes participated in the pilot study. In addition to their genetic predisposition for type 2 diabetes, the majority of the children (70%) also had at least one environmental and/or physiological risk factor for developing the disease, most commonly obesity as determined by body mass index (BMI). The program included eight, 1-hour activity-oriented sessions, with a focus on nutrition, exercise, and diabetes education. In addition, pre- and post-program health screenings were administered. Evaluations of the program indicated that it had a positive impact on parents and children in their eating, shopping, and exercise habits. Ninety-four percent of parents rated the program as very helpful and informative. In particular, results of the health screenings alerted parents to the importance of changing family lifestyle patterns. Parents also reported that children eagerly shared information gained from the program with relatives, and as a result, other family members also indirectly benefited from the program.

Another pilot project, *Jump Into Action* (Holcomb et al. 1998), is a school-based intervention for Mexican American children in the fifth grade. This program encouraged children to eat low-fat foods and exercise regularly to reduce the risk of developing type 2 diabetes. Fifth graders (ages 10–12) were targeted primarily because children in this age group are at the point in their lives of developing life-long habits, can understand cause and effect relationships, and are beginning to make their own food and exercise decisions. The intervention study was based on an interdisciplinary approach to health education that combined health education with reading, writing, math, science, and physical education. Information was presented in the form of a workbook and as hands-on, participatory-style activities. Program evaluations indicated that the approach was effective in increasing knowledge and self-efficacy and in improving diet and exercise-related behavior. New knowledge and behavioral practices gained from the program were also sustained at the time of the follow-up, which was at least four weeks after the program's end.

Sustainability is an important goal of many diabetes intervention/prevention endeavors. The *Quest* program in the Gila River Indian Community (Pima tribe) is a school-based curriculum program for grades K-2 (Cook and Hurley 1998; see also chapter in this volume). The curriculum teaches children diet- and exercise-related skills necessary to maintain a healthy body weight. The four components of the program include: physiological assessments; classroom instruction on diabetes, with take-home information; an increase in the amount of physical activity during the school day; and a structured school breakfast and lunch program that supports a low-fat, controlled carbohydrate diet. Outcome data has been collected on these children but has not been published.

The *Kahnawake Schools Diabetes Prevention Project* in Quebec, Canada, was established to prevent type 2 diabetes among Mohawk children (Macaulay et al. 1998; see also chapter in this volume). The prevention project targets elementary school children, parents, teachers, and the surrounding Mohawk community of Kahnawake. The long-term goal of the project is to prevent diabetes; the short-term goal is to improve nutritional habits and to increase the level of physical activity throughout the community, with a particular focus on children, ages 6–12. Both school and community-wide activities have been developed to meet these goals. The success of this project has been indicated by positive changes in the schools (e.g., healthier snacks and increased activity levels for students), increased community awareness about diabetes, and widespread community support for the continuation of the program.

Most intervention or prevention programs are aimed at young children, but one project in New Mexico did target a high school population. The goal of the *Zuni Diabetes Prevention Program* (Teufel and Ritenbaugh 1998) was to decrease diabetes risk factors among high school youth on the Zuni Indian reservation. Modifiable lifestyle habits associated with the development of diabetes were targeted for change. To achieve its goals, the program relied on diabetes education, a school-based wellness center, active development of supportive social networks (community, faculty, and youth), and modification of available foods. Rather than taking an intrusive, directive approach to health promotion (e.g., on the model of "Just say no" to drugs), this program attempted to gently, but consistently, integrate health promotion messages into the daily lives and environments of the children, allowing for a more relaxed and gradual behavioral shift. Results of the intervention indicated a decline in soft drink consumption and an increase in the glucose:insulin ratio. This decrease in the insulin levels is an important accomplishment, especially as it lowers one of the important risk factors for type 2 diabetes.

Finally, there are other community-based prevention/intervention programs that are less well-known but have been initiated by various tribes with grant support from the Special Diabetes Program of the Indian Health Service (I.H.S.) for Indians provided under the Balanced Budget Act of 1997 ($150 million for diabetes prevention over five years). Through this resource, the I.H.S. has been able to fund tribal communities to implement tribal specific diabetes prevention programs as well as to enhance I.H.S.'s own diabetes prevention programs. A number of these programs are targeting children and adolescents, but because these programs are new, it is still too early to determine the impact these prevention or intervention efforts will have in preventing or delaying the onset of diabetes. There is no question, however, that any prevention efforts for children in rural isolated communities are welcomed and are strongly supported by the communities as well by the community leadership.

While all of these community-based diabetes prevention and intervention efforts are important, replicating these programs, despite the need, is difficult. For example, unless there are additional financial resources, most school boards and school administrations are reluctant to add to their existing curriculums or to provide for additional physical education or after-school exercise programs. Similarly, many small rural communities do not have the resources to implement such projects. Other alternatives, however, are possible for these communities, e.g., a diabetes camp.

The first diabetes camp for children with type 1 diabetes was established in 1925 in Michigan by a physician, Leonard Wendt. Since then that time, specialized camps for children with type 1 diabetes have become popular worldwide (see website, http://www.childrenwithdiabetes.com/camps), with over 20,000 children attending these camps annually. The purpose of these camps is to provide a safe environment in which children are given the opportunity to meet with one another and to share their experiences while learning to manage their diabetes. A skilled medical and camping staff help ensure safety during a camp experience that is integrated with appropriate diabetes education.

The NARTC Summer Wellness Camp

NARTC at the University of Arizona collaborated with a number of tribal communities in 1987 to host the first national conference on diabetes and American Indians. It was during this conference that a number of health care providers working with tribal communities reported that a growing number of young people were being diagnosed with type 2 diabetes. Many also indicated they had little or no resources to help these children and had to rely on treatment and education models designed for adults with

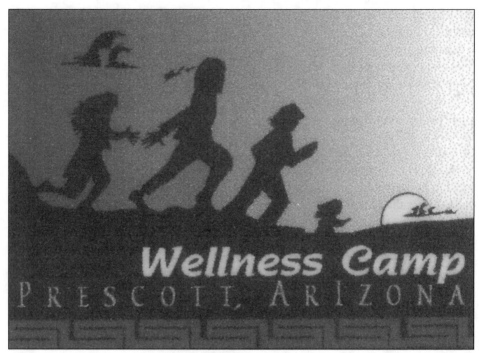

Summer Wellness Camp.

diabetes. The discussion led to the formation of a committee to explore various options. The committee decided to try a diabetes camp as an education venue, one modeled after camps supported by the ADA for children with type 1 diabetes. NARTC staff at the University of Arizona volunteered to consult with individuals in the ADA camp program and to redesign the program so that it met the needs of children with Type 2 diabetes.

The first weeklong NARTC Summer Wellness Camp for Indian Children with Diabetes was launched in the summer of 1991 with 45 campers (60% female and 40% male) plus a cadre of approximately 20 adult volunteers and faculty from the participating communities and the University of Arizona. At this first camp, the campers ranged in age from 8 to 17, an age range that subsequently proved to be too broad, i.e., the younger children had difficulty keeping up with the older ones. The age eligibility was therefore restricted the following year to children between the ages of 10 and 15.

From its inception, the Wellness Camp has been and continues to be a university and tribal community partnership. The partnership has not only allowed for equal participation, but also has kept the program cost-effective. Most importantly, the partnership allows for on-going support and follow-up for campers after they have completed the camp. The tribal health program providers who have participated in the annual camp are the best recruiters because they are able to describe to the families and their children what they should expect when their child attends the camp. These providers are familiar with what is taught at the camp and can therefore further help the children to build on their camp experience after they return home. In addition, this partnership has helped maintain a commitment and involvement of the tribal communities, especially the smaller communities that have limited resources and cannot establish their own programs for children. The commitment of all these communities is essential to the on-going success and survival of the camp for children.

The community tribal health program providers (partners) know the families in their communities and, by the fact that they are involved in diabetes prevention programs, also know who is experiencing problems with diabetes. These community partners are therefore able to identify and recruit children who would benefit from attending camp. They contact the children's parents, tell them about the camp, and work with those expressing an interest in attending by filling out the applications and helping the child schedule the pre-camp medical examination. The community partners also follow up on referrals issued by physicians.

While the community partners concentrate on working with the families and the children, the NARTC, with the help of the camp planning committee, identifies and recruits a medical team for the camp each year. NARTC staff also engage in fund raising, primarily seeking funds to help cover the camp expenses (lodging and meals) for volunteers. Fund raising activities are also undertaken by some community partners to cover or partially defray the cost of camp for the children they enroll. In addition, the community partners help recruit volunteers from their respective communities to serve as camp counselors or faculty. The university generally hires a part time camp coordinator to oversee the planning and to help coordinate day-to-day activities during camp week.

Besides the tribal communities, there are others who annually help support the camp program, including pharmaceutical companies that donate meters and strips for glucose checks. Other donors at various times have contributed funds or prizes for the camp. A couple of years after the camp program was implemented, an Indian student artist donated her skills to design a t-shirt logo for the campers. Registered dietitians employed by I.H.S. provide guidance with the camp menu as well as with nutrition education. For the first two camps, the suggested daily caloric content was limited to 1200 calories, but this was gradually increased to 2000 calories, primarily because the children were very physically active and because of the danger of hypoglycemia.

As with any diabetes camp, the medical staff is kept busy. In addition to diabetes, many of the children (up to 30%) also have other health problems, including asthma, allergies, and/or minor physical disabilities. At the end of the camp, relevant clinical or other medical information is reported back to the child's medical provider. Such reports may include the results of glucose monitoring during the week and/or any changes in diabetes medication dosages.

Issues of Cultural Sensitivity

Because all of the campers and a majority of the volunteers are American Indians or Alaska Natives, the camp gives special attention to the importance of tribal as well as childhood cultures. The curriculum and activities at the camp are especially geared towards children and, to the extent that it is possible, are delivered through culturally familiar mediums such as story telling, demonstrations, visual examples, group projects, and games. In addition, the camp becomes a tribal community of sorts as the camp grounds are taken over by the group. The walls of the common areas be-

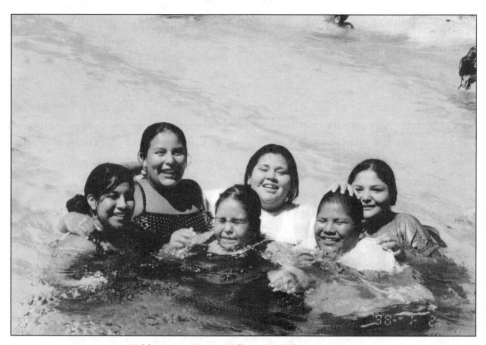

Field trips at Camp Wellness include swimming.

come blanketed with posters carrying different health messages against a colorful backdrop of tribal artwork and photographs. Each morning, a different tribal flag is raised by one of the participating tribal communities. The flags are ceremonially unfolded and raised by the children from the respective community, who also explain or tell a story about the flag. Most designs on the flags symbolize tribal history or culture. At the end of the day, a fireside activity is planned, which provides a time for story telling, singing, or tribal dancing. Tribal ghost stories are especially popular as are singing contests.

Physical Activities and Diabetes Education

The goal of the Wellness camp is to provide child-oriented and culturally sensitive diabetes education in a comfortable and fun environment. Each morning begins with all campers experiencing a new physical exercise, i.e., aerobics, weight training, or running/hiking. Other types of physical activities are also scheduled throughout the day and include hikes or team tournaments for group sports such as volleyball, basketball or, when a skilled coach is available, traditional tribal games. Approximately two field trips are also included during the week to add other exercise activities that are not available at the camp, such as swimming or paddle boating.

Formal diabetes education sessions start with a nutritional component that not only covers nutrient values of various foods, but also emphasizes why food is an important part of managing diabetes. These sessions also involve hands-on activities such as teaching the children how to make a healthy snack and how to read food labels. The sessions also provide visual illustrations of the fat and sugar content of some of the popular fast food products and sodas. Attention is paid to portion sizes as well as to food preparation. The nutrition classes also include discussion of some traditional Arizona tribal foods that are familiar and nutritious, such as mesquite beans and cholla buds.

The camp environment provides for both formal and informal diabetes education. The informal education often occurs one-on-one, with the campers asking questions of the medical staff or other volunteers. At each camp, a number of the volunteers who themselves have diabetes are a valuable resource for the children. The formal diabetes education classes commence with a brief history of diabetes and its impact (medically, socially, and culturally) on tribal communities. The session also includes a basic review of human anatomy and physiology, especially the functions of key organs such as the pancreas, and the role of insulin and glucose. How diabetes is diagnosed, treated, and the types of treatments utilized are also covered in the formal sessions, which also include a discussion on how some of the common diabetic medications work. Why and how diabetic related complications occur and are treated are also discussed.

While at camp, the children have an opportunity to demonstrate what they have learned by planning and participating in a mini-health fair. Invariably, the children select a number of games and prizes as a part of their exhibits. For example, one exhibit might have a colorful game board displaying a collection of inflated balloons, with each balloon containing a diabetes-related question on a strip of paper. Darts are provided for willing customers who, after bursting one balloon, must save the paper strip, read the question, and then provide the correct answer. A correct answer is awarded with a prize. Another game might be to ask participants to guess the sugar content in various food items, i.e., sugared cereal, diet soda, a donut, etc.

Child-oriented incentives are also integrated into the various activities. The awardees are honored at the award dinner and dance, which is held during the last night of camp. Prizes are given in various categories, usually to those who receive the most votes from peers or volunteers. Some awards are for the "the camper with most improvement in glucose management" or for the "most helpful camper," etc.

Certain camp outcomes are shared with families, health programs, and with the child's health care providers. The volunteers who accompany the campers from their respective communities are usually asked to give verbal progress reports to the parents as well as to the staff from the health programs they represent. For their part, the tribal health care providers who provide transportation and/or who accompany the children to camp continue to work with the children after completion of the camp and may refer a child back to camp in a subsequent year should there be a need. Each year a few of the campers over age 15 return to camp, where they are welcomed back as junior counselors to assist other volunteers.

The Campers

Between 1991 and 2002, 416 American Indian children and youth from 14 different tribes participated in the NARTC Summer Wellness Camp. Of this number, 62%

have been female; average age of the campers was 12.6 years. Most of the children attending camp are overweight, with BMI's > 85th percentile range. The average BMI for boys is 31.2 compared to 27.7 for girls. Close to 68% of the children have either one or both parents who are being treated for diabetes. This percentage increases to 77% when grandparent(s) with diabetes are included. In addition, approximately 28% of the children were born to mothers with diabetes.

Although camp places have been allocated primarily to children diagnosed with diabetes (both types 1 and 2), the campers, until recently, have also included children at high risk of developing diabetes. The criteria for identifying high-risk youth include: 1) impaired glucose tolerance, 2) strong history of diabetes in the family, 3) obesity, and 4) birth to a mother with diabetes. During the first camp in 1991, only 24% of the children were diagnosed with diabetes; in 2002, 95% of the camp attendees were diabetic. Approximately 30% of the children attending the 2002 camp were either on insulin or on insulin in combination with oral medication.

Most of these children were diagnosed with diabetes when they were between the ages of 12 and 13. With few exceptions, the most common intervention initially attempted with these children emphasized diabetes education, diet management, and exercise. If this intervention was not successful, oral medication or insulin was prescribed. Generally parents or guardians are given the responsibility for diabetes management, frequently without additional resources, assistance, or follow-up. Children do receive some diabetes education, but usually such sessions are directed more to the parents or guardians than to the child. Providers referring children to camp often indicate the child has a poor understanding of their health problem.

Personal and Psychosocial Consequences

It is clear that early onset of diabetes and prolonged unmanaged glucose control places children with type 2 diabetes in a vulnerable position, i.e., they are at risk for early onset of diabetic complications, have low self-esteem, and experience a poorer quality of life. Quality of life for these youth, unfortunately, has yet to receive research attention, so what is known is primarily anecdotal. For the group of children and youth who have attended Summer Wellness Camp, it is clear that the impact of the disease is devastating for many of them. For example, one camper in each of the last 2 camps had a history of suicide attempts. Another camper explained during an informal discussion that he did not want to have diabetes, and he has tried to do the opposite of what everyone tells him. He said he thought that if he did not follow the diet or take the medication, it would hasten an end to what he called "a no-life."

Girls with type 2 diabetes, in particular those who are now entering adolescence, say they do not like to talk about the future. Some say they feel they will probably not get married because of the diabetes. One young adolescent who served as a junior counselor said she thought no one would want to marry someone [like her] with insulin "needle tracks." In contrast to the girls, the young men are less talkative about the impact of diabetes on their lives although some of the consequences of having the disease are expressed in other ways, e.g., the reluctance to make friends outside the fam-

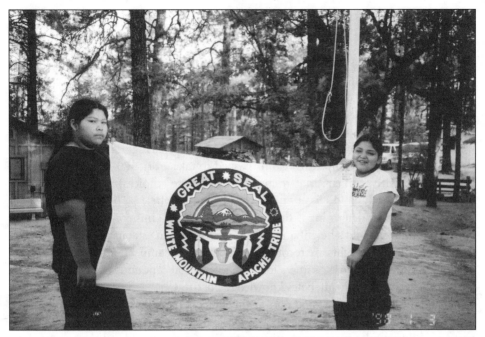

Participants in Camp Wellness.

ily circle or outside of those who already know the youth has diabetes. When asked why, one young man reported that he did not want to have to explain to strangers that he has diabetes. Another said he did not want to be treated differently, so he never talks about his diabetes, but he observed, "Even at home, we do not talk about diabetes." The latter revelation is particularly interesting as both of this young man's parents have diabetes.

The negative consequences of living with diabetes are expressed in other ways by some of the campers. For example, when asked to write what diabetes means to them, some responses were: "Something bad—it has to do with your blood sugar." "It is like a disease or sickness." "That it can kill us because it is some kind of sickness." [It] "is like a card game—I can't do anything, or play sports sometimes." Others only note that diabetes is something "bad." It is not clear how these perceptions have evolved, but some of them can be attributed to the threatening ways the negative consequences of diabetes are introduced to these children in their initial diabetes education sessions. For example, when asked where they learned to think about diabetes in this way, some replied that this was what they were told. It is obvious that many of these children have received a heavy dose of the negative consequences they would suffer should they neglect to manage their diabetes wisely. This emphasis on the negative consequences, however, seems to leave little room for presenting a more positive perspective, namely that diabetes is a condition that can be successfully managed if the patient is motivated to change some of the lifestyle behaviors that contribute to the exacerbation of the disease process.

Evaluating Outcomes

Because this camp is only a week long, there are limits to what evaluation endpoints are feasible and/or can be collected. At the present, only three markers are examined to determine the overall success of the camp, and these same measurements are also utilized to determine the impact of the camp on the individual child. The markers include 1) changes in diabetes knowledge (results of pre- and post-tests), 2) BMI (mainly weight loss), and 3) glucose readings (degree of positive change).

On the first day of camp, each child is asked to take a brief 20-item pretest (items are presented with familiar child-friendly "true or false" choices). The test is used to help determine each child's level of knowledge about diabetes. The test is repeated at the end of camp to determine if there has been a change in knowledge. On the first day of camp, each child's height and weight is recorded to establish each child's body mass index (BMI). Weights are recorded again at end of camp, and differences are calculated. On average, most campers lose between 3 and 5 pounds each and generally show improvement in the diabetes knowledge post-test.

During the week, a fasting and non-fasting glucose reading is also recorded for each camper to monitor the campers' diabetes status. This surveillance is especially important for children who may not routinely monitor their own blood sugar on a daily basis. Those who do monitor their glucose levels often perform this task 3-5 times a day in order to gauge the amount of insulin dosage needed. As a rule, most children are able to decrease their insulin dosages and/or oral medication during camp. Positive outcomes such as these help the children actually see how increased physical activity and a healthy diet impacts glucose levels.

Campers' Opinions about the NARTC Summer Wellness Camp

Each year the campers are asked about their motivation for coming to camp, to provide feedback on their camp experience, and to offer suggestions for improvement. When asked why they attended camp, several of the 2001 campers wrote that they came to have fun, to learn about diabetes, and to learn self-management strategies. A couple of campers also expressed other motivations, e.g., "to get away from my sister" and "to do something over the summer."

At the end of each camp, campers are asked to describe what was good or not so good about their camp experience. Some of the recent evaluative comments about what was good about coming to camp include the following: "You can have fun, run, and play basketball and volleyball," commented a junior counselor (LC 7/2002) who has had diabetes for 5 years. "You can exercise and go to Slide Rock," reported a 10-year old boy (VJ 7/2002) who apparently enjoyed swimming at Slide Rock. Getting up at 6 a.m., the camp food, and long hikes were mentioned as some of the things about camp that were not so good. Others stated that they enjoyed everything at camp. When asked to indicate what they have learned while at camp, most of the answers were specific to diabetes, i.e., [we] "learn how to keep our sugar down"; "to watch your sugar, watch what you eat, and take your medicine"; and " what sugar does to your body."

Summary

A diabetes education camp program for children (either at high risk or those with diabetes) is a useful educational strategy, provided the camp is used to orient those newly diagnosed or those having difficulty managing the disease. The educational goal should emphasize skills for healthy living. The teaching methods should include active, "hands-on" participation by the child, and the teaching agenda should utilize an array of teaching strategies such as story telling, demonstrations, familiar examples, etc.

Whenever possible, diabetes education should begin and end with an assessment of the child's knowledge and understanding about diabetes and diabetes management. The assessment should be given at least annually by the health care provider so that he/she can gauge the youth's knowledge and understanding of the disease.

The camp, however, is only a small part of ongoing care. The children must be monitored, assisted, and given an opportunity to continue their diabetes education after the camp is over.

Social and psychological problems that frequently accompany the daily frustrations of living with diabetes need to be recognized and addressed. Children should know that if they are frustrated or depressed, they need to consult a member of their diabetes management team, a trained counselor, or someone the child can trust to discuss confidential or troubling issues. In other instances, group or family talking circles might serve as a possible strategy for discussing either non-confidential or personal concerns. Children and youth should also be encouraged to keep a personal health journal in which they can record results of their glucose tests, BMI, and/or any other events that they believe impact their health. Such a journal might be used by the child to gauge progress and/or barriers to managing diabetes.

Periodic workshops or special sessions should also be offered to parents so that they can add to their knowledge and skill and become more effective in helping their children live with diabetes. Some discussion items could include topics such as pregnancy and diabetes, stress and diabetes, self-image, etc.

Diabetes education needs to be interesting, appropriate, and ongoing. Most importantly, it should be more than a glucose report card or the dissemination of colorful brochures.

Acknowledgments

We want to thank Robert S. Young, PhD for commenting and suggesting changes in the earlier draft of this manuscript. We also want to thank the many campers whose stories or experiences are at the heart of this chapter.

References

American Diabetes Association (ADA). 2000. Type 2 Diabetes in Children and Adolescents. Pediatrics 105: 671–80.

Blackett, Piers R, Tim Taylor, Dana Russell, Min Lu, James Fesmire and Elisa Lee. 1996. Lipoprotein Changes in Relation to Body Mass Index in Native American Adolescents. Pediatric Research 40(1): 77–81.

Brown, David. 2002. Diabetic Children Suffer as Young Adults, Study Finds. *Washington Post.* June 12:A02.

Casper, R.C. and D. Offer. 1990. Weight and Dieting Concerns in Adolescents, Fashion or Symptom? Pediatrics 86(3): 384–90.

Claus, Cynthia, Y. Sakiestewa, Shelia Murphy, M. Weahkee and Charles Wilson. 1999. Knowledge, Awareness, and Belief Issues Related to Diabetes Prevention for Native American Families. Workshop Session, Diabetes in American Indian Communities, Albuquerque, October 27–29.

Cook, Valerie V. and Joann S. Hurley. 1998. Prevention of Type 2 Diabetes in Childhood. Clinical Pediatrics 37(2): 123–29.

Dabelea, D., R. L. Hanson, Peter H. Bennett, J. Roumain, William C. Knowler and David J. Pettit. 1997. Increasing Prevalence of Type 2 Diabetes in American Indian Children. Diabetologia 41: 904–10.

Davis, C., Y. Gomez, L. Lambert and B. Skipper. 1993. Primary Prevention of Obesity in American Indian Children. Annals of New York Academy of Science 699: 167–80.

Dean, Heather J., R.L. Mundy and M. Moffatt. 1994. Non-insulin-dependent Diabetes in Indian Children in Manitoba. Canadian Medical Association Journal 147: 52–57.

Fagot-Campagna, Anne, David J. Pettitt, David J. Engelgau, Michael M. Burrows, Linda S. Geiss, Rodolfo Valdez, Gloria L.A. Beckles, Jinan Saaddine, Edward W. Gregg, David F. Williamson and Venkat Narayan. 1999. Type 2 Diabetes among North American Children and Adolescents: An Epidemiologic Review and a Public Health Perspective. The Journal of Pediatrics 136(5): 664–72.

Gilliland, Susan S., Jeanette S. Carter, Georgia E. Perez, Jackie Two Feathers, Cynthia K. Kenui, and Marjorie K. Mau. 2000. Recommendations for Development and Adaptation of Culturally Competent Community Health Interventions in Minority Populations with Type 2 Diabetes mellitus. Diabetes Spectrum 11(3): 166–74.

Gittelsohn, Joel, S.B. Harris, A.L. Thorne-Lyman, A.J.G. Hanley, A. Barnie and B. Zinman. 1996. Body Image Concepts Differ by Age and Sex in an Ojibway-Cree Community in Canada. Journal of Nutrition 126(12): 2990–3000.

Goodman, Mary Ellen. 1970. The Culture of Childhood. New York: Columbia University: Teachers College Press.

Hall, Rick. 1999. The Soda Pop Story. Electronic document <http://nutrition.about. com/health/nutrition/library/weekly/aa120199a.htm>, accessed April 12.

Harris, Stewart B., Bruce Perkins and Elaine Whalen-Brough. 1997. Non-Insulin-Dependent Diabetes Mellitus among First Nations Children. Canadian Family Physician. 42: 869–76.

Holcomb, David, Juanita Lira, Paul M. Kingery, D.W. Smith, Dorothy Lane and Jackie Goodway. 1998. Evaluation of Jump into Action: A Program to Reduce the Risk of Non-Insulin Dependent Diabetes Mellitus in School Children on the Texas-Mexico Border. Journal of School Health 68(7): 282–88.

Indian Health Service (I.H.S.) National Diabetes Program. 1999. Special Diabetes Program for Indians. Interim Report to Congress. Rockville, MD: USPHS:I.H.S.

Jain, Anjali, Susan N. Sherman, Leigh A. Chamberlin, Yvette Carter, Scott W. Powers and Robert C. Whitake. 2000. Why Don't Low-Income Mothers Worry About Their Preschoolers Being Overweight? Pediatrics 107(5): 1138–46.

Joe, Jennie R. and Robert S. Young, eds. 1992. Diabetes as a Disease of Civilization. Berlin: Mouton de Gruyter.

Jones, Kenneth Lee. 1999. Non-Insulin Dependent Diabetes in Children and Adolescents: The Therapeutic Challenge. Clinical Pediatrics 37(2): 103–10.

Kaplan, Aaron S., Babette S. Zemel and Virginia A. Stallings. 1996. Differences in Resting Energy Expenditure in Prepubertal Black Children and White Children. Journal of Pediatrics 129: 643–47.

Kitagawa, Teruo, Misao Owada, Tatsuhiko Urakami and NaokoTajima. 1992. Epidemiology of Type 1 (Insulin-Dependent) and Type 2 (Non-Insulin-Dependent) Diabetes Mellitus in Japanese Children. Diabetes Research and Clinical Practice 24 (Suppl): S7–S13.

Liddane, Lisa. 2001. Type 2 Diabetes Has a New Young Face. The Orange County Register. February 28, 2001. Accent Section C:3.

Lindner, Lawrence. 2000. Type 2 Diabetes Hits Kids. Washington Post. December 5: Z10.

Macaulay, Ann C., Gilles Paradis, Louise Potvin, Edward J. Cross, Chantal Saad-Haddadd, Alex M. McComber, Serge Desrosiers and Rhonda Kirby. 1997. Primary Prevention of Type 2 Diabetes in First Nations in First Nations: Experiences of the Kahnawake Schools Diabetes Prevention Project. Canadian Journal of Diabetes Care 22(3): 44–49.

Marlow, Elizabeth, Gail D'eramo Melkus and Anna Maria Bosma. 1998. STOP Diabetes! An Educational Model for Native American Adolescents in the Prevention of Diabetes. Diabetes Educator 24(4): 441–50.

Mazur, Marcia L., Jennie R. Joe and Robert S. Young. 1999. Why Are Children Being Diagnosed With a "Middle-Aged" Disease? Diabetes Forecast 51(12): 47–54.

McKenzie, Shirlyn, B.J. O'Connell, L.A. Smith and W.E. Ottinger. 2000. A Primary Intervention Program (Pilot Study) for Mexican American Children at Risk for Type 2 Diabetes. Diabetes Educator 24(2): 180–87.

Narayan, K.M. Venkat. 2001. Diabetes Mellitus in Native Americans: The Problem and Its Implications. Population Research and Policy Review 16: 169–92.

Neel, James V. 1962. Diabetes Mellitus: A "Thrifty" Genotype Rendered Detrimental by "Progress." American Journal of Human Genetics 14: 353–62.

Pettitt, David J., Patricia P. Moll, William C. Knowler, David M. Mott, Robert G. Nelson, Mohammed F. Saad, Peter H. Bennett and Bruce A. Kotke. 1963. Insulinemia in Children at Low and High Risk of NIDDM. Diabetes Care 16(4): 608–15.

Pinhas-Hamiel, Orit, Lawrence M. Dolan, Stephen R. Daniels, Debra Standiford, Phillip R. Khoury and Philip Zeitler. 1964. Increased Incidence of Non-Insulin-Dependent Diabetes Mellitus among Adolescents. Journal of Pediatrics 128: 608–15.

Office of Minority Health. 1965. National Standards on Culturally and Linguistically Appropriate Services in Health Care. DHHS, OMH.

Rosenbloom, Arlan L., Jennie R. Joe, Robert S. Young and William E. Winter. 1999. Emerging Epidemic of Type 2 Diabetes in Youth. Diabetes Care 22: 345–54.

Sevilla, Graciela. 1999. 20 Years of Research for What? Tribe Asks. Arizona Republic October 31:B1.

Story, Mary, Karen F. Strauss, Elenora Zephier and Brenda A. Broussard. 1966. Nutritional Concerns in American Indian and Alaska Native Children: Transitions and Future Directions. Journal of the American Dietetic Association 98(2): 170–76.

Teufel, Nicolette I. and Cheryl K. Ritenbaugh. 1967. Development of a Primary Prevention Program: Insight Gained in the Zuni Diabetes Prevention Program. Clinical Pediatrics 37(2): 131–41.

Wake. Melissa, K. Hesketh and F. Cameron. 1968. The Child Health Questionnaire in Children with Diabetes: Cross-Sectional Survey of Parent and Adolescent-Reported Functional Health Status. Diabetic Medicine 17(10): 700–7.

Walker, Mark. 1969. Obesity, Insulin Resistance, and Its Link to Non-Insulin-Dependent Diabetes mellitus. Metabolism 44(9), Suppl 3: 18–20.

CHAPTER 18

TOUCH THE HEART OF THE PEOPLE: CULTURAL REBUILDING AT THE POTAWOT HEALTH VILLAGE IN CALIFORNIA

Mariana Leal Ferreira, Twila Sanchez and Bea Nix

Songs are the source of the strength and power for the Individual Yurok Indian. Singing, particularly ceremonial singing, is the strength and power of the tribe, a manifestation of the cyclic interaction (Wesonah) of the Yurok universe.

Barbara Redner 1982

Summary of Chapter 18. This chapter discusses the history of the Potawot Health Village from the point of view of its spiritual and conceptual masters—the Yurok, Wiyot and Tolowa Indigenous Peoples of northern California. We provide social, historical, and ethical contexts and concerns for an analysis of the process of cultural rebuilding launched at the newly built Potawot Health Village in 2001. Located in Arcata, in the Humboldt County, Potawot is now the main headquarter of a complex of 12 health clinics owned and operated by the Yurok, Wiyot and Tolowa nations, and administered by United Indian Health Services (UIHS). Potawot and its satellite clinics are located on and around reservations and rancherias in the Humboldt and Del Norte counties, providing health services to 9 Indigenous nations and serving more than 13 thousand patients.[1] Cultural rebuilding at the Potawot Health Village takes Indigenous words, feelings, and actions very seriously. Here, we propose that paying close attention to Indigenous conceptions of culture allows community members, health professionals, administrators and policy makers to tackle more efficiently the social and emo-

---

1. The Indigenous population of the service area counties includes individuals from the following nations: Yurok, Wiyot, Tolowa, Wylacki, Hupa, Smith River, and Mattole. UIHS also provides services to Indigenous Peoples from across the United States residing in our service area. Rancherias and reservations in the service area include: Blue Lake Rancheria, Big Lagoon Rancheria of Smith River Indians , Cherae Heights Indian Community of the Trinidad Rancheria, Coast Indian Community of Yurok Indians, Resighini Rancheria, Elk Valley Rancheria, Rohnerville Rancheria of Bear River of Mattole Indians, Smith River Rancheria, Table Bluff Rancheria of Wiyot Indians, Yurok Tribe of California.

tional dimensions of diabetes mellitus. We discuss empowering ideas and activities, such as women support groups, music and art therapy, and the right to food that can help prevent and treat diabetes. The activities focus on two main ideas: 1) that strengthening Indigenous generosity and solidarity ties, allowing individuals—women in particular—to build self-esteem, stand up for themselves, grieve collectively in situations of distress, and seek reciprocal solutions to their problems alleviates emotional suffering; and 2) emotional well-being has the potential to soothe the nervous system, bringing heightened blood sugars down and allowing individuals to be in control of their health.[2]

ℬ   ℬ   ℬ

Introduction: The Importance of Culture for a Healthy Community

The importance of culture for a healthy community has been acknowledged by the Yurok, Tolowa, Wiyot, Karuk, Hupa, and other Indigenous Peoples in northern California for thousands of years. More recently, these communities have been investing in processes of cultural rebuilding, following the destruction of their ways of life in the last 150 years since the American invasion of California in 1848 and the Gold Rush in the 1850s. In less than one hundred years, large-scale violence and epidemics of contagious diseases wiped out 90 to 95 percent of California's Indigenous population. In the 1950s, the life-expectancy of genocide survivors was at its lowest: 36.4 years for the Yurok People and approximately the same for most local communities (Ferreira 1996, 1998, 1999).

The inauguration of United Indian Health Services (UIHS) in 1970 and its main facility, the Tsurai Health Center in Trinidad (now replaced by Potawot in Arcata), was an attempt on the part of the Yurok, Tolowa, Wiyot, Karuk, and Hupa nations to offer culturally sensitive and ethically grounded health services to communities now deeply suffering from degenerative diseases—diabetes, cancer, hypertension, and heart disease. In 2001, the Potawot Health Village was built by the Yurok, Tolowa and Wiyot Peoples in the city of Arcata, in the Humboldt Bay Area, to replace the smaller Tsurai clinic. With the opening of Potawot, access to comprehensive health care and the quality of the medical, dental, mental health, nutrition and community services improved dramatically. UIHS's nationally recognized diabetes prevention and tobacco awareness programs are featured at Potawot. Traditional healing and cultural facilities, including a sweathouse, dance pit and a wellness garden are central to the spiritual and cultural aspects of the health care provided.

Health professionals in northern California and in the United States at large, broadly speaking, have only recently started taking seriously the efficacy of culturally sensitive approaches to health and healing. Attention to socio-cultural determinants of health affecting local Indigenous Peoples, especially how trauma, poverty, and racial discrimination converge to produce inhuman health outcomes—is also just beginning.

---

2. Most information in this chapter was originally presented as a report commissioned by United Indian Health Services (UIHS) for the Evaluation Committee of the Potawot Health Village in 2001.

Many practitioners are slow to take Indigenous Peoples' knowledges and practices seriously, and embrace preventive and therapeutic ideas and activities that transcend the biomedical emphasis on the physical body. As we argue here, this prejudice stems from 1) a strong conviction that biomedicine has the answer, or the ability to find the causes of and develop therapies for all "diseases"; and 2) the use of a conservative and quite dated concept of culture based solely on "norms," "values," and "behaviors." These factors lead to 3) a solid resistance in honestly considering what Indigenous Peoples themselves feel, think, say and do about culture, history, and power relations (in the delivery of health services, for example); resulting in 4) a lack of interest in new studies about the effectiveness of cultural rebuilding in improving individual and community health.

The effects of a strict biomedical approach are disastrous: health disparities are usually seen as a result of "cultural difference" and Indigenous Peoples are blamed (genetically or otherwise) for their high rates of both contagious and degenerative diseases. Kim Humphrey brilliantly explores the impact of such a conceptualization of difference in "Culture Blindness?" (see chapter 19 in this volume), discussing the thinking of a group of health professionals who provide services to Aboriginal people in Australia's northern Territory. As medical anthropologist Paul Farmer (1996: 281) considerately put it, "otherness" allows us to detach ourselves from the causes of social suffering, making pain and misery more distant and thus less affective.

Here, instead, Yurok, Tolowa and Wiyot knowledges—their thoughts, words, feelings and actions—are taken very seriously. We propose that paying close attention to local conceptions of culture allows community members, health professionals, administrators and policy makers to address the social, emotional and political dimensions of health. Creative activities proposed in the second half of this essay address culturally sensitive preventive strategies and therapies that can improve the social well-being of Indigenous Peoples.

Everyday Life and the Power of Ethnographic Fieldwork

We want to begin by making a case for ethnographic, empirical research because this method of inquiry has the potential to reveal a completely different world, so different that we seem to be confronted by a different order of things. The "order" is distinct because individuals' life trajectories and experiences reveal novel associations or "networks of analogies" (Foucault 1975: xi) that transcend by far the common associations made between diabetes and sedentary lifestyle, diet, and genetics. The oral testimonies of Yurok, Wiyot and Tolowa men, women and children about their experiences in mining and logging camps, boarding schools, fish canneries, prisons and reservations delineate intricate connections between the classification of diseases and American family values; between the distribution of land and the transformation of "Indian" soul and conduct; between the circulation of commodities (alcohol, bullets, clothing, food and women) and the notion of civilization; and between military genocidal practices and a particular knowledge of the human body (see chapters 3 and 14 in this volume). Ethnographic fieldwork has the power to illuminate individuals' ideas and feelings about the world they live in and help construct on a daily basis. Attention to apparently small, ordinary and all too familial details of people's every day lives shows how culture is created and recreated by individuals in action. This perspective shies away from the conservative conception of culture as a complex of norms and values that determine how individuals behave, as discussed ahead. Fieldwork results covering northern California Indigenous awareness, perceptions, and expectations of the Potawot Health Village constitute the bulk of this chapter. The research process was geared towards uncovering socio-cultural knowledges and practices tribal members identify as being of key importance to advance a *theoretical basis for cultural rebuilding*. This means coming up with culturally sensitive and ethically grounded ideas and strategies that can improve community and individual health in northern California.

Ethnographic fieldwork is the research method par excellence used by anthropologists and social scientists in general to generate an understanding of individuals' perceptions of a particular social process. It is both a qualitative and quantitative method that may include surveys, participant- observation, and open-ended, semi-structured and structured interviews that can be applied to healthcare issues in numerous ways (Savage 2000). Ethnographic fieldwork is based on direct contact with the people "in the field," that is, in their homes, at work, in social gatherings, at health facilities, during leisure activities, and so on. The main idea is to understand the sensitivity individuals themselves have developed about, for instance, what a healthy community is, the reason for the widespread use of drugs, or the high incidence of diabetes. In the specific case of diabetes, this means going beyond what medical studies have discovered (or not) about the disorder (transcending the relationship between diet, sedentary lifestyle and the so-called Indian heritage), and seriously taking into consideration risk factors raised by local populations.

Mariana Ferreira conducted 95 open-ended interviews with Yurok, Tolowa and Wiyot youth, adults and elders in 2000 and 2001 at various health clinics, tribal offices, social gatherings, and in their homes and workplaces in northern California. The interviews were carried out in the context of UIHS's "Cultural Evaluation Committee of the Potawot Health Village," which hired Mariana to document the importance of cultural rebuilding for a healthy community (Ferreira 2001). The objective of the interviews was twofold: 1) to document the extent to which the administration of United Indian Health Services has integrated Yurok, Wiyot and Tolowa knowledges and practices into the process of cultural rebuilding at Potawot; and 2) to document the scope of cultural sensitivity at Potawot in mobilizing the communities for the promotion of healthy lifestyles that meet their political and ethical aspirations. Special emphasis was given to the process of unveiling thoughts and feelings community members would like to contribute towards enhancing the collective nature of the PHV, as well as advancing its potential for cultural rebuilding. Interviews gravitated around how tribal leaders, administrators, patients and their families experience and reflect about, and what they expect from the Potawot Health Village (PHV). Some of the cultural and ethical contexts and concerns addressed in this chapter are poignantly raised by Ann Macaulay and collaborators in this anthology (see chapter 16), in a formidable discussion of the Kahnawake Schools Diabetes Prevention Project of the Kanien'kéha:ka (Mohawk) community in Canada.

Interestingly, the process of ethnographic fieldwork allowed current perceptions to surface about how "culture" is defined and put to use not only by each and every nation in northern California, but also intra-nations, that is, individuals within a given society may differ in their perspectives and feelings towards culture. The strong relationship between social equality and community health became readily apparent, generating heated discussions between not only interviewees and interviewer, but also among Mariana Ferreira, Bea Nix, Twila Sanchez, and other members of the Potawot Evaluation Committee. Arguments about the prevalence and distribution of type 2 diabetes within communities and families emerged in the context of a debate linking the historical and political usages of the concept of culture, and racial discrimination. For instance, community members questioned to what extent the notion of "culture" has been used as a politically correct substitute for "race" and thus justify "genetic" and altogether "behavioral" differences that make "Indians" particularly susceptible to almost *all*—contagious and degenerative diseases alike! In this chapter, instead, type 2 diabetes is used as a case in point to discuss cultural integrity, social equality, and community health. From this perspective, the presence of diabetes is an indicator of community distress, rather than a disease in itself.

Cultural Rebuilding at the Potawot Health Village

*I appreciate the fact that UIHS [United Indian Health Services] is attempting to incorporate our **culture** and our **knowledge** into the Potawot Health Village, that they are making the building and landscape culturally relevant to us.*

…

Symbols send a message, welcome a community. The new Potawot Health Village welcomes the people because it uses symbols that are important for the people, setting the tone for that visit. Everyone around here knows that the area has a new village, and that it was built by Native Americans, for Native Americans.

…

*I see the **power** of ownership in terms of the symbolic and emotional ownership of the building—I see this power when I hear people say that they own the place, that "this is our place." People have a sense of pride about it. That can be a powerful process because people can feel comfortable in their **culture**. Potawot is a place where you feel respected and honored for your cultural and your spiritual life.*

> Jim McQuillen, on June 15, 2001. Jim is a Yurok Tribal Member and the Director of the Yurok Tribe's Education Department.

Culture, knowledge and power are key terms that closely reflect Yurok, Wiyot and Tolowa perceptions and expectations about the Potawot Health Village. The above passage is part of a larger narrative by Yurok tribal member Jim McQuillen, the former Principal of the Margaret Keating Elementary School on the Yurok Indian Reservation, and the father of three children. McQuillen illustrates the importance of a culturally sensitive health facility to local Indigenous communities. Like McQuillen, many individuals interviewed in Humboldt and Del Norte counties also assert that the incorporation of Indigenous knowledges and practices into the conception, construction and administration of Potawot improves the quality of medical care, and thus encourages people to seek health services at the new clinic. As McQuillen likes to put it, "Potawot is a place where you feel respected and honored for your cultural and your spiritual life."

Designed as a Northern Californian village, the redwood plank houses, sweat lodge, medicine garden, wellness trails, and brush dance pit at Potawot have symbolic value for the Tolowa, Wiyot and Yurok Peoples. According to several community members, these are Indigenous symbols indicating that American Indian Peoples and their respective cultures in California are not dead. Instead, they are well and alive, and Potawot welcomes us to witness the importance of cultural rebuilding to promoting wellness. Tribal members that were reluctant to seek medical care at the Tsurai Health Center in Trinidad because it was considered a non-Indigenous facility have now begun to consider the Potawot Health Village as a place where they can feel comfortable about cultural diversity. In other words, as Yurok tribal member William Einman put it, "making it more cultural in the forefront helps with healing because it makes people feel they belong there. And we actually do, because this is our clinic."

The Potawot name itself, which identifies in the Wiyot language the tract of Wiyot ancestral territory in the Humboldt Bay Area where the health village is located, is a political statement. As several interviewees pointed out, numerous landmarks in northern California, including sacred sites, such as redwood groves, coastal trails, boulders, bays and towns, carry non-Indigenous or Caucasian/European names. This is the case of Trinidad Bay, the location of the Tsurai Village in Yurok territory where Spanish navigators first arrived in the late eighteenth century. This is also the case of the Gedediah Smith Redwoods, the Harry Merlo State Recreation Area, and the Whiskey Shasta-Trinity Recreation Area in Humboldt and Del Norte counties, named after European settlers and explorers. Humboldt is a German name, and Del Norte means "of the north" in Spanish, the language of early California conquistadors. And California itself is the name of the queen of the Amazons, the mythical tribe of sex-crazed women warriors the Spaniards were constantly seeking!

Community members feel the new clinic honors Indigenous Peoples because it says out loud: "Potawot is a facility designed, built, administered and owned by Indigenous Peoples."

How do Yurok, Wiyot and Tolowa individuals define and experience culture? What does "cultural rebuilding" mean to the patients of the Potawot Health Village and to the broader community?

Yurok, Tolowa and Karuk individuals, families and community members resort to their own feelings, thoughts, actions and languages to construct, and make sense of the world they live in. In this sense, they are *agents of their own destinies*, rather than passive victims of an oppressive history between Indigenous and non-Indigenous Peoples. In the process, they produce knowledge about this world, and this knowledge is, ultimately, associated with *CULTURE*. According to local community members, knowledge encompasses the ways is which individuals think about the world, how people see and feel about themselves and others around them, and what people do in their daily lives. This is what becomes clear when we look at the following narratives about the meanings of culture:

> Culture is a state of mind almost. It includes your history, stories that are told, the ways families have done things, and the language itself, because we learn culture through the language. Culture is fluid, too, which means it is always changing. There are certain things that you need to do the same, such as cer-

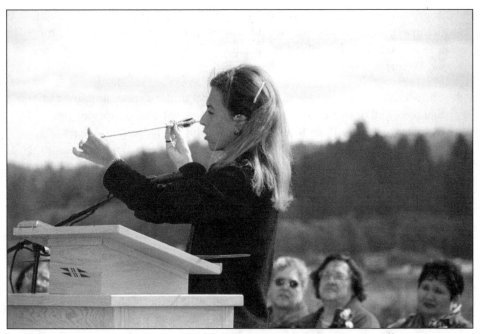

Dedication Ceremony at the Potawot Health Village in 2002. Mariana Ferreira offers an arrow sent by the Xavante Indigenous People of central Brazil to help fight diabetes, in exchange for diabetes supplies sent to the Xavante by UIHS. Photo: Rose Kidder.

emonies, but those, too, can change over time. It is the sudden change in culture that upsets people, such as the changes brought about by the Gold Rush. (William Einman, Yurok)

I wish I could tell everybody how good I feel about my culture. Actually, culture is about feeling good about yourself, [knowing] that everything you do, say or think really matters. Your ideas matter. The stuff you know matters. Your spirituality matters. Now, when you don't feel good about yourself, everything can go to hell, there's no culture left (anonymous).

Culture is a person's belief system, their traditions, the ways a certain group of people are used to doing certain things. People sharing a same culture have the same ceremonies in common, expressing the ways in which they communicate collectively. (Twila Sanchez, Yurok).

Culture to me is valuing our traditions, our prayers. I pray everyday for the Creator, so that he can bless us and always bring happiness to the people. To be truly cultural, a person has to be loving. There is love in culture, culture is about love, our Indian love. (Aileen Figueroa, Yurok)

Culture, to me, is much more than just what we eat, how we look and what we believe in. Most people I know, anthropologists included, think about Indian culture as everything that catches their eyes, things that we do different. It is a very limited way of seeing things, of explaining why things happen to us. To me, culture is much more than that, it is about what we know, our language, our medicine, our love, our spiritual life. If doctors thought about culture in a more open way, they would understand that the Potawot Clinic must have a heart, and this will be the healing power of that place. (Cheryl Sneider, Wiyot)

I think culture is a way of life, how we connect to the Creator and live a spiritual life. If all of that is gone, the Tolowa people will also disappear. I started this place here [the Table Bluff Rancheria], and I will die here. We maintain our culture alive because we feel good about who we are, and who we want to be. This is because we have the Creator in us, to keep us alive. (Betty Green, Yurok)

Culture is something that can be recreated in our daily lives, as we live on and try to understand the world we live in. It is not exactly traditions, that is, things from the past. As you and I sit here and talk about all this, we are, in a way, creating new cultural ways of going about our lives, and making ourselves understood. My family and I invest in keeping Tolowa culture alive, and this brings us good health and spiritual well-being. (Loren Bommelyn, Tolowa)

Is it possible to talk about what we are like without considering what we have gone through? What kind of idea of culture is this? Something stuck in the past? Some people say because an idea is "old," it is valuable. I don't think so. There are ideas that have survived because they are based on knowledge, and ideas that are based on feelings. Culture is a blend of both. If knowledge changes, if feelings change, culture also changes. (Bea Nix, Yurok)

These ideas form the grounding basis for modern conceptions of culture advanced by critical anthropologists and theorists of social practice interested in intersections of culture, social justice and human rights (Barth 1995; Farmer 2003; Ferreira 2004, in press; Gupta and Ferguson 1992; Pino and Ferreira forthcoming; Scheper-Hughes and Bourgois 2004; Preis 1996). Although several definitions of "culture" have been advanced in anthropology's 150 years of existence as a discipline, the classic conception of culture as a "set of values and norms that determines behavior," advanced by anthropologist Franz Boas during the turn of the twentieth century, is used consistently throughout the medical literature on type 2 diabetes that claims to take "cultural factors" into consideration (Ferreira and Nix 2000). Factors deemed "cultural" mirror those variables that researchers can easily recognize, measure and correlate according to biomedical criteria, such as weight, blood sugars and blood pressure, level of activity and family history of diseases, among many others.

The use of a dated, and quite restrictive concept of "culture" can explain why emotions and traumatic memory cannot be stated in terms of the conceptual and instrumental tools supplied by the clinical paradigm. The adoption of the classic notion of culture by the biomedical community has profound implications to the knowledge that is produced about type 2 diabetes and other ailments. Coupled with the accepted biomedical data about type 2 diabetes, which gravitates around diet, sedentary lifestyle and genetics, "cultural" norms and values are reduced to nutritional and exercise behaviors, which are ultimately connected to individuals' genotypes. Such a narrow and dated conception of culture has prevented researchers from grasping the broader and deeper conceptions of self, identity, and the body, which are at stake in determining the social and existential causes of degenerative diseases.

Furthermore, the idea that all American Indians share a universal culture, ethnic identity, and even a common genotype is widespread in the medical literature, the mass media, and the popular imagination. A singular "Indian culture/Indian identity" stance prevails in reference to the worldviews, knowledges, languages and bio-identities of nearly 800 Indigenous nations in the United States, whether federally recognized or not. Ideas and arguments made about "Indian culture" and "ethnicity" are usually based on the assumption that ethnic identity is a characteristic of primordial and tribal societies, and that only a few societies in North America and in Europe represent modernity (Ahmed 2002: 215). Modern societies have moved beyond and evolved away from religion, beliefs and customs—the characteristics that are believed to make up "Indian culture." The move from culture to heritage is guaranteed, and in the absence of a genetic component (like a diabetes gene), culture becomes the determining factor: "You are Indian, therefore you are at heightened risk for diabetes." The psychological impact of such a statement on Indigenous Peoples' identities is tremendous.

The apparently simple and innocuous statement that "Indian heritage" is a risk factor for diabetes is emotionally charged because it touches deeply upon issues of self-knowledge, body-imagery and social identity. As a Yurok outreach worker at United Indian Health Services in California recently put it, "To say I am an American Indian means I am or will be diabetic." A recent statistical analysis of the Yurok database, however, reveals that there is a weak, negative correlation between diabetes and quantum of Indian blood. Contrary to what would be expected, a close analysis of the distribution of intermarriage and of blood quantum levels among 16 extended Yurok families (sample size: $n = 544$) living in northern California since 1850 reveals that there is a small, negative correlation ($-.21811$) between Amerindian blood quantum and type 2 diabetes. (This correlation, although low, is not a chance finding, because $T = -5.2030636$, which is highly significant.) It should be noted that the so-called Amerindian blood quantum reflects the total amount of "Indian" blood, as a direct product of intermarriages between the Yuroks, and the Karuk, Tolowa, Hupa Peoples in the area. Respondents identified in the Yurok database that were listed as "full blood" evoked the same tribal identities for parents as for themselves. Individuals identified as less than full blood (for example, 1/2 Yurok and 1/2 Tolowa, or 1/2 Yurok and 1/2 Caucasian) listed different identities for their mother and father. In other words, blood quantum less than full blood is accompanied by an ethnic or tribal identification of the foreign elements in the parents' lineage. The data were analyzed by means of a Logistic Regression (a standard technique in epidemiological research), which in this case was used to predict the probability of an individual of a given blood quantum level (ranging from 0 to 1.0, that is, no Indian blood to full blood) having diabetes. Figure 1 gives a graphical interpretation to the logistic regression function, and the result of the increasing odds ratio.[3]

---

3. The odds ratio tells us the degree of increase in the chance that an individual will have diabetes for a one-unit increase in blood quantum. Here, we see the odds ratio of .853, which means

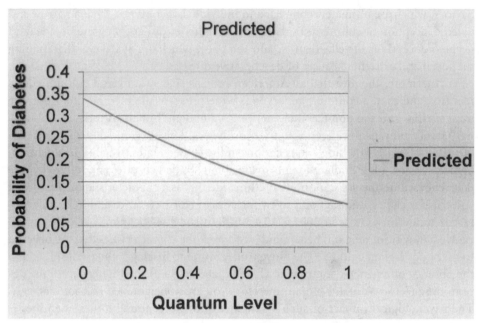

"Indian Blood " is not a risk factor for diabetes in northern California.

As shown above, there is a lower chance for people of full blood quantum, and a higher chance for individuals of mixed ancestry to develop type 2 diabetes. The most distinctive feature of this figure is the very low frequency of diabetes in "full blood" American Indians. This is important because in the past many researchers have alluded to increased risk of diabetes in full bloods. We see that at least in the Yurok case, this hypothesis does not hold true. There is an increased frequency of diabetes in more heavily admixed American Indians. The Pearson correlation between diabetes and blood quantum is -.218 (p <.0001), which indicates that as quantum increases towards full bloods, the frequency of diabetes decreases.

In short, biological "Indian heritage" does *not* appear to be a risk factor for type 2 diabetes among the Yuroks of northern California. There are several reasons that can help explain the weak correlation between blood quantum and diabetes in northern California. Being a hierarchical society, Yurok families that occupy a higher place in Yurok hierarchy have tended to intermarry less with non-Indians because of stricter rules of social conduct. These families seem to be socially and emotionally more stable, with lower rates of unemployment, suicide, domestic violence, drug abuse, and so forth. Individuals in these families tend to be successful professionally and, on average, have higher annual incomes. Interestingly enough, patterns of diet and exercise among the different families remain similar.

Families whose members have higher Indigenous blood quantum are protected against diabetes *not because of their genes* or what is very loosely and irresponsibly defined in the medical literature as "Indian heritage", but because these families are considered by the community and consider themselves to be more "traditional." Such fam-

---

that for a one-unit increase in blood quantum, there is an 8.53% increase in the odds an individual will have diabetes.

ilies are known to possess a greater degree of what is called cultural competence or cultural consonance (Dressler and Bindon 2000), adhering more strictly to long-established knowledges and practices.

This is not to say that recently re-invented Indigenous traditions are not "genuine" and therefore modern, such as fry bread and, in some cases, buffalo meat—staple post-contact components of numerous Indigenous diets today in the U.S. (see Omura, chapter 6 in this volume). In fact, social scientists have long asserted that traditions are inherently re-invented by all Peoples, Indigenous or not, and deemed traditional insofar as they are recognized by their peers as such (Hobsbawm and Ranger 1992). Such a perspective helps avoid the pervasive traditional/modern dichotomy, which automatically casts Indigenous Peoples in a remote uncivilized and ahistorical past, only to be overcome once "Indians" adhere to modernity and its ideas of rationality, secularism, and scientific and economic progress. Because modernity was located in and spread from Europe over the last two centuries it allowed Europe to become the standard-bearer of civilization, indeed of the future (Ahmed 2002). Cultural and racial superiority has ever since been implied thus making the so-called red race inherently "disease-prone" for a variety of ailments.

These finding demonstrates, among other things, that the concept of "Indian heritage" cannot be used as a general risk factor for American Indians, let alone for Indigenous Peoples globally. Yurok, Tolowa and Wiyot community leaders in northern California feel that blaming "Indian blood" is a pretext for discrimination and is ultimately racist, because the whole notion of "Indian heritage" is not explicitly defined. And more: the question is not about "blood" altogether, but indicative of a trend for diabetes to manifest itself in broken, traumatized families. They repudiate this novel and genetically based form of colonial control, which mimics the tight discipline and punishment carried out in boarding schools, reservations, labor camps, high-tech prisons and mental homes that they themselves and their close relatives—and Indigenous Peoples worldwide broadly speaking—were and still are confined to.

In fact, few medical studies actually correlate individual genetic admixture with the occurrence of diabetes, when stating that Indian blood quantum structures risk for diabetes. Most studies take "Indian heritage" for granted, and use it as a major variable to establish genetic causative links for the diabetes epidemic. The problem here is, of course, one of social identity, because it is closely related to the question "Who is an Indian"?—which appears as the most frequently asked question in the Bureau of Indian Affairs' website. While there are nations, such as the Pima of the Gila River Indian Community, which require a minimum of 1/4 "Indian blood" for tribal membership, in other groups who have "open enrollment," such as the Cherokee Tribe of Oklahoma, there are members today who are 1/2048 Cherokee (the fractions are always multiples of 2). Genetically speaking, "Indian heritage" obviously has different meanings for enrolled members of the Pima and Cherokee nations.

It should also be noted that while genetic testing for other degenerative ailments that are most prevalent among Caucasian populations, such as Alzheimer and Huntington Disease, are carefully divulged, the medical community has no reservations about advertising "Indian heritage," however loosely defined, as a risk factor for diabetes. The medical community is cautious about publicizing "whiteness" as a risk factor for Alzheimer and Huntington Disease. There is concern that genetic testing may produce "genetic social outcastes" because issues involving health insurance, life insurance policies, employee discrimination and negative social stigma are at stake (Weir et al. 1994). Now take the "thrifty gene theory" (Neel 1962, 1982), for instance, suggesting the existence of a hypothetical Indian genotype prone for diabetes in a situation of modernity. Although it is widely marketed as a theory, it has failed to show the mechanisms through which a hypothetical thrifty gene, which protected the Indian body against starvation in times of great seasonal fluctuation, became maladaptive with modern patterns of food consumption and the ability to store fat, leading to diabetes.

Ultimately, blaming Indigenous Peoples' "faulty genes" helps cultivate ethnic or racial hatred, making Indigenous Peoples a prime object for biomedical and criminal interventions—what to say of the new industrial prison complex in the United States employing confinement of Indigenous Peoples and other ethnic minorities for profit? Indigenous communities become easily susceptible to the capitalistic and bureaucratic prerogatives of the pharmaceutical and medical technology industries. Political ideology and medical technology merge together to engender a continuum of violence, generating anger, hatred, despair, hopelessness not only against the colonizer, but amidst Indigenous Peoples themselves. It is the mimetic aspect of ethnic hatred that seems to partly account for the continuing genocide of Indigenous Peoples worldwide: the opposed groups, whether Indigenous or not, mirror the hatred, rhetoric, and fears of each other. Ethnic hatred "makes everyone an outsider; and it makes everyone a target. Everywhere—in the shopping arcade, at the bus stop, in the cinema, in your living room—you are vulnerable to sudden, random violence. Anger and hatred are easily generated" (Ahmed 2002: 216).

The negative effects of the "thrifty gene" and other genetic theories on the prevention, diagnosis and treatment of type 2 diabetes and other degenerative diseases among Indigenous Peoples in northern California have been discussed extensively elsewhere (Ferreira 1996, 1998, 1999, 2002a, 2002b, and chapters 3 and 14 in this book). Our research has shown the ways in which Indigenous social relationships have become increasingly forged around "biological identities" since the U.S. government enacted the *Dawes Act* or *General Allotment Act* in 1887, officially stipulating "blood" as a criteria for Indianess and thus—believe it or not!—entitlement for land ownership of Indian reservations. The 19th and 20th centuries were indeed marked by an explosion of biological techniques exercised by colonizers across the globe to subjugate Indigenous bodies and control their populations, marking the beginning of an era of "bio-power" (Foucault 1978). As a result, Indigenous Peoples in northern California tend to structure their personal interactions taking blood quantum and genetic makeup into consideration (Ferreira 1998 and chapter 3 in this anthology). Couples consider fractions of "Indianess" in their marital decisions and adoptions—a high degree of Indian blood, for instance, puts them at higher risk for, say, diabetes, while a low degree might not make them eligible for health care and other federal benefits. Teenagers sometimes end up using bio-identities as excuses for "Indian" failures, and on occasion deny their Indigenous ancestry and mobilize against each other after relentless media and academic representations of the genetically flawed "Indian people." Adults tell one another to watch out for sugar, fat, alcohol and drugs, because "your blood tells on you: the doctor can tell right away what you've been up to." This attitude leads to another important impact of genetic paradigms on individuals' self-knowledge: Patients and their families reason that if diabetes is genetic or in their blood, "there is nothing that can be done about it." Why undergo a strict diet, vigor-

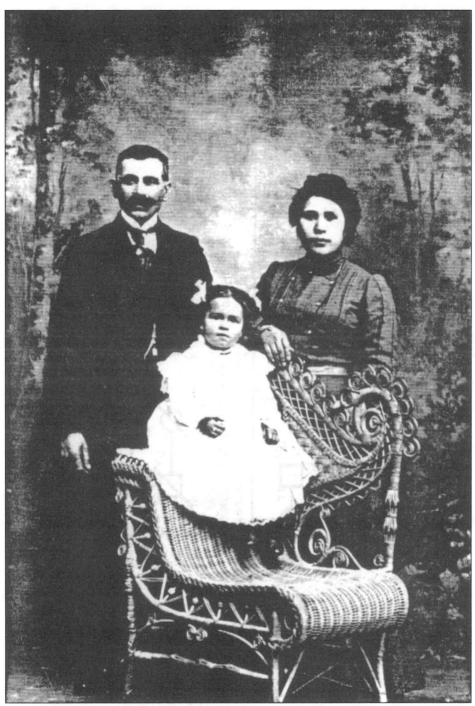

Yurok women married non-Indian, often foreign men in the late 1800s and early 1900s. Here, Sen yu teis na (later called Agnes Tom Mattz), her Portuguese husband Manoel Mattz and their son Emery Mattz in the year 1900. (Courtesy Lavina Bowers)

ous exercises, and frequent blood screening if the disorder is a hereditary ailment? These findings have made health professionals at United Indian Health Services (UIHS) and most recently at the Potawot Health Village stop blaming the "thrifty gene" as a risk factor for diabetes. In "Diabetes as a Metaphor," Terry Raymer (chapter 12 in this volume) competently addresses, from a physician's viewpoint, the benefits of the shift from a clinical, genetic perspective to a critical, spiritual approach to diabetes mellitus in his work at Potawot.

Considerable efforts in trying to find a genetic cause for type 2 diabetes have remained unsuccessful. Although recent data (Williams et al. 2000) collected among the Pima Indians of the Gila River Indian Community in Arizona (who reportedly have the highest rate of type 2 diabetes in the world) suggest "strong genetic components" in type 2 diabetes, the nature of such genetic components have *not* been determined. In this respect, and under its mandate to eliminate health disparities, HEALTHY PEOPLE 2010, a national health promotion and disease prevention initiative of the Department of Health, makes the following statement about "Race and Ethnicity:"

> Current information about the biologic and genetic characteristics of African Americans, Hispanics, American Indians, Alaska Natives, Asians, Native Hawaiians, and Pacific Islanders does *not* explain the health disparities experienced by these groups compared with the white, non-Hispanic population in the United States. These disparities are believed to be the result of the complex interaction among genetic variations, environmental factors, and specific health behaviors (US DHHS 2000: 12–13; our emphasis).

Back to the main point we are trying to make in this chapter: The adoption of a modern concept of culture allows emotional experience to become variably important in structuring risk for diabetes because emotions are an essential aspect of knowledge— and therefore, of culture. We are *not* talking about "belief systems" or "Indian beliefs," but of Indigenous *sciences*—that is, highly structured systems of knowledge, which have their own internal logic. The equivalency of Indigenous taxonomies to scientific taxonomic categories was very well established in studies initiated in the late 1940s by the illustrious French anthropologist Claude Lévi-Strauss (1969 [1949]), launching much research in what became known as the ethnosciences. Furthermore, linking culture, knowledge and emotions offers fundamental insights into the association between the endocrine and the nervous systems—the autonomic nervous system in particular. Physiologically speaking, the relationship between emotional suffering as generated by traumatic experience, and elevated blood sugars—an important symptom of diabetes—has been established for over 100 years. Increased pituitary-adrenal and autonomic responses to stress and trauma have been linked to the onset of diabetes mellitus since the French physiologist Claude Bernard first showed, in 1877, that diabetes originates in the nervous system (Bernard 1877). The subjective aspects of emotions— sensations and feelings—intensify the activity of the autonomic nervous system (ANS), which produces alterations in cardiac frequency, blood pressure and concentration of blood sugars. Traumatic events and traumatic memory itself can result in a marked and eventually sustained hyperglycaemia, as clearly discussed by Jo Scheder, and Angele McGrady and Kim Gower-Dowling (see chapters 1, 11 and 15 in this volume).

Electing *knowledge*[4] as a major modality of culture (rather than norms, values, and behaviors) promotes an understanding of how distinct peoples experience the world and act upon it, including their feelings and thoughts about health and illness. The adoption of a modern concept of culture can help Indigenous Peoples devise analytic models with explanatory and predictive power, to understand what the factors that play a role in rendering them vulnerable to type 2 diabetes are. It can also help propose activities that strengthen Indigenous generosity and solidarity ties, allowing individuals—women in particular—to build self-esteem, stand up for themselves, grieve collectively in situations of distress, and seek reciprocal solutions to their problems alleviates emotional suffering. The suggested activities outlined below are also centered around the idea that emotional well-being has the potential to soothe the nervous system and bring heightened blood glucose levels down, combating the diabetes epidemic and allowing individuals to be in control of their health.

Touch the Heart of the People: Suggested Activities for a Theory of Cultural Rebuilding

What are the Yurok, Tolowa and Wiyot cultural knowledges and practices that can help promote social well-being at the Potawot Health Village? How can such wisdom be articulated with other health care models so as to enhance their preventive and therapeutic effects? Tolowa, Wiyot and Yurok community members have repeatedly requested that their collective strengths and remarkable qualities be continuously acknowledged at the Potawot Health Village.

Underlying all the activities here presented is the idea that the health of individuals is directly connected to the health of the land. The Potawot Restoration Area or *Ku'-wah-dah-wilth* ("Comes Back to Life," in the Yurok language) was designed to restore and protect wetlands, provide wildlife habitat, restore native plant communities and provide open space for cultural education and practices, passive recreation, organic food production, medical and basketry material gathering and spiritual meditation. *Ku'-wah-dah-wilth* preserves cultural and natural landscapes not only for the UIHS community but also for all people of California's North Coast region.

It is important to point out that before the inauguration of the Potowat Health Village in 2001, UIHS had already begun investing in a more holistic approach to health promotion based on "cultural health activities" since the early 1990s. Building upon "traditional Tribal teachings and activities," coalitions that have carried out activities among rural and urban communities in Northern California include: the Smith River Coalition, when Yurok and Tolowa elders showed participants how to catch and dry surf fish on sand beds, how to gather and prepare seaweed, and how to cook sand bread on the gravel and coals of the fire; the Klamath Coalition, in which knowledge regarding the gathering of traditional foods and materials for regalia and basketmak-

---

4. For historical and cultural information about the Yurok, Tolowa and Wiyot Peoples, see Collins 1997; Heizer & Mills 1991; Keeling 1993; Kroeber 1910, 1948, 1976, 1978; Nelson Jr. 1978; Pilling 1978; Thompson 1991; Waterman 1993.

ing was shared, as well as how boarding school experiences impacted the lives of tribal members; and the McKinleyville/Arcata Coalition, when stories on how ancestors took special care of themselves physically, mentally and spiritually were narrated during an "intergenerational walk and run" (Ferreira 1996). What we propose, here, is an intensification of these and other activities in a more systematic way, so as to promote emotional liberty based on Wiyot, Tolowa and Yurok expertise.

We hope the strategies outlined below efficiently replace the highly medicalized approach to health and disease that prevails in most medical facilities, with a more holistic, culturally sensitive and politically meaningful one. A theory of cultural rebuilding *empowers* the local people because it makes them an integral part of the healing process. A natural side-effect of such empowering programs is the automatic reduction of medical and pharmaceutical intervention, bringing a decrease in the amount of medications patients take on a regular basis. In the process, the notion of a healthy community moves away from the clinical and the industrial settings, back into where it belongs: *in the heart of the people.*

1. Women Support Groups[5]

Throughout history and across cultures, and religions women have been in the forefront as leaders in their communities. Native American Women are no exception; they are in the forefront, making changes to better their lives and the lives of their family and community.

When women come together in a "Women's Support Group," changes can be made. It is a wonderful experience to sit and talk among other women who are having similar life experiences and we can communicate openly without fear of judgment or embarrassment. We share a common ground and very often share the same hopes for our family and community.

Women Support Groups are exactly that, support for women. We come together on various levels: education, income, family units, life experiences, etc. The bonding that can take place in a support group is both wonderful and meaningful. The relationships that come together during a support group can last a lifetime. I remember, as a child in the summer, women young and old would gather at the creek to stay cool. They would be busy making baskets, cleaning berries, crocheting and listening to each other, sharing their knowledge and their lives. It was not called (at that time) a Woman's Support Group, but that is what it was.

> Twila Sanchez, Yurok Tribal Member and Support Group Facilitator. UIHS Diabetes Awareness Program, September 2000.

The recent history of Indigenous Peoples in northern California has shown that since the early 1900s, most households have become female headed. Yurok, Tolowa, Wiyot and other Indigenous women have been given the major responsibilities of making ends meet out of virtually nothing, and of dealing with the escalating problems of unemployment, drug abuse and domestic violence. Although rates of violence and drug abuse have increased for both males and females, the situation is especially alarming among single Indigenous mothers living in poverty. Adverse life conditions, in turn, lead to an

---

5. This section on Women's Support Groups draws on material originally presented at the 5th International Conference on Diabetes and Indigenous Peoples in Christchurch, New Zealand, in October 2000 (Sanchez & Ferreira 2000).

overall deterioration of Indigenous health and generate a myriad of social ailments, such as type 2 diabetes itself, domestic violence, depression, substance abuse and suicide.

Depressive disorders are of momentous concern for Indigenous Peoples. The governmental Indian Health Service program "Mental Health and Social Services" has recently recognized that "the level of psychosocial and emotional distress is high" in Indigenous communities.

> The improvements in physical health status for Indian populations have not been paralleled in the mental health and social services area. The workloads reported by field staff reflect serious mental and social problems in many AI/AN communities on reservations and in urban settings (IHS 1999).

Indian Health Service also asserts that mental health and social problems are associated with more than one-third of the demands made on health facilities for services. Depression, anxiety and post- traumatic stress disorder are emotional problems that are reported frequently in the agency's workload data. There are several indicators of the severity of the problem. Suicide rates rank about 2.4 times the national average for American Indian/Alaska Native males aged 15 to 34. The rate of homicide, and accidental death in young Indigenous males is about twice the national average. The homicide mortality rate for American Indian females 25 to 34 years of age is about 1.5 times that for the general U.S. population. Problems of alcohol abuse, depression and anxiety frequently underlie and complicate treatment for physical disorders and traumatic accidents, requiring considerable attention from caregivers (IHS 1999).

In northern California, current indicators of psychosocial stress point to the urgent need for further research among the Yurok, Karuk, and Wiyot nations that can lead to culturally sensitive and ethically grounded intervention and prevention services. For Humboldt and Del Norte counties American Indian youth, mental health issues of immediate concern are: a) school failure, b) the risk of removal from home, c) out-of - home placement in non-Indian foster care, d) the risk of violence, dysfunctional families who are dealing with depression, alcoholism, substance and tobacco abuse, spousal and/or sexual abuse, and e) the risk of suicide (UIHS 2000). The need for support groups is critical. Women are especially in need of support systems because they are the ones who end up bearing the burden of heading huge households and dealing with domestic violence, unemployment, etc. Because of their prominent positions in the last 50 years as tribal chairwomen, environmental leaders, health advocates and social justice and human rights defenders, they are the ones intensively dedicated to preserving and recreating cultural knowledges and practices, including teaching their own Indigenous languages to the children.

Recent studies have demonstrated that early adverse experiences play a preeminent role in the development of neurological disorders in adult life, thereby contributing to vulnerability to mental illness (Heim et al. 2000, Mullen et al. 1996, Nemeroff 1999, Stein et al. 1996). Women with a history of childhood sexual or physical abuse, for instance, exhibit more symptoms of depression and anxiety, and more frequently attempt suicide than women without a history of childhood abuse (Heim et al. 2000). Childhood abuse also predisposes to the development of anxiety disorders in adulthood, including panic disorder and generalized anxiety disorder (Pérez-Sales et al. 2000; Portegijs et al. 1996; Stein et al. 1996). Early parental loss, whether due to parental

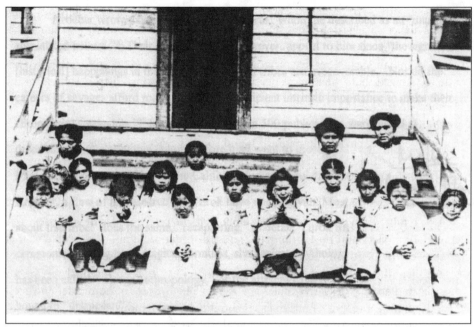

Yurok and Hupa girls at the Hoopa Boarding School in 1907. (Courtesy Mollie Ruud)

separation or premature death has also been found to increase the risk for major depression in case control and epidemiological studies (Agid et al. 1999; Brown & Dollery 1984; Furukawa et al. 1999; Mullen et al. 1996; Okley-Browne 1995; Roy 1985). In all these studies, nervous system hyperreactivity appears as a persistent consequence of childhood abuse that may contribute to the predisposition for type 2 diabetes.

In northern California, too, there is a strong, positive association between individuals who have experienced traumatic events, and individuals who have been diagnosed with type 2 diabetes, as we have demonstrated elsewhere (see chapters 3 and 14 in this book). The strong association between emotional suffering and the onset of type 2 diabetes has taken United Indian Health Services to promote women support groups at the Potawot Health Village and its satellite clinics. Diabetes patients, pregnant women and young mothers get together to strengthen solidarity ties, discuss preventive strategies and build community support for their own projects and initiatives. Such support groups are highly desirable because they allow the women to discuss their feelings, providing the bases for them to manage or "navigate" their emotions (Dressler and Bindon 2000). It makes women feel that what they think, say and do is important, and that other people care for them. "It makes us feel good about who we are and understand our desires," as Twila Sanchez, the organizer of women support groups at UIHS, recently put it. "If we want to create social well-being, we necessarily need to start by surveying women's current needs and aspirations. In order to propose solutions to diabetes and other problems, we definitely have to go back to the community and start from the bottom up, and not from the top."

Twila Sanchez, Bea Nix, Lavina Bowers, Susan Masten and other Indigenous women with extensive experience organizing and facilitating support groups for battered women in northern California, highly recommend the formation of such groups to generate emotional well-being and combat diabetes, depression, alcoholism and other ailments. Here is Twila Sanchez again, in 2003:

> **I cannot stress enough the importance** of offering a community diabetes support group at your health care facility. As a co-facilitator, participating in a support group, I have experienced a whole new perspective on ways people deal with their diabetes.
>
> A support group is multi-faceted. It can be a talking circle, a gathering place or a get together. It can be structures or unstructured. When to meet, where to meet, how often, how long—these are a few of the decisions the group can make. The participants set the rules or guidelines for the meetings. Our group has changed the norms many times, with confidentiality being respected by everyone.
>
> A support group gives folks a venue to express and recreate their feelings, concerns, fears, anxieties, and worries in the presence of other community people dealing with the same issues. They laugh, cry, console, advise, scold and coach each other on a regular basis. The friendships that grow from a support group and the support given and received cannot be measured in scientific terms but we know it works.
>
> Some people need to attend a support group once a week, others may drop in once a month, still others may attend twice a year.
>
> Attitudes and emotions are very important in dealing with diabetes and life style changes. A support group can help women and men understand they are not alone. Other people in the community have the same struggles, hardships, failures, successes and concerns.

2. Music Therapy: Sacred Songs and Chanted Prayers

Music is said to soothe the savage beast. Whether it be to soothe a snake back into a basket or to provide us with a night of entertainment, music has been with us in every shape, way and form since ancient times. What is it about music that makes it so appealing to us? If it were merely a cacophony of sounds, then it surely would not have lasted this long. It seems that music is something more, something that is capable of touching us on some deeper, almost spiritual level. What kind of music is able to do this well is up to the individual and the community—for some it could be Mozart, for others it could be Steppenwolf, and yet for others it could be Alvin and the Chipmunks. This creates an interesting question for us: If music can touch us in such ways, what else can it do for us? Better yet, how can music aid us in coping with our daily lives? This question is being partially dealt with by a new realm of therapies for the mind and the body, and one such therapy is music therapy.

> Amir Arman, poet and activist, 2000.

Music therapy is not really a new realm of research, and obviously not a novel way of creating sentiments with the use of melodies. Music therapy has been widespread throughout the world for millennia, predating ancient Greece and pervasive in China,

---

Potawot Health Village Diabetes Support Group/ Talking Group—Now Extended to Men!

Purpose: To bring people with diabetes together, in an informal setting, for support and education; and to deal with the emotional/psychological and practical issues of diabetes and its complications.

Method: The support group meets weekly for an hour and a half in a quiet and comfortable setting. The group is co-facilitated by an Indigenous member of the diabetes team and a clinical counselor. We begin each meeting seated in a circle for "socializing" and a healthy snack. Then each person does a "check-in," sharing events of the past week and describing such concerns as "blood sugars," and other diabetes related information. Participants also contribute successes and failures, strengths and goal setting. We share a lot of laughter and sometimes fears. Other family members who either provide support at home or are at risk for developing the signs and symptoms of diabetes are also part of the group. The facilitators are there to help keep the group moving, offer information, set a tone for positive conversation, but not to dominate. The group is like a family.

Results: People in the group feel like they are not alone in their distress and in their experience with diabetes. Participants learn new ways to cope with adversity, as well as have a "good" life despite (or even because of) diabetes. They gain in strength and in the desire to help others. A four-part professionally produced video called "Living with Diabetes" is just being completed, and it was the group's idea and energy from start to finish. It is intended to be shown in Indian country and will also be shown on our local public TV station in northern California.

Conclusion: A support group/talking circle focused on diabetes is powerful and helpful, as it combines education, culturally respectful approaches and resources, care and support to allow individuals with a chronic ailment to live a good life and teach others how to prevent complications or diabetes altogether.

India, Germany, and in Indigenous communities across the globe. Tolowa, Wiyot and Yurok community members in northern California maintain that sacred songs and chanted prayers have always exerted physical and social therapeutic effects in

---

STARTING A SUPPORT GROUP:

- Find a person willing to take a leadership role (**You** could be that person_)
- Make a request to initiate a support group to your health care facility/Diabetes Co-ordinator
- Talk to community people that suffer from diabetes about the support group
- Ask your community health representatives and other clinic staff to get the word out to the community
- Set deadlines
- Make a commitment to stay with it—sometimes the support activities can go on for months or even longer
- Be consistent in your day, time and meeting place
- Learn and enjoy the group!

Twila Sanchez, Administrative Assistant, Diabetes Awareness Program, and David Schaffer, Child and Family Services, United Indian Health Services, Inc., 2002.

their lives. The healing power of music in northern California has been documented in a few anthropological studies (Ferreira 1996; Keeling 1993, 1997; Lang 1993; Margolin 1993). These studies attest that for centuries, Yurok, Wiyot, and Tolowa peoples have resorted to music in their daily lives as well as in specific therapeutic rituals, such as Brush Dances and World Renewal Ceremonies. However, the systematic use of songs and chanted prayers in everyday life suffered a great blow when 1) American Indian children were not allowed to speak their languages (and violently punished if they did so) during the period in which they were confined in boarding schools (approximately from 1890 to 1940); and 2) when American Indian religious practices were discriminated against and prohibited in California and all over the United States, for that matter, with the *Major Crimes Act* in 1885 (Wilkins 2002). Today, the process of cultural rebuilding at the Potawot Health Village includes a special effort to restore the daily and ceremonial use of songs and chanted prayers in community life.

The use of music therapy in a clinical setting, at patients' homes, and at social gatherings broadly speaking can greatly enhance the project of cultural rebuilding, as well as exert a therapeutic effect on patients and in the community at large. In the medical literature, music, and more specifically music therapy appears as a therapeutic technique that reduces anxiety and stress levels, and lowers blood sugars (Alexander 2001; Howard 2001; Khalfa et al. 2003; Knight 2001; Salamon et al. 2003). Music influences human action by affecting the brain and subsequently other bodily structures in ways that are observable, identifiable, measurable, and predictable, thereby providing the necessary foundation for therapeutic applications. Such types of psychoacoustic treatments have only recently begun to receive serious consideration from the medical establishment as an effective way to lower cortisol levels—a hormone that has been linked to depression, heart disease, hypertension, diabetes and various other ailments of the industrialized world. Music therapy is a culturally significant technique and an inexpensive one that has great potential to help restore the equilibrium of healthy Indigenous lifestyles that were dramatically damaged in the past 150 years in northern California and all over the world, for that matter.

Music Therapy Websites

An interesting website to visit is The American Music Therapy Association. The mission of the American Music Therapy Association is to advance public awareness of the benefits of music therapy and increase access to quality music therapy services in a rapidly changing world. <www.musictherapy.org>.

Other websites of note on music therapy include:

- Native Reign. A Northern Cheyenne performing group that combines traditional Indigenous dances, skits, with contemporary music to celebrate the history and traditions of the Cheyenne nation.
  <www.loc.gov/bicentennial/propage/MT/mt_s_baucus4.html>.

- VOICES. A World Forum for Music Therapy <www.voices.no>.

- Center for Music Therapy <www.centerformusictherapy.com>.

- Music Therapy Info Link <http://hometown.aol.com/kathysl/index.html>.

- British Society for Music Therapy <www.bsmt.org>.

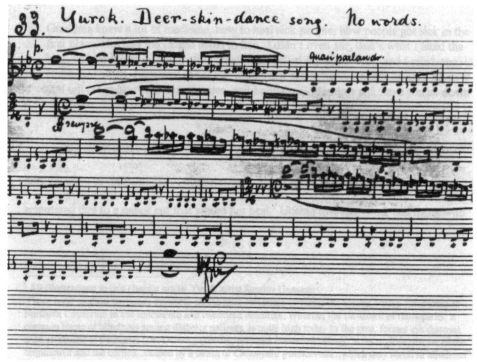

Yurok Deer Skin Dance song. No words. (Courtesy Mollie Ruud)

- Music as Therapy <www.m-a-t.freeserve.co.uk>.
- Music Therapy Education <http://music-therapy-education.com>.
- Music Therapy.cc <www.musictherapy.cc>.

3. Art Therapy: Basket Weaving, Beading, and Abalone Carving

The salutary force of traditional artistic productions, such as basket weaving, beading, abalone carving, among other sacred Indigenous creations can also exert a beneficial effect on the physical and emotional well-being of local community members. These and other artistic creations are culturally significant to the Tolowa, Wiyot, and Yurok peoples and have the power to promote and/or elevate the self-esteem of children, adults, and elders. Art therapy is the therapeutic use of art making, within a professional relationship, by people who experience illness, trauma, or challenges in living, and by people who seek personal development. Through creating art and reflecting on the art products and processes, people can increase awareness of self and others, cope with symptoms, stress, and traumatic experiences, enhance cognitive abilities, and enjoy the life-affirming pleasures of making art (Parvy 2004; Tavares 2003; Weinstein 1998).

Interesting websites on Indigenous Art, with many ideas for workshops and creative artistic activities, include the following:

- Indian Arts and Crafts Association <www.iaca.com/update/frames2.htm>.

- Native Tech. Native American Technology and Art <www.nativetech.org>.
- Native American Indian Art <www.kstrom.net/isk/art/art.html>.
- Native American Fine Art <www.3mesas.com>.
- Native Music and Arts Organizations <www.nativeculture.com/lisamitten/ music.html>.
- Native American Art Show <www.nativeamericanartshow.com>.
- Native American Art <http://stepintothegarden.com/links/nativeamericanart.html>.

The following websites bring valuable information on the benefits of art therapy:

- Art Therapy—Institute of the Redwoods <www.pacificsites.com/~arttherapy>.
- Midwest Festival of Expressive Arts Therapies <www.dcs.wisc.edu/pda/ex-pressive-therapies/?source=overture>.
- American Art Therapy Association <www.arttherapy.org>.
- The British Association of Art Therapists <www.baat.org>.
- Arts in Therapy Network <www.artsintherapy.com>.

4. History Telling

We suggest enhancing the practice of history telling for different audiences: internal workshops at Potawot and UIHS satellite clinics, as well as for the more general public in local schools, cultural centers, etc. Showing outsiders the cultural strengths and political engagement of local communities promotes a positive image of Indigenous Peoples. In turn, internal workshops focused on historical testimonies about the gold rush, boarding school experiences, termination policies, and racial discrimination, for example, can provide community members with opportunities to grieve in more efficient ways, and generate discussion about effective coping mechanisms. Various recent studies show the psychological benefits of identifying the most meaningful characters in the social imaginary and narrating its experience, in the sense that "stories are weapons against disease," as the Swiss writer W. M. Diggelmann put it (De Oliveira et al. 2003; Schmid 2001).

Interesting websites that deal with the importance of Indigenous Peoples' history telling, as well as the process of collecting and archiving the products of the Native press and materials related to Native press history; collecting and documenting the works of Native writers, and constructing bibliographic guides to Native writing and publishing, include the following:

- Storytellers. Native American Authors Online. <www.hanksville.org/story-tellers>.
- OYATE. A Native organization working to see that our lives and histories are portrayed honestly (Includes workshop on oral history) <www.oyate.org>.
- American Native Press Archives <www.anpa.ualr.edu>.
- Wordcraft Circle of Native Writers and Storytellers. <www.wordcraftcircle. org>.

> **THE RIGHT TO FOOD: KEY FACTS**
>
> **Rome Declaration on World Food Security, 1996**
> "We, the Heads of State and Government…reaffirm the right of everyone to have access to safe and nutritious food, consistent with the right to adequate food and the fundamental right of everyone to be free from hunger."
>
> **International Covenant on Economic, Social and Cultural Rights, 1966**
> "The States Parties to the present Covenant recognize the right of everyone to an adequate standard of living…including adequate food…" and agree to take appropriate steps to realize this right. *Article 11(1)*
>
> **Universal Declaration of Human Rights, 1948**
> "Everyone has the right to a standard of living adequate for the health and well-being of himself and of his family, including food…" *Article 25 (1)*

- A Spirit Talk Gathering. Dedicated to The Continued Advancement of World Health Through Healing Body, Mind, & Spirit of All Creators Manifestations! <www.spiritalk.net>.

- The National Council on Alcoholism and Drug Dependence. Cultural Enhancement Through Story Telling. <www.ncadd.org/programs/treatment/ cets.html>.

- Native American Public Telecommunications. Empowering, Educating and Entertaining through Native Media <www.nativetelecom.org>.

- Native American Journalists Association <www.naja.com>.

5. The Right to Food: Traditional Food Gathering and Preparation

Access to quality, nutritious food has become a human rights issue for Indigenous Peoples globally since everyone has the fundamental right to be free from hunger and undernutrition. There are profound contradictions between the dominant economic and clinical visions of what a "healthy diet" is, and the situation of hunger and scarcity that prevails in Indigenous communities, as clearly documented in Part 2 of this book (see chapters by Omura, Roy, Smith Morris, Lang, and Korn & Ryser). The curing power of food gathering and preparation can only be effective if Indigenous Peoples' Right to Food is respected. The realization of this fundamental right requires not only equitable and sustainable food systems, but also entitlements relating to livelihood security such as the right to work, land reform and social security.

In addition, the therapeutic force of traditional foods becomes more effective if and only if individuals have access to sacred and practical knowledges about these foods, and to the practices of gathering and preparation. From local to international levels, there is a growing understanding of how culturally important Indigenous Peoples' traditional subsistence foods are to the overall well-being of their communities. Health professionals usually consider only nutritional standards and sometimes economic aspects when prescribing "healthy" diets. Cultural standards are frequently ignored or deemed unhealthy, especially for individuals suffering from or at risk for diabetes. The political and spiritual aspects of food are rarely taken into consideration in biomedical settings. This right to food and the so-called taste of necessity (Bourdieu 1986), as discussed by several authors in Part II of this book, are essential to reframe the diabetes question from the perspective of Indigenous Peoples themselves. Taking the Right to Food into consideration in clinical settings allows health professionals to make informed and safe recommendations about the nutritious, curative and spiritual powers of Indigenous foods. Gathering trips, experimental kitchens, the confection of cookbooks, and the video documentation of traditional dietary practices for a healthy lifestyle are activities that can readily be implemented to improve Indigenous Peoples' social and emotional well-being.

The Right to Food. Indigenous Peoples International Consultations on the Right to Food

[...] The spiritual and physical relationship of Indigenous Peoples to their lands as a human right is a basic principle in international human rights law that is recognized universally. Indigenous Peoples have relied for millennia on their lands and natural resources for their means of subsistence and for their cultural, physical and spiritual survival. There is no need to expand on the physical, spiritual and cultural reliance and relationship of the Gwichi'n and Sammi Peoples on caribou and reindeer, the Macaw on their whales, the Maya on their corn, the Masai on their cattle. It is found in our traditions and song, in our ceremony, in our relationship with the natural world. This relationship is recognized in international human rights instruments, the studies of experts, and in many declarations, all calling for the recognition, protection and enjoyment of Indigenous Peoples' right to their lands and the practice of their cultures, languages and religions.

It is true that in parts of the world, Indigenous Peoples have grown to rely on wages within the dominant economy and culture for food and the basic necessities of life. Forced from their lands through outright theft of land, loss of territory, and ruination of their environment, urbanization of Indigenous Peoples is a trend that is in full rigor. But in most parts of the world where Indigenous Peoples still live in community, practicing their own cultures, languages and traditions, they still rely on traditional means of subsistence in harmony and relationship with our mother Earth. They produce their own food and provide for themselves their major means of subsistence. For Indigenous Peoples this is a collective endeavor. As Fernando Cardenal once wrote, the first act of culture is the sharing of food. [6]

Many Indigenous Peoples recognize that change must come and that their societies and cultures will have to change, to adapt to the modern world. But the determination to remain who they are, to fully enjoy their human rights and fundamental freedoms as Indigenous Peoples, is constant. The struggle for our human rights is not against change but only against that change that takes and destroys our lands, change that is imposed upon us forcibly and violently. The struggle continues to be against the gross and massive violations of our human rights as Peoples. Article 1 in Common[7] recognizes that Indigenous Peoples have a right to

---

6. Fernando Cardenal is a Nicaraguan Jesuit and the first Minister of Education in the Sandinista government in Nicaragua [authors' note].

7. "Article 1 in Common" is Article 1 of both the UN International Covenant on Civil and Political Rights and the International Covenant on Economic, Social and Cultural Rights. It is identical in both Covenants: 1. All peoples have the right of self-determination. By virtue of that right they freely determine their political status and freely pursue their economic, social and cultural development. 2. All peoples may, for their own ends, freely dispose of their natural wealth and resources without prejudice to any obligations arising out of international economic co-operation, based upon the principle of mutual benefit, and international law. In no case may a people be deprived of its own means of subsistence. 3. The States Parties to the present Covenant, including those having responsibility for the administration of Non-Self-Governing and Trust Territories, shall promote the real-

freely determine their own priorities in development and their own pace of development. We only struggle against violations of our human rights and fundamental freedoms that break the relationship with our lands and territories and destroy our identity, not only as individuals, but more importantly as Peoples. It is as Peoples that we are Indigenous.

Indigenous Peoples are Peoples. The right to food for Indigenous Peoples is tied to their right to their lands and the resources the land provides. As Peoples, they cannot be deprived of their means of subsistence. We struggle as Peoples to implement our own vision of development, our own process of development and our own right to food. [...]

From International Indian Treaty Council (IITC 2002); excerpt reproduced with permission. See <www.treatycouncil.org> for more information on the Right to Food.

Interesting websites that deal with Indigenous rights and practices about food, include the following:

- International Indian Treaty Council (IITC), Right to Food. Includes the IITC Right to Food Bulletin, and various links to IITC interventions to the United Nations, such as the Permanent Forum on Indigenous Issues, First Session, in New York, May 2002, on the Right to Food, Food Security and Food Sovereignty. <www.treatycouncil.org/new_page_5241.htm>.
- Indigenous Environmental Network, "Right to Food and Food Security" <www.ienearth.org/food_security.html>.
- Declaration of the World Food Summit <www.fao.org/worldfoodsummit>.
- Traditional Food, Health and Nutrition <www.kstrom.net/isk/food/foodmenu.html>.

Selected references on American Indian Foods and Indigenous cookbooks:

- Food and Culture, references http://lilt.ilstu.edu/rtdirks/NOAMERIND.html
- Selected references on American Indian Foods, Smithsonian Institute <www.nmnh.si.edu/anthro/outreach/food.html>.
- Native Way Cookbook. Cookbook of the Grandmothers. <www.wisdomkeepers.org/nativeway>.
- Native American Cooking Books <www.accessory-finder.com/native-american-cooking-books.asp>.
- Delicious Foods and Recipes from American Indian Peoples <www.cookingpost.com>.
- Native American Indian Cooking. Recipes from the Southwest and more. <www.omega23.com/books/s5/s11i0299nativeamericancooking.html>.
- NATIVETEC: Native American Technology and Art <www.nativetech.org/food>.

---

ization of the right of self-determination, and shall respect that right, in conformity with the provisions of the Charter of the United Nations.

Final Thoughts

The emotional aspects of culture bring tremendous insights into how we think about individual and community health. The theoretical basis for cultural rebuilding, in the opinion of community members, should be centered around the notions of emotional liberty and emotional suffering, taking into consideration a politically meaningful history of emotions of California peoples (here discussed in detail in Chapter 14).

Showing how emotions change over time, and how they relate to projects of sovereignty and liberation, in the context of oppression and domination can be instrumental in building a conceptual and theoretical framework for cultural rebuilding in the context of individual and community health. Such a theory should, from the very start, acknowledge the importance of the construction and management of emotion among individuals and communities in northern California. Adopting a conception of culture that values knowledge and power as its major components encourages us to attend to the pragmatic, political and historical dimensions of emotional experience, focusing on the ways in which power relations and discourses of emotion are tied together. This means, among other things, revealing not only what can, cannot or must be said about self and emotion, what is taken to be true or false about them, and what only some individuals can do about them, but also how emotion discourses establish, assert, challenge, or reinforce power or status differences. By following anthropologists interested in ethnopsychology (Averill 1994; De Sousa 1987; Lutz 1985, 1990; Lutz and Abu-Lughod 1990), emotion is here conceived as to offer culture and individual specific interpretations of social action, and to provide culture and specific motivations for social action—all in a language that is strongly bound in relations of power.

In sum, if we adopt Tolowa, Wiyot and Yurok conceptions of culture, emotional experience becomes of key importance in the process of rebuilding culture. The adoption of such modern conceptions of culture can help Indigenous Peoples—in both North and South America, and all over the world, for that matter—devise analytic models with explanatory and predictive power for understanding what are the factors that play a role in rendering Indigenous Peoples vulnerable to diabetes, cancer, hypertension, heart disease and other disorders. A theoretical model for cultural rebuilding should necessarily help Indigenous populations provide for the social well-being of their communities and thus regain control of their health situation.

By sponsoring cultural activities at Potawot, community solidarity ties have been strengthened and the basis for the recreation of a system of reciprocity laid out. The Potawot Health Village is now further investing in the promotion of social and emotional well-being in the Indigenous communities it services in northern California. This involves, among other things, creating opportunities for community members to share cultural knowledges and practices within the Potawot complex. Programs need to be built on spiritually and scientifically grounded theories and models, rather than on speculations about putative genetic or biologic features that Indigenous Peoples share in the U.S. or elsewhere. Furthermore, the explanatory and predictive power of any analytic model needs to be grounded in the ethics of social justice.

In order to elucidate the links among domination, demoralization and disordered emotional experience, which afflict American Indian communities in the U.S., Indigenous health initiatives should, in our opinion, (1) reconsider the diabetic experience within a broader semantic domain that extends well beyond the narrowly defined biologic and genetic condition into the realms of social relations, history and Indigenous identity, which can lead us to (2) consider type 2 diabetes as a *reaction* of the organism to adverse life conditions, rather than a morbid or pathological phenomenon superimposed on the organism. [8] In this respect, and if we consider emotional experience—especially traumatic memory—as variably important for structuring risk for type 2 diabetes, we strongly believe that it will take *emotional liberty*, among other things, to free Indigenous Peoples from the deleterious effects of the diabetes epidemic. As defined by anthropologist W. Reddy (1999), emotional liberty is the freedom to change goals in response to bewildering, ambivalent situations, and to undergo conversion experiences and life-course changes involving numerous contrasting incommensurable factors. What emotional liberty means for Indigenous Peoples and individuals at risk for diabetes and correlated illnesses, however, will depend on what each and every one of them define as social and emotional well-being.

Acknowledgments

We want to thank Yurok, Tolowa and Wiyot community members who have dedicated much of their time and wisdom to the process of cultural rebuilding at the Potawot Health Village. We also want to thank health professionals, especially Dr. Terry Raymer, the Board of Directors of United Indian Health Services (UIHS) and Jerry Simone, Executive Director of UIHS, for their support. Thanks are also due to the California Endowment, which has continuously supported United Indian Health Services and the construction of the Potawot Health Village. The authors greatly appreciate all the effort that Gretchen Lang, the co-editor of this book, put into this chapter. Last but not least, To all our relations!

References

Agid, O., B. Shapira and J. Zislin. 1999. Environment and Vulnerability to Major Psychiatric Illness: A Case Control of Early Parental Loss in Major Depression, Bipolar Ddisorder and Schizophrenia. Molecular Psychiatry 4: 163–72.

Ahmed, Akbar. 2002. "Ethnic Cleansing': A Metaphor For Our Time? *In* Genocide. An Anthropological Reader. Alexander Hinton, ed. Malden, MA: Blackwell Publishers.

Alexander, M. 2001. The Charms of Music. Step by Step Prescription for Patients. North Carolina Medical Journal Mar–Apr. 62(2): 91–94.

---

8. This is what the French physiologist Claude Bernard (1877) proposed more than 100 years ago, when he went against theories of his day and argued that the symptoms of diabetes (*excessive* urination, thirst and sugar in both the blood and the urine), save for their *intensity*, are known to the normal, physiological state.

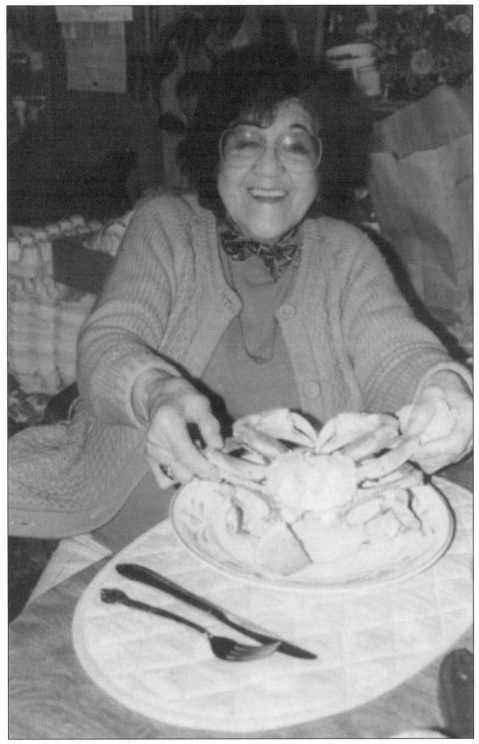

Aileen Figueroa, Yurok singer and teacher of the Yurok language, in 1996. Photo: Mariana L. Ferreira.

Averill, J. 1994. Emotions Unbecoming and Becoming. *In* The Nature of Emotions: Fundamental Questions. P. Ekman and R. Davidson, eds. Oxford: Oxford University Press

Barth, Fredrik. 1995. Other Knowledge and Other Ways of Knowing. Journal of Anthropological Research 51: 65–67.

Bernard, Claude. 1877. Leçons sur le Diabète et la Glycogenèse Animale. Londres; Madrid: Librairie J.-B. Baillière et Fils.

Bourdieu, Pierre. 1986. Distinction: A Social Critique of the Judgement of Taste. New York: Taylor & Francis Books.

Brown, M. J. and C. T. Dollery. 1984. Adrenaline and Hypertension. Clinical Experiments in Hypertension 6(1-2): 539–49.

Collins, James. 1997. Understanding Tolowa Histories: Western Hegemonies and Native American Responses. New York: Routledge.

De Oliveira, C., F. B. de Oliveira, M. L. Fortunato and A. O. Silva. 2003. Madness in Freedom: Experiences in Crato-CE (1930–1970). Revista Brasileira de Enfermagem Mar-Apr; 56(2): 138–42.

De Sousa, R. 1987. The Rationality of Emotion. Cambridge, MA: MIT Press.

Dressler, William and James Bindon. 2000. The Health Consequences of Cultural Consonance: Cultural Dimensions of Lifestyle, Social Support, and Arterial Blood Pressure in an African Community. American Anthropologist 102(2): 244–60.

Farmer, Paul. 2003. Pathologies of Power. Health, Human Rights, and the New War on the Poor. Berkeley, Los Angeles & London: University of California Press.

———1996. On Suffering and Structural Violence: A View from Below. Daedalus. Special Issue on Social Suffering 125(1): 261–83.

Ferreira, Mariana K. Leal. 2004(in press). The Color Red. Fighting with Fruits and Flowers in Xavante Territory, Central-Brazil. *In* Art and Music in a Globalizing Latin America. M. Ferreira, M. Suhrbier and U. Prinz, eds. Indiana (journal), Special Issue [Ibero-American Institute, Berlin].

———2002a. Tupi-Guarani Apocalyptic Visions of Time and the Body. Journal of Latin American Anthropology 7(1): 128–69.

———2002b. Diabetes tipo 2 e povos indígenas no Brasil e nos Estados Unidos. Cultura, Saúde e Doença. Londrina: Universidade Estadual de Londrina.

———2001. Cultural Integrity, Social Inequality, and Community Health. A Report to the Evaluation Committee of the Potawot Health Village. Arcata: United Indian Health Services.

———1999. Corpo e História do Povo Yurok. [Body and History of the Yurok People] Revista de Antropologia Universidade de São Paulo vol 41 (2): 17–39.

———1998. Slipping Through Sky Holes. Yurok Perceptions of the Body in Northern California. Culture, Medicine and Psychiatry 22(2): 171–202.

———1996. Sweet Tears and Bitter Pills. The Politics of Health among the Yuroks in Northern California. Unpublished Doctoral Dissertation, University of California at Berkeley and at San Francisco.

Ferreira, Mariana Leal and Bea Nix. 2000. 'Look Inside My Heart:' Applying a Modern Concept of Culture to the Study of type 2 Diabetes. Paper presented at the 5th

International Conference on Diabetes and Indigenous Peoples, Christchurch, New Zealand, Oct 3–6, 2000.

Foucault, Michel. 1978. The Right of Death and Power over Life. *In* History of Sexuality. New York: Random House.

_____1975 [1963]. The Birth of the Clinic. An Archaeology of Medical Perception. New York: Vintage Books.

Furukawa, T. A., A. Ogura, T. Hirai, S. Fujihara, T. Kitamura and R. Takahashi. 1999. Early Parental Separation Experiences among Patients with Bipolar Disorder and Major Depression: A Case Control Study. Journal of Affective Disorders 52: 85–91.

Gupta, Akhil and James Ferguson. 1992. Beyond 'Culture': Space, Identity, and the Politics of Difference. Cultural Anthropology 7(1): 6–15.

Heim, C. J Newport, S. Heit, Y. Graham, M. Wilcox, R. Bonsall, A. Miller and C. Nemeroff. 2000. Pituitary-Adrenal and Autonomic Responses to Stress in Women after Sexual and Physical Abuse in Childhood. Journal of the American Medical Association 284(5): 592–97.

Heizer, R. and J. Mills. 1991 [1952]. The Four Ages of Tsurai. A Documentary History of the Indian Village on Trinidad Bay. Berkeley, Los Angeles and London: University of California Press.

Hobsbawm, Eric and Terence Ranger, eds. 1992. Invention of Tradition. Cambridge: Cambridge University Press.

Howard, B. 2001. Sweet the Sound. Music in Medicine. North Carolina Medical Journal May-Jun; 62(3): 166–70.

Indian Health Service (IHS)/Mental Health Services. 1999. "2001 Budget Request." IHS-48 MENTAL HEALTH SERVICES Indian Health Service Clinical Services Albuquerque, NM.

International Indian Treaty Council (IITC). 2002. Briefing Paper, Indigenous Peoples International Consultations on the Right to Food. Pahajachel, Solola, Guatemala, April 17–19, 2002.

Keeling, Richard. 1993. Cry for Luck. Sacred Song and Speech among the Yurok, Hupa, and Karok Indians of Northwestern California. Berkeley and Los Angeles: University of California Press.

_____1997. North American Indian Music : A Guide to Published Sources and Selected Recordings. (Garland Library of Music Ethnology) New York: Garland Publishing.

Khalfa, S., S. D. Bella, M. Roy, I. Peretz and S. J. Lupien. 2003. Effects of Relaxing Music on Salivary Cortisol Level after Psychological Stress. Annual New York Academy of Science 999: 374–76.

Knight, Rickard. 2001. Relaxing Music Prevents Stress-induced Increases in Subjective Anxiety, Systolic Blood Pressure, and Heart Rate in Healthy Males and Females. Journal of Music Therapy. 38(4): 254–72.

Kroeber, Alfred L. 1910. Yurok. *In* Handbook of American Indians North of Mexico. F.W. Hodge, ed. Vol. 2, Bulletin 30. Washington: Bureau of American Ethnology.

_____1948. Anthropology. New York: Harcourt, Brace.

_____1976. [1925] Handbook of the Indians of California. New York: Dover.

_____1978. Yurok Myths. Berkeley: University of California Press.

Lang, Julian. 1993. Ppethivthaaneen. *In* The Way We Lived. California Indian Stories, Songs, and Reminiscences. M. Margolin, ed..Berkeley, CA: Heyday Books.

Lévi-Strauss, Claude. 1969 [1949]. The Elementary Structures of Kinship. Boston: Beacon Press.

Lutz, Catherine. 1990. Engendered Emotion: Gender, Power, and the Rhetoric of Emotional Control in American Discourse. *In* Language and the Politics of Emotion. C. Lutz and L. Abu-Lughod, eds. Cambridge: Cambridge University Press.

_____1985. Depression and the Translation of Emotional Worlds. *In* Culture and Depression. Arthur Kleinman and Byron Good, eds. Berkeley, Los Angeles and London: University of California Press.

Lutz, Catherine and L. Abu-Lughod, eds. 1990. Language and the Politics of Emotion. Cambridge: Cambridge University Press.

Margolin, Malcolm, ed. 1993 [1981]. The Way We Lived. California Indian Stories, Songs, and Reminiscences. Berkeley, CA: Heyday Books.

Mullen, P. E., J. Martin and J. Anderson. 1996. The Long-term Impact of the Physical, Emotional, and Sexual Abuse of Children: A Community Study. Child Abuse and Neglect 20: 7–21.

Neel, James. 1962. Diabetes Mellitus: A 'Thrifty' Genotype Rendered Detrimental by 'Progress'. American Journal of American Genetics 14: 353–62.

_____1982. The Thrifty Genotype Revisited. The Genetics of Diabetes Mellitus.*In* Seron Symposium, No. 47. J. Kobberling and R. Tattersall, eds., pp. 283–93. New York: Academic Press.

Nelson Jr., Byron. 1978. Our Home Forever. A Hupa Tribal History. Hoopa, CA: The Hupa Tribe.

Nemeroff, C.B. 1999. The Preeminent Role of Early Untoward Experience on Vulnerability to Major Psychiatric Disorders: The Nature-Nurture Controversy Revisited and Soon to be Resolved. Molecular Psychiatry 4: 106–8.

Okley-Browne, M.A., P.R. Joyce, J.E. Wells, J.A. Bushnell and A.R. Hornblow. 1995. Disruptions in Childhood Parental Care as Risk Factors for Major Depression in Adult Women. Australian NZ Journal of Psychiatry 29: 437–48.

Parvy, P. 2004. Art and Therapy: A Good Encounter. Soins Psychiatry Mar-Apr; (231): 35–37.

Pérez-Sales P., T. Durán-Pérez and R.B. Herzfeld. 2000. Long-term Psychosocial Consequences in First-degree Relatives of People Detained, Disappeared or Executed for Political Reasons in Chile. A Study of Mapuce and Non-Mapuce Persons. Psicothema 12: 109–16.

Pilling, Arnold. 1978. Yurok. In Handbook of North American Indians. Vol 8: 137–54. Washington: Smithsonian Institute.

Pino, Manuel and Mariana Ferreira (forthcoming). Take Our Word For It. Indigenous Peoples of Turtle Island. Wadsworth Publishing Co.

Portegijs, P.J.M., F.M.H. Jeuken, F.G. van der Horst, H.F. Kraan and J.A. Knottnerus. 1996. A Troubled Youth: Relations with Somatization, Depression and Anxiety in Adulthood. Family Practitioner 13: 1–11.

Preis, Ann-Belinda. 1996. Human Rights as Cultural Practice: An Anthropological Critique. Human Rights Quarterly 18(2): 286–315.

Reddy, W. 1999. Emotional Liberty: Politics and History in the Anthropology of Emotions. Cultural Anthropology 14(2): 256–88.

Redner, Barbara. 1982. The Wolf Chief's Son. In Our People Speak. An Anthology of Indian Writing. Students at Humboldt State University, eds. Arcata, CA: Humboldt State University/Indian Teacher Education and Preparation Program (ITEPP)/Redwood Writing Project

Roy, A. 1985. Early Parental Separation and Adult Depression. Archives of General Psychiatry 42: 987–91.

Salamon, E., M. Kim, J. Beaulieu and G. B. Stefano. 2003. Sound Therapy-Induced Relaxation: Down-Regulating Stress Processes and Pathologies. Medical Science Monitor 9(5): 96–101.

Sanchez, Twila and Mariana Ferreira. 2000. From the Bottom Up: Women Support Groups Reduce Risk for type 2 Diabetes among Indigenous Peoples. Paper presented at the 5th International Conference on Diabetes and Indigenous Peoples in Christchurch, New Zealand, October 3–6, 2000.

Savage, Jan. 2000. Ethnography and Health Care (Education and Debate). British Medical Journal Dec. 2, 2000. 321: 1400–2.

Scheper-Hughes, Nancy and Philippe Bourgois, eds. 2004. Violence in War and Peace. An Anthology. Malden, MA: Blackwell Publishing.

Schmid, H. J. 2001. Walter Matthias Diggelmann—The Healing Effect of Story Telling. Schweiz Rundsch Medical Praxis Jun 21, 90(25–26): 1148–50.

Stein, M. B., J. R. Walker and G. Anderson. 1996. Childhood Physical and Sexual Abuse in Patients with Anxiety Disorders in a Community Sample. American Journal Psychiatry 153: 235–39.

Tavares, C. M. 2003. Role of Art at the Psychosocial Assistance Centers—CAPS. Revista Brasileira de Enfermagem Jan–Feb., 56(1): 35–39.

Thompson, Lucy. 1991 [1916]. To the American Indian. Reminiscences of a Yurok Woman. Eureka, CA: Cummins Printing Co. Reprinted by Heyday Books, Berkeley, CA.

United Indian Health Services (UIHS). 2000. Department of Child and Family Services, Arcata.

U.S. Department of Health and Human Services (DHHS). 2000. Healthy People 2010 (Conference Edition, in 2 Volumes). Washington DC.

Waterman, T. T. 1993 [1920]. Yurok Geography. Trinidad, CA: Trinidad Museum Society.

Weinstein, E. 1998. Elements of the Art of Practice in Mental Health. American Journal of Occupational Therapy 52(7): 579–85.

Weir, Robert, Susan Lawrence and Evan Fales, eds. 1994 . Genes and Human Self-Knowledge: Historical and Philosophical Reflections on Modern Genetics. Iowa: University of Iowa Press.

Wilkins, David E. 2002. American Indian Politics and the American Political System. Lanham, MD: Rowman and Littlefield Publishers.

Williams, Robert, Jeffrey C. Long, Robert L. Hanson, Maurice L. Sievers and William C. Knowler. 2000. Individual Estimates of European Genetic Admixture Associated with Lower Body-Mass Index, Plasma Glucose, and Prevalence of Type 2 Diabetes in Pima Indians. American Journal of Human Genetics 66: 527–38.

CHAPTER 19

Culture Blindness? Aboriginal Health, 'Patient Non-Compliance' and the Conceptualisation of Difference in Australia's Northern Territory[1]

Kim Humphery

Can I just say too, I don't think it's just an Aboriginal problem. It's a problem in our culture too, you know…I don't like Aboriginal people or 'non-compliance' being labelled as a 'cultural thing' because, once again, doing home nursing in white culture you'd often go and find, you know, the elderly person on chronic meds and they've always missed a few, you know, and that's not an Aboriginal thing…

Remote Area Registered Nurse, Northern Territory, Australia, 1998

Summary of Chapter 19. Designed primarily as a discussion piece, this chapter briefly explores the thinking of a group of Australian health professionals in relation to the notion of 'cultural difference'—understood in common-sense rather than theoretically reflexive terms. In particular, the paper interrogates the manner in which non-Indigenous medical practitioners and registered nurses involved in the provision of services to Aboriginal people in Australia's Northern Territory (NT) tend to reduce the experienced difficulties of such work to issues of cultural disjunction. In offering such an analysis, the chapter draws on a recent qualitative study into the perceptions and experiences of both Indigenous and non-Indigenous health professionals working in the NT and offering services to Aboriginal people through various government and community-based agencies. This larger study—known as the Rethinking Compliance project—was undertaken within the Cooperative Research Centre for Aboriginal and Tropical Health centred in Darwin and grew, in part, out of earlier research under-

---

1. This paper draws extensively on research undertaken in the Northern Territory from 1997 to 2001 in collaboration with Tarun Weeramanthri and Joe Fitz under the auspices of the Darwin-based Cooperative Research Centre for Aboriginal and Tropical Health (CRCATH). I am most grateful to Tarun and Joe, and to the CRCATH, for permission to draw on this work.

taken on the lived experience of diabetes within remote NT Aboriginal communities (Humphery et al. 2001, 1998).

♣   ♣   ♣

Throughout this paper I will use the term 'Aboriginal' rather more so than 'Indigenous', in recognition of the fact that in a Northern Territory context the former term is more appropriate than the latter—since 'Indigenous' is usually utilised in Australia as a rubric term for both Aboriginal and Torres Strait Islander peoples. It is also important, right from the outset, to note some of the politics of this language. These rubric designations remain utilised by *both* Indigenous and non-Indigenous Australians as referential terms, as problematic 'namings'. Thus, within the nationwide network of Indigenous controlled, community-based health services, such groupings are routinely referred to as Aboriginal Health Services. Likewise, while strenuously emphasising the socio-cultural diversity existing amongst Indigenous Australians, many Aboriginal and Torres Strait Islander people continue to utilise this seemingly 'homogenising' terminology for important strategic political and identificatory purposes. Nevertheless, this is also accompanied by both entrenched and emergent 'namings' adopted by Indigenous Australians to signal cultural diversity. Thus, in south-eastern Australia the term 'Koori' is dominant as a way of referring to people attached to a loosely defined south-eastern geographic area (and this is increasingly being made more complex through accompanying identification by language group). In the Northern Territory, many Aboriginal people identify through their language group first and foremost, but will utilise as well the more general term: Aboriginal. The important point to note is that amongst most non-Indigenous Australians there is a continuing propensity to elide these cultural diversities when using the terms Aboriginal and Indigenous, whereas the use of these terms by Indigenous Australians does not imply such elision.

There is no attempt here to offer a concerted general overview of the Rethinking Compliance project. Instead, this piece focuses on one of the key themes emerging from the research: the manner in which non-Indigenous health professionals in their attitudes towards cross-cultural health care tend to exaggerate, even fetishise, the importance of the 'the cultural' in relation to what they perceive as Aboriginal 'health beliefs and practices', understood as a largely homogenous set of ideas universally evident within all remote Indigenous communities. Moreover, this process of exaggeration occurs in a manner which, ironically, both underestimates the importance of developing more sophisticated understandings of cultural disjunction *and* eclipses an attention to other possible factors underlying the difficulties of successful service provision and uptake, such as poverty, the institutional frameworks of medical provision, and the ramifications of a history of colonial dispossession. This tendency to 'fetishise' the cultural deserves considered attention since it illustrates a number of points about the dynamics of biomedically framed health services provision within an Australian Indigenous context.

Australian Socio-Cultural Research on Indigenous Health: Some Background

Since the 1970s in Australia, much of the socio-cultural commentary on Indigenous health has been at pains to emphasise the culturally specific manner in which health and well-being is conceptualised and approached within Australian Indigenous communities. Indeed, in face of a 'culture blind' and colonising history of western biomedical intervention, a number of social researchers and health practitioners working across a range of disciplines were, by the 1970s, giving voice to an emerging interest in the dimensions and complexity of Indigenous health cultures. As a response to the failed and highly destructive 'assimilationist' policies of successive Australian governments towards Aboriginal and Torres Strait Islander peoples, an increasing number of health researchers, drawing in part on a 'health beliefs' model, wrote of the need to better understand and engage with Indigenous ideas in relation to health and illness (Hamilton 1974; Moodie 1973; Soong and Fejo 1976; Tatz 1972, 1974).

By the 1980s, an increasing interest in the health knowledges utilised within Indigenous communities had resulted in the development of a more concerted body of research drawing on the traditions of medical anthropology and health sociology. This was evidenced by the publication of *Body, Land and Spirit* in 1982, a collection of essays edited by Janice Reid which brought together much of the existing non-Aboriginal interpretations of various Indigenous 'beliefs and practices' in relation to health and wellbeing. This collection, along with other work such as that of Taylor (1977), Tynan (1979), Soong (1983), Reid (1978, 1983) and also Nathan and Japanangka (1983) broke new ground in exploring the disjunctions between Western and Aboriginal and Torres Strait Islander understandings of ill-health.

Very broadly, these studies suggested that Indigenous health knowledges in Australia differed substantially from western conceptualisations, particularly in relation to beliefs about how sickness was caused, how it could be treated, and how the relationship between the body, society, culture and the natural environment was to be understood. Thus, researchers drew particular attention to what they saw as a commonly shared 'holistic' understanding of health within Aboriginal societies; an understanding which emphasised the mutual interdependence of self, body, kin, nature and spirit. In this, Australian research mirrored the findings of international work undertaken in similar contexts on the dynamics of Indigenous knowledge systems.

The role of 'medicine men' and traditional methods of healing had long been a theme within anthropological studies of Australian Indigenous cultures (Berndt 1964; Cawte 1974; Elkin 1945). So too had the exploration of Indigenous notions of causality in relation to illness and injury, particularly the notion of supernatural or spiritual causes. By the 1980s, however, Australian researchers were seeking a rather more complex understanding of contemporary Indigenous health knowledges in relation to the causes and treatment of ill-health. Indeed, researchers suggested that the anthropological interest in 'traditional cultures' and medicine men had led to an overemphasis on the relative importance of supernatural causes within Indigenous health cultures (Scarlett et al. 1982: 165), and an underemphasis on the role of women in health maintenance (Bell 1982). Researchers suggested that, as within non-Indigenous cultures, Aboriginal and Torres Strait

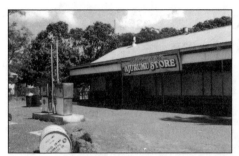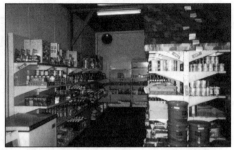

Recent social research into Indigenous health has focused in particular on the material as well as cultural circumstances underlying the rise of illnesses such as diabetes. These photos illustrate a typical 'remote community store', and the limited foods available within. (photos by author)

Islander peoples called on a range of explanations for ill-health including: environmental factors (such as the effects of heat and cold, wind and rain), natural causes (such as age), emotional factors (such as the health effects of shame, worry, grief, homesickness), magical or supernatural causes (connected with the breaking of taboos or cultural laws, and with sorcery), and emergent causes, such as alcohol and smoking (Bell 1982; Berndt 1982; Biernoff 1982; Hamilton 1976; Reid 1978, 1983; Tonkinson 1982; Waldock 1984).

Since this flowering of work in the early to mid-1980s exploration into the socio-cultural aspects of Indigenous health knowledges and practices has been rather patchy, despite the fact that an attention to 'cultural difference' and 'cultural appropriateness' has become a central facet of the rhetoric of Aboriginal health policy nationwide. There has, however, been some very useful research conducted during the 1990s into the social and cultural aspects of Indigenous health, as well as into health-threatening behaviours, particularly in the Northern Territory. This includes the work of Mobbs (1994) on the socio-cultural context of Indigenous health and wellbeing, Brady (1991, 1992) on the social dynamics of alcohol use and petrol sniffing, Saggers and Gray (1991) on the historical and political context of health services and interventions, Skov (1994) on understandings of infant health, Weeramanthri and Plummer (1994) on the meanings of mortality, Rowse (1996) on the utilisation of the concept of tradition in addressing Indigenous health issues, Devitt and McMasters (1996) on perceptions and understandings of End Stage Renal Disease (ESRD), Scrimgeour et.al. (1997) and Humphery et al. (1998) on the social relations and cultural interpretation of diabetes, and Willis (1999) on the culturally specific meanings of palliative care.

Much of this qualitative and anthropological research is more clearly focused than earlier socio-cultural work on the successful implementation of health promotion programs and health services. That is, it is focused on making the delivery of health services more effective in terms of health outcomes and more culturally and socially 'appropriate' to Aboriginal and Islander people (through, for example, facilitating greater community control of health services or greater involvement of Aboriginal health professionals in health interventions). Recent socio-cultural research thus builds on earlier analyses, at times broadening the area of discussion to include an engagement not only with an orthodox anthropological understanding of health knowledges and practices but with a critical and politically informed exploration of the material circumstances and contemporary social and cultural contexts in which Indigenous People live (Saggers and Gray 1991).

Four things can be said about this body of research. First, research on the socio-cultural aspects of Indigenous health in Australia has overwhelmingly been focused on remote area research, or on Indigenous communities which retain so called 'traditional' aspects of existence—and this continues to be the case despite the fact that most Indigenous Australians live in urban settings. Second, almost all of this work has been undertaken by non-Indigenous researchers, a situation that has been slow to change in Australia but is now showing signs of doing so with the emergence and recognition of key Indigenous health professionals, social researchers and health research organizations. Third, the focus of this research has been resoundingly one-way, with very little socio-cultural research undertaken on the beliefs, practices and broader health knowledges of non-Indigenous health professionals involved in cross-cultural service provision. Fourth, and most importantly for this discussion, the call for an attention to cultural appropriateness in the design and delivery of Indigenous health services has been, as noted above, seemingly 'successful' in that it has become a central rhetorical principle of Indigenous health policy and professional practice on both a national and state level in Australia. However, it is the dimensions and limitations of this official and professional attention to the cultural that we will explore in the remainder of this chapter.

The Uses of Culture

A number of researchers in Australia, while cognisant of the need for culturally appropriate policies and professional practices in relation to Indigenous communities, have critically explored the manner in which the concept of culture itself is differentially utilised by various actors within the broad field of Indigenous health and welfare. Thus, Franscesca Merlan (1989) writing on the objectification of culture in Aboriginal Affairs drew attention to the manner in which the full scope of Aboriginal demands is reduced by governments routinely to supporting the perceived 'cultural' rather than political and economic dimensions of those demands. Merlan illustrated also, however, how the very constitution of a distinct Aboriginal cultural domain is a matter of struggle both within Indigenous communities and between those communities and the Euro-Australian institutions with which they must deal.

In a slightly different vein, Maggie Brady (1995) has analysed the uses of the notion of culture, or more specifically 'cultural tradition', in addressing alcohol dependence within Aboriginal communities. Brady offers a complex analysis of this, interrogating both the reasons why the notion of 'tradition' has come to be used as a vehicle for addressing substance abuse issues by some Aboriginal communities and the possible valorisation of an 'imagined authenticity' involved in such appropriations. Brady thus seeks to explore in deliberately evaluative terms the *possible* rather than hoped for and/or fetishised uses of culture and tradition in alcohol treatment, noting how an exclusive attention to cultural loss and rejuvenation eclipses a consideration of the possible socio-economic, structural and psychological factors involved in substance abuse. In doing this, Brady throws out a challenge to both Indigenous and non-Indigenous understandings of 'culture'.

Similarly, Tim Rowse has pursued a number of these issues in his book *Traditions for Health* (1996). As this title suggests, Rowse's interest is in exploring, through the prism of health services and interventions, 'the dynamic and contested nature of Aboriginal traditions' (Rowse 1996: 5). Rather than treat Aboriginal cultural 'traditions', 'customs' and, indeed, 'Aboriginality' as fixed and unproblematically possessed (or, indeed, as homogenous), Rowse interprets them as artefacts of a political and historical struggle between the Indigenous and the non-Indigenous realms.

These kinds of explorations, none of which seek to deny the importance of cultural identity to Australian Indigenous Peoples or the necessity of using the concept of culture in strategic ways, suggest some productive avenues of analysis. They point in particular to the need to both historicize and critically analyse the rise and use of the concept of the cultural within fields such as Indigenous health. There has, however, been little attempt in Australia to discursively analyse the conceptualisation and use of 'culture' in such specific contexts; to document the everyday manner in which both Indigenous and non-Indigenous Peoples involved in areas such as health services provision construct and draw on notions of cultural difference (and of the cultural) in their daily work and interactions. The research conducted for the Rethinking Compliance project, on which this chapter draws, provides at least the beginnings of such a grounded analysis in relation to the words and stated actions of non-Indigenous health professionals, and it is to this research and these perceptions that we now turn.

Researching 'Patient Non-Compliance'

The Rethinking Compliance project, undertaken between November 1997 and April 2000, was designed to explore the social, medical and cultural dimensions of so called 'patient non-compliance' with western health advice and medical treatments by Aboriginal Peoples in the Northern Territory (NT). The NT is one of two Australian territorial jurisdictions that, along with the six state jurisdictions and the national, federal government, make up the Australian governmental system. The NT covers a vast geographic area of well over 1.3 million square kilometres with an often rugged and inaccessible terrain ranging from semi-arid desert lands to tropical savannas. Its sparse population numbers just over 200 thousand. However, the NT is unique in Australia in that over 28% of its population are Indigenous Australians (whereas on a national level only 2.1% of the Australian population is Aboriginal or Torres Strait Islander). This is important to realise in the context of the present chapter, since to work in the health field in the NT is necessarily to work within the field of *Indigenous health*.

This is not least the case because of the appalling disparities in health status between Indigenous and non-Indigenous Australians. These disparities are legion, but it should at least be pointed out that the average life expectancy for Aboriginal and Torres Strait Islander individuals is, at birth, 20 years lower than that for other Australians. Moreover, Indigenous Australians suffer higher death rates, and die at younger ages, from causes common to both Indigenous and non-Indigenous populations. These causes include diseases of the circulatory system, accidents, self-harm and assault, cancers, respiratory diseases and endocrine/metabolic diseases (Australian Institute of Health

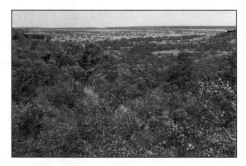

The Northern Territory is a place of environmental as well as cultural difference. These
photos illustrate the terrains of the semi-desert
and of the tropical savannah (photos by
author).

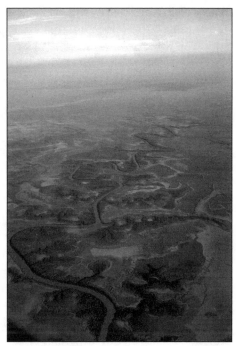

and Welfare 2002: 193–94). In the NT in particular, in part because of the remote locations of many Aboriginal communities (see air photo) and a long history of inadequate health services provision, a large burden of ill-health is thus carried by the Indigenous population, and Indigenous Territorians make up the majority of those
receiving government and community-based health services.

It is not apposite here to provide a detailed methodological account of the Rethinking Compliance project. Briefly, however, the project principally involved undertaking a qualitative study of health professionals working throughout the NT with
the intent of documenting and critically discussing their perceptions and experience
of service provision within a cross-cultural context. This research focused in particular on the issue of treatment uptake and refusal or, in current biomedical language,
'patient compliance and non-compliance'. It did so from the point of view of 'providers'
(mostly Euro-Australian) in order to reverse the usual research process, making non-
Indigenous health professionals themselves—and especially the systems and organisational frameworks they work within—the subject of searching inquiry, rather than
Aboriginal 'patients' and their cultures.

This research was undertaken using a fairly straightforward process of qualitative
group interviewing. Overall, a total of 19 semi-formal interviews involving 76 health
professionals (both Indigenous and non-Indigenous) were conducted in Darwin (the
NT capital) and in the NT centres of Katherine, Tennant Creek and Alice Springs
throughout 1998. Of those participating in the interviews, 19 were Aboriginal
Health/Liaison Workers, 7 were allied health professionals, 6 were mental health nurses,
22 were registered nurses, and 22 were medical practitioners. Interviews were conducted with health professionals working within four of the five NT hospitals, two
(community-controlled) Aboriginal Medical Services and several program units within

the NT Department of Health. The questions asked of non-Indigenous health professionals ranged from basic information regarding their work history to broader deliberation on why they chose to work in a predominantly Indigenous health context, what perceived problems they faced in doing so, if and when they utilised the language of non-compliance, how they thought about and addressed the difficulties of cross-cultural service provision or thought others (such as government agencies) should do so, and what knowledge and understanding they felt they had of the lives and background of their Indigenous 'patients'. Overall, the interviews generated over 20 hours of taped discussion and approximately 340 pages of typed transcript.

As noted previously, very little research of this type has been undertaken in Australia in the field of Indigenous health. There are to date only a handful of studies which investigate the beliefs, actions and broader health knowledges of health service providers (both non-Indigenous and Indigenous) working within a cross-cultural context or which provide some commentary on this process (Bennett et al 1995; Crawshaw and Thomas 1993; Devitt and McMasters 1998; Mobbs 1986; Nathan 1980; Rasmussen 2001; Scrimgeour et al. 1997; Tregenza and Abbott 1995). Indeed, the comparative dearth of information available in Australia on how health service providers think about their knowledge, experiences and practices in relation to interacting with Indigenous Peoples formed the backdrop to the Rethinking Compliance project. This absence of analysis is even more evident when it comes to specific areas of biomedical concern such as 'patient non-compliance', often presumed (without quantitative evidence) to be a particularly major problem within the area of Aboriginal health.

For readers unfamiliar with the language of 'non-compliance', some brief explanation of these terms may be useful. Generally, the terms 'compliance' and 'non-compliance' are used within the biomedical field to describe the degree to which patients follow the advice of and/or treatments prescribed by health service providers, particularly medical practitioners. The degree to which people *do not* act on health advice and/or *alter or refuse* treatments is spoken of, within the biomedical field, as the degree to which people are 'non-compliant'.

The language of 'patient compliance' and 'non-compliance' was adopted during the 1970s in the United States and elsewhere in order to re-describe what was long understood as a perennial problem of clinical practice—the failure of patients to 'follow doctor's orders'. Such language, however, has, at least in an international context, long been under challenge by those critical of a biomedical worldview (Learner 1997; Taussig 1980; Trostle 1988) and is now being challenged also by many working within the health field as inappropriate to contemporary conceptualisations of the medical encounter (Holm 1993; Marinker 1997). Essentially, these challenges focus on the pejorative or patient blaming nature of this language, and the manner in which such terminology tends to both draw on and reconfirm the assumed medical and social power of health professionals.

Within the broader study on which this paper is based, the use and politics of the language of non-compliance—and its embeddedness within a broader discourse of control that has become central to the self-understanding of biomedical practice—was explored and critiqued in considerable detail. In this chapter, however, our concern is more specifically focused on how notions of non-compliance were connected by those participating in the study with questions of cultural difference.

Voicing Cultural Difference

One of the core areas explored during the group interviews undertaken as part of the Rethinking Compliance study was the *perceived reasons* for the apparent non-utilisation of Western health services and non-uptake of Western treatments by some (perhaps many) Aboriginal patients. In their responses to a short, pre-interview question sheet, which was administered as part of the study, non-Indigenous participants in particular tended to emphasise cultural differences and communication difficulties between provider and patient as the key factors underlying 'non-compliance'. Additionally, participants emphasised also a perceived lack of understanding of Western culture—especially health cultures—on the part of Aboriginal people with whom they came in contact. These perceived factors, particularly that of cultural difference, dominated group discussion as well—with a litany of other factors placed underneath them. This hierarchy of factors underlying 'patient non-compliance' was articulated clearly by one medical practitioner based within an NT community controlled Aboriginal Medical Service (AMS):

> Initially, I think the main one [reason for patient non-compliance] is the mismatched worldview [between provider and patient]. Basically, I think that's the number one…and then just right down to simple things like literacy, numeracy, you know, understanding of the English language, physical impairments, hearing and social set up…

In voicing these thoughts this participant spoke for many others. Indeed, a great many of the non-Aboriginal interviewees within the compliance study sought to offer such a hierarchy of underlying causes for 'non-compliance'—even though they were not pressed to offer such a ranking. In seeking to explain the reasons underlying Aboriginal peoples' apparent unpreparedness to utilise and/or take up treatments and services, the vast majority of non-Indigenous health professionals thus prioritised a somewhat ill-defined notion of cultural difference as *the* key factor. Embedded within this notion was an equally thin understanding of culture as set of static, tradition-bound 'beliefs'.

What, then, did participants mean by cultural difference? Often any such difference was recognised by non-Aboriginal participants in terms of a series of factors generalised around concepts such as differential time consciousness, differential sense of pain and risk, and/or different conceptual systems per se. Often, too, there was a clear tension embedded within peoples' comments between acceptance of and frustration with these perceived differences in relation to, for example, the importance of keeping to appointments, the avoidance of health risks related to diet or drug use, and the acceptance or otherwise of biomedical scientific knowledge as an explanatory schema. Undoubtedly, the responses to this question relating to the reasons underlying 'non-compliance' were some of the least guarded the research team received during the project interviews. Moreover, the language people used was often rich in unselfconscious generalisation spanning a continuum from sometimes breathtaking bigotry to empathic regard. While cultural differences were often initially identified in terms of alternative social practices, many non-Indigenous participants quickly moved from such specifics to, much more problematically, offering 'statements of Aboriginality'. This can be clearly seen in the following group of comments taken from a number of separate interviews; interviews in which culture—which must surely be understood as a highly dynamic, constitutive and multifaceted phenomenon—was, as mentioned above, all to readily conflated with belief, mindset, habit, and tradition (and these comments are quite deliberately grouped here for purposes that will become later apparent):

> …a lot of it [has] to do with the way Aboriginal people think about preventative medicine…They don't think in terms of prevention…They live for here and now, how they feel now, and a lot of what we're saying [about] compliance is related to preventative things…They don't understand. It's a different way that Aboriginals think in terms of preventative medicine. And we have more of a concept of doing something now, whether it's going to affect the future. That is not the way they're brought up (Hospital-based medical practitioner).

> The other thing that I frequently find is the issue of time, is that you might suggest to someone that they come back tomorrow. Well, they don't turn up and you think, 'bloody hell, they didn't turn up'. But they might come back two days later…But time doesn't seem as important to them and, you know, we have this sort of feeling, 'well you didn't bloody well come back yesterday, so I'm not going to put myself out today for you', that attitude. Whereas, they have a different concept of time, I think, to us (Hospital-based medical practitioner).

> …the way they bring their kids up is different to us. They don't force things like that [taking medication] on them, where we do. If a kid doesn't like it, well it's just like, 'OK, the kid doesn't like it'. And that's because it's a lack of education and a lack of understanding. And it's not their way (Hospital-based registered nurse).

> They can't concept tomorrow, I think, and, you know, visualise that, O.K., if you don't do this today well then the consequences tomorrow or down the track will be there (Hospital-based registered nurse).

> It's part of their culture that you grow up and die. It's not like the Western culture where you try and remain young and fit and healthy as long as you jolly well can at any expense…In Aboriginal communities…you get born, you live and you die, the cycle of life (Hospital-based registered nurse).

> That's it, that's the one thing, they don't see it's important [health]. Whether it be through lack of education or through their cultural beliefs or whatever, it is not seen to be important…You ask them what health is. It's like, 'what do you mean what health is?'. It's just like not a known word, 'what's health and sickness?'. It's different models. We work under different models than what they do in the way that we see, you know, wellness and sickness. (Hospital-based registered nurse)

> But sometimes, like the mums on the wards, they're there and they don't really want to leave, but they've got family business, sorry business, a big funeral…It's really, it's cultural. You know, I don't know how we deal with that.

We try and deal with that and say, well their cultural thing and their family are so important that we need to accept that (Hospital-based medical practitioner).

I have presented these various statements on 'the cultural' in Aboriginal health in order to give a sense of the ideas invoked in response to our question on the underlying reasons for 'patient non-compliance' in the NT. For those readers unfamiliar with the language of qualitative interviews, particularly those undertaken in a cross-cultural context, these statements may well shock. The language here is, as mentioned above, unguarded, clumsy and, at times, unnervingly blunt, indeed brutal. We can, however, work with these statements on a number of levels. Treated empirically, these responses identify a number of perceived cultural factors observed by participants to impact on the 'non-compliance' of Indigenous patients. On this level, some of the observations indicate a number of socio-cultural forces that *may* be at play in the uptake and non-uptake of services and treatments. These observations also, to offer a slightly different reading, testify to a level of consciousness on the part of service providers about cultural issues—even though we may want, in some instances, to take considerable exception to the content and expression of this consciousness. Textually, however, these statements obviously constitute a lot more than observation, and they suggest something beyond the fact that health service providers are 'thinking about culture'.

To be sure, the above comments are, as I have already intimated, not all of a piece. Looking underneath any uniformity of language used, they in fact indicate somewhat different ways of identifying and speaking about cultural differences—and quite different levels of consciousness on the part of individual non-Aboriginal participants. One or two of the above comments are inquiring and self-reflective while many indicate what, at best, must be seen as a repressive tolerance. In this short paper, however, I want to treat these comments as an interconnected set or group of statements, leaving an individual analysis of them open to the reader. I also want to avoid a reductionist reading of them as simply racist. My point in doing so is to identify something of the general nature of health service provider commentary on culture and cultural difference—at least in a NT context—and to extract from these statements a complexity of approach.

On the most obvious level, this group of statements illustrates both a culled knowledge of (and frustration with) 'Aboriginal ways and values', as well as a real uncertainty about how to deal with or even report this knowledge. These statements also indicate two further modes of dealing with perceived cultural difference. One of these modes is the manner in which cultural differences are constantly *universalised* with these comments rather than dealt with in their specificity, constantly understood as definitional of an all-encompassing conceptual division between *homogenous* groups, rather than as specific alternative social and cultural practices underwritten by *internal* as well as cross-cultural disparities. The second mode of approach to cultural difference evident within this set of statements is the manner in which *culture* and the impact of *colonisation* is conflated—giving rise to an image of contemporary Aboriginality that wavers between seeing Aboriginal peoples as *differently cultured* to seeing them as unsuccessfully *enculturated* into a western context.

These modes of approaching cultural difference were embedded within and reinforced by participants understanding of 'culture' itself. Throughout many of the interviews undertaken as part of compliance study there were two predominant senses in which the concept of culture was invoked by non-Aboriginal participants. On the one hand, culture was overwhelmingly understood as something possessed by Aboriginal people; it was understood very much as both tradition and a mindset. On the other hand, culture was something the 'west' was seen to possess as well. Yet, in practice, 'western ways' were barely interpreted or spoken about as culture at all. As a consequence this restricted and static vision of culture seemed to relegate Aboriginal societies and individuals to being both 'locked-in' to an antiquated world view and as having ultimately to decide between tradition and modernity.

There were exceptions to this rule. Indeed, it is worth reiterating at this point that the qualitative research drawn on within this chapter yielded a complex body of information and it is not my intention to simplistically characterise health professionals in the NT as uniformly lacking in self-reflexivity or simply bigoted. On a number of occasions and at more reflective moments a handful of non-Aboriginal participants emphasised both the impact of colonisation on Aboriginal lives and the limits of their own cultural knowledge in the eyes of their Aboriginal patients. Here, cultural difference was spoken of not simply as a source of service provider frustration or as a lack of understanding on the part of Indigenous Peoples, but as reflecting a genuine gulf between provider and patient—a gulf that is confusing and frustrating to both. Here also was a move—however tentatively—towards a view of western culture *as culture*, not as norm. Three examples will suffice:

> I think also part of it comes—I think you see this wherever you work—is that people who have a sense of direction or purpose or meaning, or whatever you want to call it, in their lives, some sense of hope or some structure to live within, tend to care about themselves, you know, and about others, and are therefore more willing to take active steps to try and improve things for themselves and have a sense of the future...Whereas, I think people who lack that don't, you know, they don't see the point....And I think that is true, you know, for some groups of Aboriginal people, not all, but certainly there is, you know, a cultural loss and dislocation and hopelessness (AMS-based medical practitioner).

> But there's a real big...I find there's a big gulf between me and them. Of all this stuff that I don't really understand. And so three quarters of the time you're just going, you're just doing what you would do for a white person because you should be offering them the same sorts of treatment. But you know that your miles away from where the patient is at. You haven't even touched first base with what the real issues are...Or the compliance issues (Hospital-based medical practitioner).

> ...you are basically, you are operating with different world views. There are different understandings of illness and health, of causation and treatment... Even if there is a connection on a personal level, you still have that great gulf... I mean, sometimes I feel a little bit uncomfortable because basically it is cultural imperialism, you know. You've got some person who is receiving two theories of causation. One is from their family and perhaps from a traditional

healer and the other theory of causation is coming from us, and we're saying you have to do this...(AMS-based medical practitioner).

The Place of 'the Cultural' in Aboriginal Health Services Provision

Although only providing a glimpse of how participants in the Rethinking Compliance project utilised the concept of culture in discussing Aboriginal patients, this material offers some productive ground on which to explore current service-provider thinking. More broadly it illustrates something of the dynamics of a non-Indigenous recourse to cultural difference as an explanation for the state of Indigenous/non-Indigenous relations, and of Indigenous health.

In one sense the attention to culture evident within the comments cited throughout this piece testifies to a certain (at times admirable) acceptance among NT health professionals of the importance of cultural difference as an intervening element in the relationship between them and their Aboriginal patients. On the other hand, this very consciousness appears to eclipse the search for or recognition of alternative explanations for the unwillingness of some Aboriginal people to utilise biomedically framed health services and treatments. In short, the cultural becomes both selectively invoked/defined and resolutely exaggerated, even fetishised, as an intervening factor. To put it more plainly, and to unravel the title of this chapter, a 'culture blindness' continues to frame the provision of biomedical health services in the NT but, at the same time, service provider conceptualisations of Aboriginal people and their health-related behaviours becomes (in heavily ironic twist) somewhat 'blinded' by a culturalist reductionism.

This reductionism, in particular, can be more clearly grasped by contrasting participant's attention to culture with their relative *inattention* to other possible factors affecting the ability of Aboriginal patients to utilise biomedical services and treatments. One of the most striking aspects of the qualitative research undertaken during the compliance study was the lack of recognition on the part of most participants of the everyday socio-economic factors possibly underlying 'patient non-compliance' (such as poverty and unemployment, overcrowded and inadequate housing, lack of access to transport, and poor educational opportunities). This was matched by an equally striking failure to discuss the impact of institutional arrangements and organisational structures on the nature of service provision and its uptake. While 'the cultural' was a concept much discussed and invoked by non-Aboriginal participants, there was far less consciousness of 'the social' and 'the institutional' as factors to be dealt with in any discussion of Aboriginal health.

Very few non-Aboriginal participants, then, directly recognised poverty (and, more widely, colonisation) as a major issue in relation to Aboriginal ill-health and wellbeing. Furthermore, while a number of participants identified particular aspects of their institutional setting as potentially undermining the desire or ability of Aboriginal people to utilise biomedical services, few took this further venturing to critique in more general terms institutional and organisational structures and approaches. Most notable of all, very few of the non-Aboriginal participants raised the issue of organisational control, or the politics of health institutions in the NT being run largely by non-Indigenous health practitioners and managers—an issue that is crucial within the community controlled sector. This is a sector in which Indigenous People control and extensively staff Aboriginal Health Services (involving advocacy/research functions, on-site clinical services, and outreach health service delivery) in all the major NT population centres.

In other words, there was simply a lack of consciousness on the part of many non-Aboriginal participants of structural and institutional issues. Instead, people tended to individualise the 'compliance difficulties' they experienced precisely around the (more palatable, if confusing) notion of cultural difference. This tendency to focus predominantly on a conceptual disjunction between individuals, rather than on the broader socio-economic, institutional and organisational factors possibly impacting on the Aboriginal utilisation of health services, in many respects mirrors health sciences training in which emphasis is placed on the provider-patient dyad. Yet this predominant concern with a cultural divide mirrors also something wider than this; the manner in which attending to cultural and communicative *difference* enables, perhaps ironically and often unconsciously, the deployment of a de-politicised explanation for the *inequalities* between Indigenous and non-Indigenous Australians.

It would seem less than reflexive, however, to chide the health sciences alone for a particularistic and culturally reductionist way of understanding the contemporary 'problems' of Aboriginal health. On the contrary, social science research in the area of Indigenous health must itself take considerable responsibility for encouraging any fetishisation of the cultural in relation to the way in which non-Indigenous health professionals now conceptualise service provision issues, at least in the NT. It was, after all, as we noted at the beginning of this chapter, the fields of medical anthropology and health sociology—from the 1970s on—that increasingly drew attention to the 'cultural chasm' affecting Aboriginal health in Australia. Undoubtedly, such work has been part and parcel of the much broader 'cultural turn' within the humanities and social sciences in general, a phenomenon beyond the scope of this paper to explore. I do not wish to undermine the importance of the now considerable body of socio-cultural work on Aboriginal health knowledges and on cross-cultural service provision. Yet this work has, over the past three decades, had a rather contradictory impact on the broad field of Aboriginal health itself. On the one hand it has, quite rightly, positioned culture as a centrally important terrain of struggle in relation to the health and wellbeing of Indigenous Australian communities, and it has forced the biomedical to at least begin to think reflexively. On the other hand, it has ironically provided the biomedical field with an all too palatable framework for continuing to narrowly conceptualise the dynamics of Aboriginal ill-health. Any such culturalist framework fits rather well within a disciplinary field which has long relegated the socio-economic aspects of ill-health to minor status and which has effectively marginalised any institutional critique of its functioning. In this context, the notion of attending to 'difference' in cross-cultural service provision is easily accommodated to a liberal individualist conception of provider-patient relationships. This mentality or set of structuring beliefs and presuppositions in relation to the concept of cultural difference is evidenced directly in the interview material presented here.

Conclusion

The material presented and analysed in this chapter offers only a brief glimpse of the diversity of opinion expressed throughout the research phase of the Rethinking Compliance project. Nevertheless, by focussing on one of the key themes identified within the interview material—cultural difference—this paper alerts us to a growing concern often informally vented by those working in an Indigenous health context (particularly by Aboriginal and Torres Strait Islander commentators) but until now very poorly documented; the manner in which an attention to the concepts of 'cultural sensitivity' and 'cultural appropriateness' tends to rhetorically stand in for additional and broader reform in the provision of mainstream health services to Indigenous People in Australia. The material presented here reminds us that the now entrenched (though often shallowly understood) emphasis placed on cultural appropriateness within cross-cultural health services provision comes at a cost and that there is a continuing need to further emphasise accompanying radical reform of the economic, political, institutional and socio-structural factors underlying Aboriginal and Torres Strait Islander ill-health. Just as importantly, this material indicates that any eschewing of the political and economic aspects of Indigenous demands for better health is not only, as Merlan (1989) argues, the product of deliberate governmental strategy to attend to the most palatable 'cultural' aspects of those demands, but is structured into the everyday approach and imaginings of health professionals, of those who *work the system*, however conscientiously and/or resistantly they do so.

Acknowledgments

This paper draws extensively on research undertaken in the Northern Territory from 1997 to 2001 in collaboration with Tarun Weeramanthri and Joe Fitz under the auspices of the Darwin-based Cooperative Research Centre for Aboriginal and Tropical Health (CRCATH). I am most grateful to Tarun and Joe, and to the CRCATH, for permission to draw on this work.

References

Australian Institute of Health and Welfare. 2002. Australia's Health 2002. Canberra: AIHW.

Bell, D. 1982. Women's Changing Role in Health Maintenance in a Central Australian Community. *In* Body, Land and Spirit, J. Reid, ed. pp. 197–224. St. Lucia, Qld: University of Queensland Press.

Bennett, E., L. Manderson, B. Kelly and I. Hardie. 1995. Cultural Factors in Dialysis and Renal Transplantation Among Aborigines and Torres Strait Islanders in North Queensland. Australian Journal of Public Health 19(6): 610–15.

Berndt, C.H. 1965. The Role of Native Doctors in Aboriginal Australia. *In* Magic, Faith and Healing. A. Kiev, ed. pp. 264–82. London/New York: Free Press.

_____1982. Sickness and Health in Western Arnhem Land: A Traditional Perspective. *In* Body, Land and Spirit, J. Reid, ed. pp. 121–38. St. Lucia, Qld: University of Queensland Press.

Biernoff, D. 1982. Psychiatric and Anthropological Interpretations of Aberrant Behaviour in an Aboriginal Community. *In* Body, Land and Spirit. J. Reid, ed. pp. 139–53. St. Lucia: University of Queensland Press.

Brady, M. 1991. Drug and Alcohol Use among Aboriginal People. *In* The Health of Aboriginal Australia. J. Reid and P. Trompf, eds. pp. 173–217. Sydney: Harcourt Brace Jovanovich.

_____1992. Heavy Metal: The Social Meaning of Petrol Sniffing in Australia. Canberra: Aboriginal Studies Press.

1995. Culture in Treatment, Culture as Treatment: A Critical Appraisal of Developments in Addiction Programs for Indigenous North Americans and Australians. Social Science and Medicine 41(11): 1487–98.

Cawte, J. 1974. Medicine is the Law. Honolulu: University of Hawaii Press.

Crawshaw, J. and D. Thomas. 1993. It's Not Enough to Know About Diseases: Report of the Review of Aboriginal and Torres Strait Islander Health Care in the Darwin Area. Darwin: Danila Dilba Biluru Butji Binnilutlum.

Devitt, J. and A. McMasters. 1998. Living on Medicine: A Cultural Study of End Stage Renal Disease Among Aboriginal People. Alice Springs: Institute of Aboriginal Development Press.

Elkin, A.P. 1945. Aboriginal Men of High Degree. Sydney: Australasian Publishing Company.

Hamilton, A. 1974. The Traditionally Oriented Community. *In* Better Health for Aborigines. B.S. Hetzel et.al., eds. St. Lucia: University of Queensland Press.

Holm, S. 1993. What is Wrong with Compliance? Journal of Medical Ethics 19: 108–19.

Humphery, K, M. Dixon Japanangka and J. Marrawal. 1998. From the Bush to the Store: Diabetes, Everyday Life and the Critique of Health Services in Two Remote Northern Territory Aboriginal Communities. Darwin: Diabetes Australia Research Trust/Territory Health Services.

Humphery K, T. Weeramanthri and J. Fitz. 2001. Forgetting Compliance: Aboriginal Health and Medical Culture. Darwin: Northern Territory University Press/Cooperative Research Centre for Aboriginal and Tropical Health, Darwin.

Learner, Barron, H. 1997. From Careless Consumptives to Recalcitrant Patients: The Historical Construction of Noncompliance. Social Science and Medicine 45(9): 1423–31.

Marinker, M. 1997. 'Writing Prescriptions is Easy.' British Medical Journal 314(8 March): 747–48.

Merlan, Francesca. 1989. The Objectification of 'Culture': An Aspect of Current Political Process in Aboriginal Affairs. Anthropological Forum VI(1): 105–16.

Mobbs, R. 1986. 'But Do I Care!': Communication Difficulties Affecting the Quality of Care Delivered to Aborigines. Medical Journal of Australia, Special Supplement. 144(June 23): S3–S5.

_____1994. In Sickness and Health: The Sociocultural Context of Aboriginal Wellbeing, Illness and Healing. *In* The Health of Aboriginal Australia. J.Reid and P.Trompf, eds. pp. 292–325. Sydney: Harcourt Brace.

Moodie, P.M. 1973. Aboriginal Health. Canberra:Australian National University Press.

Nathan, P. 1980. 'A Home Away From Home': A Study of the Aboriginal Health Service in Fitzroy. Melbourne: Preston Institute of Technology Press.

Nathan, P. and D.L. Japanangka. 1983. Health Business. Melbourne: Heinemann.

Rasmussen, L. 2001. Towards Reconciliation in Aboriginal Health: Initiatives for Teaching Medical Students about Aboriginal Issues. Melbourne: VicHealth Koori Health Research and Community Development Unit, University of Melbourne.

Reid, J. 1978. Change in the Indigenous Medical System of an Aboriginal Community. Australian Institute of Aboriginal Studies Newsletter 9 (January): 61–72.

_____1983. Sorcerers and Healing Spirits: Continuity and Change in an Aboriginal Medical System. Canberra: Australian National University Press.

Reid, J., ed. 1982. Body, Land and Spirit: Health and Healing in Aboriginal Society. St. Lucia: University of Queensland Press.

Rowse, T. 1996. Traditions for Health: Studies in Aboriginal Reconstruction. Darwin: North Australia Research Unit.

Saggers, S. and D. Gray. 1991. Aboriginal Health and Society: The Traditional and Contemporary Aboriginal Struggle for Better Health. Sydney: Allen & Unwin.

Scarlett, N., N. White and J. Reid. 1982. "Bush Medicines": The Pharmacopoeia of the Yolngu of Arnhem Land. *In* Body, Land and Spirit. J. Reid, ed. pp. 154–91. St. Lucia: University of Queensland Press.

Scrimgeour, D., T. Rowse and A. Lucas. 1997. Too Much Sweet: The Social Relations of Diabetes in Central Australia. Alice Springs: Menzies School of Health Research.

Skov, S. 1994. Childhood Diarrhoea in a Central Australian Aboriginal Community: Aboriginal Beliefs and Practices in the Context of the Ecology of Health. Masters of Public Health Thesis, University of Sydney.

Soong, F.S. 1983. Role of the *Margidjbu* (Traditional Healer) in Western Arnhem Land. Medical Journal of Australia 1: 474–77.

Soong, F.S. and W. Fejo. 1976. Health Education Approaches in Aboriginal Communities in the Northern Territory: What We Have Learned. Medical Journal of Australia, Special Supplement (November 27): 1–5.

Tatz, C. 1972. The Politics of Aboriginal Health. Politics, Supplement vii(2), November.

_____1974. Innovation Without Change. *In* Better Health for Aborigines? Report of a National Seminar at Monash University. B. Hetzel et. al, eds. pp. 107–20. St. Lucia: University of Queensland Press, St. Lucia.

Taussig, M.T. 1980. Reification and the Consciousness of the Patient. Social Science and Medicine 14B: 3–13.

Taylor, J.C. 1977. A Pre-Contact Aboriginal Medical System on Cape York Peninsula. Journal of Human Evolution 6: 419–32.

Tonkinson, M. 1982. The Mabarn and the Hospital: The Selection of Treatment in a Remote Aboriginal Community. *In* Body, Land and Spirit. J. Reid, ed. pp. 225–41. St. Lucia: University of Queensland Press.

Tregenza, J. and K. Abbott. 1995. Rhetoric and Reality: Perceptions of the Roles of Aboriginal Health Workers in Central Australia. Alice Springs: Central Australian Aboriginal Congress.

Trostle, J.A. 1988. Medical Compliance as Ideology. Social Science and Medicine 27(12): 1299–1308.

Tynan, B.J. 1979. Medical Systems in Conflict: A Study in Power (Thesis). Department of Anthropology, University of Sydney.

Waldock, D.J. 1984. A Review of Aboriginal Health Beliefs and Their Incorporation Into Modern Aboriginal Health Delivery Systems. The Australian Health Surveyor (December 15), 16: 3–14.

Weeramanthri, T. and C. Plummer. 1994. Land, Body and Spirit—Talking About Adult Mortality in an Aboriginal Community. Australian Journal of Public Health 18(2): 197–200.

Willis, J. 1999. Dying In Country: Implications of Culture in the Delivery of Palliative Care in Indigenous Australian Communities. *Anthropology and Medicine* 6(3): 523–35.

STRIVING FOR HEALTHY LIFESTYLES: CONTRIBUTIONS OF ANTHROPOLOGISTS TO THE CHALLENGE OF DIABETES IN INDIGENOUS COMMUNITIES

Dennis Wiedman

Summary of Chapter 20. Working among Indigenous communities and minority groups throughout the world anthropologists have actively contributed to the theoretical, applied, and practical knowledge about diabetes. This chapter highlights medical anthropologists who over the past quarter century have made significant contributions at the community level to diabetes research and intervention. An understanding and appreciation of anthropological insights would enable Indigenous communities to take actions to reduce diabetes, or prevent it from occurring, by striving for "healthy lifestyles."

ﯤ ﯤ ﯤ

Introduction

Over the past quarter century anthropologists documented that diabetes control and prevention requires much more than clinical interventions and self-care. To reduce diabetes requires healthy lifestyles attainable only through community-wide action by tribal organizations, governments, health care professionals and voluntary organizations. Biomedical professionals are just now beginning to realize this. Writing in *The New England Journal of Medicine*, Tuomilehto (2001) reports on a large-scale longitudinal study in Finland showing that lifestyle changes can reduce the incidence of diabetes. Recently, in 2003, anthropologists Cheryl Ritenbaugh, Nicolette Teufel-Shone and Jennie Joe, Jr. were among the first to document changes at the community level that can reduce diabetic risk (Ritenbaugh et al. 2003). Diabetes and associated metabolic disorders were believed by many to be inevitable consequences of genetics and the modern lifestyle. We now know that by striving for healthy lifestyles, Indigenous communities can reduce the diabetes rate and possibly prevent it from occurring.

Anthropologists have contributed to the biological, social, and cultural knowledge about diabetes since Russell Judkins' 1975 publication on food and diabetes among the Iroquois (Judkins 1975; Judkins 1978). Since then over 40 anthropologists have published more than 200 journal articles, books and chapters specifically on diabetes. To facilitate research these were accumulated and published as a bibliography on the Internet in 2002 (Wiedman 2002). An historical perspective on this accumulation of work demonstrates anthropology's dedication to addressing the problem of diabetes among Indigenous Peoples and minority groups.

Anthropological efforts to understand diabetes have involved populations throughout the world. By far, Canada has received the most comprehensive and systematic anthropological attention of any region of the world. In the 1970s, when it was realized that diabetes was of epidemic proportions among Native Americans in the US, systematic efforts were made in Canada to initiate research and interventions to thwart the coming epidemic. Overall, the most comprehensive work is by the biological anthropologist and physician T. Kue Young, now at the University of Toronto. His many publications, which began in 1979, report on diabetes among Native Canadians and focus on prevalence rates and causal factors of obesity (Young 1979).

Australia and Oceania have also drawn significant anthropological attention. For American Samoa, Douglas Crews' publication on mortality and modernization appeared in 1982 (Crews and Mackeen 1982), and James Bindon's work on modernization appeared from 1991 through 1998 (Bindon 1988; Bindon et al. 1991).

Research in the United States is the next most studied region. Native Americans are by far the group receiving the greatest anthropological attention in terms of numbers of publications. Hispanic Americans have a good number of anthropological studies, primarily Mexican Americans along the border in Texas and migrant farm workers. Work with African Americans has focused on educational and health care services (Frate et al. 2000). Another area of focus is on the physicians and health care providers serving these populations (Larme and Pugh 2001; Stein 1992).

Anthropologists have an opportunity to work with populations in many world regions where diabetes is predicted to become an epidemic, especially in China, Russia, the Middle East, India, Africa, Central America, South America, and the Caribbean. Anthropologists have much to contribute by working with communities and designing healthy lifestyles that could lessen or even prevent the predicted diabetes epidemic.

Sessions specifically devoted to diabetes first appeared in the early 1970s at the meetings of the American Anthropological Association (AAA), the oldest and largest professional organization of anthropologists. The first session, organized by Gretchen Chesley Lang and Jo C. Scheder in 1984 at the AAA, led to the publication of the special issue of the journal "Medical Anthropology" edited by Maria Luisa Urdeneta (Urdaneta and Krebiel 1989). More recently, sessions that Dennis Wiedman organized in 2000, 2001 and 2002, once again called together the leading researchers to address the diabetes epidemic. The 2002 session titled "Healthy Lifestyles and Communities: Future Scenarios to Reduce the Diabetes Epidemic" developed a foundation for this book. Gretchen Lang was a discussant, and Carolyn Smith-Morris, and Daniel Benyshek were session participants. My overview of the anthropological contributions to diabetes research, concluded with ways in which anthropologists could work with communities to address the diabetes problem, namely action research and interventions. To be most effective, anthropological contributions could focus on:

1. Empowering groups and leadership with knowledge.
2. Influencing healthy choices of foods in community stores and more access to healthy foods.
3. Enhancing activity levels with design of transportation systems, work and exercise facilities.
4. Promoting efforts to influence health and food policies.

This chapter builds upon the insights gained from these sessions and my own diabetes research beginning in the 1970s among the Oklahoma Delaware and Cherokee, and more recently among Alaska tribal villages. I was the second anthropologist to receive a Ph.D. for research devoted to type 2 diabetes; Cheryl Ritenbaugh, whose work is highlighted later, was the first (Ritenbaugh 1974). My dissertation focused on the diabetes epidemic among Oklahoma Native Americans (Wiedman 1979). Diabetes was unknown to this population prior to 1940, although Oklahoma Whites and Blacks had reported cases since the 1910s. At the time I started my research, Dr. Kelly West, epidemiologist and physician at the University of Oklahoma Health Sciences Center, was just publishing his WHO study of a dozen populations around the world in which he showed that sugar consumption did not correlate with diabetes increases; rather, adiposity or percent body fat did (West 1978). His work supported the theory that diabetes was a "Disease of Civilization" associated with a modern lifestyle. Other studies at the time noted that Indigenous Peoples of the South Pacific had high diabetes rates; however, Pacific islands where people still lived a traditional lifestyle had low rates. Similarly, other studies showed that diabetes increased as groups migrated from rural to urban settings in Australia, Israel, and Africa. So my 1979 doctoral dissertation focused on understanding why diabetes among Okalahoma Native Americans began around 1940. Living among the Cherokee in a remote valley of the Ozark Mountains of Eastern Oklahoma, I conducted a survey of historic living sites and collected oral histories of who was related to whom, and who lived where and when. I combined this information with historical records and censuses to produce a 150-year history of land use and lifestyles. Briefly stated, after arriving from the Southern Appalachians in 1835, the Cherokee continued their agricultural way of life on small farms dispersed over the hills, valleys and mountains. Beginning in 1936 subsistence farms began to fail, and by 1946 the last family in the valley moved off their farm. They moved out of the area to California, or they moved to the gravel road that was built through the valley. They began working for the cattle ranchers who had purchased the land. Except for small gardens, they no longer produced their own food; instead, they purchased food from stores. This major demographic and economic change supported the explanation for diabetes as a "Disease of Civilization," and the modern lifestyle (Wiedman 1987, 1989). A major change with a transition to the modern lifestyle is food processing, preparation and consumption. "Frybread" is a near universal food that developed during this transition among Native North Americans. Considering its pervasive use for over 100 years, nutritional educators and clinic physicians had little information about frybread's nutritional content. By gathering frybreads from Seminole Fair vendors, Janell Smith and I reported on our laboratory analyses of the fat content and suggested several alternatives for cooking and dietary education (Smith and Wiedman 2001).

In the summer of 2001, I traveled with several nutritionists to four remote tribal villages in Alaska. Roads to larger towns did not connect these Indigenous communities; small planes and occasional barges brought in supplies. Men and women were physically active in hunting, fishing and the processing and storage of a wide array of subsistence foods: Inupiat primarily harvest whale and caribou, Athabascan pursue moose and salmon, Aleut focus on salmon and crab, while Tlingit seek salmon and halibut. Small stores in each village provided access to a limited amount of basic food items. Given that diabetes was rare, these are models of Indigenous communities living healthy, diabetes-free lifestyles (Smith et al. in press).

This brief example of my research illustrates the array of methods used by anthropologists. Contributions by anthropologists to better understand diabetes cover the full range of anthropological inquiry: genetics, metabolism, physical functioning, cultural explanations, stress, nutritional change, modernization, technological change, patients and health care provider interactions, community interventions, national health care policy, and world systems of health care and food distribution. The anthropological perspective, by incorporating the smallest gene segment to the largest world system, is the broadest of all the academic disciplines. The history of diabetes research presented in this chapter demonstrates that anthropology truly does seek to understand the whole panorama of human existence in geographic space and evolutionary time.

In this chapter the life work of anthropologists Rebecca Hagey, Linda Garro, Joel Gittelsohn, Linda Hunt, and Cheryl Ritenbaugh is highlighted. These individuals serve as examples of the broad range of ways that anthropologists have contributed to community level research, interventions and understanding. Many others could have been profiled, especially T. Kue Young (Young 1979; Young et al. 2002), Emöke Szathmary (Szathmary 1985, 1994), Kenneth Weiss (Weiss 1995; Weiss et al. 1984) and Robert Williams (Williams 1983; Williams et al. 2000). Their research has contributed to the biological, metabolic, genetic and epidemiological understanding of diabetes. For example, T. Kue Young, a medical doctor/epidemiologist with a British Ph.D. in physical anthropology, is the most prolific publisher of books and journal articles devoted to diabetes. In this paper, I have highlighted the work of medical anthropologists whose research has focused on or advocated for interventions at the individual and community level among Indigenous or minority communities. Unless another discipline is specifically noted, individuals discussed in this chapter are professionally-trained anthropologists. A rich set of citations to publications is also included so community members can easily locate additional knowledge and resources to help reduce the diabetes epidemic.

Increasingly, more individuals and Indigenous organizations are becoming actively involved in the planning, implementation and evaluation of health care delivery in their communities. With more knowledge and a sense of hope, Indigenous communities can become influential change agents in the provision of health care, the physical design of their communities, and the kinds of food and drinks that are readily accessible. With empowerment come creative and innovative ways to address diabetes that best fit a community's local beliefs and healthy life ways, thereby enhancing the overall quality of life.

Cultural Sensitivity through Community and Clinical Collaborations

Rebecca Hagey, a nurse anthropologist working with First Nations in Toronto during the early 1980s, was an early contributor whose work influenced many later anthropologists, nurses and Indigenous health service providers. She worked to develop a Native Diabetes Program with Ojibway and Cree leaders and the faculty of Nursing at the University of Toronto. A key to the success of the program was the development of the story "Nanabush and the Pale Stranger," which places diabetes into a "Native" perspective. By generating metaphors, symbols, stories, dances and ceremonies, the program made health information understandable and useful. The feared and avoided topic of diabetes was made meaningful and tolerable. Stories about Nanabush provided explanations for diabetes, answered numerous non-biological questions, resolved conflicting systems of belief, and indicated appropriate coping strategies. She brought to the medical profession's attention the fact that all information is a form of propaganda that is tied to deeper meaning structures. In their clinical interactions with patients, physicians are the architects of meaning and explanations about diabetes. Culturally sensitive clinical practice requires knowledge of both folk and professional construction of meaning (Hagey 1984, 1989).

Profile: Rebecca Hagey

Two statements characterize Rebecca Hagey's approach to community level diabetes preventions: "True self-care can result only when client's dignity and sovereignty has not been violated," and "A cooperative environment cannot be created when the authority and values of the caregivers dominate." She is the earliest anthropologist to advocate for culturally sensitive diabetes health care delivery programs. In the early 1980s she published several articles on the Native Diabetes Program at the Native Canadian Centre in Toronto. In affiliation with the Nursing Department at the University of Toronto, this Centre served the 30,000 Ojibway, Metis and Cree living in the Toronto urban area. The goal of the program was to facilitate a learning environment derived from the native culture and thereby promote self-help and a positive means of coping with diabetes. Cultural expression was explicitly considered important to the sense of community and the basis for identification and resolution of problems. In addition to collaboration and consultation with small groups of diabetes patients and their families, native political organizations and spiritual leaders were involved and Native staff and collaborated with community services agencies. Learning and teaching followed Native principles of communication, patterns of social organization and the use of cultural metaphors. Native artists helped produce banners, posters and T-shirts (Hagey and Buller 1983).

The program recognized the Ojibway rules of questioning: direct, factual or personal questions were not considered appropriate, as they would be met with either meaningless, diverting answers, or more often complete silence. Program staff also recognized the cultural meanings of body position and movements.

Cultural expression through drumming, dancing and storytelling facilitated the reorientation of knowledges and behaviors concerning diabetes. Stories about diabetes were created based on the cultural metaphor of Nanabush, the traditional Ojibway mediator between the Creator and the Indian people. Often depicted in Ojibway mythology as a hare, his split nose represents his two personalities: sometimes bumbling and other times wise. Nanabush is the embodiment of Ojibway morality, moderation and balance. Positive and negative ideas are always together, nothing can be all bad or good. Presented within Nanabush's principle of balance, information about food, exercise and insulin was more rapidly understood. The incorporation of traditional beliefs about Windigo also countered the wise Nanabush. Windigo represented out-of-control diabetes, isolation, vulnerability, victimization, blame mentality and continued breakdown of the family clan system. Nanabush represented controlled diabetes, internal strength through unity, support, freedom, responsibility, and the ultimate order and power of Indigenous Peoples as a whole (Hagey 1984).

Spiritual leaders incorporated ritual drumming, dancing and the use of the circle as in Native cosmology. For example, the program incorporated the traditional emphasis on the circle into the logo of the Native Diabetes Program; also during the talking stick ceremony each person had an opportunity to express him or herself while sitting in a circle. These cultural metaphors, ceremonies, drumming and dancing enable Indigenous Peoples to regain power and assume responsibility for taking actions to regain balance individually and as a community. Three insights summarize her work (Hagey 1984: 271):

1. Recognize that culturally specific logic constructs frameworks of meaning or explanatory systems. In both professional and folk cultures these point to illness agents and their modus and locus operandi.

2. Reconstruct meaning through cultural expressions; these facilitate negotiation of systems of belief and coping behaviors.

3. Recognize that coping is organized by cultural frameworks of meaning. The meaning CONTENT determines the coping process. This is key to facilitation.

Notable Diabetes Publications

Hagey, Rebecca and E. Buller. 1983. Drumming and Dancing: A New Rhythm in Nursing Care. Canadian Nurse 79(4): 28–31.

Hagey, Rebecca. 1984. The Phenomenon, the Explanations and the Responses: Metaphors Surrounding Diabetes in Urban Canadian Indians. Social Science and Medicine 18(3): 265–72.

_____ 1989. The Native Diabetes Program: Rhetorical Process and Praxis. Medical Anthropology 12(1): 7–33.

Cultural Models of Diabetes

Like Rebecca Hagey, other anthropologists continue to focus on the ways Indigenous Peoples talk about, explain, and adjust to the experience with diabetes. Gretchen Lang's work among the Dakota focused on ways diabetes is experienced by patients as they try to follow prescribed treatments in the home setting, and how diabetes is perceived by diabetics and their families. Dietary modification is most often problematic, involving meanings that are not immediately apparent to a cultural outsider. Lang asked people why they thought they had diabetes or what they thought about the efficacy of their current treatments. Most individuals turned the conversation to the discussion of food and eating, a recalled traditional lifestyle, and at times a commentary upon their political history and ethnic boundaries. This was a shift from the individual and singular body to Dakota identity and the collective body (Lang 1989; see also, Chs. 2 and 9 in this volume).

Similarly, Samantha Thompson's work among Australian aborigines living in urban Melbourne shows that this population does not explain diabetes as a problem with their bodies, but rather as a symptom of a life out of balance, a life of lost or severed connections with land and kin, and a life with little control over past, present or future. Her ethno-epidemiological approach analyzed lived experiences, lay meanings and models of diabetes at three levels of connectedness: the family, community, and society. Individuals whose locus of control is external to the body, do not focus on the body as the cause; thus an intervention based on body image as a motivational stimulus would not be successful because it is counter to their dominant cultural beliefs (Thompson and Gifford 2000).

This focus on the similarities and differences of the diabetes experience is not only valuable for a better understanding of diabetes; it can be valuable for a better understanding of the full range of health concerns. How do we know if an explanation for diabetes is one person's way of seeing it, or common throughout a community, a region, or the world? In other words, is a particular diabetes explanation the consensus of the village members, a particular family, or a specific individual? This variety in diabetes explanations and causes is important for health providers who wish to provide culturally sensitive and effective health care. Research methods used to formulate cultural consensus models and causal explanations for diabetes have focused on Linda Garro's work among the Anishinaabe community in Manitoba from 1987 to 1966. By using survey questionnaires, she had individuals list and rank their explanations regarding the causes of diabetes from their perspective. Building upon this she was able to identify a community's explanatory framework or explanatory model for diabetes (Garro 1995). Her work has greatly refined anthropological research methods well beyond the study of diabetes.

Profile: Linda Garro

Linda Garro has a long history of contributions to understanding Indigenous health, beginning in Mexico with her work on medical decision-making with her husband, John Garro (Young and Garro 1994; originally published in 1981). Linda Garro's work among the Canadian First Nations of Manitoba, Canada, provides community leaders and health care providers a better understanding of Indigenous explanations for diabetes: its causes, treatments and life ways. She interviewed individuals diagnosed with diabetes in communities of Anishinaabe, better known as Ojibway, Chippewa and Saulteaux. She has been able to document the collective memory, the cultural framework or model that gives individuals meaning to the occurrences of diabetes and provides a rationale for taking actions in response to an illness.

Anishinaabe talk about the causes of diabetes in various ways: as the result of individual decisions as well as from environmental and societal causes (Garro 1995). To better understand these cultural explanations, Garro focused on the merits and validity of two kinds of interview format —an open-ended, explanatory-model-type interview and a more structured, true-false interview. From the Anishinaabe responses she identified a set of explanations found in all three communities: "White Man's sickness," "Anishinaabe sickness," and "other sicknesses."

"White man's sicknesses" were unknown prior to the arrival of Europeans. They are seen as a consequence of changes occurring since that time, such as the inferiority of present-day foods compared to wild foods, the amount of sugar in new foods, chemical additives in store-bought foods, or poisons in the air and water. "Anishnaabe sickness" is thought to be caused by "bad medicine," another's use of power to cause harm, or "ondjine," something that the person did in the past, and can only be managed by an Anishinaabe healer. A third set of explanations is a sickness not attributed to the two other categories. These sicknesses run in families, or are due to a state of imbalance primarily from over consumption of foods, sugar, sweetened drinks, alcohol, or greasy foods. Anishinaabe sickness was not brought up as an explanation by anyone as a cause of diabetes. Diabetes is considered a white man's sickness. Garro contends that these explanatory models influence individual decisions about health care treatments and causes (Garro 2000).

Cultural models developed through a series of interviews can serve as an important way of communicating a community's health beliefs and practices to health care providers and policy decision makers. This research methodology enables the development of more precise, culturally sensitive, and appropriate health services, treatments, and community-wide interventions. Going beyond the subject of diabetes, Linda Garro's work has greatly influenced anthropological research methods and cultural consensus modeling. It is considered the foundation for understanding Indigenous medical knowledges, practices and decision-making.

Notable Diabetes Publications

Garro, Linda C. 1995. Individual or Societal Responsibility? Explanations of Diabetes in an Anishinaabe (Ojibway) Community. Social Science and Medicine 40(1): 37–46.

_____2000. Remembering What One Knows and the Construction of the Past: A Comparison of Cultural Consensus Theory and Cultural Schema Theory. Ethos 28(3): 275–319.

Patients and Providers

Within the clinic or health care setting, attention to cultural similarities and differences among patients and providers enables more appropriate health care delivery. These differing assumptions, expectations, and perceptions affect the interactions and health outcomes.

Rebecca Hagey clearly stated this recurrent anthropological theme: medical practitioners should recognize the metaphors and cultural values of the patients. Most notably, she found that biomedical discourse is dominated by regimens and the imposition of non-native foods and behaviors (Hagey 1984). Her collaboration with Indigenous and non-Indigenous health workers in diabetes education demonstrates how a traditional Indigenous story can be adapted to provide a culturally appropriate understanding of diabetes. Narrative and story telling as intervention, highlights the useful integration of Indigenous metaphors and concepts of illness and biomedical concepts. Here we see effective use of anthropological insights on language and culture. This is an example of purposeful cultural creation, the synthesis of two cultural models for the purpose of diabetes prevention.

At an even more detailed level, the linguistic analysis by Woolfson (Woolfson et al. 1995) found that even though patients and providers may speak the same language, English, misinterpretations continue. He documented that in the diabetes clinic, the Mohawk spoke English using Iroquois grammar and sociolinguistic patterning. These differences in the use of English lead to misinterpretation, because the health care providers did not recognize the cultural meaning associated with their use.

More recently, in 2000, Steve Ferzacca characterized the clinical encounter as focused on the cultivation of an ideal self, based on a capitalist logic that links self-discipline, productivity, and health. He shows how this shared logic produces individualized regimes of self-care. At the clinical practice level it produces hybrid medical practices that incorporate differing objectives and emphases concerned with a tolerable present or an ideal future (Ferzacca 2000).

Christina Miewald in 1997 reported on the Community Health Awareness and Monitoring Program (CHAMP) in Kentucky. She documented that even though this was a purposefully designed, relatively open, and egalitarian health care setting, the medical practices and philosophy continued to rely on white middle-class norms of patient motivation, education, and self-care. Even so, she considers that the emphasis on health education masks the economic, political and racial inequalities beyond the clinic that create barriers to self-care in everyday life. When clinics honor the white, middle class ideals of self-control and individualism, they devalue others' worldviews, especially in marginalized neighborhoods and ethnic groups where social interdependence is vital (Miewald 1997).

By focusing primarily on the knowledge, assumptions and behaviors of medical doctors and health professionals, Anne Larme (2001) turned the eye of medical anthropology from the Indigenous patient to the attitudes of the biomedical practitioner. She documented that a major barrier to care is the clinician's attitudes towards patients. In her various publications since 1998 she stressed the need for the health care system to shift from an acute disease model to a chronic disease model. She found that health professionals do recognize contextual factors as important barriers to optimal diabetes care. These barriers include physician time constraints, the economics of the private practice setting, the maldistribution of professionals in the low-income communities, the lack of health care access for low-income patients, and the insufficient focus on prevention in the U.S. health care system. Her numerous publications in biomedical journals, rather then anthropological journals, have been influential on the ways doctors interact with minorities and patients from different cultural backgrounds.

Linda Hunt's publications over the years have noted that patients and providers may initially hold distinct views of diabetes; however, after repeated and long-term interactions, patients often develop concepts of the ailment that are quite similar to the bio-medical perspective of the providers (Hunt et al. 1997, 1998a, 2000, 1998b, 1998c). Over time both come to share a common perspective on diabetes as a disease and the regimen of self-care; however, clinicians try to evaluate, motivate and educate, while patients focus on ways to modify and adapt to everyday life experiences. Hunt's "Contrasting Perspectives Model" provides a useful graphic diagram that clearly distinguishes between the clinic-world view of the practitioner and the life-world view of the patient (Hunt and Arar 2001).

Profile: Linda Hunt

Linda Hunt's work among Mexican-Americans along the Texas border provides a model of how the cultures of patients and practitioners differ and how they become more similar through time with clinical interventions and health education.

Her work is based on an ethnographic study of self-care behaviors and illness concepts among Mexican-American diabetes patients. Open-ended interviews were conducted at two public hospital outpatient clinics in South Texas with Mexican-Americans who had diabetes for at least 1 year and did not have major impairment yet. Interviews focused on their concepts and experiences in managing their illness and their self-care behaviors. She noted how patients' causal explanations of their illness connected the illness in a direct and specific way to their personal history and their past experience with treatments. While most cite biomedically accepted causes such as heredity and diet, they elaborate these concepts into personally relevant constructs by citing "Provoking Factors," such as behaviors or events. Their causal models are thus both specific to their personal history and consistent with their experiences with treatment success or failure (Hunt et al. 1998).

Medical anthropologists involved in clinical research are often asked to help explain patients' "noncompliance" with treatment recommendations. The clinical literature on "noncompliance" tends to problematize only the patient's perspective, treating the provider's perspective as an uncontroversial point of departure. Hunt focuses on the interaction between provider and patient assumptions, expectations, and perceptions in managing chronic illness. Her graphic diagram represents a useful analytical framework for contrasting patient and provider goals, strategies, and evaluation criteria in chronic illness management. This approach goes beyond contrasting patient and provider concepts and explanations of the illness itself, and examines their contrasting views within the dynamic process of long-term care. This approach is especially useful because it maintains a balanced focus on the health provider's perspectives while giving serious consideration to the patient's perspective (Hunt and Arar 2001).

Notable Diabetes Publications

Hunt, Linda M., Miguel A. Valenzuela and Jacqueline A. Pugh. 1998. Porque me toco a mi? Mexican American Diabetes Patients' Causal Stories and their Relationship to Treatment Behaviors. Social Science and Medicine 46(8): 959–69.

Hunt, Linda M., Nedal H. Arar and Laura L. Akana. 2000. Herbs, Prayer, and Insulin. Use of Medical and Alternative Treatments by a Group of Mexican American Diabetic Patients. Journal of Family Practice 49(3): 216–23.

Hunt, Linda M. and Nedal H. Arar. 2001. An Analytical Framework for Contrasting Patient and Provider Views of the Process of Chronic Disease Management. Medical Anthropology Quarterly 15(3): 347–67.

Biomedical Domination and the World System

Over the past 100 years, with the increasing authority of the medical profession, traditional medicines and healers were downplayed and often disqualified from providing health services. The professionalization of medicine based on the germ theory, surgical procedures, and injections moved health care from the country doctor, or general doctor in towns, to hospital care in metropolitan centers where specialized and costly technologies could be maintained only with high usages. Rural doctors became nearly non-existent. Political power shifted to allopathy and hospital-based care. Non-surgical, non-germ-theory-based health professions were systematically reduced in numbers and some totally eliminated. Chiropractic, Homeopathy, and Osteopathy are a few of those that remain. With this professionalization of health, local health traditions and Indigenous healers were completely ostracized and discredited. The power and politics shifted from local communities to metropolitan centers. Community members lost power, knowledge and control of their own health system and their own bodies (Helman 1994). Medical discourse became structured around the terminologies of pathological anatomy and the clinical experience (Foucault 1973). Biomedicine recognizes only observable and measurable signs and physical symptoms. The non-observable or non-measurable was deemed unimportant. Disease explanations based on social relations, spirits, breaking of taboos, traumatic life experiences, emotions, economic inequalities and cultural factors were excluded from the dominant biomedical explanations.

The emergence of biomedicine as a global medical system greatly impacted Indigenous medical systems around the world. Critical medical anthropologists, Hans Baer, Merrill Singer and Ida Susser (Baer et al. 1997) concluded that regardless of the country, "biomedicine attempts to control the production of health care specialists, define their knowledge base, dominate the medical division of labor, eliminate or narrowly restrict the practices of alternative practitioners, and deny lay people and alternative healers access to medical technology." The recent call for local control and exercise of Indigenous power was in response to this domination.

Indigenous Medicine

Traditional healing and the use of plants and natural substances is a hallmark of anthropology and the basis for traditional Indigenous communities. Although a few diabetes researchers have reported on ethnomedical remedies, for example Winkelman's work on the use of a cactus in the Baja of Mexico (Winkelman 1986, 1989), diabetes is a new illness among most populations; thus traditional terms and treatments have not had significant time to develop. As noted earlier, "Anishinaabe sickness" was not brought up as an explanation by any Anishinaabe as a cause of diabetes. Diabetes is considered a "whiteman's sickness."

Biomedical clinicians have a great concern that use of traditional healers and medicines interferes with their medical treatment and prescribed regimens. Linda Hunt examined the use of alternative treatments for diabetes with a sample of Mexican-American patients. She analyzed interview transcripts for alternative treatments named, patterns of use, evaluation of those treatments, and the use of biomedical approaches. Herbs were mentioned as possible alternative treatments for diabetes by 84 percent of the patients interviewed. However, most had rarely if ever tried herbs, and viewed them as supplemental to medical treatments. Most said prayer influences health by reducing stress and bringing healing power to medicines. None used *curanderos* (traditional healers) for diabetes. Most of those interviewed actively used biomedical treatments and were less actively involved in alternative approaches. Statistical tests of association showed no competition between biomedical and alternative treatments, and alternative treatment activity tended to be significantly lower than biomedical. Most study participants emphasized medical treatment and used alternative treatments only as secondary strategies. Patients who actively used alternative approaches also actively used biomedical methods. They were using all resources they encountered. Traditional attitudes and beliefs were not especially important to the patients in this study and presented no barriers to medical care. For these patients, it also cannot be assumed that belief in alternative treatments and God's intervention were indicators of fatalism or noncompliance. Instead consideration of individual treatment behaviors is required (Hunt et al. 2000).

The research of Susan Weller and Roberta Baer (Weller and Baer 2001) in four widely separated Hispanic communities also showed that alternative medicines and traditional healers are infrequently used to cure diabetes. Puerto Ricans living in Connecticut, Mexican Americans in Southern Texas, Mexicans in Guadalarjara, Mexico, and rural Guatamalans had very similar, predominantly biomedical, explanations for diabetes. There was a belief in the effectiveness of the herbal remedies aloe vera, cactus juice, and nopal within all four communities, and the Mexican sample had a belief in emotional causes for diabetes. The high degree of sharing with little unique variation in explanations for diabetes demonstrated the pervasiveness of modern media and the rapid communication of biomedical therapies and disease explanations.

Given the increasing numbers of people with diabetes, and the high cost of biomedical medications and treatments, we can predict the creation of more Indigenous explanatory models, treatment practices and ethnobotanical remedies. For example, within the past few years, "Historical Trauma" and "Intergenerational Grief," have quickly been accepted among Native Americans and Native health care providers as explanations for major health problems, including diabetes. The most succinct advocate is Maria Yellow Horse Brave Heart, a Lakota Indian with a Ph.D. in Social Work: "Historical trauma response is a constellation of characteristics associated with massive cumulative group trauma across generations" (Brave Heart 1999). Her many publications, beginning in 1995, focus on healing historical trauma and unresolved grief. The current generation not only experiences discrimination, poverty and feelings of worthlessness, but their lives are embedded in the past historical experiences of genocide, dispossession from their ancestral lands, abusive boarding schools, and eradication efforts to distinguish traditional language, kinship systems, and religious beliefs. Brave

Heart contends this is another form of Post-traumatic stress syndrome similar to that documented for Vietnam veterans. In his presidential address to the American Public Health Association, Michael Bird (2002), a Santo Domingo/San Juan Pueblo, also expressed his view that disparity and dispossession are at the root of Indigenous health inequalities.

Jo Scheder in 1988 made the strongest anthropological statement delineating stress as a major factor in explaining Mexican-American farm worker diabetes (Scheder 1988; reproduced in this volume, Ch. 11). Likewise, Bill Dressler and collaborators in 1996 focused on acculturational stress and diabetes for the Mississippi Choctaw (Dressler et al. 1996). His continuing work quantitatively relating stress to hypertension is a notable contribution in medical anthropology. In her examination of life history narratives of California Yurok, Mariana Ferreira (Ferreira 1998; reproduced in this book, Ch. 3) related the current diabetes epidemic to Yurok body imagery constructed from generations of misfortunes, traumatic events, violence and despair. The chapters in this book are precisely devoted to better understanding the interrelationships of stress, diabetes and overall wellness.

Modernization and Technological Change

Diabetes is beginning to be recognized not only as an epidemic among Indigenous Peoples, minorities and the poor; it is an epidemic among humans everywhere who live a modern or westernized lifestyle. Globalization, modern lifestyles and the adoption of industrial technologies come with the price of chronic diseases. My own research in the 1970s was the first anthropological support of this correlation with modernization. Diabetes began within years of the Oklahoma Cherokee abandoning subsistence agriculture in the 1930s and 40s for a wage labor, industrially produced foods and labor saving devices (Wiedman 1979, 1987). Even though Indigenous Peoples may reportedly live longer with modernization, this increased longevity and the number of people over age 40 does not account for the dramatic increases in diabetes (Wiedman 1989).

Indigenous Peoples who adopt the modern lifestyle have easy access to calorie-dense foods, and the increasing number of labor-saving devices reduces energy expenditures. Individual interventions such as weight loss and physical exercise programs have shown limited improvements. Short bouts of moderate physical activity, especially those incorporated within the daily activity, are increasingly shown to be an effective way to maintain a healthy body weight over long periods of time. Biomedical studies comparing the Pima in Arizona with the Pima in Sonora, Mexico, now suggest that activity is independent of obesity as a factor for diabetes. People who are obese can reduce their risk for diabetes by having an active daily life (Kriska et al. 2003, 2001).

Modifying aspects of the widespread material culture of modernity may be easier for Indigenous communities than modifying individual knowledges and practices through individual interventions and education, which is the customary biomedical approach. Anthropologists have worked with communities to identify constraints to increasing activity levels and make recommendations to implement locally appropriate strategies to deal with these constraints. The challenge is to identify modifications in the physical environments that are acceptable to the community.

Anthropologists Cheryl Ritenbaugh, Nicolette Teufel-Shone and Jennie Joe's diabetes interventions among the Zuni of Arizona focus on community-level changes that can reduce diabetic risk. This four-year multiple-cross-sectional study examined the specific effects of changes in a cultural setting. Working together, the Pueblo of Zuni, the Zuni Public School District and the University of Arizona collaborated in the development, implementation and evaluation of a high-school-based diabetes prevention program. The Zuni Teen Wellness Center at Zuni High School involved about 400 Native teenagers in fitness/exercise, nutrition and diabetes education. Anglo teens with no intervention served as a control group. The Zuni Pueblo had accessed local water that was high in sulfur and iron. Over the years they became reliant on sugared soft drinks as the main form of liquid in their diets. The project provided purified drinking water in coolers for students in several school locations. Vending machines that had provided only sugared soft drinks and snacks were restocked with sugar-free diet beverages and healthful snacks. Project staff worked with the school food service to increase fruits and vegetables and decrease fat in school lunches. Students and staff produced posters, displays, school announcements, and public service announcements for the local radio station. Through these means nearly every student in the school was exposed to some aspect of the diabetes prevention curriculum. These efforts produced a "cultural" shift among teens: it became acceptable to choose water or diet soft drinks. Fasting insulin levels for Zuni youth of both genders were significantly higher than Anglo youth at the beginning of the intervention and showed a downward trend each year. By year three, both Zuni males and females were similar to the Anglo comparison group (Ritenbaugh et al. 2003).

Material culture items, such as advertisements for fast food, promote the availability and consumption of energy-dense foods. Anthropologists have worked to identify culturally appropriate media and strategies for communicating health messages. Joel Gittlesohn's work among the Sandy Lake Cree led him to conclude that weaving interventions programs into the existing ethnomedical model may prove more effective than imposing an external biomedical model on the community. His work then turned towards community interventions. While dietary linkages to diabetes are recognized, physical activity as a means of controlling obesity and decreasing the risk for diabetes is often not part of the local ethnomedical model. Gittelsohn used his research among the Sandy Lake Cree to develop culturally appropriate health education interventions (Gittelsohn et al. 1996), in the Marshall Islands of the South Pacific to influence island stores to stock and advertise healthy foods, and among Black Americans to substantiate the importance and value of integrating spirituality in church-based nutrition and exercise programs (Cortes et al. 2001; Young et al. 2001). His efforts are detailed in the following profile.

Profile: Joel Gittlesohn

Beginning in the early 1990s, Joel Gittlesohn worked with Canadian First Nations, Pacific Islanders, and Black American communities on a wide array of diabetes issues. He has been very influential outside of anthropology since his publications are interdisciplinary and appear in a wide array of medical journals. His work has focused on the foods that are available to local populations: subsistence foods in Canadian First Nations as compared to store purchased foods. In the South Pacific islands, where imported foods are available primarily through small privately owned grocery stores, he has worked with store owners to influence the types and quality of foods made available as well as the marketing symbols used to promote the various products. Most recently he has turned towards influencing community interventions, weaving together Indigenous knowledges and practices with biomedical practitioners.

His first published work focused on developing culturally appropriate health education diabetes interventions among the Sandy Lake Cree, an Ojibwa-Cree Community in Northern Ontario. In 1996, he used applied ethnographic research to describe diabetes within the sociocultural context, and belief systems that affect activity and dietary behaviors. Local concepts of food and illness were dichotomized into "Indian" and "white man's" groupings, with Indian foods perceived as healthy and white man's foods as unhealthy. Diabetes was believed to result from consumption of white man's "junk foods," especially sugar and soda; some believed the disease could be avoided by eating traditional Indian foods such as moose, beaver, and duck. He found that while dietary linkages to diabetes are recognized, physical activity as a means of controlling obesity and decreasing the risk for diabetes was not part of the local ethnomedical model (Gittelsohn et al. 1996).

His research has also focused on the community's knowledge of age and sex-related patterns of body image concepts and how this can assist in the design of obesity-reducing interventions targeting specific groups. Pediatric overweight is a harbinger of future diabetes risk and indicates a need for programs targeting primary prevention of obesity in children and adolescents (Hanley et al. 2000). Through nutritional and dietary surveys he identified that dietary-fiber-depleted starchy foods are conducive to the development of diabetes mellitus. The change of foods is especially noticeable among the youth. Adolescents aged 10 to 19 years consumed more simple sugars and less protein than adults over the age of 49 and ate more potato chips, fried potatoes, hamburger, pizza, soft drinks and table sugar. Adults over age 19 retained more traditional eating habits, using more bannock (fried bread) and wild meats than younger individuals. He recommended that interventions to prevent diabetes in the community should include culturally appropriate and effective ways to improve the nutritional adequacy of the diet, reduce fat intake and increase the use of less refined carbohydrate foods (Wolever et al. 1997).

Most of these foods are relatively high in fiber and low in fat. High consumption of junk foods and the bread-and-butter group was associated with substantial increases in risk for diabetes. These foods tend to be high in simple sugars, low in fiber and high in fat. More fatty methods of food preparation are also associated with increased risk for diabetes in this population. This information was incorporated into an ongoing community-based diabetes prevention program in the community (Gittelsohn et al. 1998).

In urban and remote settings of the Marshall Islands of the South Pacific Gittlesohn helped to develop a diabetes-prevention intervention based on research methods utilizing in-depth interviews, semi structured interviews, and direct observation of household behaviors. Foods were classified into two main conceptual spheres: Marshallese foods from the islands and imported American foods. Marshall Islanders believe that diabetes, a prominent illness in their lives, is caused by foods high in fat and sugar, consumption of imported/American foods high in fat and sugar, and atomic bomb testing. Physical activity and eating a traditional diet were viewed as important for preventing diabetes. The traditional belief system links a large body with health, and a thin body with illness. These findings were used to develop a diabetes-prevention home-visit intervention currently being implemented and evaluated in Marshallese households (Cortes et al. 2001). Access to imported foods is primarily through the island stores; his survey of the stores, the foods the storeowners ordered and advertised were analyzed. Working with storeowners to provide and advertise healthy foods is an important way to control diabetes in small, isolated communities.

From his work with African-American community churches Gittlesohn produced information used to develop two culturally appropriate interventions showing that church-based nutrition and exercise programs supplemented with spiritual strategies significantly benefited the cardiovascular health of African American women (Yanek, et al. 2001).

In analyzing the motivations for successful participation in weight loss programs Gittlesohn focused on groups of African-American women who were currently physically active or currently sedentary. Motivators for the exercisers to start exercising were health concerns, weight control, stress reduction, and the influence of others. In contrast, the sedentary women reported that social support and enjoyment would be motivating (Young et al. 2001).

Notable Diabetes Publications

Gittelsohn, Joel, S.B. Harris, S. Whitehead, T.M.S. Wolever, A.J.G. Hanley, A. Barnie, L. Kakegamic, A. Logan and B. Zinman. 1995. Developing Diabetes Intervention in an Ojibwa-Cree Community in Northern Ontario: Linking Qualitative and Quantitative Data. Chronic Disease in Canada 16: 157–64.

Gittelsohn, Joel, S.B. Harris, K.L. Burris, L. Kakegamic, L.T. Landman, A. Sharma, T.M. Wolever, A. Logan, A. Barnie and B. Zinman. 1996. Use of Ethnographic Methods for Applied Research on Diabetes among the Ojibway-Cree in Northern Ontario. Health Education Quarterly 23(3): 365–82.

Young, D.R., Joel Gittelsohn, J. Charleston, K. Felix-Aaron and L.J. Appel. 2002. Motivations for Exercise and Weight Loss Among African-American Women: Focus Group Results and Their Contribution Towards Program Development. Ethnicity & Health 6(3-4): 227–45.

Policy Develoment

At the local policy level, anthropologists are now influencing companies, stores, government agencies, schools, university dormitories, cafeterias and other organizations whose decisions affect the daily activity of people through the availability of food and drink, or the design of buildings and recreational areas. Their research, publications and teaching are influencing basic nutrition research, research method refinement, and effectiveness of medical curriculum. These efforts are now influencing national and international policy.

Cheryl Ritenbaugh, a member of the International Obesity Task Force, developed policies stating that public health efforts cannot rely solely on individualized health education strategies, but that living environments need to be transformed so that they promote and support healthy eating and physical activity habits throughout the life cycle for the entire population. Furthermore, strategies need to address the underlying societal causes of obesity through transformation of thinking on transport, environment, work facilities, education, health and food policies as well as social and economic policies. These efforts require coordinated action from all relevant sectors of a nation, society, and local community (Kumanyika et al. 1998).

Profile: Cheryl Ritenbaugh

The first anthropology Ph.D. dissertation written specifically on diabetes was in 1974 by Cheryl Ritenbaugh. Since that time she has continued to devote efforts to diabetes, obesity prevention, cancer among post-menopausal women, and the refinement of nutritional research methodology. She has evaluated health among the Zuni Tribe of Arizona, the Dogrib of Canada, and Indigenous Peoples in Washington State. She has taken her knowledge and the anthropological perspective on diabetes and obesity to the highest levels of policy making by contributing to the International Obesity Task Force. Her work has led to policies and interventions restricting soda and soda machines in tribal communities and schools.

Her program evaluation efforts demonstrate that for diabetes prevention programs to succeed in Indigenous communities it is essential that they be community-based and supported. Collaborating with anthropologist Nicolette Teufel, Cheryl evaluated the most notable community-based diabetes project, the Zuni Diabetes Prevention Program. Focused on high-school-age youths, the program is designed to enhance knowledge of diabetes; increase physical activity, and fruit and vegetable intake; and reduced the consumption of soft drinks. Based in a school wellness center, interventions include diabetes education, supportive social networks, and modification of the food supply available to teens. Evaluation results show a significant reduction in soft drink consumption and improved glucose/insulin ratios, suggesting a decline in the incidence of hyperinsulinemia (Teufel and Ritenbaugh 1998).

Her earlier work examined dietary change among Dogrib Indians of the Canadian Northwest Territories, comparing the acculturated to less-acculturated settlements undergoing change from a "traditional" to a "modern" life-style. Among these settlements of subsistence hunters the traditional food base was stable and they had a low prevalence of diabetes. With acculturation, rather than the replacement of traditional foods, the new industrialized processed foods obtained through stores and government programs were added to the stable traditional diet. The addition of new food sources increased caloric intake (Szathmary et al. 1987). With acculturation, the macronutrient composition changes from that of a hunting-based diet (high protein, moderate fat, low carbohydrate) to one with relatively more carbohydrate and fat, and less protein. This pattern is especially evident among younger Dogrib (Ritenbaugh et al. 1996).

Cheryl Ritenbaugh and Carol Goodby examined the implications of a northern hunting adaptation where there is a reliance on animal foods and seasonal shortages in terms of energy digestion, absorption, metabolism and storage. They analyzed the physiologic adaptations to a high protein, moderate fat, low carbohydrate diet compared to agriculturally based subsistence systems and industrialized societies. Specific metabolic pathways were identified as fruitful areas for further research regarding genetic variants in New World populations (Ritenbaugh and Goodby 1989).

At the population level, the global obesity epidemic reflects a set of profound societal changes including modernization, economic transition to market economies, urbanization, changing occupational structures, and globalization of food markets. These have inadvertently led to a fall in spontaneous and work-related physical activity, and a readiness for over-consumption of energy dense/high fat foods. Past attempts to improve community diet and physical activity habits, however, have had little impact on body weight. Experiences in the U.S. and elsewhere have demonstrated that obesity is far more difficult to control than other chronic conditions or risk factors for non-communicable disease. This is illustrated by the case of Minnesota, where obesity levels rose despite sophisticated public health programs to improve physical activity levels and other risk factors for coronary heart disease. Suggested reasons for the apparent failure relate to over-reliance on educational strategies without attending to the environmental changes needed to encourage and support behavior change, and the lack of commitment to action from all relevant sectors of society. A multi-sectorial and broad-based public health approach to prevention is required if the dramatic rises in obesity rates seen throughout the world today are to be tackled effectively. This requires the identification of practical strategies to prevent populations in general from becoming fatter, but also complementary targeted preventive strategies for high-risk groups (Kumanyika et al. 1998).

Notable Diabetes Publications

Ritenbaugh C, N.I. Teufel-Shone, M.G. Aickin, J.R. Joe, S. Poirier, D.C. Dillingham, D. Johnson, S. Henning, S.M. Cole and D. Cockerham. 2003. A Lifestyle Intervention Improves Plasma Insulin Levels Among Native American High School Youth. Preventive Medicine 36(3): 309–19.

Ritenbaugh, C. and C. S. Goodby. 1989. "Beyond the Thrifty Gene: Metabolic Implications of Prehistoric Migration into the New World." Medical Anthropology 11(3): 227–36.

Anthropologist and Indigenous Community Collaborations

From this historical review we can see that anthropologists continue to make significant contributions to understanding diabetes, and designing effective prevention and treatment programs. This illustrates that anthropologists have an increasingly influential and important role in the health and well being of the world's populations.

Many world populations are in a pre-diabetic transition. With globalization and industrialization we can predict that the rate of diabetes will increase significantly. However, Indigenous communities learn from these insights and take actions to design healthy lifestyles.

Anthropologists can make a significant contribution to the diabetes problem by working with Indigenous community members on interdisciplinary teams to design culturally appropriate methodologies and interventions (see chapter 16, Macaulay et al., in this volume). To be proactive, anthropologists can work with Indigenous groups to create, reintroduce, or redefine traditional substances and practices that would benefit a healthy lifestyle and prevent diabetes. Innovative narrative interpretations similar to Hagey's Nanabush are an example. Elevating and honoring the running traditions of the Zuni to promote physical activity is another, as is the promotion and use of Native teas and flavored drinks to substitute for sugared and high calorie sodas. A major challenge is to design instruments that solicit motivating factors and benefits of "good health," and then to use these in ways that stimulate healthy lifestyles. Anthropologists can help influence companies, stores, government agencies, schools, university dormitories, cafeterias and other organizations whose decisions affect the daily activity of people and the availability of food and drink. Working with Indigenous communities in the design of buildings and recreational areas could significantly increase daily activity levels. By promoting the positives of "healthy communities," rather then the negatives of "disease" prevention, community empowerment could reduce the pandemic of chronic diseases associated with the industrial lifestyle.

During these 25 years of contributions to diabetes research, anthropologists have shown they can work with Indigenous communities to use these skills, insights and perspectives to influence cultural changes in support of "healthy communities." A number of anthropological insights gained over these years could be integral to Indigenous community efforts:

1. Local cultural knowledges about diabetes, its causes and treatments differ from the standard biomedical model.
2. For diabetes interventions to be long lasting and effective, local cultural systems and languages provide a framework within which interventions must be constructed.
3. Selection of appropriate forms of local vocabulary enhances health care workers' communication with individuals with diabetes and those at risk.
4. Ethnographic methods bridge the different cultural systems in a community and should be required whenever developing diabetic interventions in new or challenging cultural settings.

Acknowledgments

This entire chapter is an acknowledgement of numerous anthropologists. Written from another perspective it would have highlighted a different set of contributors. Any omissions were not intended. A full range of anthropologists and their publications are available on the Internet web page: "Anthropological Contributions to Diabetes Research and Intervention: A Bibliography." http://www.fiu.edu/~wiedmand/medan-thro/diabetesanthropubs.htm (Wiedman 2002)

I would like to especially acknowledge the Delaware elder, Nora Thompson Dean. In the 1960s she welcomed me, and my wife Felicia, to be part of the Delaware people of northeastern Oklahoma. The many ways that diabetes negatively influenced the quality of Nora's life and her family, set me off on a lifetime pursuit to enhance the health of Native Americans. Secondly, I am indebted to Kelly West, at the University of Oklahoma Health Sciences Center. His profound understanding of diabetes in the 1970s was prophetic of the diabetes epidemic in the US today. And thirdly, to my mother and father, Frances and John Wiedman, who still to this day, bring to my attention Native American issues and events. Their values continue on. But most of all, I must acknowledge my wife Felicia, who has been by my side for all these years.

References

Baer, Hans, Merrill Singer and Ida Susser. 1997. Medical Anthropology and the World System. Westport, Connecticut: Bergin and Garvey.

Bindon, James R. 1988. The Natural History of Diabetes in Samoa. Collegium Antropologicum 12(suppl): 85.

Bindon, James R., D.E. Crews and William W. Dressler. 1991. Life Style, Modernization, and Adaptation Among Samoans. Collegium Antropologicum 15: 101–10.

Bird, Michael E. 2002. Health and Indigenous People: Recommendations for the Next Generation. American Journal of Public Health 92(9): 1391–92.

Brave Heart, Maria Yellow Horse. 1999. Gender Differences in the Historical Trauma Response Among the Lakota. Journal of Health and Social Policy 10(4): 1–21.

Cortes, L. M., Joel Gittelsohn, J. Alfred and N. A. Palafox. 2001. Formative Research to Inform Intervention Development for Diabetes Prevention in the Republic of the Marshall Islands. Health Education and Behavior 28(6): 696–715.

Crews, Douglas and E. Mackeen. 1982. Mortality Related to Cardiovascular Disease and Diabetes Mellitus in a Modernizing Population. Social Science and Medicine 16: 175–81.

Dressler, William W., James R. Bindon and M. Janice Gilliland. 1996. Sociocultural and Behavioral Influences on Health Status among the Mississippi Choctaw. Medical Anthropology 17(2): 165–80.

Ferreira, Mariana K. 1998. Slipping Through Skyholes: Yurok Body Imagery in Northern California. Culture, Medicine and Psychiatry 22: 171–202.

Ferzacca, Steve. 2000. "Actually, I don't feel that bad": Managing Diabetes and the Clinical Encounter. Medical Anthropology Quarterly 14(1): 28–50.

Foucault, Michel. 1973. The Birth of the Clinic: An Archaeology of Medical Perception. A.M.S. Smith, transl. New York: Pantheon.

Frate, Dennis A., Monroe Ginn and Lela Keys. 2000. A Community-Based Case Management Model for Hypertension and Diabetes. Practicing Anthropology 22(3): 34–38.

Garro, Linda C. 1995. Individual or Societal Responsibility? Explanations of Diabetes in an Anishinaabe (Ojibway) Community. Social Science & Medicine 40(1): 37–46.

———2000. Remembering What One Knows and the Construction of the Past: A Comparison of Cultural Consensus Theory and Cultural Schema Theory. Ethos 28(3): 275–319.

Gittelsohn, Joel, S. B. Harris, K. L. Burris, L. Kakegamic, L. T. Landman, A. Sharma, T. M. Wolever, A. Logan, A. Barnie and B. Zinman. 1996. Use of Ethnographic Methods for Applied Research on Diabetes among the Ojibway-Cree in Northern Ontario. Health Education Quarterly 23(3): 365–82.

Gittelsohn, Joel, T. M. Wolever, S. B. Harris, R. Harris-Giraldo, A. J. Hanley and B. Zinman. 1998. Specific Patterns of Food Consumption and Preparation are Associated with Diabetes and Obesity in a Native Canadian Community. Journal of Nutrition 128(3): 541–47.

Hagey, Rebecca. 1984. The Phenomenon, the Explanations and the Responses: Metaphors Surrounding Diabetes in Urban Canadian Indians. Social Science and Medicine 18(3): 265–72.

———1989. The Native Diabetes Program: Rhetorical Process and Praxis. Medical Anthropology 12(1): 7–33.

Hagey, Rebecca and E. Buller. 1983. Drumming and Dancing: A New Rhythm in Nursing Care. Canadian Nurse 79(4): 28–31.

Hanley, A. J., S. B. Harris, Joel Gittelsohn, T. M. Wolever, B. Saksvig and B. Zinman. 2000. Overweight among Children and Adolescents in a Native Canadian Community: Prevalence and Associated Factors. American Journal of Clinical Nutrition 71(3): 693–700.

Helman, Cecil. 1994. Culture, Health and Illness: An Introduction for Health Professionals. Oxford: Butterworth-Heinemann.

Hunt, Linda and Nadel H. Arar. 2001. An Analytical Framework for Contrasting Patient and Provider Views of the Process of Chronic Disease Management. Medical Anthropology Quarterly 15(3): 347–67.

Hunt, Linda M., Nadel H. Arar and Anne C. Larme. 1998a. Contrasting Patient and Practitioner Perspectives in Type 2 Diabetes Management. Western Journal of Nursing Research 20(6): 656–76; discussion. pp. 677–82.

Hunt, Linda M., Nedal H. Arar and Laura L. Akana. 2000. Herbs, Prayer, and Insulin. Use of Medical and Alternative Treatments by a Group of Mexican American Diabetic Patients. Journal of Family Practice 49(3): 216–23.

Hunt, Linda M., Jacqueline A. Pugh and Miguel Valenzuela. 1998b. How Patients Adapt Diabetes Self-Care Recommendations in Everyday Life. Journal of Family Practice 46(3): 207–15.

Hunt, Linda M., Miguel A. Valenzuela and Jacqueline A. Pugh. 1998c. Porque me toco a mi? Mexican American Diabetes Patients' Causal Stories and their Relationship to Treatment Behaviors. Social Science and Medicine 46(8): 959–69.

Hunt, Linda M., Miquel A. Valenzuela and Jacqueline A. Pugh. 1997. NIDDM Patients' Fears and Hopes about Insulin Therapy: The Basis of Patient Reluctance. Diabetes Care 20(3): 292–98.

Judkins, Russell A. 1975. Diet And Diabetes among the Iroquois: An Integrative Approach. International Congress of Americanists, 41st, Mexico, 1974. Actas Del Xli Congreso Internacional De Americanistas 41(3): 313–22.

———1978. Diabetes and Perception of Diabetes among Seneca Indians. New York State Journal of Medicine 78(8): 1320–23.

Kriska, Andrea M., Mark A. Pereira, Robert L. Hanson, Maximilian P. de Courten, Paul Z. Zimmet, K. George M.M. Alberti, Pierrot Chitson, Peter H. Bennett, K.M. Venkat Narayan and William C. Knowler. 2001. Association of Physical Activity and Serum Insulin Concentrations in Two Populations at High Risk for Type 2 Diabetes but Differing by BMI. Diabetes Care 24(7): 1175–80.

Kriska, Andrea M., Aramesh Saremi, Robert L. Hanson, Peter H. Bennett, Sayuko Kobes, Desmond E. Williams and William C. Knowler. 2003. Physical Activity, Obesity, and the Incidence of Type 2 Diabetes in a High-Risk Population. American Journal of Epidemiology 158(7): 669–75.

Kumanyika, S., V. Anitpatis, R. Jeffery, A. Morabia, Cheryl Ritenbaugh and W. P. T. James. 1998. The International Obesity Task Force: Its Role in Public Health Prevention. Appetite 31(3): 426–28.

Lang, Gretchen Chesley. 1989. "Making Sense" About Diabetes: Dakota Narratives of Illness. Medical Anthropology 11(3): 305–27.

Larme, Anne C. and Jacqueline A. Pugh. 2001. Evidence-Based Guidelines Meet the Real World: The Case of Diabetes Care. Diabetes Care 24(10): 1728–33.

Miewald, Christina E. 1997. Is Awareness Enough? The Contradictions of Self-Care in a Chronic Disease Clinic. Human Organization 56(3): 353–63.

Ritenbaugh, Cheryl. 1974. The Pattern of Diabetes in a Pima Community, University of California, Los Angeles.

Ritenbaugh, Cheryl and Carol S. Goodby. 1989. Beyond the Thrifty Gene: Metabolic Implications of Prehistoric Migration into the New World. Medical Anthropology 11(3): 227–36.

Ritenbaugh, Cheryl, Emöke J.E. Szathmary, Carol S. Goodby and C. Feldman. 1996. Dietary Acculturation Among the Dogrib Indians of the Canadian Northwest Territories. Ecology of Food and Nutrition 35(2): 81–94.

Ritenbaugh, Cheryl, Nicolette I. Teufel-Shone, Mikel G. Aickin, Jennie R. Joe, Steven Poirier, D. Clay Dillingham, David Johnson, Susanne Henning, Suzanne Cole and David Cockerham. 2003. A Lifestyle Intervention Improves Plasma Insulin Levels Among Native American High School Youth. Preventive Medicine 36: 309–19.

Scheder, Jo C. 1988. A Sickly-Sweet Harvest: Farmworker Diabetes and Social Equality. Medical Anthropology Quarterly 2: 251–77.

Smith, Janell, Penelope Easton, Dennis Wiedman, Nancy Rody, Kari Hamrick, Betsy Nobmann, Emma Widmark, Diane Peck and Jennifer Cipra. (In Press) Evaluation of BMI and Body Fat Determinations as Health Indices in Women Living in Alaska

Rural Villages: Result of the WIC Healthy Mom Survey, Summer 2001. Alaska Medicine.

Smith, Janell and Dennis Wiedman. 2001. Fat Content of South Florida Indian Frybread: Health Implications for a Pervasive Native-American Food. Journal of the American Dietetic Association 101(5): 582–85.

Stein, Howard F. 1992. The Many-Voiced Cultural Story Line of a Case of Diabetes Mellitus. Journal of Family Practice 35(5): 529–33.

Szathmary, Emöke J. E. 1985. Search for Genetic Factors Controlling Plasma Glucose Levels in Dogrib Indians. In Diseases of Complex Etiology in Small Populations. E. Ranajit Chakraborty and Emöke J. E. Szathmary, eds. pp. 199–225: New York: Alan R. Liss.

_____1994. Non-Insulin Dependent Diabetes Mellitus Among Aboriginal North Americans. Annual Review of Anthropology (23): 457–82.

Szathmary, Emöke J., Cheryl Ritenbaugh and Carol S. Goodby. 1987. Dietary Change and Plasma Glucose Levels in an Amerindian Population Undergoing Cultural Transition. Social Science and Medicine 24(10): 791–804.

Teufel, Nicolette I. and Cheryl K. Ritenbaugh. 1998. Development of a Primary Prevention Program: Insight Gained in the Zuni Diabetes Prevention Program. Clinical Pediatrics 37(2): 131–41.

Thompson, Samantha J. and Sandra M. Gifford. 2000. Trying to Keep a Balance: The Meaning of Health and Diabetes in an Urban Aboriginal Community. Social Science and Medicine 51(10): 1457–72.

Tuomilehto, J, J. Lindstrom, J.G. Ericksson, T. T. Valle, H. Hamalainen, P. Ilanne-Parikka, S. Keinanen-Kiukaanniemi, M. Laakso, A. Louheranta, M. Rastas, V. Salminen and M. Uusitupa. 2001. Prevention of Type 2 Diabetes Mellitus by Changes in Lifestyle Among Subjects with Impaired Glucose Tolerance. New England Journal of Medicine 344: 1343–50.

Urdaneta, Maria Luisa and Rodney Krebiel. 1989. Anthropological Perspectives on Diabetes Mellitus Type II. Medical Anthropology 11(3): 221–26.

Weiss, Kenneth M. 1995. Implications of Genetic-Variation within and between Human Populations. Population Research and Policy Review 14(3): 315–25.

Weiss, Kenneth M., Robert E. Ferrell and Craig L. Hanis. 1984. A New World Syndrome of Metabolic Diseases with a Genetic and Evolutionary Basis. Yearbook of Physical Anthropology 27: 153–78.

Weller, Susan C. and Roberta D. Baer. 2001. Intra- and Intercultural Variation in the Definition of Five Illnesses: AIDS, Diabetes, the Common Cold, Empacho, and Mal De Ojo. Cross-Cultural Research 35(2): 201–26.

West, Kelly. 1978. Epidemiology of Diabetes and its Vascular Lesions. New York: Elsevier.

Wiedman, Dennis. 1979. Type II Diabetes Mellitus and Oklahoma Native Americans: A Case Study of Culture Change in Oklahoma Cherokee, University of Oklahoma.

_____1987. Type II Diabetes Mellitus, Technological Development and the Oklahoma Cherokee. In Encounters in Biomedicine: Case Studies in Medical Anthropology. Hans Baer, ed. New York: Gordon and Breach.

_____1989. Adiposity or Longevity: Which Factor Accounts for the Increase in Type II Diabetes Mellitus When Populations Acculturate to an Industrial Technology? Medical Anthropology 11(3): 237–54.

_____2002. Anthropological Contributions to Diabetes Research and Interventions: A Bibliography. <www.fiu.edu/~wiedmand/medanthro/diabetesanthropubs.htm>. First published November 5, 2002. Accessed March 19, 2004.

Williams, Robert C. 1983. Has the Recessive Hypothesis for Susceptibility to Insulin-Dependent Diabetes Mellitus been Firmly and Unequivocally Rejected? Diabetes 32(8): 774–76.

Williams, Robert C., J. C. Long, R. L. Hanson, M. L. Sievers and W. C. Knowler. 2000. Individual Estimates of European Genetic Admixture Associated with Lower Body-Mass Index, Plasma Glucose, and Prevalence of Type 2 Diabetes in Pima Indians. American Journal of Human Genetics 66(2): 527–38.

Winkelman, Michael. 1986. Frequently used Medicinal Plants in Baja California Norte. Journal of Ethnopharmacology 18(2): 109–31.

_____1989. Ethnobotanical Treatments of Diabetes in Baja California Norte. Medical Anthropology 11(3): 255–68.

Wolever, T. M. S., Joel Gittelsohn, J. Gao, A. J. G. Hanley, S. B. Harris and B. Zinman. 1997. Low Dietary Fiber Intake Associated with Diabetes in a Remote Aboriginal Community in Northern Ontario. Diabetes 46: 1423–23.

Woolfson, P., V. Hood, R. Secker-Walker and A. Macaulay. 1995. Mohawk English in the Medical Interview. Medical Anthropology Quarterly 9(4): 503–9.

Yanek, L. R., D. M. Becker, T. F. Moy, J. Gittelsohn and D. M. Koffman. 2001. Project Joy: Faith Based Cardiovascular Health Promotion for African American Women. Public Health Reports 116: 68–81.

Young, D. R., Joel Gittelsohn, J. Charleston, K. Felix-Aaron and L. J. Appel. 2001. Motivations for Exercise and Weight Loss Among African-American Women: Focus Group Results and Their Contribution Towards Program Development. Ethnicity and Health 6(3-4): 227–45.

Young, James, and Linda C. Garro. 1994. Medical Choice in a Mexican Village. Prospect Heights, Illinois: Waveland Press.

Young, T. Kue. 1979. Changing Patterns of Health and Sickness Among the Cree-Ojibway of Northwestern Ontario. Medical Anthropology 3: 191–223.

Young, T. Kue, P. J. Martens, S. P. Taback, E. A. C. Sellers, H. J. Dean, M. Cheang and B. Flett. 2002. Type 2 Diabetes Mellitus in Children—Prenatal and Early Infancy Risk Factors Among Native Canadians. Archives of Pediatrics and Adolescent Medicine 156(7): 651–55.

CONTRIBUTORS

Sherri Bisset, MSc

I am currently pursing a doctorate degree in Public Health at the Université of Montréal. I hold post-secondary degrees in Community Health, Epidemiology and Nutrition. My educational training over the next several years will address evaluation research, social inequalities in health and childhood development. Eventually, I would like to contribute to advancing knowledge surrounding the school as a setting for health promotion.

Jocelyn Bruyère, BA, BScN, MSc

I am an educator, researcher, and program administrator with a Masters of Science degree in Community Health Sciences from the University of Manitoba, Canada. I am a First Nation member of Opaskwayak, Manitoba. This contribution is based on Masters Thesis topic: Understandings about Type 2 Diabetes Mellitus among the Nêhinaw (Cree). As Tribal Nursing Officer at the Cree Nation Tribal Health Centre, I am Responsible to ensure nursing, medical and health services are provided to the Swampy Cree Tribal Council First Nations. Also responsible for diabetes coordination and representation. I co-chair the Manitoba First Nations Diabetes Committee (We have developed a First Nations Strategy)and also co-chair the Ministerial Advisory Committee on diabetes. Developed pamphlet in Cree and English on Diabetes for use in diabetes education in the Swampy Cree Tribal Council area. Some relevant publications include:

Margaret Cargo, PhD

I am a researcher in the Division of Population Health at the Université of Montréal Hospital Centre. My primary research interest is in uncovering the social process by which Aboriginal communities develop their collective capability to promote and protect their health and thus reduce health inequalities. Other interests include community governance, colonialism and Aboriginal health status, epistemology and theory in health research.

Treena Delormier, MSc

I am Kahnawakero:non and have been a KSDPP Community Advisory Board member since KSDPP "officially" started in 1994. I have worked as a research assistant with the project as well. I am a mother and dedicated to improving the health of Aboriginal communities. Professionally, I am a doctoral candidate in the public health program (Health Promotion option) at the Université de Montréal, hold a masters degree in nutrition and am a professional dietitian.

Mariana Leal Ferreira, PhD

I am a Brazilian anthropologist specializing in the social causes of illness, the politics of Indigenous identity, and human rights in South and North America. After working as a nurse, math teacher and coordinator of Indigenous school programs in central Brazil and in the Amazon from 1978 to1992, I completed a doctorate in medical anthropology at UC Berkeley and UC San Francisco in 1996. My dissertation, Sweet Tears and Bitter Pills. The Politics of Health among the Yuroks in Northern California is a political history of emotions, trauma and type 2 diabetes. Post-doctoral work at the U of São Paulo on poverty, violence and substance abuse on southern Brazilian Indigenous territories has now led me to compare the dramatic mental health situation (suicide in particular) of Indigenous children in Brazil and the US.. My publications include books, literary and scholarly articles, some written specifically for Indigenous schools and a broader non-academic audience on topics including the anthropology of education; the mathematics of peace and solidarity; poverty and scarcity on Indigenous territories; Indigenous children, human rights and environmental justice.

Sophie Frishkopf, BA

I was trained in medical anthropology at the University of Arizona. Following my studies I worked for four years as a Research Assistant at the Native American Research and Training Center in Tucson, Arizona. Currently, I work as project coordinator of a research project on depression at the Boston Medical Center in Boston, Massachusetts.

Kim Grower-Dowling, BA

I received my BA from Siena Heights College in Adrian, MI, with a dual major in art and management. I am currently a Research Assistant for a project on Stress Management in Type 2 Diabetes Mellitus in the Department of Psychiatry at the Medical College of Ohio.

Kim Humphery, PhD

I teach history and social theory at RMIT University, Melbourne Australia. Much of my academic work has been on the history and contemporary nature of materialism and consumption, particularly in Australia. But I have, as well, worked for many years as a qualitative social researcher, particularly in the field of Indigenous health. From 1999 to 2001 I was a Senior Research Fellow with the VicHealth Koori Health Research and Community Development Unit at the University of Melbourne, and from 1997 to 1999 I held a similar fellowship at the Cooperative Research Centre for Aboriginal and Tropical Health in Darwin. In Darwin, I started working on how diabetes was being experienced and thought about within two remote Aboriginal communities, one 'saltwater' and one 'desert' community. I moved from there to exploring in broader terms the dynamics of cross-cultural health care in collaboration with my colleagues Tarun Weeramanthri and Joe Fitz. Besides having produced a number of reports and discussion papers in the area of Indigenous health, I am author of Shelf Life (Cambridge University Press 1998) and, with Tarun Weeramanthri and Joe Fitz, Forgetting Compliance: Aboriginal Health and Medical Culture (Northern Territory University Press 2001).

Jennie R. Joe, PhD

I am a medical anthropologist who holds a professorship in Family and Community Medicine and directs the Native American Research and Training Center at the University of Arizona. As a member of the Navajo Nation, my health-related research interests include chronic diseases and its impact on American Indian/Alaska Native communities as well as other indigenous communities in Australia, New Zealand, and

Canada. Some of the specific areas of interests include diabetes, cancer, health policies, and cross-cultural perceptions of health and illness.

Leslie E. Korn, PhD, MPH

I am the granddaughter of Romanian Jewish women who healed with their hands
and their food. I embraced this cultural memory only years after I had been living in
the dry forest of Mexico wondering why I felt so totally at home in that beautiful land
touching the feet and bellies of my patients. Following 10 years in Yelapa, I returned
to complete my formal graduate training at Lesley University, (Health Psychology)
Harvard School of Public Health and Harvard Medical School (Religion and Psychology). I returned to Mexico following my PhD from the Union Institute (Traditional
Medicine and Feminist Theory) where I conducted the work outlined in this chapter.
I have a clinical/healing practice in Olympia WA. My current research is funded by the
National Institutes of Health to document the effects of Polarity Therapy on the health
of American Indian family caregivers. I am married, with three grown step-sons and
a wild dog who figures in everything.

Gretchen Chesley Lang, PhD

I am a cultural anthropologist; my research has primarily addressed health issues,
foodways, and sustainability issues. In the early 1970s, I worked with Ojibway migrants
to inner-city Minneapolis—categorized by themselves and others as "drinkers"—
whose adaptive strategies included a wide variety of casual labor jobs and services of
the first American Indian halfway house; with Dakota (Sioux) community members
and health care workers to portray varied perspectives on health, diabetes and diabetes
care at Devil's Lake Reservation, ND; and have documented the role of "kitchen gardens"—trees, plants and animals—in household food security in three villages in rural
Tamil Nadu, S. India.(1994, as Indo-American Fellow). I am Prof. Emerita, Anthropology, U of North Dakota, and continue scholarly activities including a life history
project, topics in foodways, sustainable lifeways, photographic representation, and the
use of literature and film in teaching anthropology.

Lucie Lévesque, PhD

I joined the School of Physical and Health Education at Queen's University
(Kingston, Ontario, Canada) in 2002 as Assistant Professor in Exercise and Health Psychology. My graduate training in exercise psychology (PhD from Laval University in
1997) and post-doctoral work in health promotion (Université de Montéal, 1998-2001)
bring a behavioural and ecological perspective to issues of physical activity involvement and community health promotion. As co-investigator of the Kahnawake Schools
Diabetes Prevention Project since 1998, I contribute to research activities that pertain
to community physical activity involvement.

Ann C. Macaulay, MD

I am an Associate Professor in Family Medicine at McGill University. In 1970 I was
the first family physician to be hired by the Kanien'kehá;ka (Mohawk) community of
Kahnawake, when the community began directing their own health services. I this position I became concerned about the high prevalence of diabetes in the community.
Today I am the Scientific Director of the Kahnawake Schools Diabetes Prevention Project (KSDPP) Center for Research and Training in Diabetes Prevention located in Kah-

nawake and funded by the Canadian Institutes of Health Research. This is based on an innovative partnership between Kahnawake, McGill University and Université de Montréal, for the intervention and evaluation of the primary prevention of Type 2 diabetes in Aboriginal peoples, and for training Aboriginal researchers, other researchers and community members in community–based participatory research for community mobilisation for diabetes prevention.

Alex M. McComber, MEd

Tekwanonhwará:tons. Otsehtokon niwaksennò:ten wakskaré:wake Kahnawake nitewaké:non. I am Otsehtokon (a.k.a. Alex M. McComber), bear clan from Kahnawa:ke Mohawk Territory. I have been with the Kahnawake Schools Diabetes Prevention Project since its inception in 1994 and presently work as the Training Coordinator. I hold a Bachelor of Arts in Teacher Training from St. Francis College in Brooklyn New York and a Masters in Education Administration from McGill University in Montreal. I have been a substance abuse program coordinator, and a high school teacher and principal at the Kahnawa:ke Survival School. I am current Chairman of Board of the National Aboriginal Diabetes Association, an adjunct professor at McGill's Faculty of Education and a little league coach. I have served on various Kahnawa:ke boards of directors for education and recreation and am a former volunteer firefighter and ambulance driver. My wife and three children are the most loving and patient people on Mother Earth.

Angele McGrady, PhD, MEd, LPCC

I am currently a Professor, Department of Psychiatry, and Administrative Director, Complementary Medicine Center, Medical College of Ohio, Toledo, Ohio. I received my BS from Chestnut Hill College in Philadelphia, my Masters in Physiology from Michigan State University and PhD in Biology from the University of Toledo. Later my interests shifted to psychophysiology so I completed a Masters in Guidance and Counseling. I am licensed as a Professional Clinical Counselor and certified by the Biofeedback Certification Institute of America. I am a professor in the Department of Physiology and maintain a practice in counseling and biofeedback in the Department of Psychiatry. I am also director of the Complementary Medicine Center at the Medical College of Ohio. My research and clinical specialties are stress related disorders and emotional problems associated with chronic medical illness. I have published more than 50 peer reviewed articles, seven book chapters and co-edited one book.

Bea Nix

I am currently a clinic coordinator at a medical clinic in Weitchpec, California, on the Yurok Indian Reservation. I am a member of the Yurok Tribe. Originally, I started working with the model diabetes program at United Indian Health Services. In that capacity, I worked for many years with Native Peoples and diabetes education. I have been part of the effort to help disseminate diabetes education at a national and international level, including Hawai'i and Canada.

Emily Omura, BA

During the summer of 2002, I was granted a Higher Education Consortium Urban Affairs internship at the White Earth Land Recovery Project (WELRP). Working on the Mino-Miijim project under Margaret Smith was an incredible experience, and when the summer ended I remained a volunteer and found school-related excuses to return to White Earth: a photoethnography project and my senior thesis for Macalester College. I have given both of these projects to the WELRP. My future plans include medical school; at present I am teaching English in Japan.

Louise Potvin, PhD

I obtained my doctorate in Public Health in 1986 from Université de Montréal. I am professor at the Department of Social and Preventive Medicine, Université de Montréal and researcher at the Interdisciplinary Health Research Group. Since 2001, I have held the CHSRF/CIHR Chair on Community Approaches and Health Inequalities, which aims to document how public health interventions in support of local social development contribute to the reduction of health inequalities in urban settings. My main research interests are the evaluation of community health promotion programs and how local social environments are conducive of health. I was a member of the WHO Working Group on the evaluation of health promotion.

Terry Raymer, MD

Born, raised, and lived in California my whole life (except for a couple of lengthy excursions to Europe and beyond), but as I learned at the lunch table one day, that doesn't make me a "native." I have worked at United Indian Health Services for the last 14 years as a family physician, the last 6 dedicated primarily to diabetes care. I have also worked with the Indian Health Service (IHS) National Diabetes Program and have assisted with the California Region of the IHS as an Area Diabetes Consultant. When I'm not working at the clinic, I usually wheedle away a little time with my son or daughter while trying to comprehend how these two teenage "offspring" seem to have a better grasp on life than I ever did. The rest of my precious little time is spent on my bike or occasionally in my kayak supposing I'm puzzling out some spiritual conundrum, which usually deteriorates into ruminating over mundane tragedies.

Muriel Roddier, PhD (Anthropology), State Diploma in Nursing (France)

I am a nurse and an anthropologist, and have lived and worked on l'ile de La Reunion (Reunion Island) in the Indian Ocean since November, 1991. I received my State Diploma in Nursing in 1981 and in 1999 I received my doctorate in Anthropology. My work with diabetes in La Reunion includes setting up a regional health program, followed by creating a regional network for the prevention of cardio-vascular and renal problems, and participation in many research projects in addition to diabetes, and other subjects such as toxicology. As a nursing and public health instructor, I have introduced anthropological approaches into public health training and research on Reunion Island, and have co-organized a degree program in diabetes care and patient education with University of La Reunion.

Bernard Roy, PhD

I first became interested in the question of diabetes in 1986 while I was working with the Aboriginal Innu Nation in Québec (Canada). At the time I was a registered nurse in the Innu community of Unamen Shipu of the Saint Laurence's Lower North Shore. From that moment on, I embarked on a quest of sorts in order to understand the reasons for the failures of the established approaches I was applying daily in my work as a nurse. As a result, I began an extensive research process closely linked to the Aboriginal milieu, which lead me to study health and community, applied social sciences and to a complete a doctorate in Anthropology. In 2002, I published in French, at Presse de L'Université Laval, the general principals of my research in a work entitled Sang sucré, pouvoirs codés, médecine amère. Since 1996, I have been the head of a firm of consultants in social research, "Groupe Recherche Focus" (www.grfocus.com) that specialises, in particular, in evaluation. I am also an associate professor at the Department of Anthropology at Laval University in Québec.

Rudolph C. Ryser, PhD

I grew to the age of awareness in a tiny village on the Pacific Coast surrounded by the sea, forests, long beaches and mild climate in the State of Washington—so similar to the semi-tropical comunidad in Mexico. The youngest of eight children I grew up in the Taidnapum Cowlitz way even though I knew nothing of the Indian politics that would later define so much of my life. While I received my formal education at Washington State University and the Union Institute and University my practical and fundamental education took place in the struggle to achieve the fullest expression of Indian Rights. I served as an advisor, researcher, and writer with the key leadership of US Indian tribes and later with leaders from other indigenous peoples elsewhere in the world for more than thirty years to negotiate peaceful relations with often violent and dangerous state's governments and their policies. For the last twenty-five years I have served as the Board Chair and Executive Director of the Center for World Indigenous Studies, a policy analysis, education and research organization dedicated to the advancement of indigenous peoples' rights through activist scholarship. My wife and I have three beautiful sons.

Twila Sanchez

I am a Yurok Tribal Member and the Diabetes Program Assistant at United Indian Health Services, in northern California. I help to develop, plan, implement and evaluate community based programs, and have co-facilitated diabetes support groups, youth and adult physical activity programs, diabetes shoe programs, among many others. In the past I worked with Native American health clinics by facilitating community focus groups, talking circles, and community forums throughout California. This helped to determine the communities' understanding, knowledge, and concerns in regards to diabetes.

Jo Scheder, PhD

I am a biocultural anthropologist. My research focuses on health disparities and the biopsychological effects of "stress" (discrimination, inequality, colonialism). Beginning in the late 1970s while I was a health outreach worker and graduate student immersed in neuroscience and endocrinology, my work has been carried out in a range of clinical, community, and academic settings. In 1981 I joined the Hawaii-Samoa Stress Study on an NIMH post-doctoral fellowship, which led to a series of Assistant Professorships at the University of Hawaii-Manoa. In the early 1980s, I began working in documentary video and television production in Hawai'i, which led to long-term involvement with the Native Hawaiian sovereignty movement. In the late 1980s I was an ethnographer for a NIDA-funded AIDS project, and in the 1990s began consulting with the Sex Abuse Treatment Center in Honolulu. I now teach for several departments at the University of Wisconsin-Madison, and collaborate with physicians studying Complementary, Alternative and Integrative Medicine.

Carolyn Smith-Morris, PhD

My work at the Gila River Indian Reservation has spanned my doctoral degree in anthropology, my engagement, marriage, and the birth of two fabulous daughters. So my interest in the pregnancies of Gila River women is not entirely academic but personal as well. I continue this work at Gila River while enjoying a position in the Department of Anthropology at Southern Methodist University in Dallas, Texas. That school's summer campus in Taos, New Mexico affords me the opportunity to explore health-related topics with members of the northern 8 pueblo tribes as well. I hope to begin a study of stress and diabetes using Gila River community member researchers in the coming years. This type of programming is needed and asked for by the tribe, so that tribal members can conduct more of their own research and program development.

Dennis Wiedman, PhD

Type II diabetes mellitus was the basis of my doctoral dissertation from the University of Oklahoma in 1979. My research has involved the Cherokee, Delaware, Plains Apache and urban Native Americans in Oklahoma, and the Seminole of Florida. Recent research on healthy lifestyles and diabetes in Alaska indigenous communities included the Aleut, Inupiat, Tlingit, and Athabascans. Currently, I serve in the professional/practicing seat on the Executive Board of the American Anthropological Association. At Florida International University, the public research university in Miami, Florida, I teach medical anthropology and Native American Studies. As Director of Program Review in the Office of Planning and Institutional Effectiveness, I coordinate the quality assessment of the full range of academic degrees and programs.

Index

- A -

Aboriginal and Torres Straits Islanders, 498

Aboriginal Australians, 9, 494

Aboriginal Health/Liason workers, 499

Act of eating, 19–20, 167, 173–75, 177–78, 180–81

Akimel O'odham (Pima), 9–10, 15, 20, 30–31, 78, 100–1, 149, 187, 189–98, 200, 202, 228, 287, 306, 308, 316, 325, 333, 437–39, 446, 469, 472, 492, 523, 532, 534

Alcoholism, 13, 75, 77–78, 81, 83, 89, 91, 96, 100, 103, 243, 247, 326, 363, 366–67, 372, 381, 475, 477, 482

Aldosterone, 388

Art therapy, 24, 459–60, 480–81, 490–91

Autogenic relaxation, 22, 387, 390–91, 397, 400, 406

Autonomic system, 13, 22, 251, 303, 307, 311, 354, 357–58, 372, 374, 385, 387, 390, 395, 472

- B -

Baer, Hans, 280, 521

Bernard, Claude, 16, 27, 282, 382, 472, 486, 488

Biofeedback, 272, 332, 387, 390, 395–397, 400–1, 403, 405–6, 538

Boarding schools, 73, 75, 78–79, 81–82, 86, 93, 127, 147, 155, 326, 358, 363, 366–68, 374, 376, 461, 469, 479, 522

Body imagery, 18, 29, 73, 77, 83, 91, 98, 272, 351, 395, 523, 530

Bourdieu, Pierre, 174, 181, 183, 185, 338, 350, 483, 488

Breathing therapy, 22, 387, 390

- C -

Camp Wellness, 23, 435–36, 447–48, 450–54

Canguilhem, George, 7, 11, 14, 16, 27, 76, 94, 100, 120, 375, 382

Catecholamine, 280, 283, 288, 290, 302–3, 307, 343

Center for Traditional Medicine, 231–33, 235, 237–39, 241, 245, 259, 271, 273

Chacalans, 232, 247

Children, 3, 6, 9, 23, 30, 54, 62, 66, 73, 76, 83–84, 86, 89, 91, 93, 96, 103, 109, 111–12, 124, 127, 133, 136, 142, 149, 163, 165, 192, 205, 212, 220–22, 233–34, 236, 238–39, 243–44, 246–47, 260, 263, 271–72, 294–95, 317–19, 326–27, 333–34, 339, 351–52, 355, 357, 367–68, 370, 372, 384, 407–9, 411–14, 421–25, 428, 430, 435–58, 461, 463, 475, 479–80, 490, 525, 531, 534, 536, 538, 540

Civil rights, 26, 483

Colonialism, 17–22, 27, 40–43, 46–48, 50–51, 156–57, 182, 272, 310, 337–338, 345, 347–48, 350, 357, 535, 540

Colonization, 7, 9, 34, 40, 43, 123–26, 156–58, 162, 240, 243, 248, 251, 258, 367, 381, 389

Community Health Awareness and Monitoring Program (CHAMP), 519

Community health workers (CHR's), 169, 173, 207, 537

Community support, 23, 25, 239, 259, 301, 369, 375, 379, 383, 415, 419, 423–24, 426, 446, 474, 476–78, 488, 540

Community-based participatory research, 27, 407–8, 415

Community-based program, 23, 139, 525, 527

Comunidad Indigena de Chacala, 231–32, 253–56, 270

Conceptualization of difference, 461

Conditions of existence, 22, 25, 343

Convention on the Rights of the Child, 26

Cooperative Research Center for Aboriginal and Tropical Health (CRCATH), 493, 507

Cortisol, 283, 298, 306–7, 310, 333, 337, 353, 388, 479, 489

Cree, 19, 123–27, 129, 132–33, 135–38, 172, 226, 272, 333, 515, 524–25, 535

Cultural competence, 469

Cultural consonance, 42, 49, 383, 469, 488

Cultural disjunction, 24, 62, 493–94, 506

Cultural expansionism, 17, 40

Cultural identity, 8, 63, 110, 133, 147, 151, 153, 158, 161, 174, 176, 178, 259, 269, 341, 489, 498

Cultural imperialism, 37, 504

Cultural rebuilding, 24, 81, 459–64, 473–74, 479, 485–86

Cultural sensitivity, 37, 346, 408, 435, 449, 462, 507, 511, 515

Culturization, 20, 167, 169, 174

- D -

Dakota Sioux, 9, 65, 70, 203, 207, 210–11, 229, 537

Das, Veena, 337–38, 350

Declaration of the Americas on Diabetes, 168

Demoralization, 16–17, 251–52, 485

Depopulation, 33, 39–43, 45–47, 49–51, 354, 366

Depression, 5, 30, 45, 48, 51, 79, 81–82, 156, 214, 251–52, 282, 313, 315, 318, 323–26, 331, 353, 367, 372, 374, 380, 382–85, 388–89, 401–4, 475–77, 479, 486, 489–91, 536

Devil's Lake Sioux Reservation, 54, 206–7, 214, 226

Diabetes industry, 8, 375

Domestic violence, 79, 237, 247, 363, 367, 380–81, 468, 474–75

Domination, 16, 183, 338, 348, 380–381, 485, 511, 521

Douglas, Mary, 51, 136, 174, 177, 184, 229, 512, 530

Draft Declaration of Indigenous Peoples' Rights, 25–26

Drug abuse, 18, 73, 244, 362–63, 367, 381, 468, 474

- E -

Ecological approach, 419–21

Economic justice, 162

Embodiment, 15, 190, 516

Emotional Liberty, 3, 5, 13, 17, 21–22, 358, 367–68, 380, 385, 474, 485–86, 491

Emotional suffering, 5, 7, 13, 21–22, 25, 357–58, 363, 367, 369, 374, 380–81, 460, 472–73, 476, 485

Emotions, 13, 22, 49, 74, 87–88, 198, 280, 299, 340, 349, 357–58, 367, 369, 374, 379–82, 385–87, 389, 395, 397, 403, 466, 472, 476–77, 485, 488, 491, 521, 536

Endocrine system, 11, 13, 22, 251, 358, 374, 388, 472, 498

Environmental change, 73, 301, 437, 528

Epinephrine, 283, 303, 306, 308, 310

Ethnic identity, 8, 10, 63, 148, 150–51, 153, 158, 182, 467

Ethnographic fieldwork, 20, 53, 74, 459, 461–62

Ethnographic research, 24, 58, 137, 357, 369, 372, 461–62, 525–26, 531

Etiology, etiological explanations, 7, 13, 18–20, 24, 31, 54–55, 57, 60, 63–64, 67, 115, 118, 123, 128, 198, 206, 208–9, 220, 276, 279–80, 282, 289, 298, 305, 322, 335, 341–43, 346, 406, 437, 443, 533

- F -

Farmer, Paul, 7, 28, 36, 56, 67, 69, 135–36, 146–48, 163, 201, 220, 367, 383, 461, 466, 488

Food gathering, 141, 241, 260, 263, 327, 373, 412, 459, 473, 482

Foster homes, 79, 358, 368

Foucault, Michel, 75, 92, 101, 180, 363, 383, 489, 530

Fur trade, 125, 367

- G -

Geertz, Clifford, 55–56, 70

Generosity, 212, 218, 347, 350, 357, 376, 379, 460, 473

Genetic determinism, 3, 7, 13–14, 28

Genetic discrimination, 12

Genetics, 5, 13–14, 18, 24, 27, 30–31, 41, 73–74, 76–77, 102, 146, 164–65, 189, 229, 302, 309, 313, 315, 324, 333, 386, 433, 458, 461, 466, 490, 492, 511, 514, 534

Genocide, 7, 9–10, 17, 22, 26, 31, 49, 81, 249, 345, 357, 366–67, 460, 470, 486, 522

Gestational diabetes, 20, 187, 189–91, 193–95, 197, 200–1, 322–23, 330–33, 409, 435–36

Gila River Indian community, 15, 20, 29, 78, 187–90, 192, 446, 469, 472

Glycemic control, 114, 269, 309, 332, 334, 341, 348, 352, 354, 387, 396–97, 406

Gold mining, 84

Good, Byron, 70, 137, 202, 384, 490

Grief, 17, 22, 33–51, 68, 338, 345, 349, 374, 379, 385, 496, 522

- H -

Hawaiians, 16, 33–40, 43, 45–47, 51, 331, 337–38, 343, 345, 347, 350, 388, 472

Hoopa Valley Indian Reservation, 360

Huhukam Memorial Hospital, Diabetes Education Center, 191–92, 195

Human rights, 25–30, 57, 383, 466, 475, 482–84, 488, 491, 535–36

Hunger, 71, 138, 319–20, 323, 440, 482

- I -

Identity, 3, 5, 8, 10, 14–16, 19–20, 27, 30, 51, 57, 62–63, 69, 78, 110, 119, 131, 133, 135, 139–40, 147–51, 153, 158, 161–62, 164, 167–86, 216, 220, 225–28, 234–35, 244, 247, 254, 256, 259, 269, 337–38, 341, 370, 374–75, 381, 384, 467, 469, 484, 486, 489, 498, 517, 535

Indian Health Service Five-Sites Diabetes Program, 54, 207

Illness narratives, 18, 29, 53, 55–56, 58, 70–71, 123, 137, 164, 185, 190–91, 202, 205, 208, 225–26, 274, 357, 368–69, 532

International Labor Organization (ILO), 27

Indian policies, 12, 18, 73, 367

Innu, 8–9, 20, 167, 169–73, 175–83, 185, 539

Innui Food Guide, 170–71

International Conference on Diabetes and Indigenous Peoples, 3, 474, 489, 491

- J -

Jump Into Action Program, 446, 457

Juvenile diabetes, 9, 335

Juvenile halls, 147, 358, 368

- K -

Kahnawake School Diabetes Prevention Project (KSDPP), 23, 407, 409–410, 412, 414–430, 446, 535, 537

Kanien'kehá:ka (Mohawk), 407–28, 462

Klamath River Reserve, 360

Kleinman, Arthur, 19, 54–56, 62, 70, 116, 120, 124, 135, 137, 207, 209, 228, 338, 350, 384, 490

KSDPP Code of Research Ethics, 23, 407, 417–19, 428

Kung San, xix-xx

- L -

LaDuke, Winona, 140, 145, 150–51, 157, 163–64

Layperson accounts, 53, 56, 64, 67

Lévi-Strauss, Claude, 76, 87–88, 102, 177, 185, 255, 274, 374, 379, 384, 472, 490

Life stressors, 397

Lock, Margaret, 7, 30, 75, 103, 299, 310, 338, 350

Loss, 5, 8, 21, 34, 40–43, 45–49, 57, 59, 66, 112, 118, 129–30, 132, 134, 139, 147, 154, 156–57, 162, 177, 214, 222, 239, 251–52, 261, 266–67, 282, 285, 289, 293, 299, 317, 321, 327, 338, 345–46, 349, 372, 375, 382, 389, 409, 439, 441–42, 454,

475, 483, 486, 497, 504, 523, 526, 534

Love, 22, 46, 142, 347, 349, 357–86, 465–66

- M -

Malnutrition, 82, 112, 156, 236, 249, 323, 334, 380

Mamit Innuat Organization, 169, 171

Mauss, Marcel, 178, 181, 185, 255, 274, 379, 384

Medical anthropology, 3, 24, 29–31, 51, 69, 71, 100, 102–3, 106, 136–37, 164, 185, 190, 202, 227, 229, 274, 276, 279–80, 305, 307, 309–10, 331, 353–54, 367, 385, 433, 495, 506, 512, 514, 516, 519, 521, 523, 528, 530–34, 536, 541

Mexican-American migrant farmworkers, 21, 280, 283

Mexican-Americans, 279, 284, 287–88, 297–98, 308–9, 311, 337, 340–41, 353, 520

Migrant farmworkers, 21, 280, 282–83, 285, 307

Mino-Miijim, 139–42

Mintz, Sidney, 109, 121, 153, 164, 257, 275

Mohawks, 410–11, 420, 432

Music therapy, 24–25, 459–60, 477, 479–80, 489

- N -

NARTC Summer Wellness Camp, 435–36, 447–48, 451, 454

Native Diabetes Program (Native Canadian Centre, Toronto), 207, 226, 432, 440, 515–16, 531

Navajo, 9, 77, 137, 536

Nêhinaw Cree, 19, 123–25, 132, 135, 535

Nervous system, 11, 13, 22, 31, 88, 103, 251–52, 283, 303, 307, 309–11, 325,

354, 357–58, 372, 374–75, 379–80, 385, 387, 390, 395, 400, 460, 472–73, 476

Neuroendocrinology, 280, 337

Northern Territory, 9, 24, 360, 370, 461, 493–94, 496, 498–99, 507–9, 536

Nutritional trauma, 21

- O -

Obesity, 8–9, 23, 78, 81, 102, 109, 117, 157, 183–84, 191, 210, 228, 249, 280, 297–98, 302, 307–8, 311, 331–34, 337, 339, 353, 406, 409, 413, 433, 438–41, 443, 445, 452, 456, 458, 512, 523–25, 527–28, 531–32

Ojibwe, 139–40, 144, 150, 154–55, 160

Opaskwayak Cree Nation, 19, 123–25, 127, 133, 135–38

Oppression, 17, 20–22, 39, 146, 148, 163, 182, 279, 335, 338, 342–43, 345, 348, 357, 374, 380–81, 485

Otherness, 13, 461

- P -

Pan American Health Organization, 168, 309

Pediatric diabetes, 382, 435, 437, 525

Penal system, 93, 363

Pharmaceutical industry, 375

Physiology of oppression, 21–22, 335, 342–43, 348

Pima, 9–10, 15, 20, 30–31, 78, 100–1, 149, 187, 189–98, 200, 202, 228, 287, 306, 308, 316, 325, 333, 437–39, 446, 469, 472, 492, 523, 532, 534

Post-traumatic stress disorder, 92, 103, 374

Potawot Health Village, 23, 81, 364, 383, 386, 459–60, 462–65, 472–73, 476, 478–79, 485–86, 488

Poverty, 4–5, 11, 16, 20, 23–24, 27, 61, 63, 79, 108, 112, 117, 127, 130, 146–47, 149, 156, 163, 176, 210, 212, 228, 243, 300, 323, 327, 337, 340, 344, 351, 379–80, 439–40, 443, 460, 474, 494, 505, 522, 536

Psychoneuroimmunology, 40, 42

Psychotherapy, 389, 403, 406

Public policy, 7, 25, 430

- Q -

Quality of life, 3, 7, 250, 282, 325, 435–36, 439, 452, 514, 530

Quest Program, 446

- R -

Racial discrimination, 26, 82, 95, 340, 353, 367, 370, 460, 463, 481

Racism, 5, 12–13, 15, 20, 30, 35, 182, 327, 338, 340–41, 350–51, 354, 380, 427

Reddy, William, 17, 367, 379, 486

Relaxation therapy, 22, 25, 387, 389–390, 394, 396, 398, 400–1, 405

Research ethics, 23, 407–8, 417–19, 426, 428–30, 433

Rethinking compliance, 493–94, 498–501, 505, 507

Rethinking Compliance Project, 493–94, 498–500, 505, 507

Réunion Island, 9, 17–20, 105–21, 539

Right to food, 24, 36, 132, 459–60, 482–84, 489

Rivers, W.H.R., 56

- S -

Scheper-Hughes, Nancy, 5, 7, 30-31, 75, 99, 103, 132, 138, 299, 310, 337, 354, 367, 381, 385, 466, 491

Scientific racism, 13

Segregation, 338

Self-determination, 10, 26, 179, 231, 251, 444, 483–84

Self-esteem, 14, 242, 326, 379, 439, 442, 452, 460, 473, 480

Self-knowledge, 15, 77–78, 91–92, 95, 374, 386, 467, 470, 492

Singer, Merrill, 305, 310, 521, 530

Slavery, 47, 106, 109, 111, 338

Social change, 4, 21, 73, 133, 174, 228, 281, 304

Social equality, 21, 30, 102, 276, 279–312, 354, 463, 532

Social inequality, 3–5, 7, 12, 16–17, 21, 25–26, 40, 82, 108, 148, 280–81, 297, 304, 341, 383, 488

Social justice, 3, 27, 381, 427–28, 466, 475, 485

Social marginality, 21, 283, 286, 302

Social support, 13, 21–22, 25, 47–49, 141, 200, 280, 289, 299, 301–2, 305–6, 310, 340, 358, 367, 383, 388–89, 478, 488, 526, 539

Social well-being, 4, 7, 17, 25, 50, 378, 381, 461, 473, 476, 483, 485–86

Solidarity, 20, 74, 108, 117, 167, 177, 181, 225, 357, 376, 379, 460, 473, 476, 485, 536

Sontag, Susan, 21, 315, 334

Sovereignty, 34–37, 39, 74, 236, 253, 381, 484–485, 515, 540

Spirit Lake Nation, 54, 63, 65, 68, 206

Spirituality, 41, 125, 314, 327, 329, 411, 419, 465, 524

Stress, 16, 21–22, 33, 38, 42–43, 45, 47–51, 62, 64–65, 75, 92, 103, 137, 192, 205, 221, 231, 243–52, 254, 260, 262, 266, 272–76, 279–83, 286, 288–93, 296–300, 302–11, 313, 318, 322–25, 331–32, 337–43, 345, 350–51, 353–55, 374, 379, 382–85, 387–406, 455, 472, 475, 477, 479–80, 489, 491, 514, 522–23, 526, 536, 538, 540–41

Sugar plantations, 18, 105–6, 109, 257

Support groups, 24–25, 389, 424, 459–60, 474–76, 491, 540

Surwit, Richard, 11, 15, 31, 252, 276, 282, 311, 337, 340, 352, 354, 388, 400

Sympathetic system, 88, 283, 309–10, 325, 387, 390, 400

Szathmary, Emöke, 11, 31, 185, 297–98, 311, 375, 385, 514, 532–33

- T -

Taussig, Michael, 7, 31, 56, 71, 79, 103, 208, 229, 500, 510

The Seven Generations, 261, 407–8, 410, 428

Thrifty gene, 3, 13–15, 30, 77, 92, 316, 470, 472, 528, 532

Tolowa, 23–24, 74, 318, 327, 459–64, 466–67, 469, 473–74, 478–80, 485–86, 488

Traditional food, 21, 130, 134, 139–42, 145, 149–51, 157, 159–61, 164, 216, 225, 234, 241, 266, 274, 327, 451, 459, 482, 484, 517, 527

Transcendental meditation, 387, 393, 401–2, 404, 406

Trauma, 3, 7, 11, 16–17, 21, 33, 82, 88, 190, 192, 231, 237, 240, 245–53, 256, 259, 269, 271–76, 313, 315, 318, 322–27, 334, 337–38, 351–52, 357, 369–72, 382, 384, 394, 460, 472, 480, 522, 530, 536

Treaty of Guadalupe Hidalgo, 39

- U -

UN Genocide Convention, 26, 31, 367

Unemployment, 5, 11, 61, 82, 127, 154, 203, 212, 344, 380, 440, 468, 474–75, 505

United Indian Health Services, 12, 24, 74, 78, 81, 84, 88, 92, 99, 326, 364, 370, 376, 382–83, 385–86, 459–60,

462–63, 467, 472, 476, 478, 486, 488, 491, 538–40

United Nations, 3, 8, 10, 24–25, 31, 273, 367, 459, 467, 484

- V -

Violence, 5, 18, 28, 30–31, 34, 73, 77, 79, 82, 86, 92, 100, 139, 145–47, 237, 247, 271, 337–38, 340–41, 345, 350–52, 354, 363–64, 366–67, 372, 380–81, 384–85, 460, 468, 470, 474–75, 488, 491, 523, 536

- W -

Water rights, 36, 357

Weeramanthri, Tarun, 493, 507, 536

Wellness camp, 23, 435–36, 447–48, 450–54

Wellness garden, 460, 464

White Earth Land Recovery Project, 19, 139, 143–49, 156, 163, 538

White Earth Reservation, 139, 141, 143–45, 149, 153–56, 159, 161, 164

Wild food, 62, 130–32, 134, 149, 158

Williams, Gareth, 57, 67, 71, 208, 225–26

Wisconsin Migrant Health Project, 308

Wiyot, 23–24, 74, 327, 459–64, 466, 469, 473–75, 478–80, 485–86

World Health Organization, 277

- Y -

Yelapa, 232–33, 245, 250, 254, 256, 271, 273, 537

Yoga, 22, 387, 390, 392–93, 397, 404–5

Young, Allan, 208, 225

Yurok, 6, 9, 18, 22–24, 28–29, 73–75, 77–93, 95–103, 272, 313, 318, 320, 324, 327, 332, 351, 357–64, 366–74, 376–81, 383, 385, 459–69, 471, 473–76, 478–80, 485–91, 523, 530, 538, 540

Yurok Reservation, 6, 73–74, 88, 92–93, 96, 99, 357, 360, 362–64, 369–70, 372, 379, 463, 538

- Z -

Zuni Diabetes Prevention Program, 446, 458, 524, 527, 533

Zuni Teen Wellness Center, 524